Brown Lesions

Newborns

1. Flat
   - A. Mongolian spot, 323, 399
   - B. Café au lait spot, 321, 399-400
   - C. Junctional nevus, 327, 400
   - D. Nevus of Ota, 323
   - E. Freckles, 320
   - F. Lentigo, 321
   - G. Postinflammatory hyperpigmentation, 323
   - H. Progressive pigmentary purpura, 278-280
   - I. Acanthosis nigricans, 331-332, 401
   - J. Transient neonatal pustular melanosis, 386-387
   - K. Linear and whorled hypermelanosis, 323
2. Raised
   - A. Congenital melanocytic nevus, 325-326
   - B. Skin tags, 406

Infants and Children

1. Flat
   - A. Freckles, 323
   - B. Café au lait spot, 321
   - C. Junctional nevus, 327
   - D. Mongolian spot, 323
   - E. Postinflammatory hyperpigmentation, 323
   - F. Tinea versicolor, 91-92
   - G. Diffuse endocrine hyperpigmentation, 332
   - H. Incontinentia pigmenti, 355-356
   - I. Becker's nevus, 328
   - J. Nevus of Ota, 323
   - K. Lentigo, 321
2. Raised
   - A. Intradermal nevus, 328
   - B. Dermatofibroma, 220
   - C. Spindle and epithelioid cell nevus, 226, 330
   - D. Urticaria pigmentosa, 265-266
   - E. Juvenile xanthogranuloma, 226
   - F. Blue nevus, 328
   - G. Skin tags, 406
   - H. Melanoma, 329-331
   - I. Flat warts, 139

Yellow Lesions

Newborns

1. Carotenemia, 17
2. Sebaceous gland hyperplasia, 382-383
3. Sebaceous nevus, 402-403
4. Juvenile xanthogranuloma, 226
5. Mastocytomas, 265
6. Goltz's syndrome, 357-359

NOTE: In a baby with jaundice, any skin lesion containing fluid may be yellow.

Infants and Children

1. Jaundice, 17, 125, 126
2. Juvenile xanthogranuloma, 226
3. Urticaria pigmentosa, 265-266
4. Sebaceous nevus, 402-403
5. Mastocytomas, 265
6. Carotenemia, 17

7. Xanthomas, 226
8. Necrobiosis lipoidica diabeticorum, 225
9. Goltz's syndrome, 357-359

Red Papules and Nodules

Newborns

1. Erythema toxicum, 386, 387
2. Furunculosis, 68-70
3. Insect bites, 106-107
4. Erysipelas, 260
5. Pyogenic granulomas, 250-252
6. Acne neonatorum, 34-35, 387, 388
7. Epidermal nevus, 400-402
8. Candidiasis, 93, 94, 389-390
9. Hemangiomas (tufted angiomas), 242
10. Congenital syphilis, 77, 78
11. Eosinophilic folliculitis, 137
12. Mastocytomas, 265
13. Malignant tumors (rhabdomyosarcoma, neuroblastoma, leukemia cutis), 233-234
14. Extramedullary hematopoiesis, 113

Infants and Children

1. Insect bites, 106-107
2. Acne, 24-33
3. Viral exanthems, 113-138
   - A. Rubella, 116-117
   - B. Rubeola, 113-116
   - C. Infectious mononucleosis (Epstein-Barr virus), 122-124
   - D. Herpesvirus, 132-133
   - E. Parvovirus B19, 118-121
   - F. Echovirus, 121-122
4. Urticaria, 257-268
5. Scarlet fever, 67-68
6. Erythema multiforme, 196-198
7. Erythema marginatum, 268-269
8. Erythema annulare, 268
9. Furunculosis, 68-70
10. Candidiasis, 92-95
11. Keratosis pilaris, 57-59
12. Early lesion of papulosquamous disease, 149-178
    - A. Pityriasis rosea, 158-160
    - B. Guttate psoriasis, 149
    - C. Acute parapsoriasis (PLEVA), 86, 178
13. Neurofibroma, 222, 323
14. Keloids and hypertrophic scars, 220-221
15. Shagreen patch, 311
16. Angiofibromas, 311
17. Pyogenic granulomas, 227, 250-252
18. Granuloma annulare, 223-224
19. Secondary syphilis, 76, 77, 160-161
20. Tinea corporis, 85-86
21. Cellulitis, 64-66
22. Angioedema, 257-261
23. Cold panniculitis, 65
24. Lupus panniculitis, 168
25. Kawasaki disease, 195-196, 198-199
26. Erythema chronicum migrans (Lyme disease), 74-75
27. Cutaneous larva migrans, 108-109
28. Swimmer's itch, 109-110
29. Fibrous forehead plaque of tuberous sclerosis, 311

E. Port wine

F. Other vascular birthmarks, 394-399
G. Neonatal lupus, 168, 169
H. Harlequin color change, 384
I. Extramedullary hematopoiesis, 113

2. Nonblanching (purpuric)
   - A. Congenital infection
     - i. Toxoplasmosis, 116, 394
     - ii. Enterovirus, 115, 121-122
     - iii. Rubella, 116, 117, 394
     - iv. Cytomegalovirus, 116, 394
     - v. Herpes simplex, 116-117, 390-391
     - vi. Syphilis, 77, 78
   - B. Coagulation defects, 394
   - C. Autoimmune disorders, 204-211
     - i. Idiopathic thrombocytopenic purpura, 123
     - ii. Systemic lupus erythematosus (SLE), 166-171
   - D. Hemangioma with platelet trapping syndrome (tufted angioma), 242
   - E. Epidermolysis bullosa, 348-354
   - F. Congenital leukemia, 233-234
   - G. Neuroblastoma, 233-234

Infants and Children

1. Blanching
   - A. Hemangioma, 237-243
   - B. Urticaria, 257-268
   - C. Livedo reticularis, 270, 275
   - D. Angiofibroma, 311
   - E. Pyogenic granuloma, 227, 250-252
   - F. Spider telangiectasia, 252-253
   - G. Telangiectasia of connective tissue disease, 171
   - H. Erythema multiforme, 196-198
   - I. Erythema infectiosum, 118-121
   - J. Kawasaki disease, 195-196, 198-199
   - K. Morbilliform viral exanthems, 120, 156
   - L. Scarlet fever, 67-68
   - M. Toxic shock syndrome, 72-73
   - N. Drug eruptions, 365-379
   - O. Urticarial lesions of juvenile rheumatoid arthritis, SLE, periarteritis nodosa, dermatomyositis, rheumatic fever, Crohn's disease, ulcerative colitis, aphthous stomatitis, Behçet's disease, thyroiditis, 171-173, 264, 268-269, 275-277
   - P. Erythema chronicum migrans (Lyme disease), 74-75
   - Q. Early lesions of pityriasis rosea, 158-160
   - R. Early lesions of guttate psoriasis, 149
   - S. Syphilis, 76-78, 160

Continued on inside back cover.

Color Textbook
of Pediatric
Dermatology

Color Textbook of Pediatric Dermatology

Fourth Edition

William L. Weston, MD

Emeritus Professor
Departments of Dermatology and Pediatrics
The Children's Hospital and University of Colorado Hospital
Denver, Colorado, USA

Alfred T. Lane, MD

Chair, Department of Dermatology
Professor of Dermatology and Pediatrics
Stanford University Hospital and Clinics
Lucile Salter Packard Children's Hospital at Stanford
Palo Alto, California, USA

Joseph G. Morelli, MD

Professor, Departments of Dermatology and Pediatrics
University of Colorado
Head, Pediatric Dermatology
The Children's Hospital and University of Colorado Hospital
Denver, Colorado, USA

MOSBY

ELSEVIER

MOSBY
ELSEVIER

Mosby is an affiliate of Elsevier Inc.

© 2007, Elsevier Inc. All rights reserved.

First published 1991
Second edition 1996
Third edition 2002
Fourth edition 2007

ISBN 9780323049092

British Library Cataloguing in Publication Data
A catalogue record for this book is available from the British Library

Library of Congress Cataloging in Publication Data
A catalog record for this book is available from the Library of Congress

---

Notice

Medical knowledge is constantly changing. Standard safety precautions must be followed, but as new research and clinical experience broaden our knowledge, changes in treatment and drug therapy may become necessary or appropriate. Readers are advised to check the most current product information provided by the manufacturer of each drug to be administered to verify the recommended dose, the method and duration of administration, and contraindications. It is the responsibility of the practitioner, relying on experience and knowledge of the patient, to determine dosages and the best treatment for each individual patient. Neither the Publisher nor the author assume any liability for any injury and/or damage to persons or property arising from this publication.

The Publisher

Printed in China
Last digit is the print number: 9 8 7 6 5 4 3 2 1

 ELSEVIER your source for books, journals and multimedia in the health sciences
www.elsevierhealth.com

Working together to grow libraries in developing countries

www.elsevier.com | www.bookaid.org | www.sabre.org

ELSEVIER   **BOOK AID** International   **Sabre Foundation**

Commissioning Editor: Karen Bowler
Development Editor: Claire Bonnett
Project Manager: Rory MacDonald
Designer: Andy Chapman
Illustration Buyer: Merlyn Harvey
Illustrator: Danny Pyne
Marketing Managers (USA/UK): Lisa Damico/Clara Toombs

The
publisher's
policy is to use
**paper manufactured
from sustainable forests**

Contents

Dedication ix
Preface xi

1. Structure and Function of the Skin 1
    The Epidermis 1
    The Dermis 4
    Host Defences of the Skin 5
    Epidermal Appendages 5
    Subcutaneous Fat 6
    Development of Skin 7

2. Evaluation of Children with Skin Disease 11
    Medical History 11
    Examination of the Skin 11
    Recording of Skin Lesions in the Health Record 21
    The Problem-Oriented Algorithm 21
    Laboratory Findings 23

3. Acne 25
    Acne Vulgaris 25
    Acne Congoblata/Acne Fulminans 34
    Neonatal Acne 34
    Infantile Acne 35
    Drug-Induced Acne 36
    Perioral Dermatitis and Steroid Rosacea 37

4. Dermatitis 39
    Atopic Dermatitis 39
    Contact Dermatitis 48
    Sebhorrheic Dermatitis 55
    Nummular Dermatitis 56
    Keratosis Pilaris, Lichen Spinulosus, Follicular Mucinosis 57

5. Bacterial Infections (Pyodermas) and Spirochetal Infections of the Skin 61
    Impetigo, Ecthyma and Bacterial Intertrigo 61
    Cellulitis 64
    Necrotizing Fasciitis (Streptococcal Gangrene) 66

Scarlet Fever 67
Folliculitis, Furunculosis, and Cutaneous Abscesses 68
Staphylococcal Scalded Skin Syndrome 70
Toxic Shock Syndrome 72
Cat-Scratch Disease 73
Spirochetal Diseases 74
Mycobacterial Disease 78

6. Fungal and Yeast Infections of the Skin 81
    Dermatophytes 81
    Hair Infections (Tinea Capitis) 81
    Fungal Infection Involving the Skin Only 85
    Fungal Infection of the Nails (Onychomycosis, Tinea Unguium) 89
    Yeast Skin Infections 91

7. Infestations 97
    Human Mite Infestation 97
    Ticks 102
    Spiders 103
    Pediculoses (Louse Infestations) 104
    Papular Urticaria 106
    Helminths (Parasitic Worms) 108

8. Viral Infections 113
    Viral Exanthems 113
    Viral Exanthems: The Morbilliform Eruptions 113
    Viral Exanthems: Vesiculobullous Eruptions 127
    Virus-Induced Tumors 138

9. Papulosquamous Disorders 149
    Psoriasis 149
    Pityriasis Rosea 158
    Lues (Secondary Syphilis) 160
    Pityriasis Lichenoides 161
    Lichen Planus 163
    Lupus Erythematosus 166
    Dermatomyositis 171
    Lichen Striatus 173
    Porokeratosis of Mibelli 175
    Juvenile Pityriasis Rubra Pilaris 176

10. Sun Sensitivity 181
    Sunburn 181
    Idiopathic Photodermatoses 185
    Erythropoietic Protoporphyria 188
    Phytophotodermatitis 190
    Xeroderma Pigmentosum 191

11. Bullous Diseases and Mucocutaneous Syndromes 195
    Spontaneous Vesiculobullous Eruptions 195
    Erythema Multiforme 195
    Kawasaki Disease (Mucocutaneous Lymph Node Syndrome) 198
    Aphthous Ulcers 200
    Geographic Tongue 202
    Miliaria (Heat Rash) 202
    The Immunobullous Diseases 204

12. Skin Cysts and Nodules 213
    Skin Cysts 213
    Adnexal Tumors 217
    Skin Nodules 220

13. Vascular Lesions 237
    Vascular Tumors 237
    Vascular Malformations 246
    Acquired Vascular Lesions 251

14. Vascular Reactions: Urticaria, Erythemas, and Purpuras 257
    Urticaria 257
    Erythemas 268
    Purpuras 272

15. Hair Disorders 285
    Common Forms of Hair Loss 285
    Uncommon Forms of Hair Loss 289
    Excessive Hair 294
    Unmanageable Hair 297
    Scalp Whorls 298

16. Nail Disorders 299
    Disruption of the Nail Surface 299
    Thick Nails 299
    Thin or Atrophic Nails 303
    Paronychia 305
    Ingrown Toenails 305
    Color Changes in the Nail 307

17. Disorders of Pigmentation: the White Lesions and the Brown Lesions 309
    White Lesions 309
    Brown Lesions 320

18. Immobile and Hypermobile Skin 335
    Skin Thickenings 335
    Morphea 335
    Lichen Sclerosus 338
    Ehlers-Danlos Syndrome 339

19. Genodermatoses 343
    Ichthyosis 343
    Netherton's Syndrome 347
    Epidermolysis Bullosa 348
    Ectodermal Dysplasias 354
    Acrodermatitis Enteropathica 360

20. Drug Eruptions 365
    Stevens-Johnson Syndrome and Toxic Epidermal Necrolysis 366
    Dress Syndrome 369
    Clinical Features 370
    Differential Diagnosis 377
    Pathogenesis 378
    Treatment 379
    Patient Education 379
    Follow-up Visits 379

21. Skin Diseases in Newborns 381
    Neonatal Skin Care 381
    Transient Skin Disease 382
    Birthmarks 395
    Common Congenital Malformations That Involve Skin 406
    Major Chromosomal Abnormalities 407
    Miscellaneous Skin Conditions in the Newborn 408

22. Dermatopharmacology and Topical Formulary 413
    Percutaneous Absorption 413
    Antiinflammatory Agents 417
    A Brief Formulary for Common Pediatric Dermatology Conditions 420

Index 423

Patient Education Sheets

See Enclosed
CD-ROM

Acne
Alopecia Areata
Atopic Dermatitis (Eczema)
Aphthous Ulcers
Creams and Ointments
Dry Skin
Hair Pulling
Head Lice
Insect Repellents for Children
Keratosis Pilaris
Molluscum Contagiosum
Nickel Allergy

Papular Urticaria
Perioral Dermatitis
Pilomatricoma
Pityriasis Alba
Psoriasis
Psoriasis Scalp Care
Scabies
Scalp Ringworm (Tinea Capitis)
Sun Protection
Urticaria Pigmentosa
Vitiligo
Warts
Wet Dressings

Dedication

This book is dedicated to the memory of Alvin Jacobs, MD. Two score years ago, there were less than five pediatric dermatologists in the United States. The effect that these "pioneers of pediatric dermatology" had on the understanding of skin diseases in children has been exponential. Doctors Nancy Esterly, Sam Weinberg, and the late Sid Hurwitz are recognized for their major contributions to the field. The authors praise all the pioneers and re-dedicate this textbook to another "pioneer"—Alvin Jacobs, MD—who promoted pediatric dermatology to primary care physicians like no other. He will always hold a special place in our memory. In its formative years, pediatric dermatology struggled to find its way as a field of medicine. Al Jacobs was always there to listen, to help, and to guide. Any pediatrician worth his or her salt knows the name of Alvin Hirsch Jacobs, MD. He presented hundreds of lectures on pediatric dermatology to national, regional, and local meetings, with never a negative comment. We can think of no others in the field who can match that accomplishment. His seminars on neonatal dermatology were classic; often they were the most popular sessions at national pediatric or dermatology meetings. Those who heard Al Jacobs talk know they heard the master. There are thousands of pediatricians whose first and often only formal teaching in pediatric dermatology came from Al Jacobs.

We decided to dedicate this book to Al Jacobs for another aspect of his professional career: his work behind the scenes in pediatric dermatology. For a complete appreciation of his contributions we must first examine the man. He was born in Reno, Nevada, and spent his boyhood among the ponderosa pines and broad valleys below the Comstock lode. This was still the Wild West, an invigorating life for an ambitious young man. After receiving the gold medal at graduation from the University of Nevada in 1933, he ventured east to the famous Johns Hopkins University School of Medicine, where he received his medical degree in 1937. After internship in Pittsburgh, he spent a year in child neurology at the Neurological Institute of New York. He returned west for training in pediatrics and infectious disease at San Francisco County Hospital, then served as chief resident in pediatrics at Stanford University. It was then June 1942, his country was at war, and Dr. Jacobs joined the Navy and was assigned to Navy

Medical Research Unit Number 1. By 1946 he was a Lieutenant Commander and ready to return to the practice of pediatrics. In his private practice of pediatrics in San Francisco, Al quickly recognized that 20% of his patients had primary skin complaints and that he was poorly prepared to deal with them. He found his colleagues in pediatrics similarly unprepared and decided to remedy the situation. After a year's fellowship in dermatology at Stanford he joined the Stanford faculty and established a career in pediatric dermatology that has spanned five decades. Until his death on November 9, 2001, he was Professor of Dermatology and Pediatrics, Emeritus (active) at Stanford University.

Al Jacobs was a founder of the Society for Pediatric Dermatology and served as its first president. In many ways Al Jacobs was to pediatric dermatology what George Washington was to the establishment of the United States. It is so crucial that the leaders at the founding have the wisdom and vision to create an organization that will grow and be flexible enough to accommodate the changes needed in future generations. The advice and counsel of Al Jacobs was critical for the field of pediatric dermatology.

It was Al Jacobs the man who endeared himself to so many in pediatrics and pediatric dermatology. He avoided the arrogance that often accompanies positions of importance in academic medicine and remained the kind, considerate, warm man who always had time to listen to your needs or your problems. It was his accessibility that made the field of pediatric dermatology accessible for all who are interested. Who could resist that big smile beneath the cookie-duster moustache or those kind, twinkling eyes? Any personal encounter with Al Jacobs made you feel you were with your best friend. When you have a moment to reflect on your own careers, remember that big smile and what it meant to pediatric dermatology.

It is said that the fulfillment of life is to love, be loved, and have useful work. Al Jacobs loved his charming wife, Opal; his children and grandchildren; and his chosen field of pediatric dermatology. In turn, he was loved by the hundreds of physicians whose lives he touched.

This book is also dedicated to our families: Dr. Janet Atkinson Weston, Betsy and Kemp Weston; Maureen, Amy, Andy, Jeremy, Jordan, and Matthew Lane; Laura Wilson, Reed and Stefan Morelli.

William L. Weston, MD
Alfred T. Lane, MD
Joseph G. Morelli, MD

Preface

This fourth edition (4e) of *Color Textbook of Pediatric Dermatology* is designed for two purposes. Firstly, 4e is intended to be a practical University course on Pediatric Dermatology. Secondly, 4e is designed as a rapid access reference source for the busy clinician. In both instances, 4e is written from the perspective of what is best for the child. For the course in pediatric dermatology, new information has been added to every chapter and there is a major reorganization of chapters 11, 13, 15, 17 and 20. Chapter 2 was expanded in order to add many clinical photographs of primary and secondary lesions. For ease of interpretation, all the line drawings are in color. The latest references were added and the information incorporated into the text as original source information. As for previous editions, the authors did not wish to copy other textbooks. It is our hope that 4e will provide a format to medical educators that wish to create a course in pediatric dermatology for their trainees.

For the reference text, the problem-oriented differential diagnosis index was redone and will remain on the front and back of the book. By understanding primary and secondary lesions as described in chapter two, the clinician can rapidly create a differential diagnosis with the index. In addition, the number of clinical photographs has increased by 30% and will be available on CD-ROM. Our colleagues primarily caring for children wished to have more images of the skin conditions described. Ten new patient education sheets have been created and the others revised. The 25 patient education sheets will also be available on CD-ROM and downloadable to print out for your patients.

This fourth revision was heavily dependent on comments from primary care providers, residents and students. The Dermatology residents at the University of Colorado systematically reviewed the previous edition a chapter per week and made many valuable suggestions for improvement. As with previous editions, all three editors read each revised chapter. We emphasized the perspective of experienced clinicians in each chapter when considering new findings and new treatments.

We have many to thank for this edition. As before, the encouragement of our mentors enabled the creation of the book. This book is dedicated to the late Dr. Alvin Jacobs who was an inspiration to us all. A special debt is owed to Drs. Robert Goltz, the late C. Henry Kempe, W. Mitchell Sams, Jr. and Lowell Goldsmith for their guidance, protected time, nurture and mentorship for our careers. We also are grateful to all our colleagues in the Society for Pediatric Dermatology who have generously used this textbook in their institutions and provided enthusiastic support for our careers. There has never been a medical association with such warmth and support for each other. We are especially indebted to Claire Bonnett, our editor at Elsevier and her colleagues at the London office.

William L. Weston, MD
Alfred T. Lane, MD
Joseph G. Morelli, MD

Structure and Function of the Skin

A firm understanding of normal skin structure and function is necessary for recognition and treatment of skin disease. Those providing medical care for children should apply the principles of skin biology to the pediatric patient and master essentials of embryology and development.

THE EPIDERMIS

Keratinization

The epidermis functions as a barrier, preventing penetration from outside and retaining substances inside.[1,2] Over 95% of epidermal cells are keratinocytes. The process of keratinocyte replication and maturation is called *keratinization*. The major keratinocyte proteins are keratins, which provide scaffolding to determine keratinocyte shape. Keratin pairs form intermediate filaments by combining an acidic keratin with a basic keratin. In proliferating basal keratinocytes, keratins 5 and 14 provide the main protein structure. As differentiation occurs, keratins 5 and 14 are replaced by keratins 1 and 10 and the cells flatten. The process of keratinization begins with proliferation of new keratinocytes in the region of the basal cell layer, near the dermal–epidermal junction (Fig. 1.1). As keratinocytes differentiate, they accumulate granules called *keratohyaline granules* in their cytoplasm, and the type of keratin bundles within the cells becomes thicker. Within the granular layer the cells lose their cylindrical and cuboidal shapes and begin to flatten as they go through a specific process of terminal differentiation or programmed cell death (apoptosis) called cornification or keratinization.[1,2] Cell nuclei are lost and the keratinocytes flatten like stacks of plates. This final layer is called the *horny layer*, or *stratum corneum*. The stratum corneum cells accumulate like bricks in a wall, separated by intercellular lipids, which function like mortar. The thick corneocyte membranes are created by the formation of an inner protein envelope including the proteins profilaggrin, involucrin, and epiligrin. The intercellular and cell-surface lipids are an integral part of the epidermal barrier function.[2]

Individual keratinocytes are bound together by desmosomes and adherens junctions. The desmosomes contain membrane glycoproteins desmocollins and desmogleins, and cytoplasmic proteins desmoplakins, periplakin, and plakoglobin.

The process of keratinization is continuous within the skin. The newly formed keratinocytes of the basal layer mature and are shed from the skin over an interval of approximately 28 days. Skin diseases may be associated with variation in the speed and process of keratinization.

Epidermal Barrier

It is said that the skin is the interface between humans and their environment. Indeed, the most important functions of the epidermis are to provide a skin barrier against microorganisms and irritating chemicals and to impede the exchange of fluids and electrolytes between the body and the environment. This barrier function resides in the stratum corneum, where the terminally differentiated keratinocyte develops a tough cell envelope beneath the plasma membrane.[3] The process of envelope formation involves biochemical processing of involucrin, the major cytoplasmic protein precursor of the cell envelope. The epidermal barrier is completed by extracellular lipid layers surrounding the terminally differentiated keratinocytes.

Although the skin, including the epidermis and dermis, is 1.5–4.0 mm thick, the epidermal barrier is

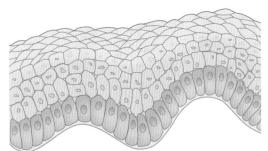

Fig. 1.1 Normal epidermis. The germinative layer with prominent nuclei is at the base of the epidermis and within the same compartment as the fully differentiated cells. As these basal cells differentiate, they migrate up toward the skin surface, shed their nuclei, become flattened, and are shed from the skin surface.

only 0.05–0.1 mm thick. By the daily shedding of one to two cell layers of stratum corneum, or scale, the epidermal barrier prevents excessive bacterial colonization of the skin surface. In addition to continuous shedding, the flattened stratum corneum cells are tightly adherent to each other, so that to obtain entrance into the lower epidermis and dermis, chemicals or microorganisms must pass between tightly compacted epidermal cells.

The water content of the environment greatly influences the epidermal barrier (see Ch. 22). Both an excessive and an inadequate water content in the epidermal barrier will cause microscopic and macroscopic breaks in the barrier.

In response to friction or other forms of repeated trauma, such as exposure to ultraviolet light (UVL) or chemical injury, stratum corneum is formed in amounts greater than usual, as can be noted on the palms and soles. The stratum corneum is thinnest over the eyelids and scrotum.

Pigmentation and Ultraviolet Light

Four biochromes in the skin are responsible for clinical pigmentation: melanin, betacarotene, oxyhemoglobin, and reduced hemoglobin.[1] The brown-black pigment melanin is the dominant pigment of the skin.[4,5] It is the pigment closest to the observer's vision and darkest in color. In dark-skinned individuals, it is difficult to recognize yellow pigment (betacarotene), red pigment (oxyhemoglobin), and blue pigment (reduced hemoglobin). Melanin is produced by the pigment-forming cell, the melanocyte, which is located in the epidermis. Different skin regions contain different numbers of melanocytes. For example, three times

as many melanocytes are found in the epidermis of the forehead as in the abdominal skin.[1] Numbers of melanocytes per unit area of skin are the same despite racial differences in pigmentation.

Each epidermal melanocyte has dendritic cytoplasmic extensions that make contact with 35 to 45 epidermal cells. This melanocyte–keratinocyte unit (Fig. 1.2) is responsible for clinical pigmentation. The brownish-black polymer melanin is produced within the melanocytes in special membrane-bound organelles called *melanosomes*. The genetic control of pigmentation is extremely complex and involves more than 150 alleles spread over 90 loci. These loci direct protein products which are structural proteins, enzymes, transcriptional regulators, transporters, growth factors, and receptors with many cellular targets and functions.[4] The enzymes, including tyrosinase, that are crucial for melanin production are contained within the melanosome membrane. Melanosomes develop in stages. Tyrosinase and other enzymes convert the colorless chemical tyrosine to an oxidized quinone compound, which in turn becomes polymerized into the brownish-black compound melanin. Clinical pigmentation depends on the stage of the melanosome produced and dispersion of melanosomes from melanocytes to keratinocytes. Keratinocytes actively phagocytize the melanosomes. In black skin, there are single units of advanced-stage melanosomes, whereas in lighter-skinned persons, the melanosomes are aggregated and of earlier developmental stages. Thus, the major difference in black and white skin is the stage of melanosome development and the ability to transfer and disperse melanin pigment, not the number of melanocytes per unit area of skin.[4]

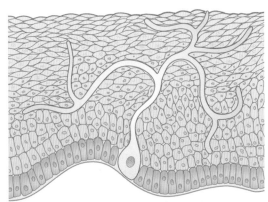

Fig. 1.2 Melanocyte–keratinocyte unit. The dendritic melanocyte, shown here as a clear cell with many branches, provides melanin pigment to many keratinocytes.

Fig. 1.3 Melanin production and transfer. Melanosomes (*inset*) are organelles formed in the rough endoplasmic reticulum and Golgi area of melanocytes. Their membranes contain the enzyme tyrosinase, which is responsible for the formation of the brown-black polymer melanin. At the end of the dendrite, the melanocytes are shown transferring pigment to the keratinocyte, where the melanin moves to form a cap of the keratinocyte nucleus as protection against ultraviolet injury.

The function of melanin is to protect the deoxyribonucleic acid (DNA) structure of epidermal cell nuclei from damage by UVL irradiation. Melanin dispersed within the cytoplasm of keratinocytes forms a protective cap over the keratinocyte nucleus when the keratinocytes are exposed to UVL (Fig. 1.3). Melanin pigment is lost by the daily shedding of stratum corneum cells. Melanin within the dermis, such as that found in dermal melanocytic birthmarks, has no such mechanism available for its elimination.

UVL from the sun increases melanin pigmentation by first oxidizing preformed melanin, increasing crosslinking of the melanin polymer and darkening the color. This effect occurs within minutes after exposure and is called *immediate pigment darkening*. During the 4–6 days after UVL exposure, both increased melanin production and melanin transfer to keratinocytes produce tanning.

Sunlight

The sun produces UVL of numerous wavelengths which, based on their biologic effects, are arbitrarily divided into three groups: ultraviolet A (UVA), ultraviolet B (UVB), and ultraviolet C (UVC) (Table 1.1). Incoming UVL from the sun is scattered by small molecules in the atmosphere and absorbed by the ozone layer; all UVL below 290 nm is absorbed, so that virtually no UVC reaches the earth's surface.

Sunburn is caused by wavelengths of light from 290 to 320 nm. Photons of UVL are absorbed by electrons of chemicals with double bonds and ring structures, such as nucleic acids, DNA, and proteins, producing excited electron states within these molecules or free radical formation. Betacarotene and melanin act by stabilizing the free radicals and are natural photoprotective chemicals found in skin. About 10% of UVB passes through the epidermis and reaches the dermis. The erythema and pain of sunburn are mediated via prostaglandins, free oxygen radicals, and other mediators.

The sunburn wavelengths of UVL are blocked by window glass. The tanning and thickening of the epidermal barrier that result from exposure to sunlight impair the penetration of UVL into the lower epidermis and dermis. Wavelengths of light from 320 to 400 nm (UVA) are responsible for the photosensitivity seen in the many drug photoallergies and psoralen phototoxicity. Light of these wavelengths passes through window glass and also is emitted from fluorescent lamps such as those used as in overhead lighting in schools.[1]

Epidermal Basement Membrane

The junction between the epidermis and dermis is the epidermal basement membrane. This structure

Table 1.1 Biologic effects of ultraviolet light

Ultraviolet (UV) group	Wavelength (nm)	Biologic effects
UVC	200–290	Cytotoxic (bactericidal, retinal injury)
UVB	290–320	Sunburn, sun tanning, systemic lupus erythematosus, skin cancers
UVA	320–400	Drug photoallergies, porphyria, phyto-photodermatitis, psoralen photoaging, PUVA therapy
PUVA, psoralen ultraviolet A-range.		

is composed of complex protein–cell and protein–matrix interactions among the basal keratinocyte, the lamina lucida, the lamina densa, the sublamina densa, and dermal collagens.[6] Keratins in the basal keratinocyte attach into the electron-dense plaques associated with the hemidesmosomes. Anchoring filaments extend from the hemidesmosome to dermal collagen fibers and have attachment sites to laminin 5 as well. The complex basement membrane anchoring interactions resists shearing forces to the skin and provides strength.

Bullous pemphigoid antigen 1 is associated with the cytoplasmic portion of the basal cell hemidesmosome, and bullous pemphigoid antigen 2 is a transmembrane portion of the hemidesmosome.[7] Laminins 5 and 6 are associated with the anchoring filaments. Laminin 1, nidogen, and type IV collagen are associated with the lamina lucida and lamina densa. The long anchoring fibrils of the sublamina densa are composed of type VII collagen. Integrins are extrahemidesmosomal attachments to the lamina densa.

Autoantibodies against basement membrane structures or genetic defects of these structures cause a variety of diseases. Correlation of the function of specific structures of the basement membrane and disease-associated defects has helped to increase understanding of the epidermal–dermal junction.

THE DERMIS

The dermis is composed predominantly of collagen fibers and elastin fibers enclosed in a gel continuum of mucopolysaccharides.[1,8,9] This fibrous complex gives the dermis its great mechanical strength and elasticity, allowing the skin to withstand severe frictional stress yet still be extensible over joints. Elastin, collagen, and mucopolysaccharide gel are all produced and secreted by fibroblasts. Types I, III, IV, and VII are the predominant collagens in the skin. Although the principal mass of the dermis consists of collagen fibers and is acellular, numerous other elements are present, including mast cells, inflammatory cells, blood and lymph vessels, and cutaneous nerves. These elements are responsible for regulation of heat loss, the host defenses of the skin, nutrition, and other regulatory functions.

Collagen, Elastin, and Mechanical Properties

Most of the mechanical strength of the skin is derived from the fibrous protein *collagen*, a macromolecule with a large hydroxyproline content.[1,8] Mature collagen structure becomes rigid with cross-linking of adjacent protein chains, and young collagen that is without significant cross-linking fails to limit skin distention. Defective collagen results in extensive and excessive distensibility of the skin, as seen in Ehlers-Danlos syndrome, or severe blisters, as seen in recessive dystrophic epidermolysis bullosa. Elastin fibers, which are composed of both an amorphous and a fibrillar portion, are responsible for the reversible distensibility that allows the skin to be restored to normal size after stretching.[1,9] Defective elastin production results in extreme wrinkling and redundant skin, as seen in cutis laxa.

Cutaneous Vasculature

Cutaneous arteries course through the subcutaneous fat and give rise to two vascular plexuses that run parallel to the epidermis. These vascular plexuses contain arteriovenous shunts to divert blood from the skin and provide nutrition to it, to regulate heat loss, and to participate in the defense against foreign substances. The epidermis contains no blood vessels and receives its nutrition via the diffusion of plasma into the intercellular epidermal spaces. The stratum corneum has no such nutritive process.

Heat Regulation and Sweating

Skin is important in the control of body temperature. Heat generated in organs and muscles is rapidly transported to the skin vasculature.[1,10,11] The cutaneous circulation acts as a radiator. Varying the rate and volume of blood flow through the skin controls heat loss from this radiator. The blood flow is controlled by the autonomic nervous system. Heat from the skin surface is lost by evaporation of water in the form of eccrine sweat. Heat loss or gain by convection or radiation depends on environmental temperature. At comfortable temperatures, body heat can be regulated by the cutaneous vasculature alone, without sweating. In hot, dry environments the core body temperature may rise slightly but is stabilized by heat loss via sweating. In hot, humid environments evaporation of water from the skin surface is restricted, and heat gain occurs in the child's body. If this condition is allowed to continue, high fever, dehydration, and sodium depletion may occur. With exercise and heat gain, sweating is critical to maintaining body temperature.[10,11] In children born with deficient numbers of eccrine sweat glands (hypohidrotic ecto-dermal dysplasia), heat gain occurs during hot weather, overheating, or exercise, and recurrent high fever is often a presenting feature of the condition.

Cutaneous Nerves

Sensory nerve endings in the skin can elicit all of the principal sensations: touch, pain, itch, warmth, and cold. The skin is supplied by both myelinated and unmyelinated branches of spinal nerves.[1,12,13] Nerve branches enter the dermis from the subcutaneous fat and form both a superficial and a deep nerve plexus. Unmyelinated branches from either plexus terminate in nerve endings that may be simple or specialized. Terminals from a single axon may serve an area as broad as 1 cm^2 and overlap with nerve endings from other axons. Inflow of cutaneous sensory information is strongly controlled and modulated by the cerebral cortex. The skin has a high sensitivity to rapid mechanical stimulation, with positional movements of less than 1 μm detectable. Sensations of cold persist continuously when skin temperature is below 30°C, and sensations of warmth persist continuously when it is above 37°C.[1] Changes in temperature of 0.03°C can be detected, especially if the skin temperature changes faster than 0.007°C/sec. Thermal sensitivity is highest on the face. At temperatures below 18°C and above 45°C, pain is produced. Pain may also be induced by pressure greater than 50 g/mm^2 and by disruption of skin.[13] A number of chemicals injected into the skin may also elicit pain. Itch is a sensation related to pain and is greatest close to transitions of mucous membranes. Histamine is considered to be the most important mediator of itch, but many other mediators are capable of producing this sensation. Itch may be exclusively central rather than cutaneous in some conditions, such as cholestasis.[14]

HOST DEFENSES OF THE SKIN

When breaks in the epidermal barrier occur, micro-organisms invade the upper epidermis. Plasma proteins, such as complement proteins and immuno-globulins that normally bathe the intercellular epidermal space, initiate an inflammatory response. In addition, antimicrobial peptides, which are synthe-sized in the skin, provide a soluble barrier that acts as an impediment to infection. These peptides, which include the cathelicidin and defensin gene families, provide rapid, broad-spectrum defense against infec-tion by acting as natural antibiotics and by parti-cipating in host cell processes involved in immune defense.[15,16] Cutaneous vasodilation (erythema) occurs early after this initial process, with diffusion of more plasma proteins, followed by the migration of neutro-phils, T lymphocytes, B lymphocytes, and monocyte-macrophages into the dermis and later the epidermis. Such cells initially accumulate around dermal blood vessels but may migrate to the epidermis through the dermal–epidermal junction and between epidermal cells. For example, in impetigo large numbers of neu-trophils accumulate just beneath the stratum cor-neum. Mast cells containing histamine, heparin, and platelet-activating factors are located around cutan-eous blood vessels and play a regulatory role in the immune response of the skin by their influence on cutaneous vascular responses.

The initial response of the skin to invasion by micro-organisms consists primarily of migration of neutro-philic leukocytes, but by 18–24 hours it is characterized by the appearance of lymphocytes and monocyte-macrophages in the dermis. Microorganisms or foreign substances not initially destroyed by neutrophils are presumably further digested by macrophages or destroyed by direct lymphocytotoxicity. A rich lym-phatic system is also found in the dermis, and foreign substances are carried to regional lymph nodes, where specific immune responses are generated by T lympho-cytes and B lymphocytes. Some antigen recognition occurs in the skin because antigen-processing cells (Langerhans cells) are found in the epidermis, and direct Langerhans–T lymphocyte contact occurs that may be important in the recognition of foreign antigens.

The epidermal barrier remains the primary defense of the skin, but microorganisms that pass through the barrier can be destroyed within the midepidermis as the skin defenses attempt to keep them out of deeper tissue.

EPIDERMAL APPENDAGES

Epidermal appendages, which are modifications of epithelium, include hair follicle structures, sebaceous glands, nails, and the apocrine and eccrine sweat glands. Hair follicles are formed through a complex developmental process.[17]

Hair Growth

The hair growth cycle has three phases: the growing phase, *anagen*; the regressing phase, *catagen*; and the resting phase, *telogen*.[1] The cells of anagen hairs have a high mitotic rate and are among the most rapidly replicating cells in humans. The hair growth originates from the hair bulb, which is located in the lower dermis.[1,17] The delta and notch genes may be involved in initiation of hair growth, along with ectodysplasin, a protein involved in ectodermal dysplasias.[18] Human scalp hair grows about 1.3 cm per month.[1] When growth of the hair ceases, the catagen phase occurs, resulting in cessation of mitosis, apoptosis, and upward migration of the hair bulb into the mid-dermis. The hair shaft becomes clubbed at the bottom, causing the catagen hair to become a telogen hair (also called *club hair*). The telogen hair remains in the follicle for 2–3 months and is pushed out when the new hair grows.

There are great differences in the hair growth cycle among the different hair types found in the various body regions. It is believed that fibroblast growth factor regulates the duration of the anagen phase and the size of the hair.[19,20] Ambisexual hair follicles are common to both sexes and are androgen dependent. At puberty, androgen converts vellus hairs to terminal hairs in the axilla and the lower pubic triangle. Conversely, conversion of terminal scalp hairs to vellus hairs occurs in the temporal area of the scalp at puberty. Male sexual hair is responsive to high androgen levels, which convert vellus hairs to terminal hairs in the beard area, ears, sternum, and upper pubic triangle. In the occipital and bifrontal areas of the scalp, androgen levels result in a conversion from terminal to vellus hairs, resulting in androgenetic alopecia.

Hair cycles are asynchronous and vary within body sites. In the scalp at any point in time, about 85% of the hairs are growing (anagen), 14% are resting (telogen), and 1% are regressing (catagen). Newborns convert most of their hairs to telogen hairs within the first 6 months of life. Some newborns take several months to develop new anagen hairs, resulting in a 'bald' baby. Other infants develop new anagen hairs so rapidly that they appear not to lose their hair. After acute febrile diseases, children or adults can have many hairs convert from anagen to telogen with a subsequent period of months with markedly thinned hair (telogen effluvium). Curly hair is in part regulated by the transcription factor DLX (distal-less) and fibroblast growth factors.[18]

Sebaceous Glands

Sebaceous glands are present everywhere on the human skin except for the palms, soles, and dorsa of the feet. Generally, they are associated with hair follicles and empty through a short duct into the canal of the hair follicle.[1] The sebaceous glands are holocrine glands that produce sebum, a semiliquid mixture of glandular cell debris containing glycerides, free fatty acids, wax esters, squalene, cholesterol, and cholesterol esters. The largest and most numerous sebaceous glands are found on the face, scalp, chest, and back.

Sebum production is androgen dependent and begins at puberty in skin regions with abundant sebaceous follicles.[1] Sebaceous gland volume, sebaceous cell size, and secretory capacity are all directly androgen dependent. Obstruction of the sebaceous gland is associated with acne in humans.

Eccrine Glands

Humans have two to five million eccrine glands. These glands function to cool the body through evaporative heat loss of eccrine sweat. In addition, these glands may help to moisten the frictional surfaces of the skin.

Apocrine Glands

Apocrine sweat glands are in the axilla, mons pubis, areola of the breast, circumanal area, and the scalp. They are located deep in the subcutaneous tissue and usually open into a hair follicle. Apocrine glands secrete a yellowish, sticky fluid after puberty. The secretion is produced in response to stress or sexual stimulation. In lower animals, these glands function as sexual attractors and territorial markers.

Nails

Nails are formed by the fifth fetal month.[1,21] The nail matrix contains epithelial cells responsible for the production of the nail plate. The nail matrix occupies an area beneath the proximal nail fold, a portion of which may be seen as the lunula. Fingernails grow approximately 1 cm in 3 months, and toenails grow more slowly. Newborn nails are spoon-shaped and thin and may remain so until 2 or 3 years of age.

SUBCUTANEOUS FAT

The subcutaneous fat lies just beneath the dermis and is composed principally of lipocytes. It serves as a cushion to trauma, a heat insulator, and a highly important source of energy and hormone metabolism.

Premature infants have poorly developed subcutaneous tissues, contributing to thermal instability and metabolic difficulties.

DEVELOPMENT OF SKIN

Periderm

Knowledge of the structure and function of developing fetal skin is invaluable in understanding abnormalities observed in newborn and infant skin. The single layer of ectodermal cells overlaying the developing fetus interacts with the mesoderm below to form the epidermis and dermis.[1,21] Through this interaction the appendages develop, and the unique properties of skin at different body sites result.

Between 4 and 5 weeks' gestation, the single layer of ectodermal cells of the fetal epidermis is covered by a layer of flattened cells called the *periderm*. The periderm cells expand across the developing epidermis by active mitosis, becoming rounded, bulging cells uniformly covered by microvilli. The stratum corneum forms beneath the periderm cells during the fifth to sixth month. At this time, periderm cells regress and become shrunken remnants that slough into the amniotic fluid and become one component of the vernix caseosa.

From the morphologic characteristics it is suggested that a transport function exists for periderm cells. The periderm may transport fluids, electrolytes, and sugars into the developing embryo.

Epidermal Development

After 8 weeks' gestation an intermediate cell layer develops between the basal cells and the periderm.[1,21] In time, this layer stratifies and adds additional cell layers. By 24 weeks' gestation, granular and cornified cells are present on almost all regions of the body. From this time until birth, the stratum corneum matures and thickens so that at birth, the term infant's skin barrier function is comparable to that of an adult. The premature infant's barrier function is more deficient the earlier the prematurity of birth.

The sequence of development of the keratins, the development of the basement membrane zone, the development of the desmosomes, hemidesmosomes, and the antigens of the epidermis have been catalogued.[1,21] The epidermis follows a sequence of development that is being intensively studied to understand the cellular interactions of normal development and the errors that occur in skin diseases.

Cells That Migrate Into the Epidermis

Although the epidermis is ectodermal in origin, cells from other sources migrate into the epidermis. Langerhans cells are present within the epidermis by 6 weeks' gestation, but they may not be functionally mature until after 12 weeks' gestation.[1,21] The melanocyte is derived from the neural crest and migrates to the epidermis before the twelfth gestational week. By 16 weeks' gestation melanocytes with melanosomes capable of synthesizing melanin are noted, and by 20 weeks' gestation the epidermis has its full complement of melanocytes. Merkel cells appear in the epidermis of the fingertips, glabrous skin, and nail beds by 12 weeks' gestation and serve as special sensory organs. These cells may develop within the epidermis rather than being an immigrant cell as previously thought.

Epidermal Appendages

Hair follicle or sweat gland development begins earlier in the scalp, palm, and sole than in other body areas. The hair germ begins in the scalp by 12 weeks' gestation as a proliferation of keratinocytes above a collection of fibroblasts.[1,21] These cells proliferate and invaginate into the dermis, forming the hair peg and the subsequent hair follicle. Granular cells are present within the hair follicle after 14 weeks' gestation, a full 6–10 weeks before they are seen in the interfollicular skin. Hair grows at an oblique angle to the skin surface such that hair will erupt caudally, causing the hair to point downward.

Anlagen of eccrine glands may be present on the sole as early as 10 weeks' gestation. The eccrine gland secretory coil forms on the sole at about 16 weeks' gestation, and the secretory and myoepithelial cells differentiate at 22 weeks' gestation. The sebaceous gland primordia develop off the hair follicle after 16 weeks' gestation. Steroid hormone stimulation of sebaceous glands is so great that these glands are considerably larger in the third trimester fetus than those of a child. Apocrine glands, the last of the appendages to develop, first appear during the sixth month of fetal development.

Nails and volar pads

Development of the fetal nail, the volar pads, skin ridges, and sweat glands are tied together in the developing digit.[1,21] These structures form simultaneously at 8 weeks' gestation, just after the digits separate from one another. By 12 weeks' gestation the proximal and distal nail folds have formed, and the volar pads are formed from mounds of mesenchyme and an increased intermediate layer of the epidermis. The distal nail fold is the first epithelial structure to keratinize, beginning at 12 weeks' gestation. A nail plate covers the nail bed by 17 weeks' gestation. Primary dermal ridges appear at 12 weeks' gestation, and secondary dermal ridges at 16 weeks' gestation.[21] Sweat gland buds appear in the fingertips at 12 weeks' gestation, but sweating does not occur until after 32 weeks' gestation.

Influences of the Dermis on Epidermal Growth and Differentiation

The fetal dermis plays a predominant role in transformation of the ectoderm into epidermis and maintenance of controlled epidermal appendage development. The continued interaction between the epidermis and dermis maintains the continued presence of the thickened skin of the palms and soles or the thinner skin of the face. The epidermal appendages are maintained by epidermal–dermal interaction, and once full-thickness injury occurs, the re-formed scar tissue appears unable to regenerate new appendages. Skin diseases associated with thickening or thinning of the epidermis may be associated with abnormal epidermal–dermal communications.

The Dermis

The primordial dermis begins as a cellular mesenchyme that is watery and without fibrous structure. By 6 weeks of age a fine meshwork of collagen fibrils underlies the dermal–epidermal junction and adheres to the dermal mesenchymal cell surfaces.[1,21] Extracellular collagen increases with age, and fibrils associate into collagen fiber bundles. Cells of the dermis become spaced farther apart, and their elongated axes become oriented parallel to the skin surface. The fine collagen network persists at the dermal–epidermal junction and ensheaths epidermal appendages as they project downward. The dermis increases in thickness from 0.1 mm at 7 weeks to 0.7 mm by 20 weeks of gestation. As the epidermal appendages project deeply into the dermis at 16 weeks' gestation, the dermis organizes two distinct regions: the papillary dermis with fine fibrillar collagen and the reticular dermis with large collagen bundles. By 20 weeks' gestation, the fetal dermis is similar to that of the adult in structure,

although still less in total thickness. Preliminary studies have demonstrated the 8-week-old fetus to contain fibronectin and types I, III, and V collagen within the dermis. By 14 weeks, recognizable fibroblasts, mast cells, endothelial cells, Schwann cells, and histiocytes are found in the fetal dermis.[21] By 60 days of gestation, anchoring filaments are associated with the basal lamina at the dermal–epidermal junction. At 22 weeks, the elastin fibers form, but well-developed elastin fiber networks are not observed until after 32 weeks, and the adult form of mature elastin fibers does not occur until after 2 years of age.

Few rigorous studies have been performed on the other components of the dermis, including vasculature, lymphatics, and nerves. Fat initially forms with discrete areas within the dermis at 16–18 weeks, then demarcation of a distinct fat layer that coincides with the development of hair follicles and their projection into the lower dermis.

Overall, newborn epidermal, hair, sweat, and sebaceous structures are nearly identical to adult structures. The dermis is less mature than adult dermis, being thinner with less organization of collagen and elastin fibers, with a less organized vascular network and cutaneous nerves.[21] The newborn dermis appears as a transition between fetal and adult structures.

REFERENCES

1. Goldsmith LA. Physiology, biochemistry, and molecular biology of the skin. 2nd edn. New York: Oxford University Press; 1991.
2. Candi E, Schmidt R, Melino G. The cornified envelope: a model of cell death in the skin. Nat Rev Mol Cell Biol 2005; 6(4):328–340.
3. Madison KC. Barrier function of the skin: 'la raison d'etre' of the epidermis. J Invest Dermatol 2003; 121(2):231–241.
4. Slominski A, Tobin DJ, Shibahara S, et al. Melanin pigmentation in mammalian skin and its hormonal regulation. Physiol Rev 2004; 84(4):1155–1228.
5. Slominski A, Wortsman J, Plonka PM, et al. Hair follicle pigmentation. J Invest Dermatol 2005; 124(1):13–21.
6. Pai S, Marinkovich MP. Epidermolysis bullosa: new and emerging trends. Am J Clin Dermatol 2002; 3(6):371–380.
7. Ghohestani RF, Li K, Rousselle P, et al. Molecular organization of the cutaneous basement membrane zone. Clin Dermatol 2001; 19(5):551–562.
8. Canty EG, Kadler KE. Procollagen trafficking, processing and fibrillogenesis. J Cell Sci 2005; 118(Pt 7):1341–1353.
9. Mithieux SM, Weiss AS. Elastin. Adv Protein Chem 2005; 70:437–461.
10. Galloway SD. Dehydration, rehydration, and exercise in the heat: rehydration strategies for athletic competition. Can J Appl Physiol 1999; 24(2):188–200.
11. Armstrong LE, Maresh CM. Effects of training, environment, and host factors on the sweating response to exercise. Int J Sports Med 1998; 19(Suppl 2):S103–S105.

12. Kanda T. Pathological changes of human unmyelinated nerve fibers: a review. Histol Histopathol 2000; 15(1):313–324.

13. Schmidt R, Schmelz M, Torebjork HE, et al. Mechano-insensitive nociceptors encode pain evoked by tonic pressure to human skin. Neuroscience 2000; 98(4):793–800.

14. Jones EA, Bergasa NV. Evolving concepts of the pathogenesis and treatment of the pruritus of cholestasis. Can J Gastroenterol 2000; 14(1):33–40.

15. Braff MH, Bardan A, Nizet V, et al. Cutaneous defense mechanisms by antimicrobial peptides. J Invest Dermatol 2005; 125(1):9–13.

16. Larson AA, Dinulos JG. Cutaneous bacterial infections in the newborn. Curr Opin Pediatr 2005; 17(4):481–485.

17. Rogers GE. Hair follicle differentiation and regulation. Int J Dev Biol 2004; 48(2–3):163–170.

18. Van Steensel MA, Happle R, Steijlen PM. Molecular genetics of the hair follicle: the state of the art. Proc Soc Exp Biol Med 2000; 223(1):1–7.

19. Schlake T. FGF signals specifically regulate the structure of hair shaft medulla via IGF-binding protein 5. Development 2005; 132(13):2981–2990.

20. Kawano M, Komi-Kuramochi A, Asada M, et al. Comprehensive analysis of FGF and FGFR expression in skin: FGF18 is highly expressed in hair follicles and capable of inducing anagen from telogen stage hair follicles. J Invest Dermatol 2005; 124(5):877–885.

21. Holbrook KA. Embryogenesis of the skin. In: Harper J, Arnold O, Prose N, eds. Textbook of pediatric dermatology, 2nd edn. Malden, Massachusetts: Blackwell Publishing; 2006:3–41.

Chapter 2 | Evaluation of Children with Skin Disease

The language of dermatology frequently inhibits students, house officers, and practitioners dealing with children from using the correct terminology for skin disease.[1] It is neither proper nor helpful to simply use the term *rash*.[1,2] This chapter describes the correct approach to the presenting features, signs, and initial laboratory findings when evaluating children with cutaneous disease. Morphology is the key to diagnosis of skin problems, and the student of dermatology should become expert in recognizing and describing morphologic features. The description of primary lesions should be memorized. Particular attention should be paid to the presence of *vesicles*, *pustules*, *scaling*, and *color changes*. These four morphologic features will allow the identification of the major morphologic groups, which is essential for proper diagnosis and differential diagnosis.[3] A problem-oriented algorithm is included in this chapter to allow determination of the morphologic groups of skin disease by their cutaneous appearance. Mastering this information will aid in communication with others delivering medical care to children.

MEDICAL HISTORY

The history obtained regarding a child's skin condition should be considered in the same fashion as a general medical history. The onset and duration of each symptom should be recorded. Associated systemic symptoms such as fever or joint pains should be sought, along with a thorough review of systems. A past medical history, complete family history, and information on recent medications should also be obtained.

Healthcare advice is primarily sought for children for three major concerns regarding their skin: itching (pruritus), scaling, and cosmetic appearance.

Pruritus

Persistent itching in the skin often provides the impetus to seek medical attention. The examiner should note whether the itching is localized or generalized and whether it is associated with skin lesions. Itching without skin lesions suggests biliary obstruction, diabetes mellitus, uremia, lymphoma, or hyperthyroidism. If the pruritus is associated with skin lesions, dermatophytosis, scabies, and the many types of dermatitis should be considered.

Scaling

Normally, one cell layer of stratum corneum, composed of flattened, nonviable remnants of keratinocytes packed with protein (keratin) is shed daily. This is not usually visible. Acute injury and resultant separation of 10–20 cell layers of stratum corneum result in clinically visible white sheets of scale, such as that seen in desquamation after a sunburn or thermal burn. Overproduction of stratum corneum by proliferating epidermis, as in psoriasis, results in visible accumulation of excess surface scale. The scale in psoriasis is thick in contrast to thin (pityriasis) scale.

Cosmetic Appearance

Parents may be concerned about the appearance of a child's skin, particularly any color change. A history of the time of appearance of skin lesions, sequence of color changes, and course of skin changes should be obtained.

EXAMINATION OF THE SKIN

The evaluation of skin lesions requires careful inspection of the entire cutaneous surface, and many skin diseases are diagnosed only by their morphologic appearance.[1-3] Examination of the skin should consist of identification of the primary lesion (the earliest lesion to appear), the size or range of the primary lesion in millimeters, secondary changes, and a description of the color, arrangement, and distribution of lesions. Often, however, one sees children with secondary skin changes without primary lesions. For correct diagnosis, a rigorous search should be made for a primary lesion. To properly evaluate the primary lesion, both visual inspection and palpation are required. Palpation should determine whether the lesion is hard or soft, and whether it moves with the skin or the skin moves over it.

Primary Skin Lesions (The Morphology of Skin)

1. A *macule* (Fig. 2.1A,B,C) is a color change in the skin that is flat to the surface of the skin and not palpable (e.g. a tan macule, café-au-lait spot, white macule, vitiligo).
2. A *papule* (Fig. 2.2A,B,C) is a solid, raised lesion with distinct borders 1 cm or less in diameter (e.g. lichen planus, molluscum contagiosum).
3. A *plaque* is a solid, raised, flat-topped lesion with distinct borders and an epidermal change larger than 1 cm in diameter (e.g. psoriasis).
4. A *nodule* (Fig. 2.3A,B,C) is a raised, solid lesion with indistinct borders and a deep palpable portion. A large nodule is termed a *tumor* (e.g. rheumatoid nodule, neurofibroma). If the skin moves over the nodule, it is subcutaneous in location; if the skin moves with the nodule, the nodule is intradermal.
5. A *wheal* (Fig. 2.4A,B,C), an area of tense edema in the upper dermis, produces a flat-topped, slightly raised lesion (e.g. urticaria).
6. A *vesicle* (Fig. 2.5A,B,C) is a raised lesion filled with clear fluid that is less than 1 cm in diameter (e.g. varicella, herpes simplex).
7. A *bulla* (Fig. 2.5D) is a raised lesion larger than 1 cm and filled with clear fluid.
8. A *cyst* (Fig. 2.6A,B,C) is a raised lesion that contains a palpable sac filled with solid material (e.g. epidermal cyst, dermoid cyst).
9. A *pustule* (Fig. 2.7A,B,C) is a raised lesion filled with a fluid exudate, giving it a yellow appearance (e.g. acne, folliculitis).

Size of the Primary Lesion

The size or range of sizes of the primary lesion or lesions should be measured in millimeters and

recorded. To expedite the examination, measure certain landmarks on the examining finger to estimate lesion size.

(A)

(B)

(C)

Fig. 2.1 **(A)** A macule is a color change in the skin that is flat to the surface of the skin and not palpable (e.g. a tan macule, café-au-lait spot, white macule, vitiligo). **(B)** A tan macule on the trunk of a child with neurofibromatosis I (café-au-lait macule). **(C)** A white macule on a child with tuberous sclerosis (ash-leaf macule).

Fig. 2.2 **(A)** A papule is a solid, raised lesion with distinct borders 1 cm or less in diameter (e.g. lichen planus, molluscum contagiosum). **(B)** Skin-colored papules on the forehead of a child with trichoepitheliomas. **(C)** A bleeding red papule on the chin of a child (pyogenic granuloma).

Fig. 2.3 **(A)** A nodule is a raised, solid lesion with indistinct borders and a deep, palpable portion. A large nodule is termed a tumor (e.g. rheumatoid nodule, neurofibroma). **(B)** Firm pink nodule on the trunk of a child. **(C)** Pink nodule on the palm of a newborn (fibrosarcoma).

Fig. 2.4 **(A)** A wheal, an area of tense edema in the upper dermis, produces a flat-topped, slightly raised lesion (e.g. urticaria). **(B)** Wheal on the forearm induced by ice in a child with cold urticaria. **(C)** Pink wheals in a child with urticaria.

Secondary Changes

1. In *atrophy* (Fig. 2.8A,B), the skin surface is depressed because of thinning or absence of the dermis or subcutaneous fat (e.g. atrophic scar, fat necrosis). If the epidermis is thinned, it appears as fine wrinkling. An *ulcer* (Fig. 2.9) with loss of epidermis and dermis may heal as an atrophic lesion (e.g. cutis aplasia, fat necrosis).

2. *Erosions and oozing* (Fig. 2.10) are moist, circumscribed, slightly depressed areas representing a blister base *(erosion)* with the roof of the blister removed (e.g. burns, dermatitis). Because the action of chewing or sucking easily removes the thin blister roof (oral mucosa lacks a stratum corneum), most oral blisters present as erosions (e.g. aphthae, herpes simplex stomatitis).

3. *Crusting* (Fig. 2.11) represents dried exudate of plasma combined with the blister roof, which sits on the surface of skin after acute dermatitis (e.g. impetigo, contact dermatitis).

4. In *scaling* (Fig. 2.12A,B,C), whitish plates are present on the skin surface (e.g. psoriasis, ichthyosis). *Desquamation* refers to peeling of sheets of scale after an acute injury to skin (e.g. burn, toxic drug reaction, scarlet fever).

5. *Excoriations* (Fig. 2.13) are oval to linear depressions in the skin with a complete removal of the epidermis, exposing a broad section of red dermis. Excoriations are the result of fingernail removal of the epidermis and upper dermis (e.g. atopic dermatitis, neurotic excoriations).

6. *Fissures* (Fig. 2.14) are characterized by linear, wedge-shaped cracks in the epidermis extending down to the dermis and narrowing at the base (e.g. palmoplantar keratodermas, warts).

Fig. 2.5 (A) A vesicle is a raised lesion filled with clear fluid (e.g. varicella, herpes simplex) that is less than 1 cm in diameter. A bulla is a raised lesion larger than 1 cm and filled with clear fluid. **(B)** Vesicle with a red base in a child with varicella. **(C)** Grouped vesicles on a red base in a child with zoster. **(D)** Bulla on the arm of a child.

Disruption of the Skin Surface

The presence of weeping, crusting, cracking (fissures), or excoriations is characteristic of disruption of the skin surface.[2] Disruption is seen in eczematous lesions but is absent in papulosquamous lesions and is an important feature in distinguishing the two.

Mobility of Skin

When grasping the skin between thumb and fore-finger, the skin should be mobile (Fig. 2.15A,B,C) Excessive stretching indicates a type of Ehlers-Danlos syndrome; immobility suggests scleroderma (see Ch. 19).

Color

The color of a skin lesion should be described as skin-colored, brown, red, yellow, tan, or blue. Particular attention should be paid to whether the red or red-brown lesion completely blanches (e.g. petechiae do not blanch). Red or red-brown color in skin is dependent on the pigment oxyhemoglobin, which is found in red blood cells within superficial cutaneous blood vessels. Compressing the superficial vascular plexus by direct pressure forces red blood cells into deeper vascular channels, and blanching of the skin is observed. If the skin does not blanch with pressure, red blood cells are outside the vascular channels and located in the adjacent dermis.

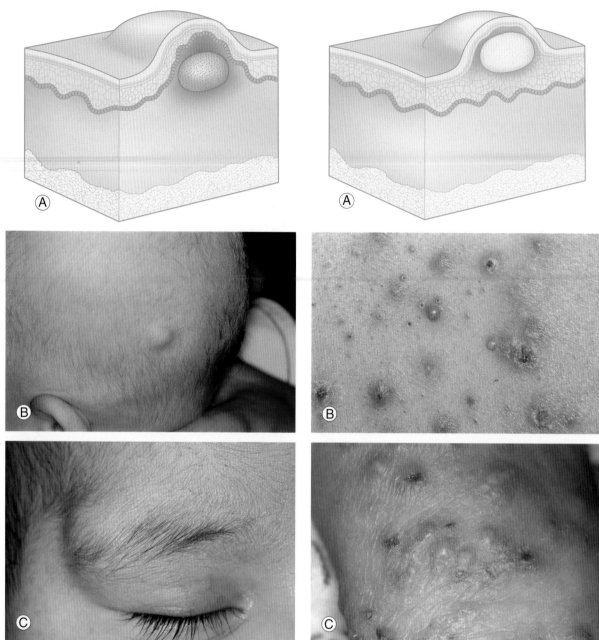

Fig. 2.6 **(A)** A cyst is a raised lesion that contains a palpable sac filled with liquid or semisolid material (e.g. epithelial cyst). **(B)** Cyst on the scalp of an infant. **(C)** Dermoid cyst on the median eyebrow of a child.

Fig. 2.7 **(A)** A pustule is a raised lesion filled with a fluid exudate, giving it a yellow appearance (e.g. acne, folliculitis). **(B)** Pustules, red papules, and open comedones in an adolescent with acne vulgaris. **(C)** Pustules of staphylococcal infection of a child with atopic dermatitis.

Fig. 2.10 Oozing in the antecubital fossa of a child with atopic dermatitis.

Fig. 2.11 Crusts on the face of a child with atopic dermatitis.

Fig. 2.8 (A) In atrophy, the skin surface is depressed because of thinning or absence of the dermis or subcutaneous fat (e.g. atrophic scar, fat necrosis). **(B)** Atrophy of a child's thigh following a subcutaneous injection.

Fig. 2.9 Ulcer within a red nodule in an infant with myofibromatosis.

Melanin is the dominant pigment in the skin. Because it is located in the outer layer of skin closest to the observer's eye, melanin may obscure other pigments located in deeper layers. In dark-skinned infants and children, one must use a disciplined approach to detect erythema, cyanosis, or jaundice. First, determine the normal skin color; then compare the involved skin area with the normal skin. Erythema will appear dusky red or violet. Cyanosis will appear black. Jaundice will appear diffusely darker, and one must examine the sclera to detect the presence of this disease. Carotenemia will appear golden-brown. The examiner may observe melanin as brown, blue-black, or black shades.

Fig. 2.12 (A) Fine scales in a child with ichthyosis. (B) Pigmented scales in a child with X-linked ichthyosis. (C) Thick, white scales on the ear of a child with psoriasis.

Fig. 2.13 Erosions (excoriations) on the foot of a child with atopic dermatitis.

Fig. 2.14 Fissure of the finger in a child with contact dermatitis.

Fig. 2.15 (A) Hypermobile skin stretched in a child with Ehlers-Danlos type I. **(B)** Lax, wrinkled skin in a newborn with cutis laxa. **(C)** Linear, tan immobile plaque in a child with morphea.

Arrangement of Lesions

1. *Discrete* lesions (Fig. 2.16) are distinct and discretely separated from one another (e.g. guttate psoriasis, varicella).
2. *Linear* lesions (Fig. 2.17) are found in a straight line (e.g. lichen striatus).

Fig. 2.16 Discrete arrangement of vesicles in a child with varicella.

Fig. 2.17 Linear arrangement of white plaque in a child with morphea.

3. Special attention should be given to *curvilinear, whorled,* or *parallel linear* lesions (Fig. 2.18A,B,C). These lesions may be seen as curved parallel lines that end abruptly at the midline.[4,5] These indicate genetic mosaicism of the epidermis and are borders between populations of normal and mutated cells.[4] These arrangements follow the embryonic lines of Blaschko mapped from epidermal nevi. The gene mutation is limited only to the affected area, and the remainder of skin does not contain the abnormal gene (e.g. epidermal nevus, nevus sebaceous, hypomelanosis of Ito, incontinentia pigmenti, Goltz syndrome, Conradi-Hunerman ichthyosis).[4,5] The presence of genetic mosaicism should prompt the examiner to assess visual and neurologic abnormalities.[4,5]

Fig. 2.18 **(A)** Curvilinear (whorled) arrangement following the lines of Blaschko (From Bologna J, Jorrizo J, Rapini R, eds. Dermatology. London: Mosby; 2003:Fig. 62.1A.) **(B)** Curvilinear (whorled) orange papules in an infant with nevus sebaceous. **(C)** Curvilinear (whorled) brown pigmentation in a child with incontinentia pigmenti.

4. *Annular* lesions (Fig. 2.19A,B) are found in a circular arrangement (e.g. granuloma annulare).
5. Vesicles, papules, or nodules found closely adjacent to each other in a localized skin area are considered to be *grouped* (Fig. 2.19C) (e.g. herpes simplex, herpes zoster).

Distribution of Lesions

It is useful to note whether an eruption is generalized, acral (hands, feet, buttocks, and face), or localized to a specific skin region, such as a dermatome.

RECORDING OF SKIN LESIONS IN THE HEALTH RECORD

Skin lesions should be described in an orderly fashion: distribution, arrangement, color, secondary changes, and primary lesion (including size). For example, gut-tate psoriasis could be written as generalized, discrete, red, scaly, 3–6 mm papules. If altered, mobility of skin, hair changes, or nail changes should additionally be recorded.

THE PROBLEM-ORIENTED ALGORITHM

After mastering the description of skin lesions the clinician can prepare a logical series of steps toward a correct diagnosis, even if the disease is initially unrecognized. Lynch has developed a problem-oriented algorithm for the nondermatologist (Fig. 2.20).[7] It can be applied to infants and children with skin disease, where it has been found to be most useful. Lynch's algorithm defines morphologic groups of dermatologic disease, which will allow the differential diagnosis and eventual correct diagnosis of a skin condition. These groups and the chapters in which they are found are listed in Table 2.1. (See also the Problem-Oriented

Fig. 2.19 (A) Annular arrangement of red, scaly papules in tinea corporis. **(B)** Annular arrangement of pink dermal nodules in granuloma annulare. **(C)** Grouped arrangement of vesicles on the ear of a child with herpes zoster.

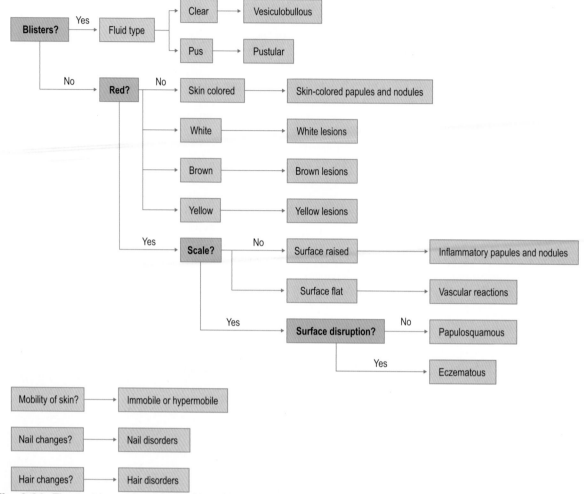

Fig. 2.20 The problem-oriented algorithm. (From Lynch PJ. Dermatology for the house officer, 3rd edn. Baltimore: Williams & Wilkins; 1994.)

Table 2.1 Groups of dermatologic disease

Morphologic group	Chapter
1. Vesiculobullous diseases	4, 5, 7, 8, 9, 11, 18
2. Pustular diseases	3, 5, 6
3. Skin-colored papules and nodules	7
4. White lesions	16
5. Brown lesions	16
6. Yellow lesions	7, 16
7. Inflammatory papules and nodules	3, 5, 6, 7, 9, 18
8. Vascular reactions	13
9. Papulosquamous diseases	9
10. Eczematous diseases	4, 18
11. Hair changes	14
12. Nail changes	15
13. Immobile and hypermobile skin	19

Differential Diagnosis Index, located inside the front and back covers of this book.)

The problem-oriented algorithm requires that three initial objective findings be determined:

Are blisters present?
Are the lesions red?
Are the lesions scaling?

A series of 10 additional determinations completes the algorithm.

The detection of blisters is the crucial initial step in this diagnostic exercise.[5] If even a single blister is detected, no matter what form of other skin lesions may be observed, the clinician should consider first the possibility of a blistering disease and proceed to determine whether the blister fluid is clear or pustular. If no blisters are observed, it should be determined if the skin lesions observed are red. If they are not red, the clinician should determine whether they are skin-colored or another color such as brown (which includes blue-black or black shades), yellow, or white.

The algorithm is particularly helpful if lesions are red.[5] If the skin lesions observed are red, it should be determined whether the individual lesions themselves are scaling or nonscaling. If they are red and nonscaling, it should be determined whether the surfaces of individual lesions are dome-shaped papules or flat. If lesions are red, nonscaling, and flat, vascular reactions should be considered. If lesions are red or raised, it should be determined whether they are firm or compressible. If compressible, vascular lesions should be considered. If firm, the morphologic group called *inflammatory papules and nodules* should be considered. If lesions are red and scaling, it should be decided whether there is surface disruption. If lesions have surface disruption, eczematous lesions should be considered. If they are red, scaly, dome-shaped papules, papulosquamous lesions should be considered.

Changes in skin mobility should be determined. This includes skin that can be stretched excessively or is fixed to the underlying fascia or deeper structures and cannot be moved. Finally, any changes to hair or nails should be described.

Starting with the three initial determinations, and then adding up to 10 more, one can place the skin disease observed into one of 13 morphologic groups. Grouping the skin disease observed in this fashion increases the likelihood of finding a precise diagnosis. Determining the proper diagnosis can be done using the Problem-Oriented Differential Diagnosis Index.

LABORATORY FINDINGS
Exfoliative Cytology

Exfoliative cytology is indicated in any blister-forming disease to detect acantholytic cells (pemphigus) or epidermal giant cells (herpes simplex or herpes zoster). *Scrape the blister base to obtain cells* with a No. 15 blade and place the sample on a glass microscope slide. Allow the sample to dry, and then apply Wright's or Giemsa stain and examine under the 40× objective of a microscope.[8,9]

Skin Biopsy

Any skin tumor, palpable purpura, persistent dermatitis, or blister that is not diagnosed by morphologic appearance should be examined by biopsy for a histopathologic diagnosis.[9]

Punch biopsy

The biopsy site should be cleansed with alcohol and then intradermally injected with 0.1–0.2 mL of lidocaine 1% using a tuberculin syringe and 30-gauge needle.[8,9] A 4 mm biopsy punch should be pressed firmly downward into the skin, which is stretched perpendicular to wrinkle lines. The punch is rotated until the soft subcutaneous fat is penetrated. The specimen is removed with forceps and scissors and placed in buffered formalin 10% for histologic examination.[8,9] For immunofluorescence testing, the specimen should be obtained from perilesional skin and frozen at −70°C or in liquid nitrogen, or placed in special skin immunofluorescence transport media.

Shave biopsy

After local anesthesia is achieved as previously described, a small elevated lesion may be shaved off with a sterile No. 15 blade or razor blade.[9]

Fungal Scraping

Any red, scaly skin or scaly scalp should be scraped to evaluate the possibility of dermatophyte infection, which can mimic a wide variety of skin disorders (see Ch. 6). Fine scales are scraped from the edge of a lesion onto a glass slide.[9] A drop of 20% potassium hydroxide added to the scale will dissolve the stratum corneum cells but not the hyphae. A coverslip is placed on the slide, and the scrapings are examined under the 10× objective of the microscope for long, thin, branching hyphae or spores.

Hair Examination

Hairs pulled from the scalp should be placed on a glass microscope slide, covered with histologic mounting media such as Histoclad or Permount and a coverslip, and examined under the 4 × objective of the microscope for hair shaft defects or telogen/anagen hair counts. Immersion oil is also helpful, but aqueous solutions are not used unless searching for fungus.

REFERENCES

1. Burton JL. The logic of dermatological diagnoses. Clin Exp Dermatol 1981; 6:1.
2. Mayer ME. The terminology of skin disorders. Primary Care 2000; 27:277.
3. Hubert JN, Callen JP, Kasteler S. Prevalence of cutaneous findings in hospitalized pediatric patients. Pediatr Dermatol 1997; 14:426.
4. Moss C. Cytogenetic and molecular evidence for cutaneous mosaicism: the ectodermal origin of Blaschko's lines. Amer J Med Genetics 1999; 85:324.
5. Paller AS. Expanding our concept of mosaic disorders of skin. Arch Dermatol 2001; 137:1236.
6. Lookingbill DP. Yield from a complete skin examination: findings in 1157 new dermatology patients. J Am Acad Dermatol 1988; 18:31.
7. Lynch PJ. Dermatology for the house officer, 3rd edn. Baltimore: Williams & Wilkins; 1994.
8. Oranje AP, Folkers E. The Tzanck smear: old, but still of inestimable value. Pediatr Dermatol 1988; 5:127.
9. Arndt KA. Manual of dermatologic therapeutics. II. Procedures and operations. Baltimore: Lippincott Williams & Wilkins; 2001.

Chapter 3 | Acne

ACNE VULGARIS

Clinical Features

The common variety of acne, acne vulgaris, is the most prevalent skin condition observed in the pediatric age group. Early lesions of acne develop primarily on the face in 40% of children aged 8–10 years. Many authorities believe acne is one of the earliest signs of puberty.[1,2] Eventually, 85% of adolescents will develop acne. Acne vulgaris peaks in late adolescence and may continue until the late twenties or early thirties.

Acne occurs in sebaceous follicles (Fig. 3.1). There are several types of follicular channels present in skin. The sebaceous follicles have large, abundant, sebaceous glands and a small vellus hair. They are located primarily on the face, upper chest, back, and penis (Fig. 3.2).

The initial lesion of acne is the microcomedone, which progresses to a comedone.[3,4] A comedone is a dilated epithelium-lined follicular sac filled with lamellated keratinous material, lipid, and bacteria. An open comedone (blackhead) has a wide patulous opening that is filled with a plug of stratum corneum cells (Fig. 3.3). Open comedones are the predominant clinical lesion in early acne vulgaris. The black color results from oxidized melanin within the stratum corneum cellular plug, not from dirt. Open comedones do not often progress to inflammatory lesions.

A closed comedone is a small white papule without surrounding erythema (Fig. 3.4). Closed comedones are the precursors to inflammatory acne. Children 8–10 years of age often have closed comedones for many months before red papules or pustules are observed (Fig. 3.5) If open (Fig. 3.6) and closed comedones are the predominant lesions seen in acne vulgaris, it is designated as *comedonal acne*.

Inflammatory lesions in acne prompt the adolescent to seek medical attention. These lesions include firm red papules, pustules, nodules, cysts (Fig. 3.7), and, rarely, interconnecting draining sinus tracts. Most adolescents at the time of examination will have a mixture of open and closed comedones, superficial red papules, and pustules (papulopustular acne) (Fig. 3.8). A small proportion will have deep nodules and cysts (nodulocystic acne) (Fig. 3.9). Excoriation of acne papules and comedones is common (Fig. 3.10) and scarring may result. Usually, multiple shallow erosions or crusts are found.

Inflammatory acne can be classified as mild, moderate, or severe. Mild inflammatory acne consists of a few to several inflammatory papules, pustules, and no nodules. Patients with moderate inflammatory acne will have several to many inflammatory papules, pustules, and a few to several nodules, whereas those with severe inflammatory acne will have numerous and/or extensive inflammatory papules, pustules, and many nodules (Figs 3.11, 3.12).[5]

Adolescents with cystic acne require prompt medical attention because ruptured cysts or sinus tracts result in scar formation (Fig. 3.13). New acne scars are highly vascular and have a red or purplish hue (Fig. 3.14). Such scars eventually regain normal skin color after several years. Acne scars may be depressed beneath the skin level, raised, or flat to the skin. In adolescents with a tendency toward keloid formation, keloidal scars can occur after acne lesions (Fig. 3.15), particularly over the sternum. Hypertrophic scars may also occur, even in those without keloids.

Several exogenous factors may affect acne vulgaris. Frictional acne from headbands, football helmets, baseball caps, tight bras, or other tight-fitting garments occurs predominantly under the skin area

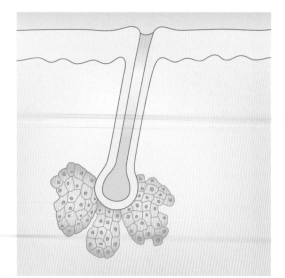

Fig. 3.1 Normal sebaceous follicles. Large sebaceous glands excrete sebum into cylindrical sebaceous channel.

Fig. 3.3 Open comedone. Wide, patulous opening of sebaceous channel with plug of stratum corneum cells in follicular mouth.

Fig. 3.2 Distribution of sebaceous follicles.

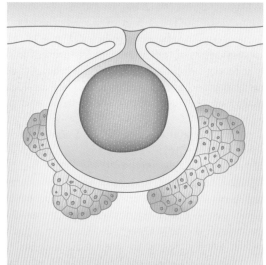

Fig. 3.4 Microcomedone (closed comedone). Obstruction of the follicular channel just beneath the opening.

where the garment is worn. Oil-based cosmetics may also be responsible for a worsening of acne over the areas where it is applied. Hair sprays and oil-based mousse cause worsening of the acne along the scalp hair margin.

Fig. 3.5 Comedonal acne. Multiple microcomedones on the forehead of an 8-year-old female.

Fig. 3.8 Inflammatory acne with red papules and pustules on the face.

Fig. 3.6 Comedonal acne with dozens of open comedones (blackheads).

Fig. 3.9 Acne cyst on the face.

Fig. 3.7 Mild inflammatory acne. Several inflammatory papules and pustules on forehead.

Fig. 3.10 Excoriated acne. Atrophic scar from attempted fingernail removal of acne lesion.

Fig. 3.11 Nodulocystic acne. Deep nodules and cysts on the face of an adolescent.

Fig. 3.13 Acne cyst healed with hypertrophic scar.

Fig. 3.14 Red-purple depressed scars on cheek of adolescent with scarring acne.

Fig. 3.12 Severe inflammatory acne. Extensive papules, pustules, and nodules on the back.

Fig. 3.15 Keloidal scarring on back of neck of adolescent with severe nodulocystic acne.

Differential Diagnosis

Conditions to be considered in the differential diagnosis of acne are listed in Box 3.1. Rosacea in children can be confused with acne vulgaris. In addition to acne papules and pustules, prominent telangiectasia and a persistent flush to cheeks, nose, or chin are observed. In many instances rosacea in children results from the use of topical glucocorticosteroids on the face (see Fig. 3.14).

Flat warts occurring on the face are sometimes confused with acne. They are papular, flat-topped, and skin-colored to slightly darker. The angiofibromas seen in tuberous sclerosis may be confused with acne. They are erythematous, soft papules seen in the nasolabial folds and on the cheeks and chin. The onset of these lesions is typically at 2–4 years of age. The absence of comedones is an important clue to the diagnosis of angiofibroma, as is the presence of ashleaf-shaped white macules, seizure disorders, and connective tissue nevi.

Molluscum contagiosum may occasionally be mistaken for acne lesions, but careful inspection will reveal the central umbilication at the top of the papule characteristic of this disease.

Pathogenesis

It is accepted that the primary event in acne vulgaris is the development of the microcomedone.[3,4] Four primary factors contribute to the development of acne vulgaris. These include: abnormal desquamation of keratinocytes in the lining of the pilosebaceous unit, an increase in sebum production, overgrowth of *Proprionibacterium acnes*, and inflammation.[3,4] This phenomenon is androgen dependent in acne vulgaris. The sebaceous follicles contain an enzyme, testosterone 5α-reductase, which converts plasma testosterone to dihydrotestosterone (DHT). DHT is a potent stimulus for sebaceous follicle cell differentiation and excessive cell and sebum production. Thus, acne requires the presence of both circulating androgens and the converting enzyme. The interplay of circulating and skin factors is believed to be crucial to the genesis of clinical acne vulgaris. However, the majority of patients who have only acne vulgaris do not have endocrinologic abnormalities.

The pathogenesis of inflammatory acne is less well understood. Spontaneous inflammation may occur in obstructed follicles. Inflammatory acne vulgaris lesions are characterized by an overgrowth of *P. acnes*. The response of the patient to *P. acnes* controls the degree of inflammation. Cellular products from *P. acnes* stimulate antibody, complement, and cell-mediated immune responses. The inflammation may lead to disruption of the follicular barrier and the release of sebum and *P. acnes* into the dermis.[3,4] Release of these contents into the dermis induces a foreign-body reaction, which may heal with fibrosis. Undoubtedly, manipulation of a closed comedone could lead to rupture of the cavity contents into the dermis, with a subsequent inflammatory response (see Fig. 3.5).

Treatment

See Tables 3.1 and 3.2 for a summary of initial acne treatment and selected acne treatment products.

Topical retinoids

The mainstay of antiacne vulgaris therapy is the use of topical retinoids applied to the skin to inhibit

Table 3.1 Quick Guide to Initial Acne Therapy

Clinical appearance	Treatment
Comedones only (Fig. 3-6)	Once daily retinoid before bed
Red papules, few pustules (Fig. 3-7)	Once daily retinoid before bed plus benzoyl peroxide 5% gel in the morning
Red papules, many pustules (Fig. 3-8)	Once daily retinoid before bed plus benzoyl peroxide 5% gel in the morning and a topical antibiotic twice a day or an oral antibiotic twice daily
Red papules, pustules, cysts, and nodules (Fig. 3-11)	Once daily retinoid before bed plus benzoyl peroxide 5% gel in the morning and an oral antibiotic twice daily

Table 3.2 Selected Acne Treatment Products

Product	Form	Size
TOPICAL KERATOLYTICS (apply once daily)		
Retinoids		
Tretinoin	0.05% solution	28 ml
	0.025% cream	20 g, 45 g
	0.05% cream	20 g, 45 g
	0.1% cream	20 g, 45 g
	0.01% gel	15 g, 45 g
	0.025% gel	15 g, 45 g
	0.1% micro gel	20 g, 45 g
	0.04% micro gel	20 g, 45 g
Adapalene	0.1% lotion	30 ml
	0.1% gel	15 g, 45 g
	0.1% pledgets	60
Tazarotene	0.05% gel	30 g, 100 g
	0.1% gel	30 g, 100 g
	0.1% cream	30 g
TOPICAL ANTIBIOTICS (apply once or twice daily)		
Benzoyl peroxide	2.5%, 3%, 4%, 5%, 6%. 8%, 10% gel	30 g, 45 g, 60 g, 90 g
	2.5%, 4%, 5%, 8%, 10% lotion	30 ml, 150 ml
Clindamycin phosphate	1% solution	30 ml, 60 ml
	1% gel	30 g, 42.77 g, 60 g
	1% pledgets	60
Clindamycin/ BPO	1% gel/5% gel	25 g, 45 g, 50 g
Azelaic acid	20% cream	30 g
SYSTEMIC ANTIBIOTICS (one or two capsules twice daily)		
Tetracycline hydrochloride		250- and 500-mg capsule
Erythromycin		250- and 500-mg capsule
Minocycline		50- and 100-mg capsule
Doxycycline		50- and 100-mg capsule
ORAL RETINOIDS (40-mg capsule twice daily for 16–20 weeks)		
Isotretinoin		10- and 40-mg capsule

formulations include gel, cream, and lotions. Retinoids should be applied to the acne-bearing areas of the skin once daily in the evening. Topical retinoids alone will control the majority of adolescent comedonal acne vulgaris. Dryness and irritation to the skin are the main side effects of topical retinoid therapy. The dryness and irritation may lead to discontinuation of therapy. Strategies designed to reduce dryness are use of a noncomedogenic moisturizer such as Moisturel, Purpose lotion, Cetaphil lotion or Neutrogena Moisture after application of the retinoid, then every other day rather than daily use of the retinoid, and the use of a cream formulation rather than a gel. Topical retinoid therapy is recommended as the primary therapy for comedonal and mild papular forms of acne. Continuous use for several months is often required. No increase in birth defects was noted in children whose mothers used tretinoin in the first trimester of pregnancy,[6] but tazarotene is rated pregnancy category X and should be used with caution in females of childbearing age.

Combination therapy

All acne vulgaris patients who have more than minimal inflammation should be started on combination therapy.[3,4] Combination therapy is the use of a retinoid with either benzoyl peroxide, topical or oral antibiotics, or azaleic acid. Combination therapy is more effective than monotherapy in the reduction of inflammatory lesions.[3,4]

Benzoyl peroxide (BPO) is the most potent topical antimicrobial. Also, microorganisms are not able to develop resistance to BPO. BPO is available in many formulations and strengths. In general, 5% is sufficient. The gel formulations are superior, but like the retinoids are more drying. Washes and cleansers are useful in covering large areas such as the back and chest. Also, BPO, being a peroxide, will bleach any colored fabric that it contacts.

Topical antibiotics are indicated in mild inflammatory acne. Due to the resistance of most *P. acnes* to erythromycin, clindamycin phosphate 1% is the now most efficacious of all topical antibiotics. Some percutaneous absorption may rarely occur with this drug, resulting in diarrhea and colitis. Topical antibiotics are less drying than the retinoids or BPO, but the development of antimicrobial resistance limits their use. They are best used in combination with BPO. This decreases the development of antimicrobial resistance and enhances efficacy.

microcomedone formation.[3,4] Retinoids normalize desquamation of the follicular epithelium and also have antiinflammatory properties. The retinoids include tretinoin, adapalene, and tazarotene. Retinoid

Oral antibiotics should be used in combination with a topical retinoid and topical BPO for the management of moderate to severe inflammatory acne vulgaris. Tetracycline, minocycline, doxycycline, and erythromycin are very effective in inflammatory acne; however, bacterial resistance to erythromycin is common. The usual dose is 500 mg to 1 g of tetracycline or erythromycin or 100–200 mg of minocycline or doxycycline taken daily divided into two doses. Tetracycline should be taken on an empty stomach for reliable absorption. Doxycycline is the most photosensitizing. Oral antibiotics should be discontinued as soon as the inflammatory lesions are under good control. Therapy for a period of at least 6–12 weeks is required for clinical improvement. Routine laboratory monitoring is unnecessary during antibiotic therapy.[7]

Following discontinuation of oral or topical antibiotics and BPO, maintenance therapy with a retinoid should be continued. If this is not done, it is likely that the primary process will restart and acne vulgaris will recur.

Oral retinoids

The oral retinoid isotretinoin (13-*cis*-retinoic acid) is very efficacious in the treatment of nodulocystic acne and severe inflammatory acne resistant to standard therapeutic regimens (see Fig. 3.11).[4,8] Isotretinoin is neither designed for nor efficacious in the treatment of comedonal acne or other mild forms of acne.[4,8] The precise mechanism of action is unknown, but decreased sebum production, follicular obstruction, and skin bacteria, in addition to general antiinflammatory activities have been described. The initial dosage is 40 mg once or twice daily (0.5–1.0 mg/kg/day) for 4–6 months, then the drug is stopped. Dosages below 0.5 mg/kg/24 hr or a cumulative dose of less than 120 mg/kg are associated with a significantly higher rate of treatment failure and relapse.[4,8] At the end of a course of isotretinoin, 40% are cured, 45% require the reinstitution of standard therapy, and 20% will need an additional course of isotretinoin.[4,8] In some patients the acne vulgaris will get worse during the first month of therapy. Side effects include dryness and scaliness of the skin, dry lips, and occasionally dry eyes and nose. Up to 10% of patients experience mild hair loss, but it is reversible. Elevated levels of liver enzymes and blood lipids may occur. Oral retinoids are the most efficacious treatment for severe cystic acne. Teratogenicity of isotretinoin is the main concern in females of childbearing potential.[4,8] The isotretinoin teratogen syndrome is characterized by malformations of the central nervous system, and has been reported in 25% of women who became pregnant while taking isotretinoin. Usage in young women of childbearing age requires strict adherence to the contraceptive recommendations and pregnancy testing guidelines.[4,8] Physicians prescribing accutane and patients taking the drug must be registered with the iPLEDGE pregnancy prevention program. Case reports suggest an association between isotretinoin and depression and suicide. Although the incidence of depression in patients taking accutane is not increased compared to the general population, this association should be discussed at the first visit and alterations in mental status assessed at follow-up visits.[4,8–10] Treatment for longer than 6 months is not recommended. At least a 3–4-month rest period from the drug is recommended before a second treatment course is considered.

Other acne treatments

There is no convincing evidence that dietary management, mild drying agents, abrasive scrubs, oral vitamin A, ultraviolet light, cryotherapy, or incision and drainage have any beneficial effects in the management of acne.

Azaleic acid 20% cream also has mild antiinflammatory properties.

Oral contraceptives have been shown to be effective in the treatment of acne vulgaris in females.[4] Other types of oral hormonal therapy should be reserved for patients with documented endocrine abnormalities or hirsutism. The presence in females of unusual acne, hirsutism, premature pubarche, or androgenic alopecia, especially when associated with obesity and/or menstrual irregularities, should prompt an endocrine evaluation.[11,12] The most common causes of hyperandrogenism in females are functional ovarian and functional adrenal hyperandrogenism. Laboratory screening for hyperandrogenism is evaluated by obtaining blood levels of total testosterone, free testosterone, luteinizing hormone/follicle stimulating hormone ratio, prolactin, dehydroepiandrosterone, and 17-hydroxyprogesterone. If any of these are elevated, referral to an endocrinologist is suggested. Treatment options for hyperandrogenism include oral contraceptives, low-dose glucocorticoids, and antiandrogens.[4]

Blue-light therapy has also been employed for the treatment of mild to moderate inflammatory acne. Eight 10–20 minute treatments given over a period of 4 weeks decreases inflammation at 8 weeks and 12 weeks after beginning therapy. It is slightly more effective than 1% clindamycin alone, but it does not treat noninflammatory lesions.[13]

Factors That Aggravate Acne Vulgaris

Acne can be aggravated by a variety of external factors, resulting in further obstruction of partially occluded sebaceous follicles. Avoidance of oil or propylene glycol-based cosmetics, hairstyling mousse, face creams, and hair sprays may alleviate acne 4–6 weeks after use of the cosmetics is discontinued. A list of nonacnegenic cosmetics and moisturizers is found in Box 3.2. Change of habits, such as not wearing tight-fitting garments, may be helpful.

Patient Education

Acne therapy requires that adequate time and explanation are part of any treatment program. It is important to explain the mechanism of acne and the treatment plan to the adolescent patient. The clinician should specifically explain that not much improvement can be expected for 4–8 weeks. Time should be set aside at the first visit to answer the patient's questions about acne. The clinician should be certain to inquire what the patient's peers, relatives, and others have advised. Written patient education handouts (see CD-ROM) and lists of useful moisturizers and cosmetics (see Box 3.2) are extremely valuable. The presence of excoriations should prompt an explanation regarding how attempted fingernail removal of acne usually results in scars that are permanent (see Figs 3.9 and 3.10). Suggestions such as applying a noncomedogenic moisturizer to the lesions rather than picking are useful.

Follow-up Visits

Follow-up visits should initially be every 8–12 weeks. Fifty percent improvement at 8 weeks is considered good initial improvement. The criterion for ideal control is a few new lesions every 2 weeks. The clinician and patient should not expect to completely prevent any new acne lesions from appearing. The clinician should also re-explain what the prescribed medications are intended to achieve and question the patient to determine whether the medications are being used properly. At the first visit a baseline evaluation grading comedones, papules, pustules, and cysts in each affected skin region should be entered on the patient's record to assist with objective measurement (Tables 3.3 and 3.4). At each subsequent visit the same scoring system should be used for comparison. Objective and subjective evaluations are more likely to differ than correlate in acne patients, and the clinician must rely on objective findings to properly evaluate response to therapy. Most authorities recommend treatment with oral antibiotics for at least 2–3 months. At the follow-up visit a decision to stop oral antibiotics is made when 90% improvement in

---

Box 3.2 Selected Noncomedogenic Cosmetics and Moisturizers

COSMETICS
Allercreme
  Matte-Finish Oil Free
Almay
  Fresh-Look Oil-Free Makeup
Clinique
  Pore Minimizer Makeup, Fragrance- and Oil-Free
Covergirl
  Fresh Look Oil-Free
Dermage
  Sheer Foundation Base
  Opaque Foundation Base
Elizabeth Arden
  Extra Control Oil Free
Lancome
  Maquicontrol, Oil-Free
Maybelline
  Shine-Free Oil-Control Liquid Makeup
Max Factor
  Maxi Shine Oil Free
Neutrogena
  Healthy Oil Free
Revlon
  New complexion Oil-Free
Ultima II
  Smoothing Oil-Free Foundation

MOISTURIZERS
Cetaphil moisturizing lotion
Cetaphil moisturizing cream
Moisturel
Neutrogena moisturizer for sensitive skin
Purpose lotion

Table 3.3 Grading System for Acne

Location	Baseline grade* (date)	FOLLOW-UP GRADE*		
		1 (date)	2 (date)	3 (date)
Face				
Comedones				
Papules				
Pustules				
Cysts				
Chest				
Comedones				
Papules				
Pustules				
Cysts				
Back				
Comedones				
Papules				
Pustules				
Cysts				

*0 = no lesions; 1 = 1–19 lesions; 2 = 20–39 lesions; 3 = 40 or more lesions. Grade each category (comedones, papules, pustules, cysts) for each location (face, chest, back).

Table 3.4 Evaluation of Acne Patients (Example)

Location	Baseline grade* (1/1/06)	FOLLOW-UP GRADE*		
		1 (3/1/06)	2 (5/1/06)	3 (7/1/06)
Face				
Comedones	2	1	1	0
Papules	1	1	0	0
Pustules	0	0	0	0
Cysts	0	0	0	0
Chest				
Comedones	0	0	0	0
Papules	0	0	0	0
Pustules	0	0	0	0
Cysts	0	0	0	0
Back				
Comedones	1	1	1	1
Papules	2	2	2	1
Pustules	1	0	0	0
Cysts	0			

*0 = no lesions; 1 = 1–19 lesions; 2 = 20–39 lesions; 3 = 40 or more lesions. Grade each category (comedones, papules, pustules, cysts) for each location (face, chest, back).

red papules and pustules is observed and documented by the scoring system listed in Tables 3.3 and 3.4. When oral antibiotics are stopped, improvement can be maintained by the continued use of a topical retinoid along with BPO alone or in conjunction with a topical antibiotic. At each follow-up visit, the clinician should emphasize that therapeutic response is slow in acne and is evaluated over weeks to months, not days. He or she should also be certain that the red purple scars, which require 6–12 months to fade, are not the lesions that determine alterations in treatment strategy. Scars are not influenced by antibiotics or keratolytics. Patient should be referred to a dermatologist if unresponsive to the initial treatment plan.

ACNE CONGOBLATA/ACNE FULMINANS

Clinical Features

Acne congoblata is severe, acute onset, eruptive nodulo-cystic acne without systemic symptoms. It is almost always seen in males. It may be seen as part of the follicular occlusion triad (acne congoblata, dissecting cellulitis of the scalp, hidranitis supprativa).

Acne fulminans is sudden-onset hemorrhagic and ulcerative acne associated with systemic symptoms. It may be seen as part of the SAPHO syndrome (synovitis-acne-pustulosis-hyperostosis-osteitis). It is also almost always seen in males.

Differential Diagnosis

The acute onset and severity of these problems makes their diagnosis relatively straightforward.

Pathogenesis

The pathogenesis of these entities is unknown.

Treatment

Treatment of acne congoblata is with isotretinoin as previously described. Treatment of acne fulminans is with the combination of isotretinoin and systemic glucocortcosteroids.[14] Recently, an anti-TNF agent has been used in the SAPHO syndrome in a patient unresponsive to isotretinoin and systemic glucocort-costeroids.[15]

Patient Education

The severe nature of these diseases should be discussed with patient. Treatment protocols need to be carefully reviewed.

Follow-up Visits

Follow-up visits should be biweekly until the disease is under control and then monthly until the treatment course is complete.

NEONATAL ACNE

Clinical Features

Neonatal acne (Fig. 3.16) is characterized by lesions primarily on the face, upper chest, and back, in a distribution similar to that in adolescent acne. The

Fig. 3.16 Neonatal acne on the face of a 3-month-old infant.

cheeks are most commonly affected. The individual lesions seen are the same as described for acne vulgaris. Inflammatory lesions are more common than comedones. The average age of onset is 3 weeks and mean duration of the disease is 4 months, with most cases resolving by 6 months of age.[16]

Differential Diagnosis

Nevus comedonicus, which may be confused with neonatal acne, is a birthmark consisting of a linear arrangement of open comedones (Fig. 3.17). It is present from birth and is usually unilateral, but bilateral lesions have been described. The anatomic abnormality of nevus comedonicus may also result in obstruction of the sebaceous follicle, with resultant red papules, pustules, or cysts, with inflammatory lesions restricted to the birthmark (Figs 3.18, 3.19).[17]

Fig. 3.17 Linear comedones in nevus comedonicus.

Fig. 3.18 Inflammatory nodules, open comedones, and hypertrophic scars within linear nevus comedonicus.

Fig. 3.19 Depressed scars in previously inflammatory linear nevus comedonicus.

Miliaria may also mimic neonatal acne, although the lesions are transient, lasting less than 48 hours, in contrast to neonatal acne lesions, which persist for weeks. Neonatal cephalic pustulosis begins in the first few weeks of life and may even be present shortly after birth. It is predominantly pustular with some papules, but no comedones. It resolves in a matter of days to a few weeks, with or without treatment with antifungals.

Pathogenesis

It is likely that neonatal acne is related to the effects of androgens on sebaceous glands. Neonatal sebaceous gland function correlates with maternal sebaceous gland function, but then declines rapidly.[18] This correlates with the spontaneous improvement in a matter of months. The role of *Malassezia* species in neonatal acne and whether or not neonatal acne and neonatal cephalic pustulosis are related entities remain matters of debate.[19,20]

Treatment

In the majority of cases, treatment is not necessary. Topical retinoids, BPO, and topical erythromcin have all been used.

Patient Education

Parents should be told of the benign nature of the disease and likely spontaneous resolution in a matter of 4–6 months.

Follow-up Visits

Follow-up visits should be monthly for the rare infant that requires treatment. Otherwise, follow-up visits are necessary only for those infants who have not improved by 6 months of age.

INFANTILE ACNE

Clinical Features

Infantile acne begins between 6 and 16 months of age with an average age of initial presentation being 9 months.[21] As with acne vulgaris, comedones, inflammatory papules, pustules, nodules, and cysts may be seen. The disease is more common in males (5:1). Infantile acne always affects the face, with the cheeks being the most severely involved area. Mean time to clearance is 18 months, with some patients requiring over 3 years to resolution.

Differential Diagnosis

The differential diagnosis is the same as for acne vulgaris.

Pathogenesis

The pathogenesis of infantile acne remains unknown, although the clinical appearance is quite similar to acne vulgaris. Screening for endocrine abnormalities with free testosterone and DHEAS is recommended, but without other clinical signs and symptoms is usually negative.

Treatment

Treatment runs the same spectrum as for acne vulgaris.[21] Mild disease requires only topical therapy. More severe disease will require oral antibiotics and in this age group erythromycin is used rather than tetracycline or its derivatives. Isotretinoin has been used in severe cases.[21,22]

Patient Education

Parents should be informed that this type of acne can have varying degrees of severity and, like acne vulgaris, treatment is based on the level of disease activity. It is thought that affected children are more likely to have severe acne vulgaris during adolescence.

Follow-up Visits

Follow-up visits should be the same as for acne vulgaris.

DRUG-INDUCED ACNE

Clinical Features

Drug-induced acne should be suspected if there is the sudden onset of a monomorphous papular and pustular eruption with involvement of the abdomen, lower back, arms, and legs (Figs 3.20, 3.21) in addition to the usual acne areas.[23]

Fig. 3.20 Steroid acne. Pustules all in the same stage on the chest of an adolescent treated with systemic steroids.

Fig. 3.21 Steroid acne on arm of adolescent.

Differential Diagnosis

Monomorphous papules and pustules in atypical locations along with a history of using a drug known to cause an acneiform eruption will separate this from acne vulgaris.

Pathogenesis

Numerous drugs including ACTH, androgenetic hormones, anticonvulsants, corticosteroids,[24] danazol, disulfiram, halogens, lithium, oral contraceptives, tuberculostatics, and vitamins B_2, B_6, and B_{12} have been reported to cause an acneiform eruption. There is no consolidating theory on the mechanism of action of the wide array of drugs.

Treatment

Treatment of choice is withdrawal of the offending drug. If this is not possible, therapy as for acne vulgaris may be instituted, but response is variable.

Patient Education

Patients should be informed that the eruption is caused by one of their medications and that the best treatment for the condition is, if possible, to stop taking the medication.

Follow-up Visits

A follow-up visit 6–8 weeks following cessation of the offending agent is recommended to see if the eruption is clearing.

PERIORAL DERMATITIS AND STEROID ROSACEA

Clinical Features

Erythema, slight scaling, and red papules characterize these closely related conditions.[25,26] In perioral dermatitis and steroid rosacea, lesions are found in the nasolabial folds, just beneath the nose, and on the chin (Figs 3.22, 3.23). Often, lesions begin as red macules with a slight scale and are misdiagnosed as dermatitis. A topical steroid is used, and the lesions get progressively worse, with redder, telangiectatic skin and red papules or pustules seen. Frequently, the child received the steroid from a relative in the healthcare field or used an over-the-counter steroid. Superpotent topical steroids are most often associated with steroid rosacea after a few weeks of use, but low-potency steroids will also induce the condition in susceptible children. The condition is most common in the preschool child.

Occasionally, pustules and red papules will be found on the lower eyelids in addition to the perioral

Fig. 3.23 Perioral dermatitis in 6-year-old boy. Note how it mimics dermatitis.

Fig. 3.24 Lower eyelid lesions in a child with perioral dermatitis.

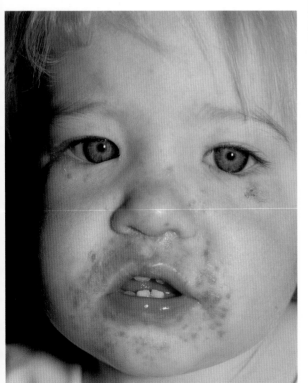

Fig. 3.22 Perioral dermatitis aggravated by topical steroid use. Toddler with perioral red papules and pustules from prolonged daily therapy with topical steroid.

skin (Fig. 3.24). Rarely, the perioral lesions will have a granulomatous histology and reveal closely spaced, red-brown micronodules in a perioral distribution.[27,28]

Differential Diagnosis

At the onset of disease, a dermatitis such as seborrheic or contact dermatitis is suspected, although careful examination will not detect disruption of the skin surface. This misdiagnosis leads to therapy that worsens the condition. Acne vulgaris may also be restricted to the perioral skin, but the presence of comedones, which are usually absent in rosacea, will help differentiate. Rarely, tinea faciei (see Ch. 6) will involve perioral skin. Scrapings for microscopic identification of fungus and fungal culture will differentiate.

Pathogenesis

Although many authorities believe that perioral dermatitis and steroid rosacea are related to acne, the pathogenesis is unclear. Sebaceous gland hyperplasia, obstructed sebaceous follicles, and prominent telangiectasias are pathologic features. In steroid rosacea the role of topically applied steroids is well established, although the exact mechanism is unknown. Although there is speculation that yeast species have a role, it is as yet unproven.

Treatment

Topical steroid preparations must be discontinued, recognizing that the condition will initially worsen. In mild cases topical antibiotics alone will suffice. With many red papules and pustules present, oral erythromycin for 4–6 weeks may be required.[25] Topical metronidazole 0.75% gel has also been shown to be effective.[26] The granulomatous form may take 6 months to clear.

Patient Education

Many patients are reluctant to stop topical steroids, because their skin is improved for 2 or 3 hours after each application. The clinician should insist that topical steroids be stopped and advise that the child's skin will worsen before it begins to improve. Patients should be cautioned not to use steroids to treat the predicted worsening. It is important to emphasize that this will respond to treatment that is similar to acne treatment. Providing advice that only certain children are susceptible is useful. For a Patient Education Sheet on Perioral Dermatitis, see CD-ROM.

Follow-Up Visits

A visit in 4 weeks to evaluate the response to therapy is recommended.

REFERENCES

1. Lucky AW, Biro FM, Simbartl LA, et al. Predictors of severity of acne vulgaris in young adolescent girls: results of a five-year longitudinal study. J Pediatr 1997; 130:30.
2. Lucky AW, Biro FM, Huster GA, et al. Acne vulgaris in early adolescent boys. Arch Dermatol 1991; 127:210.
3. Harper JC. An update on the pathogenesis and management of acne vulgaris. J Amer Acad Dermatol 2004: 51(Suppl 1):536–538.
4. Gollnick H, Cunliffe W. Management of acne: a report from a global alliance to improve outcomes in acne. J Am Acad Dermatol 2003; 49:S1–S38.
5. Brown SK, Shalita AR. Acne vulgaris. Lancet 1998; 351:1871;
6. Jick SS, Terris BZ, Jick H. First trimester topical tretinoin and congenital disorders. Lancet 1993; 341:1181.
7. Driscoll MS, Rothe MJ, Abrahamian L, et al. Long-term oral antibiotics for acne: is laboratory monitoring necessary? J Am Acad Dermatol 1993; 28:595.
8. Goldsmith LA, Bolognia JL, Callen JP, et al. Amercian Academy of Dermatology consensus conference on the safe and optimal use of isotretinoin: summary and recommendations. J Am Acad Dermatol 2004; 50:900–906.
9. Hull PR, D'Arcy C. Acne, depression, and suicide. Dermatol Clin 2005; 23:665–674.
10. Magin P, Pond D, Smith W. Isotretinoin, depression and suicide: a review of the evidence. Br J Gen Prac 2005; 55:134–138.
11. Rosenfield RJ, Lucky AW. Acne, hirsutism, and alopecia in adolescent girls: clinical expressions of androgen excess. Endocrinol Metab Clin North Am 1993; 8:347.
12. Lucky AW. Hormonal correlates of acne and hirsutism. Am J Med 1996; 98:89S.
13. Gold MH, Rao J, Goldman MP, et al. A multicenter clinical evaluation of mild to moderate inflammatory acne vulgaris of the face with visible blue light in comparison to topical 1% clindamycin antibiotic solution. J Drugs Dermatol 2005; 4:64–70.
14. Seukeran DC, Cunliffe WJ. The treatment of acne fulminans: a review of 25 cases. Br J Dermatol 1999; 141:307–309.
15. Iqbal M, Kolodney MS. Acne fulminans with synovitis-acne-pustulosis-hyperostosis (SAPHO) syndrome with infliximab. J Am Acad Dermatol 2005; 52:S118–120.
16. Katsambas AD, Katoulis AC, Stavropoulos P. Acne neonatorum: a study of 22 cases. Int J Dermatol 1999; 38:128–130.
17. Vasiloudes PE, Morelli JG, Weston WL. Inflammatory nevus comedonicus in children. J Am Acad Dermatol 1998; 38:834.
18. Henderson CA, Taylor J, Cunliffe WJ. Sebum excretion rates in mothers and neonates. Br J Dermatol 2000; 142:110–111.
19. Niamba P, Weill FX, Sarlangue J, et al. Is common neonatal cephalic pustulosis (neonatal acne) triggered by Malassezia sympodialis. Arch Dermatol 1998; 134:995–998.
20. Bergman JN, Eichenfield LF. Neonatal acne and cephalic pustulosis. Is Malassezia the whole story. Arch Dermatol 2002; 138:214–215.
21. Cunliffe WJ, Baron SE, Coulson IH. A clinical and therapeutic study of 29 patients with infantile acne. Br J Dermatol 2001; 145:463–466.
22. Barnes CJ, Eichenfield LF, Lee J, et al. A practical approach for the use of oral isotretinoin for infantile acne. Pediatr Dermatol 2005; 22:166–169.
23. Plewig G, Jansen T. Acneiform dermatoses. Dermatology 1998; 196:102–107.
24. Fung MA, Berger TG. A prospective study of acute onset steroid acne associated with administration of intravenous corticosteroids. Dermatology 2000; 200:43.
25. Weston WL, Morelli JG. Steroid rosacea in prepubertal children. Arch Ped Adol Med 2000; 154:62.
26. Laude TA, Salvemini JN. Perioral dermatitis in children. Semin Cutan Med Surg 1999; 18:206.
27. Frieden IJ, Prose NS, Fletcher V, et al. Granulomatous perioral dermatitis in children. Arch Dermatol 1989; 125:369.
28. Smitt JH, Das PK, Van Ginkel JW, Granulomatis perioral dermatitis (facial Afro-Caribbean childhood eruption [FACE]). Br J Dermatol 1991; 125:399.

Dermatitis

Dermatitis is inflammation of the superficial dermis and epidermis, leading to disruption of the skin surface. The characteristic disruption of the skin surface is recognized as crusting, weeping, excoriation, and cracking (fissures). The terms *dermatitis* and *eczema* are used interchangeably, although eczema was initially used to refer to blistering dermatitis, being derived from a Greek term meaning to boil over. Dermatitis may vary in intensity from an acute condition, with vesicle formation, oozing, and crusting, to a chronic form, with epidermal thickening; a shiny, flattened epidermal surface; and exaggerated skin creases. In an intermediate form, called *subacute dermatitis*, both vesiculation and epidermal thickening are present. *Acute dermatitis* implies an intense stimulus, whereas *chronic dermatitis* suggests a stimulus of low potency repeatedly occurring over time. All forms of dermatitis characteristically involve the epidermis, with inflammation and disruption of epidermal integrity.

The categories of dermatitis are traditional and imprecise. Except for irritant, allergic contact, and dry skin dermatitis, the pathogenesis is unknown. Therefore, it may be best simply to describe the lesions as dermatitis rather than to apply modifying adjectives, such as atopic, when the etiology is unclear. Some traditional terms are used in this section to avoid confusion with the previous medical literature.

ATOPIC DERMATITIS

Clinical Features

Atopic dermatitis is a hereditary disorder characterized by dry skin, the presence of eczema, and onset under 2 years (Box 4.1).[1,2] The term *atopy* was first employed in 1923 by Coca and Cooke to denote inherited human hypersensitivity as exemplified by asthma and hay fever. A variety of terms has been used in the literature to designate the condition. *Atopic eczema, allergic eczema, Besnier's prurigo, eczema,* and *circumscribed neurodermatitis* are terms less acceptable and less widely used than atopic dermatitis. Children with more severe atopic dermatitis are more likely to have respiratory manifestations, such as allergic rhinitis or extrinsic asthma.[2] Very rarely does a patient have all three.

The diagnosis of atopic dermatitis is a clinical one. The clinical appearance of atopic dermatitis may represent a phenotype resulting from different mechanisms. There is no single diagnostic criterion for the phenotype we appreciate as atopic dermatitis; rather, a combination of features must be considered. The major features listed in Box 4.1 are useful in the diagnosis. Although many other features may be noted, such as facial pallor, Denny's lines under the eyes, intolerance to wool or occlusive clothing, associated ichthyosis, cataracts, elevated serum immunoglobulin E levels, and eosinophilia, they are not considered diagnostic of the disease or necessary for the diagnosis.[1,2]

Atopic dermatitis usually begins before age 2 and commonly begins before the age of 6 months. At the onset the distribution is primarily on the scalp, face, trunk, and extensor surfaces of the arms and legs (Fig. 4.1). The earliest lesions appear on the scalp

Box 4.1 Cardinal diagnostic features of atopic dermatitis in children
Presence of a dermatitis
Dry skin
Onset under age 2 years
History of flexural dermatitis

Fig. 4.1 Age-dependent distribution of atopic dermatitis. Involvement of the face, scalp, trunk, and extensor surfaces of extremities as seen in infants, flexural skin in toddlers, and hands and feet in preteens and adolescents.

(Figs 4.2, 4.3) and the face (Figs 4.4, 4.5) Frequently, the dermatitis seen in the first months of life is a subacute dermatitis characterized by thickened skin and oozing (Fig. 4.6). The exact prevalence is unknown, but most authorities agree it has risen to the range of about 20% of children.[2] It is the most common dermatitis of childhood.

Itching has long been recognized as a significant feature of atopic dermatitis (Fig. 4.7). It commonly occurs in paroxysms and can be severe. In most patients itching is most severe in the evening, and scratching continues while the child is sleeping. The threshold for itching in atopic dermatitis patients is lowered, and their itching is more prolonged than that in normal persons. Scratching frenzies may be reported. The propensity for itching and the resultant trauma from scratching are central to the clinical appearance of atopic dermatitis (Fig. 4.8).

The distribution of dermatitis is largely age dependent (see Fig. 4.1).[2] Infantile atopic dermatitis, distributed largely on the face, trunk, and extensor surfaces of extremities, evolves into the childhood phase, with dermatitis on the feet and in the flexural areas, such as the antecubital fossa, popliteal fossa (Figs 4.9, 4.10), and neck. By adolescence the distribution has become that seen in older adults, with bilateral involvement of the flexural areas and hand dermatitis (Fig. 4.11). Involvement of the eyelids is common in all phases of atopic dermatitis and may help to make the diagnosis. Foot dermatitis is com-

Fig. 4.2 Onset of skin involvement in infants is frequently on the scalp.

Fig. 4.4 Early redness, scaling and dryness to cheeks in infant with initial presentation of atopic dermatitis.

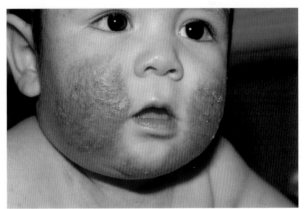

Fig. 4.5 Acute dermatitis of the cheeks with oozing and crusting in an infant with atopic dermatitis.

Fig. 4.3 Scalp involvement with 'rub alopecia' with accelerated hair loss from rubbing inflamed scalp.

Fig. 4.6 Moist crusts on red cheeks in infantile atopic dermatitis.

Fig. 4.7 Itching frenzies may be severe.

Fig. 4.9 Lichenification of the popliteal fossa from chronic rubbing of the skin in atopic dermatitis.

Fig. 4.10 Flexural involvement of popliteal fossa in atopic dermatitis.

Fig. 4.8 Severe itching in childhood atopic dermatitis.

Fig. 4.11 Dermatitis of hand and palm in adolescent with atopic dermatitis.

Fig. 4.12 Sparing of diaper area in infant with atopic dermatitis.

Fig. 4.14 Dry pinpoint red and white discrete papules on the extensor surface of the arm and keratosis pilaris.

mon in school-age children and adolescents and may be associated with atopic dermatitis or juvenile plantar dermatosis (JPD).

The primary clinical lesion of atopic dermatitis has not been described. Most of the visible skin lesions in atopic dermatitis are secondary to scratching; however, infants may develop dermatitis in areas that they cannot scratch or rub. The buttock of diaper protected skin of infants is often clear, possibly because it is inaccessible to scratching or because it is humidified by the occluding diaper (Fig. 4.12). Intense erythema and oozing are observed on the face and scalp in infancy but are otherwise absent except in patients with secondary bacterial infection. During exacerbation, dark-skinned patients may demonstrate follicular papules (Fig. 4.13), especially on the trunk. In black skin, hyperpigmented, lichenified nodules are commonly found on the lower arms and legs in addition to flexural involvement (see Fig. 4.6).

Fig. 4.15 Hypopigmented, slightly scaly patch of mild dermatitis on extremities is referred to as *pityriasis alba*.

Dry skin is a constant feature with atopic dermatitis[1,2] and may be noticed soon after birth, before the dermatitis is present (see Fig. 4.13). Patients with atopic dermatitis have reduced water content of the stratum corneum despite greater water loss through the skin and decreased water-binding ceramides on the skin surface. Dry skin and horny follicular papules (keratosis pilaris) are common findings, particularly on extensor surfaces (Fig. 4.14). Secretion of sebum and sweat may be suppressed in some patients with atopic dermatitis. Microscopic fractures of the stratum corneum during drying result in loss of the epidermal barrier and increased susceptibility to irritants and infection. There is little doubt that dryness of the skin during the winter months in cool climates is a significant factor in exacerbation of atopic dermatitis. Dry, slightly scaly, hypopigmented patches seen in mild atopic dermatitis are called *pityriasis alba* (Fig. 4.15). In pityriasis alba, histology shows mild inflammation in the hypopigmented areas.

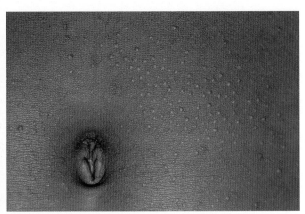

Fig. 4.13 Follicular hyperkeratosis seen on the abdomen of an adolescent with atopic dermatitis.

Box 4.2 Factors that aggravate atopic dermatitis

Drying of the skin

Soaping of the skin

Sweating

Contact sensitivity

Stress and anxiety

Secondary bacterial infection

Secondary herpes simplex virus infection

Fig. 4.17 Fissures and many breaks of the skin in atopic dermatitis, with secondary bacterial infection.

There are a number of factors that aggravate atopic dermatitis (Box 4.2). Children with atopic dermatitis may be extremely sensitive to certain contact irritants. They may experience bouts of itching and subsequent exacerbation of dermatitis when wool or an irritant chemical contacts the skin. Frequent soaping of the skin often result in prolonged itching. Sensitivity to contactants may partially explain localization of dermatitis in certain areas, particularly on the hands and feet.

Emotional stress indisputably leads to increased scratching. This occurs frequently in children, from either heightened awareness of itching or a habit of scratching. The child experiences transient relief after a scratching frenzy. Atopic dermatitis worsens during such episodes.

Secondary skin infection with bacteria such as *Staphylococcus aureus* may worsen the dermatitis (Figs 4.16–4.18) and worsen itching. Eczema herpeticum may present with fever and monomorphic papules and vesicles which may become eroded pits (Fig. 4.19).[3]

Fig. 4.18 Staphylococcal abscess of finger in child with atopic dermatitis.

Fig. 4.16 Secondarily infected atopic dermatitis with multiple pustules and areas of crusting.

Fig. 4.19 Numerous vesicles and erosions from herpes simplex virus infecting atopic dermatitis (*eczema herpeticum*).

Differential Diagnosis

Differential diagnosis should include any disorder manifested by dermatitis. Thus, contact dermatitis of the primary irritant and allergic type, seborrheic dermatitis, nummular eczema, scabies, molluscum contagiosum dermatitis, JPD, polymorphous light eruptions, the dermatitis of human immunodeficiency virus (HIV) infection, or the hereditary immunodeficiencies and tinea constitute the major considerations in the differential diagnosis of atopic dermatitis in childhood. In infants, seborrheic dermatitis may be impossible to distinguish from atopic dermatitis.

Pathogenesis

Although there are a number of hypotheses as to the mechanism of the generation of atopic dermatitis in children, the exact pathogenesis is unknown. There is no evidence to substantiate food or other allergies as the cause of atopic dermatitis.[4,5] Substances involved in both epidermal barrier dysfunction and immunity, such as the serine protease inhibitor SPINK-5 and interleukin-4 mutations, have been implicated in the pathogenesis.[6] Filaggrin is a protein that facilitates terminal differentiation of the epidermis and formation of the skin barrier. Recent data have suggested that loss-of-function genetic variants in the filaggrin gene are associated with atopic dermatitis.[7] Atopic dermatitis has been associated with various forms of both antibody and cellular immunodeficiency, abnormal β-adrenergic receptors and responses, food allergies, and aeroallergens such as house dust mites, but there is no convincing evidence to substantiate any of these hypotheses.[4] Defects in the innate immune response and production of antimicrobial peptides may also be involved.[8] The dermatitis can be exacerbated by drying or soaping of the skin, sweating, frictional irritation of the skin, or epicutaneous application of a contact irritant or allergen.

Treatment

Atopic dermatitis is a chronic disease that is frustrating for both child and parents. It may be disruptive to family dynamics and an economic burden on the family.[9,10] Weeks of effective control can be followed by a sudden, severe relapse. It is tempting for the clinician to focus on one or several factors as causes and to regard their elimination as curative. The patient or the family should be told that there is no immediate cure for atopic dermatitis but that spontaneous remissions do occur, and that this disorder can be controlled by therapy.

Initial therapy should be simple. The mainstays of initial therapy are topical steroid creams or ointments and lubrication. Depending on the climate and humidity, the treating physician may prefer the greasier

---

Box 4.3 Systemic therapy for atopic dermatitis

1. Use of hydroxyzine (1 mg/kg in a single daily dose) may decrease the sensation of pruritus. One dose given 1 hour before bedtime may be most effective. For severe pruritus, addition of cetirizine 2.5 mg for children under 6, or 5 mg for children over 6 years in the morning is helpful.

2. For crusted, oozing, infected-appearing lesions, antistaphylococcal oral antibiotics are beneficial (e.g. dicloxacillin, 12–25 mg/kg/day, or cephalexin, 25–50 mg/kg/day) three to four times a day for 10–14 days.

3. For eczema herpeticum, i.v. or oral acyclovir may be necessary for 5–10 days.

Box 4.4 Topical steroids for use in childhood atopic dermatitis

Low potency
Hydrocortisone 2.5%

Desonide 0.05%

Moderate potency (start with moderate potency)
Fluocinolone acetonide 0.025% (Fluonid, Synalar)

Mometasone furoate 0.1% (Elocon)

Triamcinolone 0.1% (Kenalog, Aristocort)

Box 4.5 Instructions for topical maintenance care of atopic dermatitis

1. Wet the skin for 5–10 minutes once a day.

2. Towel off the beads of water and quickly apply the steroid preparation to wet skin. Apply the steroid only on the area of dermatitis. Repeat the steroid application a second time 8–16 hours later.

3. Apply a lubricant to the entire body immediately after the topical steroid has been applied. The lubricant may be applied over the steroid if the steroid is a cream. The lubricant should be applied twice a day over the topical steroid.

4. Reapply the lubricant throughout the day if the skin appears dry.

5. As the skin improves, continue the lubricant twice a day or more frequently. Decrease the topical steroid to once a day, or less frequently as needed. One may also be able to decrease the potency of the topical steroid.

6. With further improvement, the frequency of lubrication can be decreased.

Box 4.6 Instructions for wet dressings

Materials needed
1. Prescription for moderately potent steroid ointment or cream.
2. Two pairs or more of cotton or mostly cotton sleepers or long johns.
3. Warm water in a sink or basin.

Technique
1. Apply steroid ointment to affected area.
2. Wet one pair of cotton sleepers in warm water.
3. Wring out thoroughly until barely damp.
4. Place damp sleeper on child and then put the dry sleeper over the damp one.
5. Be certain room is warm enough (not too hot) and child does not chill.

Duration of treatment (use 1 or 2)
1. Use overnight for 5–10 nights.
2. Change every 6 hours for 24–72 hours (e.g. reapply steroid; redampen damp sleepers).

Box 4.7 Alternative instructions for maintenance care of atopic dermatitis for busy households

1. Reduce bathing to every 3 or 4 days.
2. Apply moisturizer several times a day to dry skin.
3. Use antihistamines such as hydroxyzine at bedtime for itching as necessary.
4. If flare-up occurs, retreat as described in Boxes 4.4 and 4.5.

---

topical steroid ointments or the less greasy creams covered with a lubricating ointment, cream, or lotion. The addition of an antihistamine taken before bedtime for a 2-week period may also be helpful (Box 4.3). Topical steroids (Box 4.4) should be initially applied twice daily followed by a lubricant if a topical steroid cream is used. As the patient improves, the lubrication should be continued at least twice daily and the topical steroid applied only once a day (Box 4.5). If the dermatitis is severe, wet dressings can be used overnight (Box 4.6). Parents may exhibit an irrational fear of topical steroids, but careful studies of daily long-term use of moderate-strength steroids show no adverse effects.[11,12] If lichenification is present, topical steroids may need to be used daily for 4–6 weeks on the thickened areas.

Secondary bacterial infection by *S. aureus* or *Streptococcus pyogenes* resulting from the frequent breaks in the skin and the excoriations caused by scratching is treated with systemic antibiotics (see Box 4.3). Staphylococcal septicemia has been reported.[13] Methicillin-resistant *S. aureus* can complicate atopic dermatitis and require parenteral therapy.[14]

Secondary infection by herpes simplex virus may result in widespread vesicles and fever (see Ch. 8). Eczema herpeticum should be treated with antiherpes agents (see Box 4.3).

Use of large quantities of emollient has been well documented to improve atopic dermatitis.[15] Once improvement has been accomplished, parents may

substitute lubricants for the topical steroid to improve skin barrier function.[16,17] Also, patients and family should be instructed to pay careful attention to avoidance of factors that aggravate atopic dermatitis, which are listed in Box 4.2. On the follow-up visit, maintenance care instructions may be instituted (Boxes 4.5, 4.7). Busy households may find it impractical to follow the frequent bathing instructions listed in Box 4.5, and infrequent bathing strategies outlined in Box 4.7 may be employed.

Dry skin can be managed by rehydration of the skin with water and covering the skin generously with a lubricant. Irritant contact sensitivity can be managed by decreasing bathing to every third or fourth day and by washing infants without soap when possible. When using soap, contact with the skin can be limited by rinsing the child quickly after the soap has been applied. A soap substitute, such as Cetaphil or Moisturel cleansers, may be used. These are applied to the skin, then gently patted dry with a soft cloth instead of being rinsed off.

Sweating and heat intolerance can be managed by avoiding occlusive clothing, airtight occlusive dressings such as Saran Wrap, and overheating (Box 4.8). Direct contact with wool clothing, home cleaning agents, or irritating chemicals should be avoided.

Stress and anxiety can be difficult to manage. Stress increases the sense of pruritus. Parents usually do not intentionally accelerate stress for their children, and all stresses cannot be removed. The

---

Box 4.8 General instructions for long-term management of atopic dermatitis

Keep the skin lubricated

Wear loose-fitting cotton clothing

Keep fingernails trimmed short

Avoid overheating of skin

Always use a soap substitute

Limit time of soap-substitute exposure to the skin and pat dry – don't rinse off stress and anxiety of the atopic dermatitis condition may require therapeutic intervention and discussion with parents who already blame themselves for the child's condition. The clinician should emphasize to the parents that the primary problem is the skin condition. Removal of stress may be beneficial, but treatment of the skin is most important.

Relief of itching is the cornerstone of therapy for atopic dermatitis. Itching may be relieved by removal of the factors aggravating atopic dermatitis, or by the use of topical glucocorticosteroids of low or moderate potency or antihistamines.

Management of Acute Severe Dermatitis

Steroids and wet dressings

Acute weeping dermatitis is best treated by the application of wet dressings, the methodology for which is outlined in Box 4.6. Patients with this type of dermatitis often have multiple excoriations, crusting, and secondary bacterial infection; thus, when wet dressings are required antibiotics may also be necessary. A moderate-potency steroid ointment (see Box 4.4) should be applied to affected areas and covered with a damp cotton dressing followed by a dry cotton dressing. A handout on patient instructions for application of wet dressings is provided on the CD-ROM. The keys to successful wet dressings are to thoroughly wring out the clothing until it is barely damp and to be firm with the child. Systemic antistaphylococcal antibiotics should be administered to treat secondary infection, and oral antihistamines can be used to relieve pruritus. Therapy should be simple, and the routine use of lubricants is not recommended in the initial care of acute severe dermatitis.

Long-term management of atopic dermatitis

In addition to the methods of skin care listed in Boxes 4.5 and 4.7, cetyl alcohol lotion cleanser can be used as a soap substitute or in place of the bath. Additional lubricants can be applied throughout the day as needed.

Topical steroids and lubricants are discussed in detail in Chapter 22. Boxes 4.4 and 4.9 give a short list of commonly used products. In very humid climates lotions and creams may be effective. In drier climates greasy lubricants and ointments are more effective.

Referral for special therapy

Children who are not responding to treatment may be referred to a dermatologist for further treatment.

Box 4.9 Lubricants useful for atopic dermatitis
Hydrophilic petrolatum (Vaseline)
Aquaphor
Cetyl alcohol cream (Cetaphil)
Eucerin
Moisturel
Vanicreme

Often, therapeutic failures result from not following the treatment plan or the presence of unrecognized and untreated secondary bacterial or viral infection or scabies. A detailed history of the treatment times and individuals responsible for treatments will be useful in ascertaining compliance. Simplifying the regimen may be all that is necessary for success.

Topical tacrolimus ointment and pimecrolimus cream are calcineurin inhibitors and they may be effective in older children with limited areas of skin involvement, such as chronic facial dermatitis.[18,19] The high cost, burning and stinging on application, and the fear that they may lead to an increase of cancer limit their use to the short term, especially in children less 2 years of age.[20] The calcineurin inhibitors are about as potent as low- or medium-potency topical steroids.[21] Tars are effective in the treatment of atopic dermatitis, but they stink and stain. Phototherapy with narrow-band ultraviolet B (NB-UVB) or UVA1 sunlamps, or photochemotherapy with psoralen and ultraviolet light (PUVA) may be efficacious in children with atopic dermatitis who have failed standard therapy. Phototherapy should be supervised by trained, experienced dermatologists. In severe cases, systemic immunosuppression with ciclosporin or mycophenolate mofetil may help.

Alternative therapies

Although many parents or physicians are convinced that foods induce exacerbation of atopic dermatitis, scientific evidence to reproduce dermatitis by foods is unconvincing for most children, and delaying introduction of solids beyond the age of 6 months of life is not effective.[22] This should not become an emotional issue between parents and the treating physician. Restrictive diets have no long-term benefits in atopic dermatitis and may result in nutritional deficiency if too restrictive.[23] Evening primrose oil, desensitization shots, interferon, Chinese herbs, and a number of other remedies have been advocated, but there is no compelling evidence for their efficacy or long-term safety. Oral steroids may produce temporary benefits, but high doses are required, and they have no role in management of a chronic disease because of side effects with long-term use.

Patient Education

It is helpful to instruct the child and parents in the method of application of the topical medications (for Patient Education Sheets on Atopic Dermatitis [Eczema], and Wet Dressings, see CD-ROM). A clinician may choose to explain that the child has 'immature, sensitive' skin and that heredity plays a role in determining this tendency but the cause is not known. The clinician should emphasize to the parents the extreme pruritus associated with this condition. The severity of the itching sensation is so great that the child will produce painful, deep excoriations in an effort to relieve the pruritus. It should be stressed that a cure is not possible, but that good control can be achieved, so that the child can live a comfortable and normal life. Measures to prevent further skin irritation are also helpful (see Boxes 4.2, 4.8), especially soap avoidance, as is emphasis on the factors aggravating atopic dermatitis, particularly secondary bacterial skin infection. The patient and the parents should be told that the principle underlying good control is the liberal use of lubricants (see Box 4.9) to restore moisture to the skin and protect it from contactants. Using lubricants in this manner avoids the necessity for high-potency topical glucocorticosteroids and long-term steroid medications. The clinician should not make the patient or parents feel guilty if a flare of the eczema occurs. Active treatment should be immediately reinstituted. Therapy should be directed at relieving pruritus, not focusing pressure on stopping the child from scratching.

Follow-up Visits

The first follow-up visit should be within 7–14 days so that therapy can be reviewed. It is often helpful at this time to have the parents or child demonstrate how medication is applied and to determine how much was used. Use of the finger tip unit (FTU) is an effective and practical method to estimate the amount of topical steroids needed and used each day.[24] An FTU is the amount of ointment or cream expressed from the 5 mm diameter nozzle of the tube of medication applied from the distal skin crease at the DIP joint of the index finger to the end of the finger (Fig. 4.20). Two FTUs are about 1 g of medica-

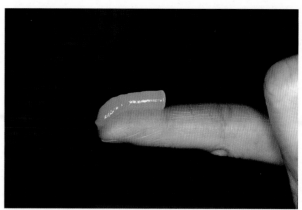

Fig. 4.20 Fingertip unit (FTU). Amount of cream or ointment from distal finger crease to tip.

tion. One FTU covers a surface area equal to the area of two palms of a flat adult hand.[24] One may also have the prescribed medication brought back for each visit so as to document the quantity used. Evaluation of the response to antihistamines and the need for antibiotics can be completed at the first follow-up visit. Thereafter, monthly visits will suffice until the patient is using lubricants only, after which he or she should be reevaluated every 3–6 months. Clinicians should be certain patients and their families know that the clinician will be available when flares occur, and the children should be examined for secondary infection at the visit related to the flare-up.

CONTACT DERMATITIS

Contact dermatitis, or dermatitis resulting from substances coming in direct contact with the skin, is divided into two subtypes: primary irritant contact dermatitis and allergic contact dermatitis.

Primary Irritant Contact Dermatitis

Strong chemicals that penetrate the epidermal barrier readily, weaker chemicals that penetrate a faulty epidermal barrier, or substances that remove intercellular lipids produce inflammation of the skin (primary irritant contact dermatitis). The form most commonly seen in pediatrics is diaper dermatitis. Dry skin dermatitis and JPD are other forms commonly seen in children.

Diaper dermatitis

Clinical features: The exact incidence of diaper dermatitis is unknown, but roughly 20% of all infants under age 2 years are believed to develop this con-

Fig. 4.21 Chafing type of diaper dermatitis.

Fig. 4.23 Candidiasis in the diaper area. A positive culture for *Candida* can be obtained from satellite pustules.

dition at some time.[25,26] Four clinical forms are recognized. The most frequently observed is chafing dermatitis, in which involvement of the convex surface of the thighs, buttocks, and waist area is common (Fig. 4.21). Chafing diaper dermatitis most frequently is observed at 7–12 months of age, when the baby's urine volume exceeds the absorbing capacity of the diaper, including the superabsorbent diapers. In the second form, the dermatitis is limited to the perianal area (Fig. 4.22). This form is particularly observed in newborns or in children who have experienced diarrhea. The third form is characterized by discrete shallow ulcerations scattered throughout the diaper area, including the genitalia. In the fourth form, beefy-red confluent erythema involving the inguinal creases and the genitalia, with satellite oval lesions about the periphery, is seen (Fig. 4.23). This fourth form is observed when sec-

ondary invasion with *Candida albicans* occurs. Despite major differences in clinical appearance, all four forms share a similar pathogenesis.

Differential diagnosis: Atopic dermatitis or the other forms of dermatitis may begin in the diaper area. Rarely, psoriasis, Langerhans cell histiocytosis, or the eruptions associated with hereditary immunodeficiencies or HIV infection may occur in this area. In perianal forms of diaper dermatitis, perianal cellulitis must be distinguished and a bacterial culture obtained.

Pathogenesis: Diaper dermatitis is a result of prolonged contact of urine and/or feces with diaper-area skin.[25-27] Feces are responsible for perianal distribution, urine for thigh and waistband lesions. Airtight occlusion of feces and urine by diaper covers increases the penetration of these alkaline substances through the epidermal barrier. Prolonged contact with water is central to the genesis of the dermatitis. Ammonia by itself is not responsible for the dermatitis. If diaper dermatitis is present for longer than 3 days, there is likely to be secondary C. *albicans* invasion of the inflammatory areas of the skin.

Treatment: The basis for all treatment programs is to remove the contactants (urine and feces) from the skin surface and eliminate maceration by keeping the diaper area dry.[28] Lubrication of diapered skin with a greasy ointment decreases the severity of diaper dermatitis and may protect the skin from urine and feces. Very frequent diaper changes, followed by application of ointment, limit maceration and decreases recurrences. Diaper changes several hours after the

Fig. 4.22 Perianal redness and shallow erosions in diaper dermatitis secondary to diarrhea.

baby goes to sleep for the night and reducing fluids just before bedtime may be beneficial. Plastic and rubber pants should be avoided when possible. Letting the diaper-area skin air dry when practical may be helpful, but moisture and maceration followed by dry air or hot, dry air such as from a hair dryer should be avoided. When contamination by urine and feces occurs, the skin should be rinsed gently with warm water. A minimum of soap should be used in this area. Care should be taken to not 'overtreat' the diaper area, because excessive washing and drying techniques can produce an irritant dermatitis.

Candidiasis in the diaper area requires topical antiyeast therapy such as nystatin or an imidazole. Use of topical steroid creams or ointments for diaper dermatitis is discouraged because of the development of striae or granuloma gluteale infantum.[29] Until toilet training is achieved or diaper care procedures are changed, recurrences may be frequent. The incidence of diaper dermatitis decreases with eight or more diaper changes per day.

Patient education: Reducing the amount of contact of urine and feces with skin is essential. Very frequent diaper changes and lubrication of the skin constitute the best prevention, with careful attention to overnight care. Having the baby sleep on a rubber sheet without a diaper cover may be helpful. Determining the person actually responsible for diaper changes during the daily routine is very helpful in planning a therapy program. In the 7–12-month-old, the parent should check the diaper for wetness several hours after bedtime and change the baby if wet. Restriction of fluids in the hour just before bedtime may also be helpful for the toddler. Parents should be told that successful toilet training is the ultimate cure.

Follow-up visits: The routine visits for pediatric care are sufficient for follow-up, but in cases of severe diaper dermatitis, a revisit in 2 days may be useful.

Dry skin dermatitis

Clinical features: A dry, rough skin surface with rectangular scales that have erythema on the scale borders is seen in dermatitis caused by dry skin (Fig. 4.24). Horny follicular papules on the proximal extremities and buttocks (keratosis pilaris) are also usually seen. Occasionally, the dermatitis will coalesce,

Fig. 4.24 Dry skin dermatitis. Infant with redness and scale secondary to excessive washing of skin.

Fig. 4.25 Lip-licker dermatitis associated with constant licking of dry lips.

and the patient will present with diffuse erythema. Lip-licking will result in dry skin dermatitis (Fig. 4.25).

Differential diagnosis: The differential diagnosis includes all other forms of dermatitis, the ichthyoses, and scabies. Children with atopic dermatitis have very dry skin.

Pathogenesis: Environmental humidity of less than 30% is the most important factor. Frequent soaping of the skin, removing skin lipids with alcohol or acetone, or the use of drying lotions predisposes children to dry skin dermatitis.

Treatment: Therapy is designed to restore moisture to the skin by liberal use of water followed by application of lubricants. Generally, application of water-in-oil emulsions (see Ch. 22) two or three times per day is sufficient.

Patient education: The value of a home humidifier in an area of low environmental humidity and of avoiding frequent soaping of the skin is important to convey to the patient or family (see Patient Education Sheet for Atopic Dermatitis [Eczema], CD-ROM). Children with dry skin require daily lubricant therapy.

Follow-up visits: One visit in 4 weeks' time to evaluate the therapy program is often sufficient.

Juvenile plantar dermatosis

Clinical features: Redness, cracking, and dryness of the weight-bearing surface of the foot are characteristic of juvenile plantar dermatosis (JPD). The great toes are often the first area involved. Involvement of the entire forefoot may occur and can mimic tinea pedis (Fig. 4.26). Involvement is usually quite symmetric. Many, but not all children with JPD exhibit features of atopic dermatitis.

Differential diagnosis: Tinea pedis often mimics JPD. However, JPD is quite common in preadolescence, whereas tinea pedis is uncommon; JPD involves weight-bearing areas, whereas tinea pedis involves the instep. Direct microscopic examination of scale with potassium hydroxide (KOH) and fungal culture will help to distinguish the two conditions. Allergic contact dermatitis usually involves the dorsum of the foot rather than the weight-bearing surface.

Treatment: The use of ointment bases such as Aquaphor or petroleum jelly applied two or three times per day is most useful. The ointment should be applied as soon as shoes are taken off to avoid heat and humidity in a shoe and xerosis in bare feet. Socks may need to remain over lubricated feet to prevent slipping and greasing of floors. Attempts to dry the feet often aggravate the condition because the feet are already dry and chapped. Topical glucocorticosteroid ointments of moderate potency may be required if inflammation is severe.

Patient education: Emphasis that this is neither a fungal infection nor the result of excessive sweating of the foot is important. The patient should recognize that the excessive dryness is similar to chapping of the skin.

Follow-up visits: A visit 2 weeks after therapy is begun is most useful in evaluating compliance and response to therapy.

Allergic Contact Dermatitis

Clinical features: The exact incidence of allergic contact dermatitis in children is unknown, but some authorities estimate it at 5–10% of all dermatitis.[30–33] By age 5, 10–20% of children have already been sensitized to at least one contact allergen, and sensitization is likely to have occurred in infancy.[34–36]

In childhood, allergic contact dermatitis usually presents as acute dermatitis with erythema, vesiculation, and oozing (Fig. 4.27). The dermatitis is limited to the area of contact with the external substance, such as the metal snaps on pants,[37] or the

Fig. 4.26 Red, shiny distal sole and toes associated with juvenile plantar dermatosis.

Fig. 4.27 Allergic contact dermatitis caused by poison ivy, with redness and linear blister formation.

Fig. 4.28 Linear blisters in allergic contact dermatitis to plants.

Fig. 4.30 Allergic contact dermatitis to nickel caused by metal snap on blue jeans.

Fig. 4.29 Chronic dermatitis on dorsa of feet and toes caused by potassium dichromate allergy from chronic exposure to leather tennis shoes.

Fig. 4.31 Nickel allergy from metal fasteners on jeans.

stem or leaf of a plant (see Fig. 4.16). Less often, children are exposed repeatedly to weaker chemical allergens, resulting in development of the features of subacute or chronic dermatitis (Fig. 4.28). Usually, the contactant is obvious, although considerable detective work is occasionally required to determine the cause. Once the response occurs and dermatitis is generated, as seen with a strong allergen such as poison ivy, it lasts for 3 weeks, even though the child has not had repeated exposure to the allergen.

Distribution of the dermatitis may provide an important clue to the contact allergen. For example, one may see involvement of the dorsa of the feet in shoe dermatitis (Fig. 4.29); of the subumbilical skin from metal snaps on pants (Figs 4.30, 4.31), earlobes, neck from necklace or chain (Fig. 4.32), wrists, and fingers caused by rings (Fig. 4.33) in metal allergy (e.g. caused by nickel); of the face and eyelids in

Fig. 4.32 Chronic dermatitis of neck from nickel allergy caused by necklace.

cosmetic allergy; of the axilla in deodorant allergy (Fig. 4.34); of the ear canal from medication; of the perioral area from toothpaste or lipstick; or of areas of

Fig. 4.33 Nickel allergy from metal ring.

Fig. 4.35 Dermatitis on top of feet from allergy to rubber chemicals (mercaptothiabendazole).

Fig. 4.34 Axillary redness and scale from allergic contact dermatitis to deodorants (formadehyde).

Box 4.10 Common sources of contact allergens in children

Plants: poison ivy, oak, and sumac (urushiol)

Clothing snaps, earrings, bracelets (nickel)

Shoes (potassium dichromate and rubber additives)

Topical medications, creams, lotions (neomycin, thimerosal, formaldehyde, quaternium 15 and other formaldehyde-releasing preservatives, wool alcohol [lanolin])

Perfumes, soaps, cosmetics (balsam of Peru, colophony, 'fragrances')

---

clothing from exposure to formaldehyde (Box 4.10). Once sensitization occurs, repeated exposure to the antigen may result in a widespread papulovesicular dermatitis or so-called 'id reaction.' This is particularly observed in nickel allergy.[30,32,37] Other areas, such as under soccer shin guards, may appear to be allergic contact dermatitis but absence of documenta-tion of allergic contact dermatitis suggests that these lesions are contact irritant reaction.[38]

Differential diagnosis: Although all other forms of dermatitis may mimic allergic contact dermatitis, it is usually localized to one area of skin. A sudden onset of dermatitis limited to the hands or feet in children and adolescents is most likely to be contact derma-titis (Fig. 4.35). Patch testing (described under Follow-up visits) may detect the chemical allergen and help distinguish allergic contact dermatitis from other forms of dermatitis.

Pathogenesis: Allergic contact dermatitis is a form of cell-mediated immunity. The process is divided into two distinct but interrelated phases: the sensitization phase, and the elicitation phase.[30,32] The antigens involved in allergic contact dermatitis are incomplete antigens called *haptens* (Box 4.11). The hapten applied to the skin surface penetrates the epidermis, com-bines with the antigen-binding site of the epidermal Langerhans cell, and is carried via the lymphatics to the regional lymph node. There the antigen is pro-cessed by macrophages and presented to T lympho-cytes. Recognition occurs, as does proliferation of the T lymphocytes specifically programmed to recognize that antigen. These T lymphocytes leave the lymph node and enter the bloodstream, migrating back to the skin. The sensitization phase takes 5–7 days to

---

Box 4.11 Characteristics of contact allergens

1. They are haptens.
2. They can penetrate the epidermis.

complete in the case of strong chemical allergens; with weak allergens, it may take from weeks to months.

In the elicitation phase, antigen-specific T lymphocytes are present in the skin. The next time the allergen comes in contact with the skin surface and penetrates the epidermis, the T lymphocyte combines with the allergen in the skin and releases inflammatory mediators, causing erythema and the accumulation and activation of mononuclear cells, which results in the dermatitis. This phase begins 6–18 hours after the antigen is applied.

A great variety of chemicals is responsible for causing allergic contact dermatitis, varying from the simple metal nickel to complex chemicals such as dinitrochlorobenzene. Common sources of contact allergens in children are listed in Box 4.10. However, they have certain features in common, as seen in Box 4.11.

Treatment: Antiinflammatory agents such as glucocorticosteroids are the therapy of choice in allergic contact dermatitis. In localized areas topical glucocorticosteroid ointments of moderate potency (see Box 4.4 and Ch. 22) applied three times per day may clear the dermatitis and decrease the discomfort. In generalized skin involvement, or in acute vesicular involvement, wet dressings and super-potent topical glucocorticosteroids for 2–3 days give dramatic relief. This is followed by application of moderate-potency topical glucocorticosteroids three times per day until the pruritus resolves. When the face or genital area is involved, or when greater than 10% of the skin surface is involved, oral glucocorticosteroids are used, such as prednisone, 1 mg/kg in a single dose every morning for 1 week and then tapered over 7–14 days. The popular steroid dose packs do not maintain their antiinflammatory effects for a sufficiently long time and often result in a rebound exacerbation of acute allergic contact dermatitis.

Patient education: Knowledge and avoidance of the offending antigen are central to the care of the child with allergic contact dermatitis. Poison ivy/oak dermatitis is the most common allergic contact dermatitis in the United States.[30,32,33] The next most common is nickel allergy. Nickel allergy often begins in infancy.[30,32,34,37] Other common contact allergens such as fragrances[39] are listed in Table 4.1. The clinician should emphasize that treatment requires 2 or 3 weeks of daily therapy.

Table 4.1 Most prevalent allergens in children

Allergen	Sensitized (%)
Plant (poison oak, ivy)	80*
Nickel	10
Neomycin	8
Potassium dichromate	8
Thimerosal	3
Balsam of Peru	2
Formaldehyde	1
Quaternium 15	1
Colophony	1
p-tert-Butylphenol formaldehyde	1
Wool (lanolin) alcohol	1

*In endemic areas of North America.

Follow-up visits: In 3–4 weeks, after the allergic dermatitis has subsided, epicutaneous (patch) testing (Fig. 4.36) to identify the offending allergen may be desirable in children in whom the cause is obscure. This is not necessary in acute poison ivy or plant-related dermatitis. Epicutaneous testing has been standardized and is reliable in detecting the suspected allergen. The test is made on the upper back. The suspected antigens are placed on the chambers, and vertical rows of three to five strips are placed on the upper back and firmly secured with nonirritating occlusive tape. The area is taped securely, so that it is airtight, and the patches are left on for 48 hours without allowing the area to become wet. The patient removes the patches and tape, and the tests are read 72–96 hours after initial application. Erythema and

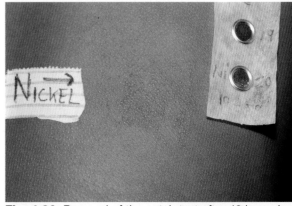

Fig. 4.36 Removal of the patch test after 48 hours in child with positive reaction to nickel.

vesiculation are observed in an allergic reaction, the same clinical and histologic features that are seen in allergic contact dermatitis. In allergic reactions the papules extend beyond the chamber margins, whereas they are limited to the chamber in irritant reactions. The angry back syndrome of hyperreactivity has not been reported in children. Standardized allergens have been developed by the North American Contact Dermatitis Group and may be obtained from the American Academy of Dermatology. Prepackaged patch testing materials such as TrueTest (Allerderm Laboratories) have been safely used in children.[34] Patch testing should be performed by a physician experienced in the interpretation and pitfalls of the procedure.

SEBORRHEIC DERMATITIS
Clinical Features

Chronic dermatitis accompanied by overproduction of sebum may occur on the scalp, face, midchest, or perineum in two age groups: the neonate and the adolescent. The scalp appears greasy, with accumulation of scales entrapped in the sebum. In some infants it is limited to the scalp, with a greasy accumulation of scales adherent to the scalp (seborrhea capitis). Many infants also have flexural dermatitis as seen in atopic dermatitis. Infants with a tendency to have seborrheic dermatitis may have severe worsening of their dermatitis if they develop persistent diaper dermatitis. In adolescents, erythema and greasy scales in the nasolabial folds and the scalp may be seen. In HIV-infected patients, seborrheic dermatitis may be an early sign of acquired immunodeficiency syndrome (AIDS). Widespread infantile seborrheic dermatitis associated with failure to thrive and recurrent infections should bring to mind a hereditary immunodeficiency disorder (Fig. 4.37).

Differential Diagnosis

Because physiologic overproduction of sebum occurs in many infants during the first 6 months of life, any dermatitis occurring at this age may be mistakenly called seborrheic dermatitis. There is considerable confusion over whether it is necessary to distinguish between atopic dermatitis, contact dermatitis, and seborrheic dermatitis in infants. Most infants with dermatitis eventually demonstrate features consistent with atopic dermatitis, especially if the involvement of the extremities and trunk accompanies the more

Fig. 4.37 Seborrheic dermatitis in an infant. Greasy scale and erythema in scalp with spreading to neck and trunk.

characteristic lesions of the scalp and face. Scabies may also mimic seborrheic dermatitis in this age group, and identifying mites by scraping unscratched burrows will confirm scabies. Seborrheic dermatitis with petechiae is often seen in Langerhans cell histiocytosis, and this diagnosis may also be excluded by skin biopsy. The hereditary immunodeficiency diseases, such as Leiner's disease, severe combined immunodeficiency, and the immunodeficiency that accompanies HIV infection, may be considered by the presence of signs and symptoms of failure to thrive, severe pulmonary or gastrointestinal infection accompanying the eruption, or the appropriate immunologic or serologic evaluation.

Multiple carboxylase deficiency and other biotin-responsive dermatoses also mimic seborrheic dermatitis, and serum biotin levels may be required to confirm the diagnosis.

Seborrheic dermatitis limited to the scalp (seborrhea capitis) must be distinguished from the diffuse form of tinea capitis caused by *Trichophyton tonsurans* and from cradle cap. A KOH examination of scalp scrapings plus a fungal culture will distinguish tinea capitis, whereas the absence of redness characterizes cradle cap.

Adolescent seborrheic dermatitis occurs in the nasolabial folds, midface, postauricular area, scalp, and chest. It may be difficult to distinguish from atopic or contact dermatitis, perioral dermatitis, or psoriasis.

Pathogenesis

Although seborrheic dermatitis has been attributed to excessive sebum accumulation on the skin surface, the mechanism is unknown. Overgrowth of *Pityrosporum orbicularis* occurs in sebum-rich environments and some authorities believe the host response to these yeasts may account for the inflammation.[40] Similarly, the pathogenesis of the seborrheic-like dermatitis of immunodeficiency or HIV infection is unknown. Although there are many carboxylase enzymes in skin, and biotin may be a cofactor for many skin enzymes, the mechanism of dermatitis is unknown.

Treatment

Topical steroid ointments of low potency applied twice daily for several days and then occasionally will often clear the dermatitis and treat recurrences. Keratolytic or antifungal shampoos on the scalp are usually not needed. They will be painful if they wash into the infant's eyes, and they may worsen the dermatitis. Tear-free shampoos should be adequate. The shampoo can remain on the scalp for several minutes while the scalp is lightly scrubbed with a soft brush or toothbrush to remove the scale and crust. The low-potency topical steroid ointment can be applied immediately after the shampoo is rinsed out. This process can be repeated daily until adequate improvement or resolution occurs. Oral biotin therapy should be used if biotin-responsive dermatoses are suspected. On the face, topical steroids should be of low potency and used twice daily for several days and then moisturizers substituted. If perioral dermatitis is suspected, antiacne therapy as outlined in Chapter 3 is used.

Patient Education

Patients and parents should be advised that the cause of this disorder is unknown. Although it is tempting to use rigorous methods to remove scale from the scalp, it is unnecessary. Gentle therapy repeated several days in a row is more effective.

Follow-up Visits

A visit in 1 week to review diagnostic tests and to evaluate response to therapy is recommended. If the lesions remain thick and crusted, the diagnosis of seborrheic dermatitis is probably incorrect and requires reevaluation of the condition. Thereafter, the child should be seen only if the dermatitis does not resolve.

NUMMULAR DERMATITIS

Clinical Features

Symmetrically distributed areas of dermatitis 1–10 cm in diameter are seen primarily on the extremities in this condition (Fig. 4.38). The Latin word *nummulus*, meaning 'little coin,' is used to describe the shape of the lesions. Two forms occur in children: the wet form, with oozing and crusting, and the dry form, with erythema and scaling (Fig. 4.39). Both forms are persistent, lasting for months if untreated. Most patients volunteer that the lesions are intensely pruritic, and they frequently are scratching the affected skin. Occasionally, a patient will deny touching the lesions.

Fig. 4.38 Two oozing coin-shaped areas of dermatitis in nummular eczema.

Fig. 4.39 Redness and scale in dry form of nummular eczema.

Differential Diagnosis

Nummular dermatitis is important because it frequently mimics two common pediatric conditions: impetigo and tinea corporis. The wet form is frequently confused with impetigo, and multiple courses of antibiotics are given before the diagnosis is suspected. Biopsy of the lesion readily distinguishes it from impetigo. The dry form can be distinguished from tinea corporis by a KOH examination of skin scrapings or a fungal culture. At times, nummular lesions will occur in otherwise typical atopic dermatitis or contact dermatitis. Presence of lichenification confirms rubbing and scratching of the lesions when the patient's history suggests absence of trauma to the lesions.

Pathogenesis

The cause is unknown. Mercury compounds can be implicated in a few patients, but are unlikely to be involved in the majority of cases.[41]

Treatment

The treatment is the same as for atopic dermatitis, although high-potency topical steroids are often required. A sedating antihistamine in the evening and a nonsedating antihistamine in the morning will reduce the pruritus. Lesions are difficult to resolve, and treatment programs require considerable effort before improvement is seen. Four to 6 weeks of therapy are required to reverse the thickening.

Patient Education

Patients should be informed of the chronicity of nummular eczema and its tendency to recur. They should be told that the cause is unknown.

Follow-up Visits

The child should be seen initially in 2 weeks to evaluate the initial response to therapy, and bimonthly follow-up for 6–12 months may be required.

KERATOSIS PILARIS, LICHEN SPINULOSUS, FOLLICULAR MUCINOSIS

Clinical Features

Keratosis pilaris is a common skin condition in childhood.[42,43] In keratosis pilaris, prominent follicular plugs are noted over the extensor aspects of the extremities, the buttocks, and the facial cheeks (Figs 4.40, 4.41). Individual lesions represent plugs of stratum corneum in individual follicular openings (Fig. 4.42). Dermatitis may surround the plugs. The affected skin surface feels rough and dry. Keratosis pilaris on facial skin is often accompanied by telangiectatic erythema, especially on the cheeks and occasionally the eyebrows (Fig. 4.43).[42] Keratosis pilaris is

Fig. 4.40 Keratotic follicular papules on cheeks in keratosis pilaris

Fig. 4.41 Keratosis pilaris.

Fig. 4.42 Keratotic follicular papules on extensor arm in keratosis pilaris.

Fig. 4.44 Two areas of lichen spinulosus associated with prominent white follicular plugs.

Fig. 4.43 Keratotic follicular papules within telangiectatic area on cheeks.

Fig. 4.45 Hypopigmented plaque of follicular mucinosis with associated follicular plugging and absence of hairs.

worsened by drying of skin and is frequently associated with dry skin, ichthyosis vulgaris, and atopic dermatitis. However, some children may present with extensive keratosis pilaris with no evidence of the other conditions. In these children keratosis pilaris is extensive and often involves the forearms, lower legs, and much of the face. Keratosis pilaris lesions often improve in a humid climate and become more extensive in a drier climate.

Lichen spinulosus represents grouping of hair follicles with prominent follicular plugs (Fig. 4.44). The lesions are usually hypopigmented and demonstrate fine scale on the intrafollicular skin.

Follicular mucinosis, also called *alopecia mucinosis*, presents with lesions that appear to be lichen spinulosus but have absent hairs (Fig. 4.45).[44] The intrafollicular skin demonstrates scale and may be indurated, giving the appearance of hairless plaques with follicular prominence.

Differential Diagnosis

Keratosis pilaris may be confused with microcomedones of acne, molluscum contagiosum, warts, milia, psoriasis, or occasionally folliculitis. Inflamed keratosis pilaris is often erroneously diagnosed as dermatitis. Because it is not seen at birth, it should be easily distinguished from neonatal acne and erythema toxicum. Lichen spinulosus may resemble lesions of keratosis pilaris, but they group together involving every follicle in one or several skin areas. Follicular mucinosis lesions are more indurated, localized, and have a more plaquelike appearance. Skin biopsy will distinguish between the two.

Pathogenesis

The pathogenesis is unknown. Some authorities regard keratosis pilaris as a disorder of keratinization.

They believe that the keratinous plug is produced through abnormal keratinization of the follicular channel. Others believe it is a response to drying of the skin surface, which results in a dry plug of scale lodged in follicular openings. It is more severe in cold, dry climates. Skin biopsy will separate these conditions because follicular mucinosis will demonstrate mucin in sebaceous glands and the outer root sheaths of affected hair follicles. Follicular mucinosis is occasionally associated with lymphoma in adults, and may uncommonly be associated with cutaneous T-cell lymphoma in children.[45]

Treatment

In the very mild forms of keratosis pilaris, the use of lubricants applied to wet skin may be sufficient to improve the condition because total resolution is often not possible. In more extensive keratosis pilaris, topical keratolytics may be required, frequently in combination with lubricants. Lactic acid 12% cream (Lac-Hydrin), a 10% urea cream, or a cream with both lactic acid and urea (Eucerin Plus Creme) applied several times a day is frequently beneficial. All treatment strategies require many weeks of therapy to see improvement. Therapy must be continued after improvement is seen. Topical tretinoin (Retin-A) or other retinoids are also effective but may cause significant irritation to the skin, particularly if the child has ichthyosis or associated atopic dermatitis. Often, when the child moves to a more humid climate the condition spontaneously improves. The facial telangiectasia, often a source of embarrassment to the child, may be treated with the vascular pulsed dye laser.

Lichen spinulosus may require low-potency topical steroid ointments in addition to lubrication for improvement. The plaques of follicular mucinosis require more potent topical steroid ointments and lubrication. Both conditions are difficult to resolve completely.

Patient Education

The patient and family should be informed of the nature of this disease and its likelihood of becoming chronic if untreated and even if treated (see Patient Education Sheets for Keratosis Pilaris and Creams and Ointments, on CD-ROM). They should also be advised of the slow response to therapy, the necessity of long-term treatment, and the usual eventual improvement or resolution of these conditions.

Follow-up Visits

A follow-up visit in 4–8 weeks to determine response to therapy is usually indicated. Thereafter, follow-up during routine evaluations is sufficient.

REFERENCES

1. Williams HC. Clinical practice. Atopic dermatitis. N Engl J Med 2005; 352(22):2314–2324.
2. Simpson EL, Hanifin JM. Atopic dermatitis. Med Clin North Am 2006; 90(1):149–167, ix.
3. Wollenberg A, Wetzel S, Burgdorf WH, et al. Viral infections in atopic dermatitis: pathogenic aspects and clinical management. J Allergy Clin Immunol 2003; 112(4):667–674.
4. Halbert AR, Weston WL, Morelli JG. Atopic dermatitis: is it an allergic disease? J Am Acad Dermatol 1995; 33(6):1008–1018.
5. Weston WL. Point-counterpoint: 'Allergy in atopic dermatitis: more harm than good?' J Cutan Med Surg 1999; 3(4):199–200.
6. Leung DY, Boguniewicz M, Howell MD, et al. New insights into atopic dermatitis. J Clin Invest 2004; 113(5):651–657.
7. Palmer CN, Irvine AD, Terron-Kwiatkowski A, et al. Common loss-of-function variants of the epidermal barrier protein filaggrin are a major predisposing factor for atopic dermatitis. Nat Genet 2006; 38(4):441–446.
8. Braff MH, Bardan A, Nizet V, et al. Cutaneous defense mechanisms by antimicrobial peptides. J Invest Dermatol 2005; 125(1):9–13.
9. Su JC, Kemp AS, Varigos GA, et al. Atopic eczema: its impact on the family and financial cost. Arch Dis Child 1997; 76(2):159–162.
10. Emerson RM, Williams HC, Allen BR. What is the cost of atopic dermatitis in preschool children? Br J Dermatol 2001; 144(3):514–522.
11. Ellison JA, Patel L, Ray DW, et al. Hypothalamic-pituitary-adrenal function and glucocorticoid sensitivity in atopic dermatitis. Pediatrics 2000; 105(4 Pt 1):794–799.
12. Charman C, Williams H. The use of corticosteroids and corticosteroid phobia in atopic dermatitis. Clin Dermatol 2003; 21(3):193–200.
13. Hoeger PH, Ganschow R, Finger G. Staphylococcal septicemia in children with atopic dermatitis. Pediatr Dermatol 2000; 17(2):111–114.
14. Gosbell IB. Methicillin-resistant Staphylococcus aureus: impact on dermatology practice. Am J Clin Dermatol 2004; 5(4):239–259.
15. Cork MJ, Britton J, Butler L, et al. Comparison of parent knowledge, therapy utilization and severity of atopic eczema before and after explanation and demonstration of topical therapies by a specialist dermatology nurse. Br J Dermatol 2003; 149(3):582–589.
16. Loden M, Andersson AC, Lindberg M. Improvement in skin barrier function in patients with atopic dermatitis after treatment with a moisturizing cream (Canoderm). Br J Dermatol 1999; 140(2):264–267.
17. Orchard D, Weston WL. The importance of vehicle in pediatric topical therapy. Pediatr Ann 2001; 30(4):208–210.
18. Reitamo S, Harper J, Bos JD, et al. 0.03% Tacrolimus ointment applied once or twice daily is more efficacious than 1% hydrocortisone acetate in children with moderate to severe atopic dermatitis: results of a randomized double-blind controlled trial. Br J Dermatol 2004; 150(3):554–562.

19. Paul C, Cork M, Rossi AB, et al. Safety and tolerability of 1% pimecrolimus cream among infants: experience with 1133 patients treated for up to 2 years. Pediatrics 2006; 117(1):e118–e128.

20. Aaronson DW. The 'black box' warning and allergy drugs. J Allergy Clin Immunol 2006; 117(1):40–44.

21. Ashcroft DM, Dimmock P, Garside R, et al. Efficacy and tolerability of topical pimecrolimus and tacrolimus in the treatment of atopic dermatitis: meta-analysis of randomised controlled trials. Br Med J 2005; 330(7490):516.

22. Zutavern A, Brockow I, Schaaf B, et al. Timing of solid food introduction in relation to atopic dermatitis and atopic sensitization: results from a prospective birth cohort study. Pediatrics 2006; 117(2):401–411.

23. Liu T, Howard RM, Mancini AJ, et al. Kwashiorkor in the United States: fad diets, perceived and true milk allergy, and nutritional ignorance. Arch Dermatol 2001; 137(5):630–636.

24. Long CC, Mills CM, Finlay AY. A practical guide to topical therapy in children. Br J Dermatol 1998; 138(2):293–296.

25. Ward DB, Fleischer AB Jr, Feldman SR, et al. Characterization of diaper dermatitis in the United States. Arch Pediatr Adolesc Med 2000; 154(9):943–946.

26. Visscher MO, Chatterjee R, Munson KA, et al. Development of diaper rash in the newborn. Pediatr Dermatol 2000; 17(1):52–57.

27. Darmstadt GL, Dinulos JG. Neonatal skin care. Pediatr Clin North Am 2000; 47(4):757–782.

28. Boiko S. Treatment of diaper dermatitis. Dermatol Clin 1999; 17(1):235–240, x.

29. De Zeeuw R, Van Praag MC, Oranje AP. Granuloma gluteale infantum: a case report. Pediatr Dermatol 2000; 17(2):141–143.

30. Bruckner AL, Weston WL. Beyond poison ivy: understanding allergic contact dermatitis in children. Pediatr Ann 2001; 30(4):203–206.

31. Mortz CG, Andersen KE. Allergic contact dermatitis in children and adolescents. Contact Dermatitis 1999; 41(3):121–130.

32. Weston WL, Bruckner A. Allergic contact dermatitis. Pediatr Clin North Am 2000; 47(4):897–907, vii.

33. Sasseville D. Phytodermatitis. J Cutan Med Surg 1999; 3(5):263–279.

34. Bruckner AL, Weston WL, Morelli JG. Does sensitization to contact allergens begin in infancy? Pediatrics 2000; 105(1):e3.

35. Clayton TH, Wilkinson SM, Rawcliffe C, et al. Allergic contact dermatitis in children: should pattern of dermatitis determine referral? A retrospective study of 500 children tested between 1995 and 2004 in one U.K. centre. Br J Dermatol 2006; 154(1):114–117.

36. Cetta F, Lambert GH, Ros SP. Newborn chemical exposure from over-the-counter skin care products. Clin Pediatr (Phila) 1991; 30(5):286–289.

37. Gawkrodger DJ, Lewis FM, Shah M. Contact sensitivity to nickel and other metals in jewelry reactors. J Am Acad Dermatol 2000; 43(1 Pt 1):31–36.

38. Weston WL, Morelli JG. Dermatitis under soccer shin guards: allergy or contact irritant reaction? Pediatr Dermatol 2006; 23(1):19–20.

39. Katsarou A, Armenaka M, Kalogeromitros D, et al. Contact reactions to fragrances. Ann Allergy Asthma Immunol 1999; 82(5):449–455.

40. DeAngelis YM, Gemmer CM, Kaczvinsky JR, et al. Three etiologic facets of dandruff and seborrheic dermatitis: *Malassezia* fungi, sebaceous lipids, and individual sensitivity. J Investig Dermatol Symp Proc 2005; 10(3):295–297.

41. Adachi A, Horikawa T, Takashima T, et al. Mercury-induced nummular dermatitis. J Am Acad Dermatol 2000; 43(2 Pt 2):383–385.

42. Lateef A, Schwartz RA. Keratosis pilaris. Cutis 1999; 63(4):205–207.

43. Dogra S, Kumar B. Epidemiology of skin diseases in school children: a study from northern India. Pediatr Dermatol 2003; 20(6):470–473.

44. Gibson LE, Muller SA, Peters MS. Follicular mucinosis of childhood and adolescence. Pediatr Dermatol 1988; 5(4):231–235.

45. Anderson BE, Mackley CL, Helm KF. Alopecia mucinosa: report of a case and review. J Cutan Med Surg 2003; 7(2):124–128.

Bacterial Infections (Pyodermas) and Spirochetal Infections of the Skin

Bacteria constantly colonize the skin surface and occasionally invade the epidermal barrier to replicate within the skin. The majority of skin microorganisms in healthy children are nonpathogenic. The two major pathogens found on children's skin are *Staphylococcus aureus* and *Streptococcus pyogenes*.[1-3] The former is found in 5% of children and the latter in 1%. However, during epidemics and in endemic areas, either of these organisms may be recovered from the skin of 50–80% of children. In warm, humid climates, and in those with poor skin hygiene, pyodermas are common in childhood.[1,3] Bacterial toxin-induced syndromes, such as scarlet fever, scalded skin syndrome, and toxic shock syndrome (TSS), are uncommon in childhood and result from skin injury by circulating toxins rather than direct bacterial invasion of skin.

IMPETIGO, ECTHYMA AND BACTERIAL INTERTRIGO

Clinical Features

Erosions covered by moist, honey-colored crusts are suggestive of impetigo (Figs 5.1–5.3).[1-9] Impetigo begins as small (1–2 mm) vesicles with fragile roofs that are quickly lost. Multiple lesions are often present, and exposed areas, such as the face, nares, and extremities, are the most common sites of involvement. The term *bullous impetigo* has been used to describe lesions with a central moist crust and an outer zone of blister formation (Figs 5.3, 5.4).[2] The blister is translucent, with a flaccid roof that is easily shed (see Fig. 5.4), such that bullous impetigo may be seen as shallow erosions with an outer rim of desquamation.[2] Whether blisters are small or large, *impetigo* is the preferred term. Impetigo has a high attack rate, and its spread is enhanced by crowding and poor socioeconomic conditions.[1,4] In contrast, ecthyma is

characterized by a firm, dry, dark crust with surrounding erythema and induration (Fig. 5.5).[2] Direct pressure on the crust results in the extrusion of purulent material from beneath the crust.

Both ecthyma and impetigo may occur simultaneously in the same patient. The clinical features are so characteristic that bacterial culture is not routinely performed.

In bacterial intertrigo, confluent, oozing areas are found in areas of skin folds such as neck, axilla, and groin (Figs 5.6, 5.7). The skin is tender, although the infant or child may not appear ill.[10]

Differential Diagnosis

Subacute dermatitis, such as nummular dermatitis, herpes simplex infections, and a kerion resulting from dermatophyte infections, may have moist crusts and mimic impetigo. Nummular dermatitis has dozens of symmetrically distributed lesions, as opposed to impetigo, which has a few asymmetric lesions. The periphery of nummular dermatitis is usually lichenified. Herpes simplex is usually a distinct group of lesions that even when crusted demonstrate a group of individual papules or vesicles beneath. Viral culture, fluorescent antibody testing of smears, or examination of Tzanck smear may be required to differentiate. A potassium hydroxide (KOH) examination or fungal culture may be required to distinguish a kerion from impetigo. Bullous impetigo must be differentiated from second-degree burns, fixed drug eruption, or the uncommon immunobullous diseases seen in childhood, such as linear immunoglobulin A (IgA) dermatosis, bullous pemphigoid, and bullous forms of erythema multiforme. A crusted second-degree burn, cutaneous diphtheria, or cutaneous anthrax may be confused with a solitary lesion of ecthyma. Bacterial

Fig. 5.1 Impetigo. Honey-colored, moist crust just above the upper lip.

Fig. 5.4 Bullous impetigo in a newborn. Multiple areas of flaccid blisters and shallow erosions on a red base.

Fig. 5.2 Impetigo. Spread of infection to top of nose from beneath the nose in an infant with impetigo.

Fig. 5.5 Dry crust with indurated border in a child with ecthyma.

Fig. 5.3 Bullous impetigo. Flaccid blister with thin border of desquamation on the abdomen of an infant.

Fig. 5.6 Bacterial intertrigo. Red oozing skin of neck folds in infant with streptococcal infection.

Fig. 5.7 Bacterial intertrigo. Red, oozing skin of popliteal fossa in infant with streptococcal infection.

culture of the purulent material beneath the crust may be required. Candidal intertrigo may be confused with bacterial intertrigo. A bacterial culture will differentiate.[10]

Pathogenesis

Invasion of the epidermis by pathogenic *S. aureus* or group A streptococci occurs in impetigo and ecthyma.[1,4] The depth of invasion in impetigo is superficial (into the upper epidermis), whereas the entire epidermis is involved in ecthyma (Fig. 5.8). Microscopic breaks in the epidermal barrier, such as the trauma of scratching dermatitic skin, predispose to impetigo, whereas staphylococci or streptococci penetrate the lower epidermis in ecthyma after injury to the mid and upper epidermis. Often, colonization of the skin

Fig. 5.8 Difference between impetigo and ecthyma. Superficial neutrophilic collection in midepidermis (shaded area on left) in impetigo in contrast to full-thickness epidermal involvement (shaded area on right) in ecthyma.

surface with the two major pathogens occurs several days to a month before the appearance of clinical lesions.[1] It is now recognized that in many areas of North America, community-acquired methicillin-resistant staphylococcus aureus (MRSA) are more likely to be responsible for impetigo than streptococci and account for 70–80% of childhood impetigo.[2,4–6] For impetigo secondary to an underlying skin disease, such as dermatitis, scabies, psoriasis, or varicella, staphylococci are virtually always responsible.[2,5] Poststreptococcal glomerulonephritis may follow such infections of the skin if nephritogenic strains of streptococci are involved.[6] Colonization of the skin surface occurs in bacterial intertrigo, and a positive culture can be obtained from the skin surface.

Treatment

Systemic antibiotics to eradicate staphylococci and streptococci are the treatment of choice for impetigo, ecthyma, and intertrigo.[2,5,9,10] To treat both pathogens, dicloxacillin, 15–50 mg/kg/day; cephalexin, 40–50 mg/kg/day; or cloxacillin, 50–100 mg/kg/day orally for a total of 10 days, may be used. Erythromycin, 40 mg/kg/day orally for 10 days, is an alternative, but in many areas of North America, strains of staphylococci resistant to erythromycin have been encountered.[2,5,6] If MRSA is recovered, bacterial sensitivities should guide therapy. In general, oral rifampin plus trimethoprim-sulfamethoxasole may be required to treat the MRSA.[4,5] Topical mupirocin for 1–5 days may be used , but mupirocin-resistant strains of staphloccoci have been observed.[4,5] If streptococci are cultured, penicillin V, 125–250 mg two times daily for 10 days, may be used.[4–8] Use of most topical antibiotics may result in partial clinical improvement but may also prolong the carriage state of the pathogen on the skin.[1,2,5] Topical mupirocin ointment is as efficacious as oral cephalexin.[7] Removal of crusts and scrubbing the impetigo skin lesions with antibacterial soaps have not been shown to be effective.[2] Hand washing with a surgical soap and simple measures of good hygiene may reduce the likelihood of spread.

The risk of nephritogenic strains of streptococci varies considerably throughout North America, but an active program in which both patients and contacts are treated will significantly reduce the incidence of acute glomerulonephritis in endemic areas.[2,6]

Patient Education

Good hand-washing techniques for the caregivers and the infected child, and good general personal hygiene, are useful in preventing further infection of contacts and reducing the chances for future infections. The child should begin treatment with antibiotic therapy at least 24 hours before returning to school or day care.[4] The highly contagious nature of these infections should be strongly emphasized, and contacts should be examined if feasible.

Follow-up Visits

A visit 10 days to 2 weeks after therapy has begun is useful to determine the therapeutic response and possible spread of the organism to contacts. In recurrent or persistent infections, bacterial culture should be performed to determine if an unusual or antibiotic resistant organism is present.

CELLULITIS

Clinical Features

Tender, warm, erythematous plaques with ill-defined borders are seen in cellulitis.[4,9–12] Occasionally, linear red macules proximal to the large plaque are seen. Regional lymphadenopathy and fever are common findings. A preceding puncture wound or other penetrating trauma to the skin is often noted (Figs 5.9, 5.10). Cellulitis of the fingertips in infants is called *blistering dactylitis* (Fig. 5.11), and several fingers may be involved. Perianal cellulitis in infants is increasingly recognized in North America and is characterized by tender perirectal erythema and pain on defecation (Figs 5.12, 5.13).[13] Superficial erosions of the perianal skin may be seen (see Fig. 5.13). Lesions may extend beyond perianal skin and involve perivaginal skin (Fig. 5.14). Infants and toddlers with perianal cellulitis often present with constipation. Perianal cellulitis in infants is virtually always caused by streptococci.

Cellulitis over large joints such as the hip, shoulder, or knee may be observed in infants and toddlers.[11] Extension into the joint cavity and bone is seen with cellulitis overlying a joint, particularly in infants. A bluish hue within the lesion in infants is particularly seen with *Haemophilus influenzae* cellulitis, but is also

Fig. 5.10 Cellulitis following self-manipulation of acne pustule.

Fig. 5.11 Blistering distal dactylitis.

Fig. 5.9 Puncture wound with surrounding cellulitis of the cheek.

Fig. 5.14 Streptococcal perivaginal cellulitis. Child also had perianal cellulitis.

Fig. 5.12 Streptococcal perianal cellulitis. Acutely tender red perianal skin.

Fig. 5.13 Streptococcal perianal cellulitis. Superficial erosions and erythema of perianal skin.

observed in cellulitis caused by other bacteria. Cellulitis of the cheeks (buccal cellulitis) or over joints in children ages 3 months to 3 years is predominantly caused by *H. influenzae* infection, whereas in older children it may result from streptococci or staphylococci.[4,9–11] *Haemophilus influenza* is now less common in North America since the introduction of the vaccine.[4] Streptococcal cellulitis spreads rapidly, within hours, in contrast to staphylococcal cellulitis. Septicemia may follow cellulitis in untreated patients.[4] Periorbital cellulitis is of great concern because of its potential for spread to the brain.[10–12]

Differential Diagnosis

Erythematous swellings overlying an unrecognized bony fracture may mimic cellulitis, although they may not feel warm. Similarly, pressure erythema, giant urticaria, and contact dermatitis in the early stages may be difficult to distinguish from cellulitis, but they do not produce tenderness. The redness and swelling over a septic joint may also mimic cellulitis. Acute cold injury to the fat of the cheeks of infants (popsicle panniculitis) may mimic facial cellulitis. Herpetic whitlow may mimic blistering distal dactylitis and diaper dermatitis, or painful rectal fissures may mimic perianal cellulitis.

Pathogenesis

Invasion of bacteria into the deep dermis and subcutaneous fat, with subsequent spread via the lymphatics, is responsible for the clinical features of cellulitis. Pathogenic streptococci account for most cases of cellulitis; *H. influenzae* and *S. aureus* including MRSA may also be responsible.[5,9–11] Blood cultures are most likely to reveal the responsible bacteria.[14] Aspiration of the center or advancing edge of the cellulitis is rarely positive.[14]

Treatment

In an acutely ill child or a child with periorbital cellulitis, hospitalization should be considered. Prompt administration of antibiotics is essential. If a streptococcal infection is suspected, systemic penicillin is given, either as benzathine penicillin, 600 000–1 200 000 U intramuscularly, or oral penicillin V, 30–60 mg/kg/day for 10 days.[4] In an acutely ill febrile infant or child, hospitalization and intravenous penicillin, up to 2 million U/day, is recommended. If staphylococcal cellulitis is suspected, oral dicloxacillin, 50–100 mg/kg/day, is recommended. If MRSA is recovered, intravenous vancomycin or triple therapy with clindamycin, trimethoprim-sulfamthoxazole, and rifampin will be required.[4,5] With blue cellulitis suggestive of infection with *H. influenzae*, a blood culture should be obtained before starting antibiotics. Common treatment regimens include cefotaxime, 75–100 mg/kg day or ceftriaxone, 50–75 mg/kg/day intramuscularly or intravenously, or ampicillin, 100–200 mg/kg/day given intravenously in combination with chloramphenicol, 50–85 mg/kg/day.[4]

Patient Education

The serious and potentially life-threatening nature of cellulitis should be explained to the patient and family. A thorough understanding of the portal of entry of bacteria is required. Instructions on the prompt cleansing of wounds should be given.

Follow-up Visits

If it is decided not to admit the child to a hospital, a visit within 24 hours is mandatory to assess the response to therapy and observe for signs of toxicity. Daily visits may be required until the child is recovering.

NECROTIZING FASCIITIS (STREPTOCOCCAL GANGRENE)

Clinical Features

Diabetic children with ketoacidosis and immunosuppressed children are susceptible to streptococcal gangrene.[15–17] This condition is rare, but public awareness is increasing in North America as stories about the 'flesh-eating bacteria syndrome' make headlines. Prompt recognition of necrotizing fasciitis may be lifesaving. The lesion begins as cellulitis, with tender erythematous plaques, usually on the leg. Within 2 hours bullae appear on the erythematous surface, accompanied by severe pain. A purulent center dev-

Fig. 5.15 Central black, painless necrosis; painful, yellow, purulent lake and surrounding erythema in necrotizing fasciitis in the leg of a diabetic adolescent.

elops, followed by the appearance of a black eschar and the subsidence of the acute pain (Fig. 5.15). The decrease in pain correlates well with destruction of the cutaneous nerves as they course through the fascia and subcutaneous tissue. Shock may develop. Over the next 2 days frank gangrene may be observed. Usually a clinical diagnosis is sufficient, but when difficulty distinguishing between cellulitis and necrotizing fasciitis occurs, magnetic resonance imaging (MRI) may be helpful.[17–17] In newborns, the most common location for necrotizing fasciitis is on the abdominal wall, where the first sign is redness and swelling of the periumbilical skin, and the diagnosis of omphalitis is considered. Culture of the deep tissues or blood yields group A streptococci.

Pathogenesis

Invasion by group A streptococci through the dermis and subcutaneous fat into the deep fascial compartments occurs because of the faulty host defenses of the immunosuppressed or diabetic patient. Often, trauma to the skin precedes the appearance of these lesions. Rapid spread and destruction of tissue occur. Compromise of blood flow occurs in deep fascial or muscular compartments, and infarction of large areas of skin and subcutaneous tissue occurs.[17]

Differential Diagnosis

Cellulitis may mimic necrotizing fasciitis early in the disease, but the rapid evolution of necrotizing fasciitis to form necrotic areas within hours after the onset helps distinguish the two. With the development of gangrene, arterial embolism or thrombosis should be considered. Metastatic calcification with occlusion of major skin vessels may also mimic necrotizing fasciitis, but its slow onset and lack of acute pain are important differentiating features.

Treatment

Prompt surgical debridement down to the fascia is essential and is the most important aspect of therapy.[4,16,17] Fluid management to maintain adequate venous return is essential, along with intravenous antimicrobial therapy at maximal doses for age, with a β-lactamase resistant bactericidal cell-wall

Fig. 5.16 Red, rough eruption of arm in streptococcal scarlet fever.

inhibitor plus a bacterial protein synthesis inhibitor such as clindamycin.[4] Correction of the metabolic abnormalities of diabetic ketoacidosis is important. For infection refractory to several hours of aggressive therapy, intravenous immunoglobulin may be considered.[4] Even with prompt surgical intervention, mortality is high.

Patient Education

The clinician should emphasize to the patient and family that good control of diabetes and proper personal hygiene are essential to prevent such episodes. Prompt cleansing of cuts or skin abrasions and application of topical antibiotics are suggested, and the patient should be strongly advised to seek prompt medical attention when the early signs of infection appear. Persons who have close contact with the affected child should contact their physician regarding prophylaxis with antibiotics.[4]

Follow-up Visits

After the patient is discharged from the hospital, a follow-up visit a week later is most helpful to evaluate the patient's progress. Weekly visits may be required to assess healing of the devitalized skin and deeper tissues.

SCARLET FEVER

Clinical Features

Scarlet fever occurs most often in children between 2 and 10 years of age.[4,18,19] The portal of entry of the streptococci may be either the pharynx or a skin wound. The exanthem appears 24–48 hours after infection and consists of erythematous macules and papules, beginning on the neck and spreading downward over the trunk to the extremities (Fig. 5.16).[4,19] In severe cases the exanthem may be petechial, and a positive tourniquet test is common. Petechiae in a linear pattern are seen along the major skin folds in the axillae and antecubital fossa (Pastia's sign). The palms and soles in scarlet fever are characteristically uninvolved, and a facial flush with circumoral pallor is common. Tongue involvement (a dry tongue with hypertrophied red papillae) is helpful in the differential diagnosis because a strawberry tongue is seen with streptococcal but not staphylococcal scarlet fever (Fig. 5.17). Generalized lymphadenopathy is common, with the inguinal lymph nodes particularly

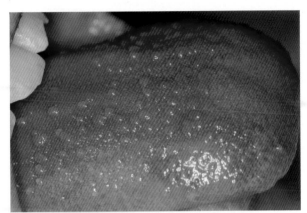

Fig. 5.17 Bright red (strawberry) tongue with prominent papillae in streptococcal scarlet fever.

enlarged. Desquamation occurs as the eruption fades, progressing in the same manner as it began. In black skin, tiny, slightly erythematous papules resembling gooseflesh are found. Although it is difficult to observe the erythema and the papular nature of the eruption in dark-skinned children, scarlet fever in these children is identical to that seen in white children.

Recent outbreaks of severe septicemic scarlet fever in North America have been noted. Hypotension and a toxic shock-like syndrome are reported. This severe disease is less likely in children than in adults.[4,19]

Differential Diagnosis

The scarlatiniform eruption is seen in other infectious diseases, such as that appearing in the early stages of viral hepatitis, infectious mononucleosis, Kawasaki disease, TSS, measles, and rubella. Drug-associated eruptions may also mimic scarlet fever. Drugs that result in scarlatiniform eruptions include the sulfonamides, penicillin, streptomycin, quinine, and atropine. Drug eruptions are more likely to produce mucosal erosions and crusts, which may be a helpful distinguishing sign.

Pathogenesis

Three immunologically distinct scarlet fever-producing toxins have been identified from cultures of *Streptococcus*.[4,19] Toxin release from streptococci is mediated by viral infection of the streptococci. The mechanism of action by the toxin on the skin is believed to depend on receptor-mediated activation of skin cells. Severe scarlet fever has been associated with the appearance of M protein type 1 and 3 strains of *Streptococcus* of an increased virulence.

Treatment

Penicillin, in the same doses as used for impetigo and streptococcal pharyngitis, is the treatment of choice for scarlet fever.[4,8] Erythromycin is used in penicillin-allergic patients. If staphylococcal scarlet fever is suspected, dicloxacillin, 15–50 mg/kg/day orally for 10 days, is recommended. Prompt treatment virtually eliminates the complications of scarlet fever, such as bacteremia, rheumatic fever, pneumonia, and meningitis.

During the later stages of desquamation, bland ointments applied to wet skin will restore the skin surface integrity and reduce cutaneous pain.

Patient Education

The association of scarlet fever with rheumatic fever is of great concern to patients and their families. It is important to reassure them that prompt treatment has virtually eliminated this association. Identification and cultures of patient contacts are essential.

Follow-up Visits

Approximately 7–10 days after the first visit, another visit is helpful to observe the response to therapy and to assess further any other sources of streptococcal infection in the household.

FOLLICULITIS, FURUNCULOSIS, AND CUTANEOUS ABSCESSES

Clinical Features

The manifestations of infection of the hair follicle vary clinically with the depth of bacterial invasion. Infection at the follicular orifice (superficial folliculitis) appears as tiny pustules, 1–2 mm in diameter (Fig. 5.18).[4] Folliculitis may be accompanied by impetigo (Fig 5.19).[20,21] Furunculosis (deep folliculitis) appears as tender erythematous nodules (Fig. 5.20).[22] Confluence of several adjacent areas of furunculosis produces a tender, erythematous tumor that becomes soft and fluctuant after several days. Abscesses are commonly found on the buttocks and trunk but may appear in any location (Fig. 5.21). Other household members may be affected.[20,22–24] *S. aureus* is regularly cultured from furuncles and abscesses, although Gram-

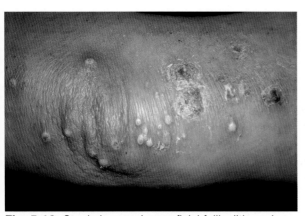

Fig. 5.18 Staphylococcal superficial folliculitis and ecthyma.

Fig. 5.21 Bacterial abscesses. Staphylococcal infection of the cheek of a child.

Fig. 5.19 Staphylococcal superficial folliculitis. Multiple pustules on a red base.

Fig. 5.22 Superficial folliculitis (left) with inflammation of the follicular mouth compared with deep folliculitis (right) with involvement of the base of the follicle and adjacent deep dermis.

Fig. 5.20 Deep bacterial folliculitis (furunculosis) on arm.

negative organisms may occasionally be found, such as in *Pseudomonas* folliculitis, associated with the use of hot tubs.[25] Superficial folliculitis is often found to contain the normal skin flora. Bacteremia from furun-

culosis or abscess may occur in an unpredictable fashion, particularly after manipulation of the lesion.

Differential Diagnosis

Acne pustules and chemical folliculitis from tars and other compounds contacting the skin may mimic superficial folliculitis. Occasionally, dermatophyte infections caused by animal ringworm or *Candida albicans* infections will produce follicular pustules.

Pathogenesis

Invasion of the follicular wall by bacteria is the usual cause of the disease (Fig. 5.22). Obstruction of the follicular orifice is an important factor in the development of the bacterial infection, particularly with staphylococcal folliculitis. Transmission of staphylococci including MRSA among household members may occur.[5,20] Occlusion of the skin or prolonged submersion in water contaminated with bacteria also predisposes to folliculitis.[22]

Treatment

Superficial folliculitis may be treated by topical antibiotics, applied twice daily for 10–14 days, and good skin hygiene. Furunculosis and abscesses are best treated by incision and drainage.[21,22] Systemic antistaphylococcal antibiotics, such as dicloxacillin, 15–50 mg/kg/day orally, or cephalexin, 40–50 mg/kg/day for 7–10 days, may be required in more severe cases. If MRSA is cultured, then rifampin plus trimethoprim-sulfamethoxasole may be required.[5] In chronic recurrent furunculosis, attention to nasal and skin carriers of staphylococci is required. Mupirocin 1% nasal ointment, with half of the prescribed amount applied to each nares daily for 5 days, and chronic antibiotic treatment with trimethoprim-sulfamethoxasole and rifampin may be necessary if good personal hygiene fails.

Patient Education

Good personal hygiene is important in preventing follicular skin infections. Thorough hand washing and daily skin cleansing with an antibacterial soap are most useful. It is advisable to instruct all household members in good hand-washing techniques. Avoiding chemicals that have resulted in follicular obstruction is beneficial. In *Pseudomonas* or Gram-negative folliculitis resulting from contaminated tubs or pools, proper chlorination or other treatment of the water should be emphasized.

Follow-up Visits

Poor personal hygiene is the most likely cause in children with recurrent episodes of furunculosis. Reemphasizing good hygiene for the entire household at the follow-up visit is most important.[22,24] Evaluation for diabetes mellitus and immunodeficiency is not warranted without recurrent or systemic infection of other organ systems such as the lungs (e.g. pneumonia), central nervous system (CNS) (e.g. encephalitis), or bone.

STAPHYLOCOCCAL SCALDED SKIN SYNDROME

Clinical Features

A spectrum of clinical presentations of staphylococcal scalded skin syndrome (SSSS) is now recognized, ranging from purely localized forms (bullous impetigo) to generalized involvement. In the generalized form, after an upper respiratory tract infection, a faint erythematous eruption begins on the central face (Fig. 5.23), neck, axillae, and groin.[4,26–28] The skin rapidly becomes acutely tender, with crusting around the mouth, eyes, and neck (Fig. 5.24). Mild friction to the skin results in epidermal separation, leaving a shiny, moist, red surface (Figs 5.25, 5.26).[26,27] In infants and preschool children the lesions are usually limited to the upper body, but in the newborn the entire cutaneous surface may be involved (Ritter's disease) (Fig. 5.27).[26,27] SSSS is uncommon over 5 years of age.

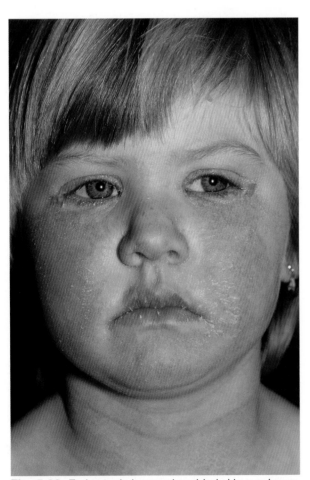

Fig. 5.23 Early staphylococcal scalded skin syndrome (SSSS) in a child, with erythema of cheeks.

Fig. 5.24 SSSS, with periorbital and perioral crusting.

Fig. 5.26 SSSS in an infant. Erythema and shallow erosions, with desquamation of the back.

Fig. 5.25 SSSS in a toddler. Erosion, with skin separated during examination by pushing on the skin surface.

Fig. 5.27 Diffuse erythema and extensive peeling in a newborn with neonatal SSSS (Ritter's disease).

Differential Diagnosis

Toxic epidermal necrolysis, which is often drug induced, may be differentiated from SSSS by skin biopsy and by a preceding history of urticarial or target lesions occurring 2–3 days before the appearance of bullae.[26,27] Pathologic examination of tissue from a patient with toxic epidermal necrolysis shows full epidermal necrosis, with a prominent perivascular dermal infiltrate of inflammatory cells. SSSS shows no epidermal necrosis or inflammatory cells on microscopic examination. In the newborn, diffuse cutaneous mastocytosis may mimic Ritter's disease. Occasionally SSSS may resemble exfoliative erythroderma, sunburn, thermal burn, TSS, or streptococcal scarlet fever.

Pathogenesis

S. aureus of phage group II[27,28] elaborates a toxin (Staphylococcus exfoliatin A), a serine protease that is carried via the circulation to the skin, where it acts on the cell surface of the epidermal granular cells and activates serine proteinases.[27] Injury to these keratinocytes results in intraepidermal separation of the cells within the granular layer and subsequent shedding of the entire granular layer and stratum corneum when a minor trauma occurs.

Treatment

Oral dicloxacillin, 15–50 mg/kg/day, is the treatment of choice. Newborns require intravenous antistaphylococcal antibiotics.[4] The skin should be handled minimally, especially during the first 24 hours. Newborns may require burn-therapy protocols, with careful attention to fluid and electrolyte losses and prevention of secondary infection of affected skin.[4,26] During the desquamation stage, bland ointments used twice a day may be helpful in restoring the skin surface and reducing cutaneous pain. Occasionally, pain during the first 24 hours is so severe as to require narcotics.

Patient Education

It is important that clinicians emphasize to patients and family that such lesions are not like a burn and that they heal without scarring. In children with normal host defenses, neutralizing antitoxins to the staphylococcal exfoliatin are rapidly formed, and the child recovers promptly. It should also be stressed that only certain staphylococci are capable of producing this condition, and that household carriers should be investigated.[4] Asymptomatic carriers may transmit the organism.[27] Nursery outbreaks require prompt investigation and culturing of all those entering the nursery, cohorting of infants and staff, empha-sis on hand washing with an antibacterial soap, and alleviating overcrowding and understaffing.[4,20]

Follow-up Visits

Routine follow-up care in regular pediatric visits is recommended.

TOXIC SHOCK SYNDROME

Clinical Features

A typical presentation of toxic shock syndrome (TSS) would involve a menstruating adolescent female who presents with a high fever, a scarlatiniform rash, and hypotension, with systolic blood pressure less than 90 mmHg or orthostatic syncope.[4,28] Prominent desquamation of the palms and soles follows the acute onset of the eruption by 1–2 weeks. These four features are the major diagnostic criteria for diagnosis of TSS (Box 5.1).[4,28]

Vomiting and diarrhea frequently precede the hypotensive state, and laboratory signs of liver, kidney, or muscle injury may be present. Diffuse redness of the

---

Box 5.1 Case definition of toxic shock syndrome

Fever (temperature higher than 39.9°C)

Rash (diffuse macular erythroderma)

Desquamation 1–2 weeks after the onset of illness, particularly of the palms and soles

Hypotension (systolic blood pressure less than 90 mmHg for adults or below the fifth percentile for children, or orthostatic syncope)

Involvement of three or more of the following organ systems:

Gastrointestinal (vomiting or diarrhea at onset of illness)

Muscular (severe myalgia or creatine phosphokinase level greater than two times normal)

Mucous membrane (hyperemia)

Hepatic (total bilirubin, serum glutamate oxaloacetate transaminase [SGOT], serum glutamate pyruvate transaminase [SGPT] two times normal)

Hematologic (platelets less than 100 000/mm³)

Renal (BUN or creatinine greater than two times normal)

CNS (disorientation or alterations in conscious-ness without focal neurologic signs when fever and hypotension are absent)

Negative results:

Blood, throat, and CSF cultures

Serologic tests for Rocky Mountain spotted fever, leptospirosis, or measles

Blood urea nitrogen (BUN), SGOT, SGPT

conjunctival, oral, and vaginal mucosa may be present.[28] Swelling of the hands and feet may be prominent. Severe myalgias or arthralgias and disorientation, meningismus, seizure, or coma may appear.[28] Although the majority of cases have been described in adolescent females, TSS was first noted in infants and children of either sex. In nonmenstrual TSS, pharyngitis or conjunctivitis lasting more than 5 days is observed, and the onset of fever and scarlatiniform rash is early in the course of disease. Nonmenstrual TSS has less frequent CNS manifestations, more frequent musculoskeletal involvement, and less anemia than that reported for menstrual TSS.[28] The circulatory collapse may be mild or severe, and a fatality rate of 10% has been reported.[28]

Differential Diagnosis

Rocky Mountain spotted fever, meningococcemia, and leptospirosis may each present with high fever, dizziness, and a rash. In each, the eruption is acral and purpuric and not scarlet fever-like. Blood cultures and specific serologic tests will help to distinguish these conditions. SSSS and TSS have many overlapping cutaneous features. The presence of skin tenderness and a positive Nikolsky sign (extension of skin separation with lateral pressure) favor SSSS. Streptococcal TSS and streptococcal scarlet fever may mimic SSSS and can be distinguished by pharyngeal and blood cultures. Kawasaki disease is more likely to occur in patients under age 5, lacks hypotension, and has prominent mucous membrane involvement. The fever in Kawasaki disease lasts for a week or more rather than the 2 or 3 days in TSS. The scarlatiniform skin eruption and desquamation may be the same in both TSS and Kawasaki syndrome.

Pathogenesis

S. aureus infection of the vagina or other tissues, such as the upper respiratory tract and sinuses, initiates the disease.[4,28] Prolonged tampon use, with positive cultures obtained from tampons, in adolescent females is very frequent.[25,28] Blood cultures positive for S. aureus may be obtained. Most authorities consider the staphylococcal toxin designated TSS-1 or enterotoxin C as responsible for the skin eruption and the systemic symptoms.[25,28] Both of these distinct exotoxins have been implicated.

Treatment

Prompt replacement of fluids to correct the hypotension is recommended, as are other general supportive measures for shock.[4,25] Treatment with a β-lactamase-resistant antistaphylococcal antibiotic, usually given intravenously, is recommended. Enzyme and toxin production by the bacteria can be inhibited with the addition of clindamycin. Bland lubricants may be used on the desquamating skin.

Patient Education

It is important for the clinician to emphasize the conditions that might favor the growth of the pathogenic organism. In adolescent females, discontinuing the use of tampons is advisable. It is unknown whether other antibacterial measures to reduce skin or mucous membrane colonization of staphylococci are useful.

Follow-up Visits

The hypotension and acute illness at the onset usually result in hospitalization. Daily examination, with documentation of the sequence of events, is often necessary to confirm the diagnosis. A follow-up visit at 1 week after discharge is advisable, as is a visit during the next anticipated menses for follow-up bacterial cultures.

CAT-SCRATCH DISEASE
Clinical Features

A primary inoculation papule on skin or mucous membrane 3–10 days after the scratch of a cat is found in 58% of children who develop cat-scratch disease (Fig. 5.28).[29,30] Inoculation of the ocular conjunctivae occurs in 5% of children, which will produce conjunctival granuloma. Persistent tender regional lymphadenitis of the lymph nodes draining the site of the cat scratch is observed in virtually all patients.[30] The lymph nodes become swollen 14–50 days after the scratch and remain enlarged for about 3 months, but may be enlarged for up to 1 year later. Spontaneous suppuration of lymph nodes occurs in 30% of cases.[4] About one-third of patients will experience a few days of fever, but occasionally fever persists for several weeks. Fatigue, headache, anorexia, vomiting, splenomegaly, sore throat, morbilliform exanthem, purulent conjunctivitis, and parotid swelling are uncommon findings in children with cat-scratch

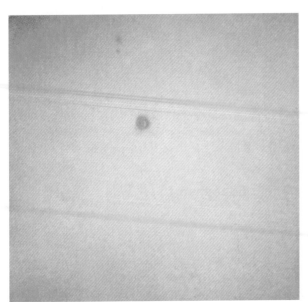

Fig. 5.28 Solitary papule at the site of a cat scratch in cat-scratch disease.

disease.[30] Quite rare are Parinaud's oculoglandular syndrome, encephalitis, and erythema nodosum.

Differential Diagnosis

Bacterial lymphadenitis caused by *S. aureus*, *S. pyogenes*, atypical mycobacteria, *Francisella tularensis*, or *Brucella* species may mimic cat-scratch disease. Biopsy of a papule or lymph node with Warthin-Starry silver impregnation stain will reveal the cat-scratch bacillus within areas of necrosis or granulomas. Molecular diagnosis by amplifying deoxyribonucleic acid (DNA) obtained from a papule or lymph node by the use of the polymerase chain reaction (PCR) is available in a few centers.[31] Other causes of persistent lymphadenopathy in children include lymphomas, cytomegalovirus (CMV), Epstein-Barr virus (EBV), mycobacterial infection, human immunodeficiency virus (HIV), toxoplasmosis, and deep fungus infection. Kerion caused by dermatophyte infection will produce local lymphadenopathy, but the kerion is much larger than an inoculation papule of cat-scratch disease.

Pathogenesis

The domestic cat is the primary reservoir of cat-scratch disease. A cat scratch (found in 80% of children with cat-scratch disease), bite, or other contact may inoculate the bacteria into the skin.[30] In 4% of cases the contact is a dog. The Gram-negative pleomorphic bacillus responsible for cat-scratch disease is *Bartonella henselae*, and may be detected in the dermis of inoculation papules or the microabscesses of enlarged lymph nodes if obtained within 1 month of the onset of symptoms. The host response may obscure the bacillus in long-standing disease. Skin test antigen for cat-scratch disease also contains the organism.[29] This organism is also believed to be responsible for bacillary angiomatosis.[30]

Treatment

In most patients spontaneous resolution of the disease occurs in 2–4 months.[4,30,32] Antibacterial therapy with rifampin, ciprofloxacin, azithromycin, gentamicin, or trimethoprim-sulfamethoxazole has been reported to be effective.[4,30,32] The optimal duration of therapy is unknown, but in immunosuppressed patients, relapses are common, and 2 months' therapy may be required for the immunosuppressed child. [4] Needle aspiration of a tender lymph node abscess is preferable to incision and drainage. Surgical excision of the lymph node is often done, especially when the diagnosis is in doubt.

Patient Education

Disposal of the healthy cat suspected of being the vector is not recommended.[30] About 5% of household contacts may develop cat-scratch disease, usually within 3 weeks of the first case. There is no evidence that the infection can be transmitted from human to human. Children should avoid rough play with a cat, and children with immune deficiencies should avoid contact with cats that scratch or bite.[4]

Follow-up Visits

Follow-up 1 week after the first visit is useful to ascertain the growth rate of enlarged nodes or to discuss biopsy results. Further visits are dictated by the child's recovery.

SPIROCHETAL DISEASES

Lyme Disease

Clinical features

The earliest feature of Lyme disease is the unique skin eruption called *erythema chronicum migrans* (ECM). ECM begins 4–20 days after the bite of a tick,

Fig. 5.29 Lyme disease. Annular erythema and central tick-bite papule.

although only one-third of patients distinctly recall a tick bite.[33,34] A red papule begins at the site of the tick bite, then slowly enlarges over several weeks to form an annular ring with a flat red border that clears in the center (Fig. 5.29). Sometimes the center remains a red, edematous plaque that feels hot. Fifty percent of patients will develop multiple secondary annular rings, which begin 1–6 days after the primary lesion appears.[33,34] Untreated ECM lasts about 3 weeks, then spontaneously resolves but may recur for up to 1 year or more, accompanied by arthritis or other symptoms. Skin lesions are associated with headaches, fatigue, myalgias, and low-grade fever.[33,34] Sometimes nausea, vomiting, sore throat, and lymphadenopathy will accompany ECM. A red nodule may appear on the ear, chest, or axillary fold, which represents borrelial lymphocytoma. Joint, CNS, and cardiac abnormalities begin about 4 weeks after the tick bite, after the ECM has resolved.[33,34] Fifty percent of untreated Lyme disease patients will develop arthritis.[33,34] The onset of arthritis is abrupt and usually monarticular (knee, shoulder, elbow, temporomandibular, ankle, wrist, or hip), and the affected joint is warm, swollen, and tender, but not red. The first episode lasts 1 week, but up to three recurrences are common. CNS disease occurs in 10–15% of untreated patients, with the classic triad of meningitis, cranial nerve palsies, and peripheral radiculoneuropathy. The meningitis is characterized by an excruciating headache and stiff neck and may include changes in behavior. The seventh nerve is most frequently involved, with recurrent episodes of facial palsy. Neuritic pain or focal weakness is seen with the peripheral radiculoneuropathy of Lyme disease. Less than 10% of patients experience cardiac involvement,

with atrioventricular block or myopericarditis reported. A great variety of additional neurologic and other organ symptoms is occasionally reported. The erythrocyte sedimentation rate (ESR) is usually elevated, but other routine laboratory studies are variable.

Differential diagnosis

Erythema chronicum migrans may mimic ringworm or be diagnosed as erythema multiforme or erythema marginatum. Tinea infections demonstrate disruption of the epidermis, but ECM does not. ECM evolves slowly, over days; erythema marginatum is transient, often changing hourly. A negative KOH examination and a skin biopsy will help distinguish. In ECM, a dense mononuclear cell accumulation around blood vessels and adnexal structures without epidermal changes is seen. A two-test approach using serologic tests for Lyme disease, with an enzyme immunoassay for immunoglobulin M (IgM) and a Western immunoblot test, is recommended when noncutaneous symptoms develop.[4,33,34] Ordering serologic tests for Lyme disease for patients with non-specific symptoms such as fatigue or arthralgia is not recommended.[4] Diagnosis using the PCR amplification of spirochetal DNA is not widely available. The organism can be cultured on modified Kelly's medium, but yields are too low for practical use.

Pathogenesis

The spirochete *Borrelia burgdorferi* is carried by a variety of ticks, predominantly the deer tick, *Ixodes dammini*. The ticks may be carried by rodents or house pets, or they may attach themselves to grasses or bushes. Humans are incidental hosts. The spirochete has irregular coils, is 10–30 μm long, and is found worldwide, although most cases come from northern Europe or the eastern, mid-Atlantic, or upper midwestern regions of the United States.[33–35] Subtypes of *B. burgdorferi* differ in North America and Europe by molecular typing, and this may account for the differences in prevalence. Within a few days after a tick bite, the spirochete migrates within the skin or enters the bloodstream. The incubation period is usually 7–14 days.[4] It appears that all symptoms and signs are directly related to the presence of the spirochete in affected tissues or the immune response to the organism.

Treatment

Some authorities advocate antibiotic treatment at the time of a deer-tick bite rather than observation, but this recommendation remains controversial and is not endorsed by the Committee on Infectious Diseases of the American Academy of Pediatrics.[4] For children over 8 years of age, oral doxycycline, 100 mg twice a day for 3 weeks, is the treatment of choice.[4,36] Younger children are treated with oral amoxicillin, 25–50 mg/kg/day divided in two doses for 14–21 days.[4] With systemic symptoms, ceftriaxone 75–100 mg/day i.v. or i.m. for 14–21 days or penicillin 200 000 units/kg/day i.v. for 14–21 days is required. [4] The ECM will disappear within 3 days with successful treatment, and secondary complications are almost always prevented. For mild secondary complications without heart block, the same oral regimens for early disease are recommended. If cerebrospinal fluid (CSF) pleocytosis or complete heart block is present, intravenous therapy with ceftriaxone, 75–100mg/kg daily for 14–21 days, or penicillin G, 300 000 U/kg/day for 2–4 weeks, may be required.[4]

Patient education

Avoidance of the tick vector is the basis of prevention.[35,36] Avoiding high-risk areas, such as wooded, grassy areas during tick season; wearing protective light-colored clothing with long sleeves and caps; using insect repellent; and periodic examination for ticks are required.[35,36] For children with ECM, parents should be advised about the possibility of secondary complications of arthritis or neurologic disease. The importance of completing the 3 weeks of therapy to avoid complications should be emphasized.

For children living in endemic areas who are 15 years of age or older, Lyme disease vaccine may be considered.[4,35,36]

Follow-up visits

After successful treatment, monthly visits for 3 months are useful to observe for late complications. A second antibiotic course may be required should secondary symptoms occur.

Syphilis

Clinical features

Acquired syphilis and congenital syphilis are uncommon, yet increasing, in industrialized countries, and common in Third World countries.[37,38] Acquired syphilis has three distinct stages.[4,37] Primary acquired syphilis is characterized by the chancre, a painless, shallow ulcer surrounded by a red indurated border that appears about 3 weeks after exposure (Fig. 5.30).

Fig. 5.30 Syphilitic chancre. Painless scrotal ulcer with indurated borders in an 11-year-old boy.

Fig. 5.31 Secondary syphilis. Ham-colored palmar macules on an adolescent with secondary syphilis.

If untreated, the chancre heals spontaneously in 1–2 months. Secondary syphilis is usually seen as a morbilliform generalized eruption accompanied by lymphadenopathy, fatigue, headache, and, sometimes, low-grade fever.[4,37] Involvement of the palms and soles is frequently observed (Fig. 5.31). Nodular, pustular, annular, and papulosquamous lesions are occasionally seen. Mucous patches are seen as weeping erosive areas on oral or genital mucosa. Tertiary stages are rare in childhood.

Congenital syphilis is usually asymptomatic in the newborn period, but may be observed as a persistent rhinorrhea that develops during the newborn period, or in severe cases, as hydrops fetalis or stillbirth.[4,37,38] The newborn with syphilis is usually small for gestational age and has mild hepatosplenomegaly.[4,37,38] Serologic testing of the mother is critical to the diagnosis because usually the newborn's symptoms are so mild they are overlooked.[4,39,40] Signs of late congenital syphilis may be the first clue to maternofetal transmission of syphilis. Late signs begin around 6 years of age and include cloudy corneas (interstitial keratitis) accompanied by photophobia and pain, bilateral eighth nerve deafness, notching of small central and lateral incisors (Hutchinson's teeth), painless swelling of the knees (Clutton's joint), perforation of the nasal septum leading to a saddle-nose deformity and perforated palate, saber tibia, and radial scarring about the mouth (rhagades).

Differential diagnosis

Syphilis is known as the great mimic, and a high index of suspicion for syphilis should be maintained. The primary chancre of acquired syphilis must be distinguished from bacterial ulcers, herpes simplex infections, chancroid, or lymphogranuloma venereum. The absence of pain is a useful distinguishing feature, and identification of *Treponema pallidum* by dark-field microscopic examination of smears of the ulcer base is definitive. Secondary acquired syphilis must be distinguished from pityriasis rosea, infectious mononucleosis, many other viral exanthems, and a number of papulosquamous diseases. Biopsy of a secondary syphilis lesion will reveal numerous plasma cells within a perivascular dermal infiltrate and swelling of the vascular endothelium.[40]

Both a nontreponemal and a treponemal serologic test for syphilis or PCR testing are required to make a presumptive diagnosis.[4,37,39,41] Nontreponemal tests include the Venereal Disease Research Laboratory (VDRL) test, the rapid plasma reagin (RPR) test, and the automated reagin test (ART). Treponemal tests include the fluorescent treponemal antibody absorption (FTA-ABS) test, the microhemagglutinin for *T. pallidum*, Western immunoblotting for *T. pallidum* antigen, and the *T. pallidum* immobilization test. In congenital syphilis the newborn presents a particularly difficult diagnostic problem because of maternally transferred immunoglobulin G (IgG).[39] In congenital syphilis the maternal syphilis serology should be positive, and the Western IgM immunoblotting test to *T. pallidum* antigen should be positive in the affected

infant. The IgM enzyme-linked immunosorbent assay (ELISA) test and the FTA-ABS should be positive in 80% of the affected babies.[39] HIV testing of the mother should be considered in babies with congenital syphilis.

Hydrops fetalis caused by congenital syphilis must be differentiated from blood group incompatibility and the rhinorrhea from upper respiratory tract bacterial and viral infections. Hepatosplenomegaly and intrauterine growth failure in newborns must be distinguished from other congenital infections, such as herpes simplex, CMV, rubella, and toxoplasmosis.

Pathogenesis

T. pallidum is the spirochete responsible for syphilis. It is spread primarily through sexual contact and invades the bloodstream in the early phase of infection.[37,40,41] The incubation period is 10–90 days.[4] The chancre of primary syphilis develops at the time the blood-borne infection is maximal; the morbilliform rash of secondary syphilis represents spirochetes that have left the bloodstream and entered the skin. Congenital syphilis represents a more massive infection than acquired syphilis, being blood borne in the fetus from the fourth month of pregnancy onward.[4,37,39,40] Rhinorrhea represents tissue infection of the nasopharynx, and late signs of congenital syphilis represent effects on developing tissues or osteomyelitis caused by *T. pallidum*.[41]

Treatment

Penicillin is the treatment of choice. Parenteral penicillin given intramuscularly weekly in the form of benzathine penicillin, in doses of 50 000 U/kg/day up to a total of 2.4 million U in a 3-week period, is recommended for children and adolescents with primary or secondary syphilis.[4] If the patient is allergic to penicillin, tetracycline, 500 mg four times a day for 14 days, or doxycycline, 100 mg twice daily for 4 weeks, is recommended. Aqueous crystalline penicillin G, 100 000–150 000 U/kg/day given intravenously every 8–12 hours for 10–14 days, is recommended for neonates with congenital syphilis.[4] If more than 1 day of therapy is missed, the entire course should be repeated. Retreatment is indicated if the clinical signs persist or recur, or if a sustained fourfold increase in a serologic test titer occurs, or if an initial high-titer serologic test fails to show a fourfold decrease within 6 months.

Patient education

Children and adolescents with primary or secondary syphilis should be thoroughly educated on transmission of the disease as recommended by the National Syphilis Elimination Program of the Centers for Disease Control and Prevention.[41] All recent sexual contacts of a child or adolescent with acquired syphilis should be identified, examined, serologically tested, and receive treatment if appropriate. Sexual abuse must be suspected in any young child with acquired syphilis. Routine serologic testing for syphilis in early pregnancy, and the importance of prenatal care for prevention, should be emphasized for congenital syphilis. It should also be emphasized that untreated syphilis in pregnancy results in death of the affected babies in 40% of cases.[4] Pregnant women at high risk for syphilis should also have serologic testing at 28 weeks of gestation. The clinician should emphasize to the pregnant woman that in congenital syphilis the long-term prognosis for the infant is good with prompt treatment, but delayed treatment may result in developmental delays and the complications of late congenital syphilis.[37,41]

Follow-up visits

After treatment, children should be seen monthly for 6 months to observe for recurrence and to monitor serologically. In congenital syphilis, serology tests should be obtained at 3, 6, and 12 months of age. Otherwise, follow-up during routine well-child care will suffice.

MYCOBACTERIAL DISEASE

Mycobacterial infections of the skin in children are uncommon. Of the mycobacterial infections, the one most likely encountered is *Mycobacterium marinum* infection, although *Mycobacterium chelonei* and *Mycobacterium avium-intracellulare* are increasingly identified as causes of lymphocutaneous syndromes.[42–45] Most mycobacterial infections cause cervical lymphadenitis in children, but cutaneous granulomas and necrotizing granulomas resulting in skin ulcers are increasingly seen.[42–45]

Mycobacterial Granulomas

Clinical features

Atypical mycobacteria, particularly *M. marinum*, produce a chronic granulomatous infection of the skin after direct inoculation through injured skin.[42–45] Contaminated fresh or salt water of warm temperatures (30–32°C), such as tropical fish tanks or hot swimming pools, is the usual source of infection in child-

Fig. 5.32 Red nodule on the finger of an adolescent male with *M. marinum* infection (swimming pool granuloma, fish tank granuloma).

Fig. 5.33 Multiple red nodules in *M. marinum* infection.

ren. The first appearance of red papules or nodules occurs at the site of abrasion or skin injury within 3–4 weeks (Fig. 5.32). The papules or nodules may ulcerate, or more likely coalesce to form a red-brown plaque or nodule (Fig. 5.33). The surface of the plaque may become verrucous. The plaque may persist for months to years if untreated. The arm and dorsum of the hand account for 80% of lesions, with the remainder on the knee. Usually the lesions are solitary, although a pattern of ascending skin nodules on an extremity has been described (sporotrichoid pattern). No lymphadenopathy is found. Adolescents are most commonly infected, but toddlers may also be infected.

Differential diagnosis

Verrucous plaques need to be distinguished from warts, psoriasis, or other granulomatous diseases such as sarcoidosis, tuberculosis, or foreign-body granulomas. The sporotrichoid pattern must be distinguished from sporotrichosis, and the ulcerative lesions must be distinguished from Langerhans cell histiocytosis, leishmaniasis, and bacterial or fungal ulcers. A skin biopsy stained for acid-fast organisms will help, but culture of the biopsy for atypical mycobacteria and deep fungal organisms will be definitive. History of exposure to a tropical fish tank or swimming in warm waters is helpful.

Pathogenesis

Abrasion or disruption of the skin, plus exposure to warm water containing the organism, is required for infection by the slender, aerobic, acid-fast rod *M. marinum*.[43,45] The organism induces a granuloma with a mixture of lymphocytes, macrophages, and epithelioid giant cells. The verrucous lesions also feature epithelial hyperplasia. Other mycobacteria may be found in soil.

Treatment

Spontaneous resolution has been reported, but it may require 1 or 2 years, and most authorities recommend antibiotic therapy. There are no blinded trials of therapy for *M. marinum* cutaneous granulomas. Treatment with rifampin, clarithromycin, doxycycline, trimethoprim-sulfamethoxazole, or ciprofloxacin has been most successful.[4,46] If *Mycobacterium chelonei* is isolated, then two drugs are required, usually clarithromycin plus one of amikacin, imipenem, trimethorpim-sulfamethoxasole, cefoxitin, ciprofloxacin, garifloxacin linezolid, or doxycycline.[4] In vitro sensitivity testing may be required. Surgical excision of the area, if feasible, is also recommended. Adjunctive therapy with recombinant cytokines such as interleukin-2 (IL-2), interferon-γ (IFN-γ), and granulocyte-macrophage colony-stimulating factor (GM-CSF) is now under study.[47]

Patient education

The clinician should emphasize that the skin abrasion is vulnerable to infection, and the child should not swim or immerse his or her skin in a tropical fish tank when a cut or abrasion is present. Cleaning the fish tank and changing the water may help, but the organism is difficult to remove from contaminated fish tanks.

Follow-up visits

After initiating antibiotic therapy, a follow-up visit at 2 weeks to monitor side effects of the therapy is indicated. If tolerated well, monthly visits are indicated until antibiotics are discontinued. Most authorities recommend continuing treatment for 1 month after the lesion has cleared.

REFERENCES

1. Ferrieri P. The natural history of impetigo. J Clin Invest 1972; 51:2851.
2. Brook I, Frazier EH, Yeager JK. Microbiology of nonbullous impetigo. Pediatr Dermatol 1997; 14:192.
3. Taplin D. Prevalence of streptococcal pyoderma in relation to climate and hygiene. Lancet 1973; i:501.
4. Report of the Committee on Infectious Disease. Red book 2003. Elk Grove Village, Ill: American Academy of Pediatrics; 2003.
5. Buescher ES. Community-acquired methicillin-resistant *Staphylococcus aureus* in pediatrics. Curr Opin Pediatr 2005; 17:67–70.
6. Hedrick J. Acute bacterial infections in pediatric medicine: current issues in presentation and treatment. Paediatr Drugs 2003; 5(suppl 1):35–46.
7. Bass JW, Chan DS, Creamer KM, et al. Comparison of oral cephalexin, topical mupirocin and topical bacitracin for the treatment of impetigo. Pediatr Infect Dis J 1997; 16:708.
8. Johnson GA. Treatment of bullous impetigo and the staphylococcal scalded skin syndrome in infants. Exper Rev Anti Infect Ther 2004; 2:439–446.
9. Sladden MJ, Johnston GA. Current options in the treatment of impetigo in children. Expert Opin Pharmather 2005; 6:2245–2256.
10. Honig PJ, Frieden IJ, Kim HJ, et al. Streptococcal intertrigo: an underrecognized condition in children. Pediatrics 2003; 112:1427–1429.
11. Baddour LM. Cellulitis syndromes: an update. Int J Antimicrob Agents 2000; 14:113.
12. Yen MT, Yen KG. Effect of corticosteroids in the acute management of pediatric orbital cellulitis with subperisoteal abscess. Ophthalmol Plastic Reconstruct Surg 2005; 21:363–366.
13. Lyon M, Doehring MC. Blistering distal dactylitis; a case series in children under nine months of age. J Emerg Med 2004; 26:421–423.
14. Mogielnicki NP, Schwartzman JD, Elliott JA. Perineal group A streptococcal disease in a pediatric practice. Pediatrics 2000; 10:276.
15. Howe PM. Etiologic diagnosis of cellulitis: comparison of the aspirates obtained from the leading edge and the point of maximal inflammation. Pediatr Infect Dis J 1987; 6:685.
16. Ahmed S, Ayoub EM. Severe, invasive group A streptococcal disease and toxic shock. Pediatr Ann 1998; 27:287.
17. Frank G, Mahoney HM, Eppes SC. Musculoskeletal infections in children. Pediatr Clin North Amer 2005; 52:1083–1106.
18. Hahn RG, Knox LM, Forman TA. Evaluation of poststreptococcal illness. Am Fam Physician 2005; 71:1949–1954.
19. Feeney KT, Dowse GK, Keil AD, et al. Epidemiologic features and control of an outbreak of scarlet fever in a Perth primary school. Commun Dis Intell 2005; 29:386–390.
20. Luby SP, Agboatwalla M, Feikin DR, et al. Effect of hand washing on child's health: a randomized controlled trial. Lancet 2005; 366:225–233.

21. Ladhani S, Garbash M. Staphylococcal skin infection in children: rational drug therapy recommendations. Paediatr Drugs 2005; 7:71–102.
22. Zimakoff J, Rosdal VT, Petersen W, et al. Recurrent staphylococcal furunculosis in families. Scand J Infect Dis 1988; 20:403.
23. Kars M, van Dijk H, Salinmas MM, et al. Association of furunculosis and familial deficiency of mannose-binding lectin. Eur J Clin Invest 2005; 35:531–534.
24. Purcell K, Fergie J. Epidemic of community-acquired methicillin-resistant *Staphylococcus aureus* infections: a 14-year study at Driscoll Children's Hospital. Arch Pediatr Adolesc Med 2005; 159: 980–985.
25. Trueb RM, Gloor M, Wuthrich B. Recurrent *Pseudomonas* folliculitis. Pediatr Dermatol 1994; 11:35.
26. Farrell AM. Staphylococcal scalded-skin syndrome. Lancet 1999; 354:880.
27. Yamasaki O ,Yamaguchi T, Sugai M, et al. Clinical manifestations of the scalded skin syndrome depend upon serotypes of exfoliative toxins. J Clin Microbiol 2005; 43:1890–1893.
28. Iwatsuki K, Yamasaki O, Morizone S, et al. Staphylococcal cutaneous infections: invasion, evasion and aggression. J Dermatol Sci 2006; 42:203–214.
29. Lamps LW, Scott MA. Cat scratch disease: historic, clinical and pathologic perspective. Amer J Clin Pathol 2004; 21(suppl):S71–S80.
30. Massei F, Geri L, Macchia ,P et al. The expanded spectrum of bartonellosis in children. Infect Dis Clin North Amer 2005; 19:691–711.
31. Qian X, Jin L, Hayden PT, et al. Diagnosis of cat scratch disease with *Bartonella henselae* infection in formalin-fixed paraffin-embedded tissues by two different PCR techniques. Diag Mol Pathol 2005; 14:146–151.
32. Zangwill K. Therapeutic options for cat-scratch disease. Pediatr Infect Dis J 1998; 17:1059.
33. Buckingham SC. Tick-borne infections in children: epidemiology, clinical manifestations and optimal management strategies. Paediatr Drugs 2005; 7:165–176.
34. Weisshaar E, Schaefer A, Scheidt RR, et al. Epidemiology of tick bites and boreliosis in children attending kindergarten or so called 'forest kindergarten' in Southwest Germany. J Invest Dermatol 2006; 126:584–590.
35. Committee on Infectious Diseases, American Academy of Pediatrics; Prevention of Lyme disease. Pediatrics 2000; 105:142.
36. Eppes SC. Diagnosis, treatment and prevention of Lyme disease in children. Paediatr Drugs 2003; 5:363–372.
37. Woods A. Syphilis in children: congenital and acquired. Semin Pediatr Infect Dis 2005; 16:245–257.
38. Soninathon U, Hannam S, Fowler A, et al. Detection and followup of infants at risk for congenital syphilis. Arch Dis. Child 2006; 91:620.
39. Wicher K, Horowitz HW, Wicher V. Laboratory methods of diagnosis of syphilis for the beginning of the third millennium. Microbes Infect 1999; 1:1035.
40. Godschalk JC, van der Sluis JJ, Stolz E. The localization of treponemes and characterization of the inflammatory infiltrate in skin biopsies from patients with primary or secondary syphilis or early infectious yaws. Genitourinary Med 1993; 69:102.
41. Pandhi D, Kumar S, Reddy BS. Sexually transmitted diseases in children. J Dermatol 2003; 30:314–320.
42. Pzniak A, Bull T; Recently recognized mycobacteria of clinical significance. J Infect 1999; 38:157.
43. Aubry A, Chosidan O, Caumes E, et al. Sixty-three cases of *Mycobacterium marinum* infection: clinical features, treatment and antibiotic susceptibility of causative isolates. Arch Int Med 2002; 162:1746–1752.
44. Smego RA Jr, Castiglia M, Asperilla MO. Lymphocutaneous syndrome: a review of non-sporothrix causes. Medicine 1999; 78:38.
45. Vu TT, Daniel SJ, Quach C. Nontuberculous mycobacteria in children: a changing pattern. J Otolaryngol 2005; 34(suppl):S40–S44.
46. Cummins DL, Delacerda D, Tausk FA. *Mycobacterium marinum* with different responses to second-generation tetracyclines. Int J Dermatol 2005; 44:518–520.
47. Holland SM. Cytokine therapy of mycobacterial infections. Adv Intern Med 2000; 45:431.

Fungal and Yeast Infections of the Skin

DERMATOPHYTES

Dermatophytes are fungi that invade and proliferate in the outer layer of the epidermis (stratum corneum). In addition to invading the stratum corneum, some species may also invade the hair and nails. Dermatophyte infections are common and increase in frequency with increasing age; in hot, humid climates; and in crowded living conditions. For example, tinea capitis is quite prevalent in children, especially in urban areas.[1–3] In one area of the United States, 4% of asymptomatic children had a positive fungal culture for scalp dermatophytes, and 50% of children with tinea capitis had a household member who was culture positive.[4]

HAIR INFECTIONS (TINEA CAPITIS)

Clinical Features

Scalp hair involvement is usually seen in prepubertal children and in North America is currently predominantly due to infections with *Trichophyton tonsurans*.[1,3–6] *Microsporum canis* is responsible in only 5% of children.[5,6] Causative agents are changing in Europe and North America as a result of immigration and increased world travel and in some locales dermatophytes such as *T. soudanese* and *T. violaceum* are found with increasing frequency.[2,3] Children with tinea capitis have a noninflammatory stage lasting 2–8 weeks, followed by an inflammatory stage. Hair loss is a regular feature of tinea capitis. *M. canis* infections are characterized by one or several patches of broken-off hairs that appear thickened and white (Fig. 6.1). The hairs fluoresce yellow-green under Wood's light examination. In contrast, *T. tonsurans* produces several distinct clinical presentations: a noninflammatory stage in which hairs break off at the follicular orifice in a circumscribed area of the scalp, which leaves small, dark hairs in the follicles, or so-called *black-dot ringworm* (Fig. 6.2); and four inflammatory stages, including (1) diffuse fine scaling of the scalp without obvious broken-off hairs (Fig. 6.3); (2) multiple scaly, pustular bald areas with indistinct margins (Fig. 6.4); (3) multiple kerions; or (4) a seborrheic dermatitis-like pattern (Fig. 6.5). The widespread inflammatory stages are more commonly seen than the black-dot form and usually are associated with regional lymphadenopathy. The presence of enlarged suboccipital or posterior cervical lymph nodes in association with hair loss should make one consider first the diagnosis of tinea capitis, although dermatitis of the scalp may also be responsible.[1] Infants under 1 year[7] and even newborns[8] are reported with tinea capitis.

The diagnosis in the noninflammatory stage should be confirmed by the following three steps: (1) Wood's light examination, (2) potassium hydroxide (KOH) examination, and (3) fungal culture.[1–10]

Wood's light examination

Wood's light examination is best performed with a hand-held ultraviolet black lamp with two fluorescent bulbs. The lamp should be held within 6 inches of the scalp to observe for yellow-green fluorescence of the thickened scalp hairs. Lint from clothing fluoresces white from the addition of optical brighteners, and scale entrapped in sebum appears a dull yellow. These may be confused with fungal fluorescence. *M. canis* fluoresces, but the epidemic form of tinea capitis caused by *T. tonsurans* does not. The Wood's light examination cannot be used to exclude the diagnosis of tinea capitis or for screening children during epidemics.

Fig. 6.1 Circumscribed patch of scalp hair loss with thick scales caused by *M. canis* infection.

Fig. 6.3 Diffuse scaling in a dandruff-like pattern in *T. tonsurans* infection.

Fig. 6.2 Circumscribed area of hair loss without scalp change and with hairs broken off at the follicular orifice. This is the black-dot pattern of *T. tonsurans* infection.

Fig. 6.4 Numerous triangle-shaped patches of hair loss accompanied by pustular kerion formation and enlarged lymph node in *T. tonsurans* infection.

Potassium hydroxide examination

Potassium hydroxide examinations for dermatophytes are simple procedures that can be performed in the office or clinic, but interpretation may be difficult for the inexperienced clinician.[7–9] If a clinician is experienced with KOH examinations, the KOH examination should be performed in every case of hair loss associated with broken hairs and in children with diffuse scaling of the scalp. If the hair fluoresces, the clinician should hold the Wood's lamp in one hand

and a curette in the other and gently remove the fluorescent hairs for KOH examination and culture by scraping the scalp with the curette. The involved hairs are loosened in the follicles and will be included in the scrapings. Scrapings should not be painful to the child. If the hair does not fluoresce, the clinician should use the curette or a cotton swab to scrape the follicular openings in the involved area of the scalp hair loss. If a kerion is present, scrape the border of the lesion, not the inflammatory center. The scrapings

Fig. 6.5 Scaling and hair loss in the seborrheic dermatitis-like pattern of *T. Tonsurans* scalp infection.

Fig. 6.6 Photomicrograph of hair dissolved in KOH. Hyphae and spores of *T. tonsurans* appear as chains within the hair shaft. There are no spores coating the hair.

Fig. 6.7 Photomicrograph of hair dissolved in KOH. Mats containing billions of small spores coat the outside of hair, with hyphae seen within the hair shaft in *M. canis* infection.

that include infected hair are placed on a glass microscope slide, partially dissolved in KOH 20%, and placed under a coverslip. After 20–40 minutes, the clinician should examine the specimen under the 10× and 40× lenses. In nonfluorescent hairs, hyphae and spores are seen within the hair shaft (Fig. 6.6).

In fluorescent hairs the outer surface of the hair is coated with mats containing thousands of tiny spores (Fig. 6.7), and hyphae may be seen within the hair shaft.

Fungal culture

Fungal culture is the most reliable test in the diagnosis of tinea capitis and should be routinely performed in children with suspected tinea capitis. Fungal culture also should be considered for household contacts because 50% of children have a culture-positive household member, including adults. A modified Sabouraud dextrose agar (dermatophyte test medium [DTM]) makes this procedure simple. Broken hairs or scrapings obtained by a sterile curette or cotton swab are inoculated so as to break the agar surface. The bottle cap is loosely applied and the culture bottles are left at room temperature. If a dermatophyte is present, the agar medium turns from yellow to red in 4–5 days, and a fuzzy white or tan growth appears on the agar surface. However, some organisms such as *T. tonsurans* may require 30 days to grow. More rapid identification by molecular techniques has been reported,[11] but these tests are yet not widely available. A positive culture can be subcultured on Sabouraud dextrose agar for precise identification.

Inflammatory lesions produce a kerion, which is an erythematous, boggy nodule with multiple superficial

Fig. 6.8 Multiple boggy, red scalp nodules with multiple pustules in newborn with multiple kerions with pustules.

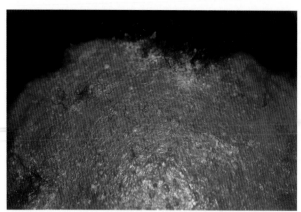

Fig. 6.9 Scarring hair loss in child with previously undiagnosed tinea capitis and kerion.

Table 6.1 Organisms responsible for tinea capitis

Feature	M. canis	T. tonsurans
Source	Cats and dogs	Other children
Fluorescence	Yellow-green	None
Human-to-human spread	No	Yes
Hair loss	Yes	Yes
Kerion	Yes	Yes
Children infected	Rural and suburban	Urban
Clinical patterns	Thickened hairs	Black-dot, dandruff-like, or multiple areas of alopecia

pustules (Fig. 6.8).[1,4,5,7] These lesions are almost completely devoid of hair and will lead to scarring and permanent hair loss if untreated (Fig. 6.9). A kerion will appear 2–8 weeks after infection begins and represents an exaggerated host response to the invading fungus. Up to 40% of untreated tinea capitis caused by *M. canis* or *T. tonsurans* may eventuate in a kerion. Scrapings for KOH examination and fungal culture should be obtained from the edge of lesions, not the inflammatory center.

Differential Diagnosis

Alopecia areata and hair pulling are the major considerations in the differential diagnosis of tinea capitis in children. Alopecia areata may be distinguished by the total absence of hair in a circumscribed patch, without any associated scalp change. In hair pulling, odd patterns of hair loss, scalp excoriations, perifollicular petechiae, and hairs broken off at differing lengths are the distinguishing features. Seborrheic dermatitis or even atopic dermatitis may mimic the diffuse forms of *T. tonsurans* scalp infection.[1]

In inflammatory tinea capitis (kerion), bacterial pyodermas are often mistaken for kerion. The pustules in kerion are sterile, however, and incision produces only serosanguinous fluid. Bacterial culture of the skin surface may yield *Staphylococcus aureus* and lead to the incorrect diagnosis of pyoderma, but one should recall that *S. aureus* frequently colonizes the skin surface, and such cultures would not detect bacterial invasion. Less commonly, traction alopecia, scleroderma, lichen planus, psoriasis, lupus erythematosus, dandruff, or porokeratosis of Mibelli may be confused with tinea capitis.

Pathogenesis

M. canis is harbored by cats, dogs, and certain rodents, and children handling such animals are susceptible to infection. Humans appear to be a terminal host for *M. canis*, and human-to-human transmission does not occur. When there is delayed hypersensitivity to the organism, a kerion may develop. Histologic study of this lesion shows a mononuclear cell infiltrate consistent with that seen in delayed hypersensitivity reactions. *M. canis* accounts for much of the tinea capitis in suburban and rural areas (Table 6.1). *T. tonsurans* is transmitted from human to human and is currently epidemic in North America. It is most prevalent in areas of crowding and accounts for virtually all tinea capitis in inner-city children in North America.[1,4–6] Transmission is predominantly from sharing hats, caps, scarves, combs, or brushes with infected individuals.[1,4–6]

Treatment

In suspected *T. tonsurans* infection, oral griseofulvin in a micronized form, 20 mg/kg/day for a minimum of 4 weeks, is the treatment of choice.[5–8,12,13] Often, treatment for 2–3 months is required with griseofulvin. Terbinafine 3 mg/kg/day orally for 2–4 weeks is an alternative, though less effective if *M. Canis* is the responsible organism.[5] Itraconazole and ketoconazole are far less effective against *T. tonusrans* than griseofulvin or terbinafine.[5] Topical antifungal agents cannot reach the hyphae within the hair shaft and are ineffective. In *M. canis*, with successful treatment the lesions become nonfluorescent within 2 weeks after the administration of griseofulvin is begun. Although griseofulvin has many rare, severe side effects, including agranulocytosis and aplastic anemia, it is a relatively safe drug in children. Absorption is enhanced by a fatty meal; taking griseofulvin once or twice a day with ice cream or whole milk is a popular prescription. In addition to oral griseofulvin, many authorities advocate an antifungal shampoo such as selenium sulfide 2.5% shampoo or ketoconazole 2% shampoo, used twice weekly on the scalp, to reduce infectivity and to hasten the child's return to school or childcare setting.[14] Kerion responds well to griseofulvin alone. The addition of antibiotics or steroids is not required.[13]

If *M. canis* infection is suspected (and a Wood's light examination is positive), either griseofulvin, 20 mg/kg/day for 4 weeks, or itraconazole, 5 mg/kg/day for 2 weeks, is recommended.[5–8, 13]

Patient Education

If *M. canis* is found, animal sources should be identified and the animal treated by a veterinarian to prevent infection of other children. In *T. tonsurans*, identification of the likely contacts is necessary. Household contacts should be cultured if possible. Children should not share combs, brushes, or head wear. School and day-care contacts should be referred for evaluation if scaling hair loss is present. Screening of contacts with a Wood's lamp is of no value because the epidemic strains in North America are not fluorescent. Patients should be instructed that hair regrowth is slow, often taking 3–6 months. If a kerion is present, some scarring and permanent hair loss may result. For a Patient Education Sheet on Scalp Ringworm (Tinea Capitis), see CD-ROM.

Follow-up Visits

A visit in 4 weeks is helpful to ascertain the effectiveness of the griseofulvin or terbinafine therapy. Reexamination for fluorescence, a KOH examination, and a repeat culture will serve as guidelines for increasing the therapeutic dosage. If the lesions are fluorescence negative, KOH negative, and culture negative at 2 weeks, a total of 6 weeks therapy with griseofulvin or 2 weeks with terbinafine may be all that is required. With griseofulvin therapy, treatment 4–6 weeks after the lesions are culture negative is a useful rule of thumb. Once treatment is initiated with antifungal shampoos plus griseofulvin or terbinafine, the child can return to school.[5,14] Shaving the head, short hair cuts, or wearing a cap to school is

unnecessary.[5,14] A follow-up visit every 2–4 weeks until hair growth begins is advised to assess for treatment failures. Asymptomatic carriers may be treated with sporicidal shampoos, such as ketoconazole or selenium sulfide, used twice weekly for 4 weeks. Asymptomatic carriers may be more likely to spread tinea capitis in school or day care than overtly infected children.[4]

FUNGAL INFECTION INVOLVING THE SKIN ONLY

Tinea Corporis

Clinical features

Dermatophyte infections on the body often consist of one or several circular erythematous patches (Fig. 6.10). The patches may have a papular, scaly, annular border and a clear center (see Fig. 6.10), or they may be inflammatory throughout, with super-

Fig. 6.10 Annular, red, scaly borders with clear center in tinea corporis.

Fig. 6.11 Red, scaly plaque with partial clearing in center in tinea corporis caused by *M. canis*.

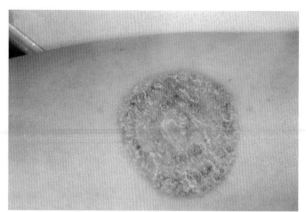

Fig. 6.12 Plaque, red throughout, with prominent pustules, in tinea corporis caused by the cattle ringworm, *T. verrucosum*.

Fig. 6.15 Multiple follicular pustules in a leukemic child with Majocchi's granulomas caused by *T. rubrum*.

Fig. 6.13 Annular, red, scaly patch surrounding the left nipple, with partial clearing in the center and red follicular papules.

ficial pustules (Figs 6.11–6.13). A most common pattern is a red, scaly patch with partial clearing and follicular pustules (Fig. 6.14). Multiple annular lesions may be seen. In immunosuppressed children, including those with cancer, or those who use potent topical steroids, invasion of the follicular orifice by the dermatophytes may predominate the clinical appearance. This produces a folliculitis pattern known as *Majocchi's granulomas* (Fig. 6.15). *M. canis*, *T. mentagrophytes*, *T. tonsurans*, *T. verrucosum*, *M. gypseum*, *Epidermophyton floccosum*, and *T. rubrum* are the most common dermatophytes responsible for tinea corporis.[6,10,15,16] Epidemics of tinea corporis have occurred in wrestlers (tinea gladiatorum) as a result of contaminated wrestling mats.[15] Misdiagnosed tinea corporis treated with potent or superpotent topical steroids will not display scaling, and the annular border may be obscured (tinea incognito).[16] Diagnosis is confirmed by KOH examination of scrapings of thin scales obtained from the border of the lesion. Cultures are not usually done routinely.

Differential diagnosis

Any skin eruption that produces an annular configuration can mimic tinea corporis. The herald patch of pityriasis rosea may mimic tinea corporis, as may any of the forms of dermatitis. The herald patch clears in the center but has central scale rather than scale at the edge. It is not unusual to confuse the annular nodules of granuloma annulare for tinea corporis. In granuloma annulare, there is no scale or surface disruption. Psoriasis, parapsoriasis, figurate erythemas, sarcoidosis, secondary syphilis, and lupus erythematosus can also mimic tinea corporis.

Fig. 6.14 Tinea incognito. Multiple follicular pustules with partial loss of annular border in adolescent mistreated with potent topical steroids.

Fig. 6.16 Annular erythema with vesicles on instep of large adolescent male foot. Tinea pedis caused by *T. rubrum*.

Fig. 6.17 Erosions and blisters on the instep of an adolescent's foot in bullous tinea pedis.

Tinea Pedis (Athlete's Foot)
Clinical features

There are three clinical forms of tinea pedis. All are found predominantly in the postpubertal adolescent and are less common in early childhood.[6,9,17–19] The most common form consists of vesicles and erosions on the instep of one or both feet (Figs 6.16, 6.17).[18,19] The dermatophyte may be identified by removing the vesicle roof, scraping the underside of the roof, and examining the scrapings under the microscope for hyphae. Occasionally, fissuring between the toes, with scaling and erythema in the surrounding skin, is seen. Rarely, diffuse scaling of the weight-bearing surface of one or both feet, with exaggerated scaling in the skin creases, the so-called moccasin foot tinea pedis, is seen. The most common organisms

responsible for tinea pedis in North America are *T. rubrum* and *T. mentagrophytes*.

Differential diagnosis

Atopic dermatitis mimics tinea pedis in prepubertal children. Contact dermatitis and other forms of dermatitis may also mimic tinea pedis. Contact dermatitis usually involves the tops of the feet, whereas tinea pedis involves the weight-bearing surface. Juvenile plantar dermatosis (JPD) is characterized by redness, dryness, and fissures of the weight-bearing surface of the foot and may be easily confused with tinea pedis. Fungal scrapings and culture are needed to distinguish tinea pedis from JPD. Scabies, granuloma annulare, and psoriasis may also mimic tinea pedis.

Tinea Faciei
Clinical features

Dermatophyte infections on the face occur commonly in children. It is often from a pet held against the child's face. Tinea faciei is erythematous, scaly, and may have a 'butterfly' distribution (Fig. 6.18). In other children the lesions may be unilateral (Figs 6.19–6.21). KOH examination of the scaly border will confirm the diagnosis. *M. canis* and the cattle ringworm, *T. verrucosum*, are the most commonly involved fungi of tinea faciei in children.

Differential diagnosis

Tinea faciei may mimic lupus erythematosus and other collagen vascular diseases. A KOH examination for hyphae should always be performed in children in

Fig. 6.18 Annular, red, scaly lesions of the nose and malar skin of a girl misdiagnosed as having lupus erythematosus. Tinea faciei caused by *M. canis*.

Fig. 6.19 A red, scaly plaque below the eye in tinea faciei caused by *M. canis*.

Fig. 6.20 Two red annular scaly plaques on the chin of an adolescent with *T. verrucosum* infection.

Fig. 6.21 Red, scaly ear and preauricular skin in a boy with tinea faciei.

whom the butterfly rash of lupus is considered. Atopic dermatitis, contact dermatitis, and seborrheic dermatitis should also be considered.

Tinea Cruris

Clinical features

An erythematous, scaly eruption on the inner thighs and inguinal creases characterizes tinea cruris.[5] Sometimes an elevated, papular, scaly border is present to suggest the diagnosis. KOH examination of the border for hyphae will confirm the diagnosis. Tinea cruris is unusual before adolescence. *T. mentagrophytes* and *E. floccosum* are the organisms most often responsible.

Differential diagnosis

Diaper dermatitis and candidiasis may mimic tinea cruris, but these usually occur in infants. Yeast infection in the perineal area may be distinguished by involvement of the scrotum. Several forms of dermatitis also occur in this area. Rarely, erythrasma, a superficial bacterial infection caused by *Corynebacterium minutissimum*, will be confused with tinea cruris. Wood's light examination in erythrasma produces a coral-red fluorescence but is negative in tinea cruris.

Pathogenesis

Dermatophyte invasion of the stratum corneum, but not the remainder of the epidermis or dermis, is responsible for superficial dermatophyte infections. The exact mechanism of the inflammation is not known, but toxins released by the dermatophyte are thought to be important in initiating the inflammatory response.

Treatment

For fungal infections that do not involve hair or nails, topical therapy is the treatment of choice (Table 6.2).[6,15] The fungicidal and fungistatic preparations are all efficacious against 90% of dermatophyte species. The allylamines are more efficacious and more expensive than the imidazoles. They are applied twice daily, either as a cream or solution, to the entire area until the lesions have cleared. This often takes 2–4 weeks of therapy. Topical terbinafine may produce clinical and mycologic clearing within 1 week.[5] Rarely are oral terbinafine, griseofulvin, itraconazole, fluconazole, or other systemic antifungal agents required.

Table 6.2 Topical antifungal agents

Class	Agent	Brand Name	Action
Allylamines	Terbinafine	Lamisil	Fungicidal
	Butenafine	Mentax	Fungicidal
	Naftifine	Naftin	Fungicidal
Hydroxypyridones	Ciclopirox	Loprox	Fungicidal
Imidazoles	Clotrimazole	Lotrimin, Fungoid, Mycelex	Fungistatic
	Econazole	Spectazole	Fungistatic
	Ketoconazole	Nizoral	Fungistatic
	Miconazole	Micatin, Desenex, Monistat-Derm	Fungistatic
	Oxiconazole	Oxistat	Fungistatic
	Sulconazole	Exelderm	Fungistatic
Polyenes	Nystatin	Mycostatin, Nilstat	Fungistatic*
Thiocarbamates	Tolnaftate	Tinactin, Aftate, Ting Tolnaftate	Fungistatic†

*No activity against dermatophytes.
†No activity against yeast.

Patient Education

Knowledge that these fungi are found in soil or animals may help identify the source and prevent other family members from being infected. The clinician should be certain to instruct the patient to treat the entire lesion plus about a 1 cm border beyond it. Efforts to keep the affected skin area dry after successful treatment, and changing habits regarding family pets, such as keeping the pets out of the child's room and not allowing the child to carry the pet, may be useful in preventing reinfection until the pet is cured. When epidemic dermatophytes are involved, examination of contacts and fungal culture of suspicious lesions is recommended.

Fig. 6.22 Marked scaling of skin creases in adolescent with tinea pedis and toenail involvement.

Follow-up Visits

A visit 2 weeks after therapy is started is helpful to ascertain its efficacy. If no response has occurred, either the diagnosis is incorrect or a resistant dermatophyte has been encountered. At this point it is useful to culture the lesion and perhaps change to a different class of topical antifungal agent. Further follow-up visits may be needed.

FUNGAL INFECTION OF THE NAILS (ONYCHOMYCOSIS, TINEA UNGUIUM)

Clinical Features

Distal thickening and yellowing of the nail plate are regular features of onychomycosis (tinea unguium) (Figs 6.22–6.25).[5,20–24] The yellowing represents separation of the distal nail plate from the nail bed,

Fig. 6.23 Thickening and scaling of fourth toenail in prepubertal child with onychomycosis due to *T. rubrum*. Child's father had untreated athlete's foot.

Fig. 6.24 Yellow, wedge-shaped thickening of great toe (dermatophytoma) and distal thickening of third toe in adolescent with onychomycosis due to *T. rubrum*.

Fig. 6.26 Multiple fungal hyphae from KOH examination of toenails seen in Fig. 6.25.

Fig. 6.25 Onychomycosis. Distal thickening and yellowing of four toenails in an adolescent.

and entrapment of air between these two structures. Usually only one or two nails (see Fig. 6.23), most often the great toenails, are involved. It is uncommon to find onychomycosis in early childhood, but it is becoming more common, and it is more frequent in the adolescent. Usually, there is a family member with untreated or recurrent athlete's foot. With toenail involvement, a concurrent tinea pedis is usually present (see Fig. 6.22).[20–24]

Differential Diagnosis

Psoriasis also causes distal yellowing and thickening of the nail, but eventually all 20 nails are involved, and superficial nail pitting is also present. Lichen planus and trachyonychia (20-nail dystrophy) also usually involve all 20 nails. Hereditary nail disorders asso-

ciated with ectodermal defects, such as pachyonychia congenita, are sometimes confused with onychomycosis. Bacterial and candidal nail involvement characteristically results in proximal rather than distal nail plate disease. A KOH examination (Fig. 6.26) or fungal culture will distinguish. At least 20 minutes may be required for KOH to dissolve the thick nail material in order to microscopically visualize fungus.

Pathogenesis

Some dermatophytes may invade nails and the stratum corneum as well. They proliferate within the nail plate, destroying its integrity.

Treatment

Successful therapy of onychomycosis is difficult. Clinical and mycologic cures have been obtained with oral treatment.[21,23] Itraconazole pulse therapy at 5 mg/kg/day orally for 1 week each month for 3–5 months has resulted in long-term clinical and mycologic cures (up to 4 years) and is the recommended treatment if there are no contraindications.[23] Itraconazole and other azoles have significant hepatic side effects and liver function tests that are minimized by pulse-dosing. If continuous therapy is used, liver function tests should be monitored monthly. In contrast, only 17.5% of treated patients responded after 6–12 months of daily griseofulvin therapy. The clinician should weigh the consequences of prolonged therapy with griseofulvin against the poor success rate. Oral terbinafine (95%), ketoconazole (80%), and itraconazole (71%) used daily for 4–8 weeks have somewhat higher reported success rates, but there are few data for long-term relapse rates. Topical agents, with the possible exception of ciclopiroxamine nail lacquer, generally are not successful in long-term cures unless used in combination with systemic antifungal agents.[21]

Patient Education

The difficulty in obtaining a cure with this disease should be thoroughly explained to the patient and the parents. The hepatic and other side effects of the oral antifungal agents and drug interactions should be explained. They may not desire oral antifungal therapy simply to achieve temporary improvement.

Follow-up Visits

Visits at 6-month intervals are useful to follow the course of the illness and observe for the possible involvement of other nails. If oral antifungal agents are used in a continuous regimen, evaluation for side effects, including laboratory tests at 1-month intervals, is recommended.

YEAST SKIN INFECTIONS

Tinea Versicolor

Clinical features

In tinea versicolor, multiple oval macules with a fine scale are found on the neck, chest, upper back, shoulders, face, and upper arms of children and adolescents (Fig. 6.27).[5,24] Occasionally, the lesions are confluent and present as a continuous sheet. Their color depends on the state of pigmentation. In well-tanned or darkly pigmented adolescents, the lesions

Fig. 6.27 Multiple tan macules with a fine scale over the chest of an adolescent with tinea versicolor.

Fig. 6.28 Tan macules of tinea versicolor on a light-skinned child.

Fig. 6.29 Tan, scaly macules on back and shoulder in child with tinea versicolor.

Fig. 6.30 Photomicrograph of KOH examination of tinea versicolor. Multiple short hyphae and spores are seen.

appear as discrete hypopigmented macules. In the winter months, as normal pigment fades, the lesions may appear as tan or dark-brown macules, hence the term *versicolor* (Figs 6.28, 6.29). The infection tends to be persistent. KOH examination of scrapings reveals numerous short, curved hyphae and circular spores, the so-called *macaroni and meatballs* appearance (Fig. 6.30). Some authorities recommend application of clear tape to the skin to pull off skin surface cells followed by microscopic examination. Occasionally, Wood's light examination reveals an orange fluorescence of the lesions if the patient has not cleansed the affected area recently. Biopsy of these lesions will show periodic acid-Schiff (PAS)-positive hyphae and spores within the stratum corneum.

Differential diagnosis

Seborrheic dermatitis, contact dermatitis, and tinea corporis can mimic tinea versicolor. Vitiligo, pityriasis alba, and other hypopigmented states such as hypopigmentation of Ito are also sometimes confused with it. Direct microscopic examination of scales will distinguish tinea versicolor from other possible causes.

Pathogenesis

The yeastlike organism *Malassezia furfur*, which in its culture phase is called *Pityrosporum ovale*, invades the stratum corneum to produce the lesions of tinea versicolor. The organism thrives in hot, humid climates and commonly colonizes the skin by adolescence. It may colonize the skin of neonates as well.[8]

Treatment

Miconazole, ciclopirox, clotrimazole, terbinafine solutions, or fluconazole shampoos applied twice daily for 2 or 3 weeks may be efficacious but are costly when one considers the amount required to cover the trunk of a child or adolescent.[25,26] Applying ketoconazole shampoo or selenium sulfide 2.5% for 30 minutes daily for 1 week followed by monthly applications for 3 months is considered the treatment of choice by many.[25,26] Application of sodium hypochlorite 15% once weekly for 2 months will result in temporary clearing, but the recurrence rate is high. After initial clearing, prevention of recurrence by monthly treatment may be considered. In tropical and subtropical climates, oral ketoconazole, fluconazole, or itraconazole given in a single dose once daily for 2 weeks may be considered in difficult cases.[5,24] A single oral dose of fluconazole or itraconazole may produce acceptable results.[27]

Patient education

Patients should be instructed that repigmentation of the hypopigmented areas will not occur until they are exposed to the sun, and that a recurrence is likely.

Follow-up visits

A follow-up visit at 1 month to evaluate therapy should be considered. If oral therapy is considered, monthly visits to monitor side effects should be instituted.

Candidiasis

Clinical features

In regions of the body in which warmth and moisture lead to maceration of the skin or mucous membranes, the tissue is predisposed to invasion by the pathogenic yeast *Candida albicans*. Candidiasis in different body sites has distinct clinical features.[5,28–33] In

Fig. 6.31 Thrush involving tongue of toddler.

Fig. 6.32 White patches on red tongue of infant with thrush due to *C. albicans*.

neonates and infants, white plaques on an erythematous base (thrush) are commonly seen on the buccal mucosa and other sites in the oral cavity (Figs 6.31, 6.32).[5,28,29] In the immunosuppressed child, such as those with HIV, thrush may also involve the lips as well as oral mucosa (Fig. 6.33). In this same age group, intertriginous involvement of the body folds is also common, such as the neck, axilla, or diaper area. The use of pacifiers in infants may be permissive for oral candidiasis, including involvement of the angles of the lips (angular cheilitis).[5,31]

Fully established diaper candidiasis demonstrates beefy erythema with elevated margins and satellite red plaques (Figs 6.34, 6.35).[28,29] However, erosions, pustules, erythematous papules, and vesicles may also be features of candidiasis of the diaper area. C. *albicans* colonizes the diaper area within 3 days of the development of diaper dermatitis and should always be considered as a secondary infection in long-standing diaper dermatitis.

Paronychia caused by candidiasis is a common result of thumb sucking. The erythema and swelling around the base of the nail are usually not tender (Fig. 6.36).

Intertriginous candidiasis involving the inframammary, axillary, neck, and inguinal body folds may also

Fig. 6.34 Beefy-red central erythema with satellite pustules in candidiasis of diaper area. Positive cultures can be obtained only from satellite lesions, not from central erythema.

Fig. 6.35 Redness of scrotum and foreskin with satellite red papules in infant with diaper rash with *C. albicans* infection.

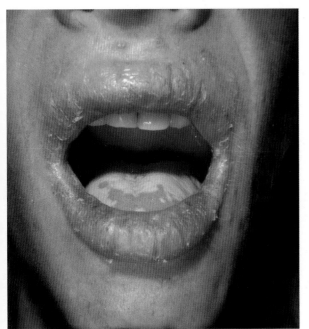

Fig. 6.33 Thick, white coating of tongue with scaling and fissuring of lips in chronic mucocutaneous candidiasis.

Fig. 6.36 Cuticular nontender swelling and erythema with thickened, disrupted nail surface in paronychia caused by *C. albicans*.

be seen in obese infants, children, and adolescents (Figs 6.37, 6.38).

A rare form of candidiasis (congenital candidiasis) acquired in utero results in generalized erythema of

Fig. 6.37 Candidal intertrigo of infant's neck.

Fig. 6.38 Candidal intertrigo of finger webs in adolescent working as dish-washer.

the newborn, with scaling and pustule formation.[30] It is particularly observed in very-low-birth-weight infants and is acquired from maternal C. *albicans* vulvovaginitis.

Vulvovaginal candidiasis appears as a cheesy vaginal discharge, with whitish plaques on erythematous mucous membranes.[31] It is most common in adolescent females but uncommon in prepubertal children.[31]

The rare candidal granulomas are oval, red plaques with a thick yellow crust. They are found on the head and neck and other areas of skin in children with defective host defenses.[5] In the syndrome of chronic mucocutaneous candidiasis (see Fig. 6.26), seen in patients with defective host defenses, persistent thrush with extensive involvement of the tongue and lips and chronic paronychia are present. Severe thrush may be observed in immunodeficient children infected with the human immunodeficiency virus (HIV). Patients on long-term glucocorticosteroid, immunosuppressive, anticancer, antibiotic, or oral contraceptive therapy (in adolescent females) appear unusually susceptible to candidiasis. Similarly, children with diabetes mellitus and reticuloendothelial neoplasms are also predisposed to candidiasis.

The diagnosis can be established by scraping the skin or mucosal lesion and observing the single budding yeast in a KOH preparation under the microscope. C. *albicans* is readily cultured on Sabouraud dextrose agar or cornmeal agar. Interpretation of a positive culture must be made with caution because C. *albicans* may reflect simple colonization.

Differential diagnosis

Herpes simplex, aphthous stomatitis, epidermolysis bullosa, geographic tongue, burns, and erythema multiforme of the oral cavity may mimic thrush. Diaper dermatitis, bacterial intertrigo, Letterer-Siwe disease, linear immunoglobulin A (IgA) dermatosis, and maceration may mimic the intertriginous forms of candidiasis.

Congenital candidiasis may be confused with severe erythema toxicum, ichthyosiform erythrodermas, immunodeficiencies, miliaria, transient neonatal pustular melanosis, infantile acropustulosis, and congenital syphilis or other intrauterine infections.

Paronychia caused by S. *aureus* may mimic candidal paronychia, but it usually has an acute onset, and the affected nail is tender and fluctuant. Psoriasis, lichen planus, and pachyonychia congenita should also be considered. Gonorrhea, *Trichomonas* infections, and chemical vaginitis may mimic vaginal candidiasis. Psoriasis, impetigo, and deep fungal infections such as sporotrichosis may be similar to candidal granulomas.

Acrodermatitis enteropathica, acquired zinc deficiency, and vitamin deficiency states may be confused with chronic mucocutaneous candidiasis.

Pathogenesis

Candida albicans may be considered a part of the normal flora of the skin and mucous surfaces in certain body areas. Colonization of the oral cavity, intestinal tract, and vagina of healthy individuals is common.[34,35] Moisture, warmth, and breaks in the epidermal barrier permit overgrowth and invasion of the epidermis by the organism. It has been demonstrated that *C. albicans* generates inflammation by activation of the complement system within the skin and attraction of neutrophils to skin sites of *Candida* invasion. Keratolytic proteases and other enzymes in *C. albicans* species allow them to penetrate the epidermal barrier more easily than other organisms.

Treatment

Topical therapy with several anticandidal agents is usually efficacious.[5] For infantile thrush the use of nystatin oral suspension four times daily for 5 days is efficacious.[5] In older children with thrush or angular cheilitis, clotrimazole troches may be useful.[5] For cutaneous candidosis, nystatin, oxiconazole, ketoconazole, ciclopirox, econazole, haloprogin, miconazole, or clotrimazole in a cream vehicle applied four times daily will result in prompt clearing of the lesions in 3–5 days. In the diaper area, application with each diaper change for 2–3 days is useful. The antifungal creams may sting or burn if there are breaks in the skin surface. Antiyeast ointments may be substituted.

Correction of the predisposing factors, such as good care of the diaper area, drying of intertriginous areas, and withdrawal of broad-spectrum antibiotics or glucocorticosteroids is also important in the management of candidiasis. Treatment of candidal vulvovaginitis or candidal infections of the nipples in nursing mothers is valuable in the therapy of thrush.

Oral therapy with fluconazole or itraconazole 5 mg/kg/day for 21 days may be required for oral candidiasis in immunosuppressed children.[5] Vaginitis in the adolescent may be treated with a single 150 mg dose of fluconazole.[5,33]

The following specific treatment protocols may be utilized:

1. *Thrush*: Apply nystatin solution topically to the area four times daily for 5 days. With recurrence, a second course of this therapy may be helpful. Simultaneous therapy of *Candida* vulvovaginitis or nipple infection in the mother is most helpful in reducing surface colonization with *C. albicans*. Discarding the infant's pacifier may help.
2. *Diaper candidiasis*: Application of nystatin (or one of the other agents listed) in a cream form with each diaper change for 2–3 days is most useful if combined with the usual measures to keep the diaper area dry and cool. Mupirocin applied 4 or 5 times a day for 5 days may also be effective.[32]
3. *Paronychia*: Nystatin cream applied nightly under occlusion (a plastic glove covered by a cotton stocking) for 3–4 weeks will often clear candidal paronychia. This should be done with caution in infants to be certain they do not aspirate the plastic into their airways.

Patient education

The patient or parents should understand that *C. albicans* is part of the normal skin flora in certain individuals and will reinvade susceptible tissue sites if the predisposing factors favoring overgrowth are not eliminated. Thus, careful attention to the treatment of intertrigo and good diaper area care are essential to achieve long-term satisfactory results. Recurrences should be retreated.

Follow-up visits

An examination 5–7 days after initiating therapy is useful to evaluate the therapeutic response and reinforce the measures to diminish warmth and moisture in intertriginous areas. Most therapy failures are due to poor compliance, not host defense defects. Widespread involvement of oral cavity, nails, and skin should trigger a suspicion of immunodeficiency.

REFERENCES

1. Williams JV, Eichenfield LH, Burke BL, et al. Scalp scaling in prepubertal children. Pediatrics 2005; 115:e1–e4.
2. Helgren J, Petrini B, Wahlgren CF. Increasing tinea capitis prevalence in Stockholm reflects immigration. Med Mycol 2004; 42:505–509.

3. Kolivras A, Lateur N, De Maubeuge J, et al. Tinea capitis in Brussels: epidemiology and new management strategy. Dermatology 2003; 206:384–387.
4. Frieden IJ. Tinea capitis: asymptomatic carriage of infection. Pediatr Infect Dis J 1999; 18:186.
5. Roberts BJ, Friedlander SF. Tinea capitis. A treatment update. Pediatr Ann 2005; 34:191–200.
6. Committee on Infectious Diseases; 2003 Red book; Elk Grove Village, Ill: American Academy of Pediatrics; 2003.
7. Gilaberte Y, Rezusta A, Gil J, et al. Tinea capitis in infants in the first year of life. Brit J Dermatol 2004; 151:886–890.
8. Smolinski KN, Shah SS, Honig PJ, et al. Neonatal cutaneous fungal infections. Curr Opin Pediatr 2005; 17:486–493.
9. Miller M, Hodgson Y. Sensitivity and specificity of potassium hydroxide smears of skin scrapings for the diagnosis of tinea pedis. Arch Dermatol 1993; 129:510.
10. Awoderu VA, Nebo GC, Otudero VO. Occurrence of dermatomycoses and in vitro therapeutic efficacy of three antifungal drugs on the growth of *Epidermophyton floccosum*. Mycopathologica 2003; 156:295–301.
11. Kamiga A, Kikuchi A, Tomita Y, et al. PCR and PCR-RFLP techniques targeting the DNA topoisomerase II gene for rapid diagnosis of the etiologic agent of dermatomycoses. J Dermatol Sci 2004; 34:35–48.
12. Honig PJ, Caputo GL, Leyden JJ. Microbiology of kerions. J Pediatr 1993; 123:422.
13. Honig PJ, Caputo GL, Leyden JJ. Treatment of kerions. Pediatr Dermatol 1994; 11:69.
14. Honig PJ. Tinea capitis: recommendations for school attendance. Pediatr Infect Dis J 1999; 18:211.
15. Kohl TD, Martin DC, Berger MS; Comparison of topical and oral treatments for tinea gladiatorum. Clin J Sport Med 1999; 9:161.
16. Romano C, Asta F, Massai L. Tinea incognito due to *Microsporum gypseum* in three children. Pediatr Dermatol 2000; 17:41.
17. Trivino-Duran L, Torres-Rodriguez JM, Martinez-Roig A, et al. Prevalence of tinea capitis and tinea pedis in Barcelona schoolchildren. Pediatr Infect Dis J 2005; 24:137–141.
18. Neri I, Piraccini BM, Guraeschi E, etal. Bullous tinea pedis in two children. Mycoses 2004; 47:475–478.
19. Geary RJ, Lucky AW. Tinea pedis in children presenting as unilateral inflammatory lesions of the sole. Pediatr Dermatol 1999; 16:255.
20. Faegermann J, Baran R. Epidemiology, clinical presentation and diagnosis of onychomycoses. Brit J Dermatol 2003; 149(suppl 65):1–4.
21. Hart R, Bell-Syer SEM, Crawford F. Systematic review of topical treatments for fungal infections of skin and nails of the feet. Br Med J 1999; 319:79.
22. Fletcher L, Hay RJ, Smeeton NC. Onychomycoses: the development of a clinical diagnosis aid for toenail disease. Part I. Establishing discriminatory historical and clinical features. Brit J Dermatol 2004; 150:701–705.
23. Huang P-H, Paller AS; Itraconazole pulse therapy for dermatophyte onychomycosis in children. Arch Pediatr Adolesc 2000; Med 154:614.
24. Truong A, Friedlander SF. Superficial fungal infections in adolescence. Adolescent Med 2001; 12:213–227.
25. Hull CA, Johnson SM. A double-blind comparison study of sodium sulfacetamide 10% lotion versus selenium sulfide lotion 2.5% in the treatment of pityriasis (tinea) versicolor. Cutis 2004; 73:425–429.
26. Lange DS, Richards HM, Guarnieri J, et al. Ketoconazole 2% shampoo in the treatment of tinea versicolor: a multicenter, randomized, double-blind, placebo-controlled trial. J Am Acad Dermatol 1998; 39:944.
27. Partap R, Kaur I, Chakrabarti A, et al. Single-dose fluconazole versus itraconazole in pityriasis versicolor. Dermatology 2004; 208:55–59.
28. Hay RJ. The management of superficial candidiasis. J Am Acad Dermatol 1999; 40:S35.
29. Chapman RL. *Candida* infections in the neonate. Curr Opin Pediatr 2003; 15:97–102.
30. Diana A, Epiney M, Ecoffey M, et al. 'White dots on the placenta and red dots on the baby': congenital cutaneous candidiasis: a rare disease of the neonate. Acta Paediatr 2004; 93:996–999.
31. Banerjee K, Certis E, de San Lazaro C, et al. Low prevalence of genital candidiasis in children. Eur J Clin Microbiol Infect Dis 2004; 23:696–698.
32. Shin HT. Diaper dermatitis that does not quit. Dermatol Ther 2005; 18:124–125.
33. Nyirjesy P. Vaginitis in the adolescent patient. Pediatr Clin North Am 1999; 46:733.
34. Hossain H, Ansari F, Schukz-Weidner NC, et al. Clonal identity of *Candida albicans* in the oral cavity and gastrointestinal tract of preschool children. Oral Microbiol Immunol 2003; 18:302–308.
35. Healey CM, Baker CJ, Zaccaria E, et al. Impact of fluconazole prophylaxis on incidence and outcome of invasive candidiasis in a neonatal intensive care unit. J Pediatr 2005; 142:166–171.

Chapter 7 | Infestations

Arthropods are constantly present in the human environment, and hundreds of species are known to cause skin disease.[1,2] Arthropods may be divided into arachnids, which have eight legs (e.g. mites, ticks, spiders), and hexapods, with six legs (e.g. lice, mosquitoes, fleas, bedbugs, ants, bees, and other insects). Biting and stinging insects may produce wheals, erythema, and even bullae from contact with the skin.[1,2] The erythematous papule with a central punctum is a common feature of insect bites. In this chapter, scabies, pediculoses, and papular urticaria are discussed in detail because they are the most common forms of infestations and often require therapeutic intervention. Cutaneous eruptions related to ticks, spiders, mites, and parasitic worms (helminths) are also considered.

HUMAN MITE INFESTATION

Scabies

Clinical features

Pruritic papules on the abdomen, dorsa of the hands, flexural surface of the wrist, elbows, periaxillary skin, genitalia, ankles, feet, and interdigital webs of the hands are seen in scabies (Figs 7.1, 7.2).[1–4] In infants, eczematous eruptions of the face and trunk are also seen (Fig. 7.3). In contrast, the head and neck regions are almost never involved in older children, adolescents, or adults. Most infants have acute dermatitis that is characterized by excoriations, erythematous papules, honey-colored crusts, and pustules. Infants have hundreds of lesions, older children and adults have few. In all children with widespread scabies, secondary impetigo is common.

Crusted nodules that may become brown with time may be apparent on the trunk of the infant with scabies (Figs 7.4, 7.5).[1] When present, S-shaped burrows are diagnostic (Fig. 7.6).[1,2] They are usually found on the wrist, palm, feet, ankles, interdigital webs, or genitalia. Nocturnal pruritus is severe. Within one household the disease may vary in severity from asymptomatic infested children to a child with a few nonpruritic papules to hundreds of lesions. Infants are likely to have dozens of lesions (Figs 7.7, 7.8), whereas older children and adults may have less than 10. A high index of suspicion should be maintained in any patient with pruritic skin disease.

Children who are unable to scratch effectively may be infested with thousands of scabies mites, which produce a diffuse hyperkeratosis and crusting of large areas of skin and lichenification that may be confused with ichthyosis.[1,3,5,6] Hyperkeratosis and scaling may be particularly prominent on the hands, feet, and genitalia.[3,5] This form of scabies is called *Norwegian scabies* (Figs 7.9, 7.10). Children with malignancies or immunodeficiencies, or those who are on immunosuppressive drugs or who suffer local immunosuppression from the use of superpotent topical steroids may similarly suffer widespread scabies infestation, with extensive scalp involvement.[1,5,6]

Differential diagnosis

The diagnosis of scabies is confirmed by scraping an unscratched burrow. The burrow is covered with a drop of microscope immersion oil, scraped with a No. 15 blade or dermal curette and the scrapings placed on a glass slide with a coverslip. Under the 10× objective of the microscope, the female mite and/or her eggs or feces should be visible (Fig. 7.11). Examination of skin scrapings obtained from the finger webs, wrists, or ankles is most likely to be positive.[1] Excoriated and crusted lesions are often negative. In children with Norwegian scabies, scraping of the thick

Fig. 7.1 Scabies. Papules and burrows on the foot of an infant.

Fig. 7.4 Scabies. Crusted nodules on the trunk of an infant.

Fig. 7.2 Scabies. Involvement of the dorsa of the hands and interdigital webs in a child.

Fig. 7.3 Scabies. Nonspecific eczematous lesions in a child's axilla.

Fig. 7.5 Scabies. Brown crusted nodules on a child's chest.

scales will often yield several viable mites.[1,3,5,6] Atopic dermatitis, lichen planus, dermatitis herpetiformis, and other severely pruritic skin conditions mimic scabies. Children with crusted scabies may be misdiag-nosed as Langerhans cell histiocytosis as skin biopsies of crusted scabies shows histiocytic proliferation and mites in the stratum corneum may be missed on biopsy.[5] Scabies should be suspected in any infant

Fig. 7.6 S-shaped burrow diagnostic of scabies. This is the preferred lesion from which to obtain a scraping.

Fig. 7.8 Scabies in an infant. Dozens of crusted nodules, red papules and eczematous changes.

Fig. 7.7 Scabies in an infant. Hundreds of red papules are present.

Fig. 7.9 Norwegian scabies. Diffuse scaling of the dorsum of the hand. Scraping of the scales revealed dozens of motile mites.

Fig. 7.10 Norwegian scabies in a child with Down syndrome. Fissures developed within thickened scales on dorsum of hand.

with a sudden onset of severely itchy dermatitis. A careful inspection for burrows and identification of household members who may have a history of itchy bumps are necessary. Seborrheic dermatitis of the scalp may mimic scabies in children with malignancy or immunosuppression.

Fig. 7.11 Photomicrograph of oval eggs and dark brown scybala in skin scraping from an infant with scabies.

Pathogenesis

Scabies is caused by the eight-legged human mite *Sarcoptes scabiei*, which may be up to 4 mm in length.[1] The female mite remains in the stratum corneum, which she traverses at a rate of 0.5–5 mm/day. She deposits her eggs during her journey and dies after 30–40 days. Her eggs reach maturity in 10–14 days, and a new cycle begins. Transmission of scabies requires human contact, although female mites can survive 2–3 days off the human body. A pandemic of scabies has followed each major war of the twentieth century. Human scabies is quite contagious because newly infested individuals may not experience itching for the first 3 weeks of infestation, and only casual contact is required for spread of mites to others.[1,2] Humans are the reservoir for scabies, and infestation of children with animal mites (e.g. dog, cat, chicken) is rare.

Treatment

Application of a scabicide, such as 5% permethrin crème, is curative.[1,2,3,7,8] In some countries, 1% gamma benzene hexachloride lotion is preferred. The lotion or cream should be dispensed as the calculated dose needed for therapy. In children and adolescents, application of 5% permethrin crème for 8–14 hours produces a 98% cure rate.[1,2,8] One 2-hour application of lindane lotion followed by a bath is curative in approximately 82% of cases; one 6-hour application cures 96% of cases.[1,2,8] Prolonged contact with the skin may result in significant percutaneous absorption. Gamma benzene hexachloride is concentrated in the central nervous system if absorbed; percutaneous absorption with central nervous system symp-toms has been reported in a few infants.[9] Some instances of lindane-resistant scabies in North America have been reported. Ivermectin at 200 µg/kg in a single oral dose has also been demonstrated to be curative.[1,2,3,6,7,8] Topical permethrin may be superior to single-dose ivermectin.[4,7,8] In children under 5 years of age and in pregnant or lactating women, gamma benzene hexachloride lotion and ivermectin are not recommended.[1,2,4,7] Permethrin crème is approved for use for infants 2 months of age or older. In any infant or toddler, covering the hands with clothing to prevent licking the scabicide from the skin is recommended. For children with only a few lesions, routine retreatment is not necessary. In infants with extensive involvement, several retreatments 7 or 8 days apart may occasionally be required. Simultaneous treatment of all household contacts is required.[1,2,7,8]

Even with the elimination of all viable scabies mites and eggs, itching may persist for 7–10 days after successful therapy. Despite the persistence of pruritus, no new lesions should be detected. Treatment failures are often the result of poor compliance or failure to treat an infested household member. In treatment failures with topical scabicides, in immunosuppressed children, or others with Norwegian scabies, single-dose ivermectin should be considered and multiple courses may be required.[1,3] Following ivermectin treatment, large sheets of hyperkeratotic scale may be shed.

Patient education

The clinician should emphasize to the patient and family the mode of transmission of scabies and identify all household contacts. Instructions on the treatment schedule should be specific; the persistence of itching even after scabicidal therapy and the importance of treating all household contacts should be emphasized. See CD-ROM for a Patient Education Sheet on Scabies.

Follow-up visits

A follow-up visit in 2 weeks is important to ascertain success or failure of therapy. Any new lesions that may have appeared should be scraped to determine whether infestation has persisted or the child is reinfested. If the mite or her products are found, retreatment is suggested. Infants, who tend to have hundreds of lesions, may require several retreatments.

Other Mite Infestations

Clinical features

Mites from nonhuman sources occasionally infest the skin of children. The canine scabies mite, usually carried on the fur of puppies with mange, may be temporarily transferred to the child.[1] The puppy will have fur loss and crusted lesions. Similarly, harvest mites or chiggers, found in grasses, grains, or overgrowth of bushes, may similarly infest children. Grain mites found in stored seeds and grains, and fowl mites found on chickens or domesticated birds such as canaries, pigeons, or swallows may also infest children. In each instance the clinical lesions are characterized by urticarial papules, sometimes with hemorrhagic puncta, and, in intense responses, blister formation. Burrows are absent. The distribution on the child's skin depends on the location of the exposed skin. Characteristically, canine scabies produces lesions on the forearms, abdomen, and thighs. Harvest mites characteristically produce lesions on the legs and around the beltline. Grain mite lesions occur on the exposed areas of the arms and legs but may be quite generalized. Fowl mites produce lesions on exposed areas of skin.

Differential diagnosis

Scabies and papular urticaria are the most important considerations in the differential diagnosis. A history of exposure to the appropriate source is most significant in the diagnosis of mite infestation. Important historical information includes the new puppy with hair loss and crusts on its skin, exposure to deep grasses and grain or stored grain, and association with birds. Exposed skin infested with fowl mites may mimic a photoeruption.

Pathogenesis

In each case the mites attach themselves to the skin to inject an irritating secretion and then fall off in a few days. Identifying the mites within skin lesions is very difficult. They do not persist on skin, however.

Treatment

Symptomatic relief with topical steroids or oral antihistamines, or both, is useful. Specific scabicides are not required.

Patient education

Prophylaxis is an important part of patient education. Treatment of the infested puppy, use of good insect repellents (Table 7.1), and staying away from those areas containing sources that are likely to produce the infestation should be emphasized. Parents and children should know that they cannot pass this eruption to others, and that itching can be quite severe, lasting for several weeks after the initial exposure.

Follow-up visits

A follow-up visit in 2 weeks to ascertain the institution of prophylaxis and the response to therapy is useful.

Table 7.1 Insect repellents for children's use

Brand	Manufacturer	% DEET
DEET-containing		
Skedaddle for Children	Minnetonka	6.5
Skeddadle for Children with sunscreen SPF 15		6.5
Off! Skintastic for Kids spray	Johnson Wax	5.0
Cutter Just for Kids	United Industries	5.0
Cutter Pleasant Protection with sunscreen SPF 15		7.0
Repel Camp Lotion for Kids	Wisconsin Pharmacal	10.0
Repel Soft Unscented gel		7.0
Plant-based repellants		
Bite Blocker (geranium oil)	Consep, Inc.	
Avon Skin So Soft Bug Guard spray (citronella 0.10%)	Avon	
Permethrin insecticide sprays		
NOTE: For clothing only! Not to be applied on skin.		
Cutter Outdoorsman Gear Guard spray (Permethrin 0.5%)	Cutter	
(Permethrin 0.5%)	Wisconsin Pharmacal	

Fig. 7.12 Tick embedded in the occipital scalp of a child.

TICKS

Clinical Features

Tick bites are usually painless and inapparent to the child. Usually, the tick is noted several days after contact with the skin when pruritus begins. Localized urticarial reactions can be found. A diagnosis is usually made by identifying the presence of the tick in particular cutaneous locations. The most common sites for tick attachment are the occipital scalp (Fig. 7.12), ear canal, axilla, groin, and vulva.[2,10] Rarely, a systemic reaction to a tick bite, characterized by fever, nausea, abdominal cramping, and headache, may occur, as may paralysis similar to Guillain-Barré syndrome, with ascending symmetric paralysis.[11] Tick paralysis may also present as ataxia. Paralysis and ataxia resolve within 24 hours of tick removal.[11] A persistent, pruritic nodule, sometimes surrounded by hair loss, may be the result of an incompletely removed tick in which

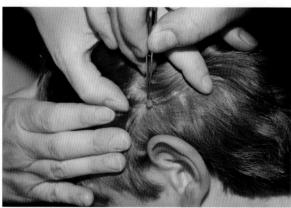

Fig. 7.13 Removal of tick by placing a forceps between the tick and the skin.

mouth parts remain in the skin. Because ticks in certain areas of North America and Europe may carry *Borrelia burgdorferi*, the spirochete responsible for Lyme disease, observation for expanding rings of erythema about the site of the bite is advised for 3 weeks after the bite (see Ch. 5).[10,12–15] The potentially severe nature of Lyme disease, and its prominence in the news media, has prompted excessive concern regarding tick bites.[2,12] Ticks also are responsible for other serious infections including Rocky Mountain spotted fever,[16] ehrlichiosis,[17] anaplasmosis,[17] tularemia, encephalitis and tick necrosis, and adenopathy syndrome.[18]

Differential Diagnosis

Most tick-bite reactions are obvious because the tick is found attached to the skin. If the mouth parts are left in the skin and a pruritic nodule remains, the diagnosis may be quite difficult to distinguish from scabies, lichen simplex chronicus, or other infestations. The expanding annular red rings of erythema chronicum migrans (ECM) may be confused with ringworm, urticaria, or other annular conditions.

Pathogenesis

Tick bites may occur when children play in the woods and when ticks are transferred from dogs or other incidental hosts to children. The tick attaches itself to the skin by its head in an effort to suck blood. The tick cuts the skin surface with chelicerae, introduces its proboscis, and secretes saliva into the wound. The saliva contains a cement substance, anesthetic, and anticoagulant, and may include the neurotoxin responsible for tick paralysis or the spirochete responsible for Lyme disease. After 24–48 hours, the tick engorges with blood from the child, which allows *Borrelia* to proliferate in the tick gut and then reenter the child from the tick saliva. A foreign body granuloma is seen in persistent nodules in the skin where tick head parts remain.

Treatment

Removal of the tick is the treatment of choice. The preferred method of removal is the insertion of a blunt instrument, such as a forceps or tweezers, between the tick head and the child's skin (Fig. 7.13). Gentle outward pressure will cause the tick to back out. This method prevents any injury to the skin and the retention of tick parts within the skin. All methods that may injure the skin, such as burning the tick or using noxious substances on the skin, should be avoided. The body of the tick should not be squeezed, and if there is a remnant in the skin, the clinician should consider simple surgical removal. If the child acquired the tick in an area endemic for Lyme disease, it should be saved in a glass jar for analysis if the child becomes ill later. Routine prophylactic administration of oral antibiotics after tick removal is not recommended.[2]

Patient Education

Prevention is the best method for tick bites. As much as possible, children should try to avoid tick habitats, such as dense brush or tall grass, and stay in the center of the path on wooded trails.[2,10] Children should wear protective clothing, such as long sleeves and caps, preferably of light color so the ticks can be easily seen. They should wear a shirt with a collar to prevent migration and tuck their pants into boots or socks. In endemic areas the regular and careful use of insect repellents (see Table 7.1) during tick season is recommended. Children and their dogs should be routinely inspected for ticks if they have been in wooded areas, and parents should be advised of the most common locations of tick bites and the preferred method of removal.[2] Clinicians should emphasize that most ticks do not carry Lyme disease. In endemic areas, Lyme vaccine may be considered for adolescents over age 15.[2,12] For a Patient Education Sheet on Insect Repellents for Children, see CD-ROM.

Follow-up Visits

A follow-up visit 2 weeks after a bite to observe for signs of ECM should be considered in areas endemic for Lyme disease.

SPIDERS

Clinical Features

Spider bites may produce local or systemic reactions. The most common is the urticarial papule from nonvenomous spiders. After a bite from a venomous spider, such as a brown recluse, hemorrhagic, painful blisters may appear on the skin and evolve over the next few days into a cutaneous infarct with skin necrosis (Fig. 7.14) and evolves to a dry, gangrenous eschar (Fig. 7.15). This reaction usually occurs on exposed

Fig. 7.14 Spider bite. Central necrosis surrounding zone of erythema.

Fig. 7.15 Spider bite. Central necrosis with eschar and surrounding desquamation.

areas of skin in a single lesion around the site of a spider bite.[19,20] The area of skin loss may be large. With black widow spider bites, systemic reactions, including headache, nausea, vomiting, chills, malaise, syncope, and coma, may develop. Thrombocytopenia, hemolysis, and hemoglobinuria, which might result in renal failure, have been reported.[20]

Differential Diagnosis

Venomous spider bites must be differentiated from pyoderma gangrenosum and from forms of vascular infarction, such as vasculitis. In pyoderma gangrenosum, the epithelial edges of the ulcer are not attached, but undermined, whereas in necrotic spider bites the epithelial edges are firmly adherent. In vasculitis, numerous lesions are present, whereas in spider bites, a single lesion is seen. Other necrotizing infections, such as ecthyma gangrenosum, caused by *Pseudomonas* infection, and streptococcal gangrene syndrome should be considered in the differential diagnosis. Lesions of herpes zoster, herpes simplex, cutaneous diphtheria, or anthrax may occasionally be confused with spider bite. In children who do not give a definite history of a spider bite, viral and bacterial cultures may be required.

Pathogenesis

Spiders with venomous jaws powerful enough to penetrate human skin, such as the Loxosceles species, produce necrotic skin reactions. In North America, the brown recluse spider *(Loxosceles reclusa)* is usually responsible for the lesion.[20] This spider is very prevalent in the midwestern United States but has occasionally been reported over many other areas of North America. The spider is small, 8–10 mm in diameter, and bears a violin-shaped band over the dorsal thorax. It is often found in old buildings. A number of toxins have been found in the venom. Neurotoxins are carried by Latrodectus spiders, including black widow spiders.[20] These spiders are responsible for systemic symptoms after a spider bite.

Treatment

With venomous spider bites, high doses of oral corticosteroids may be useful in reducing or preventing the extent of tissue damage in necrotic spider bites. Doses of 2 mg/kg/day of prednisone are usually recommended for a period of 5 days.[20] Surgical removal of the necrotic area has been performed in some instances to prevent spread of the toxin. Hospitalization may be required in severe systemic toxic reactions caused by black widow spider bites.

Patient Education

The clinician should emphasize that venomous spiders may hide in basements and that recognition of the small, thin-legged spider is important. Children should be kept from abandoned buildings, woodpiles, or other sites favored by spiders.

Follow-up Visits

A daily follow-up visit after initiation of treatment for the spider bite is necessary to evaluate for the development of systemic symptoms and progression of the individual lesion. The child should be seen until healing is observed.

PEDICULOSES (LOUSE INFESTATIONS)
Clinical Features

In human body-louse infestations, excoriated papules and pustules on the trunk and perineum are found in children and adolescents with body-louse infestations.[21,22] Often, only excoriations or their resultant hyperpigmented or hypopigmented scars are seen on the skin. The louse may be discovered by closely examining the seams of the patient's underwear or the scalp hair.

In human head-louse infestations, the gelatinous nits of the head louse appear as white, ovoid bodies tightly adherent to the hair shaft (Figs 7.16–7.18). Nocturnal pruritus is often severe with all human louse infestations.[21,22] The prevalence of louse infestations is 34 times higher in whites than in blacks.

In human pubic-louse infestations, the pubic (crab) louse may be seen crawling among the pubic hairs, or infestation with the pubic louse may present as blue-black crusted macules (maculae cerulea) in the pubic area. Nits may also be seen attached to pubic hairs.[21,22] The pubic louse may be seen in the eyelashes or the scalp of newborns.[21,22] Any 'bug' seen crawling from the newborn's eye should be considered a pubic louse unless proved otherwise.

Differential Diagnosis

Scabies, dermatitis herpetiformis, neurotic excoriations, and other highly pruritic dermatoses may be confused with pediculoses. Parents with delusions of parasitosis may transfer their delusion to their children. In certain children the retained external hair-root sheath may resemble head louse nits in the scalp. Retained hair root sheaths completely surround the

Fig. 7.16 Head lice. Numerous white nits attached to hairs.

Fig. 7.17 Head lice. Photomicrograph of nit tightly adherent to one side of a hair shaft.

hair, but the nit is attached to one side of the hair. Retained hair root sheaths may be easily removed by sliding them distally down the hair shaft, whereas the nit is tightly adherent to it. The blue-black, crusted

Fig. 7.18 Head lice. Photomicrograph of empty nit tightly adherent to one side of a hair shaft.

macules caused by pubic lice may be confused with vasculitis, folliculitis, or impetigo.

Pathogenesis

The human louse, a six-legged insect, attaches itself to the skin, ingests blood, and produces skin lesions by mechanical puncture and perhaps by injecting toxic secretions. There are two species of human lice: *Pediculus humanus*, the body louse, which has sub-species *capitis* (head lice) and *humanus* (body lice), and *Pthirus pubis*, the crab louse. The body louse, which is 2–4 mm in length, is the longest of the lice that infest humans; the pubic louse is 1–2 mm in length. The female produces new offspring every 2 weeks, and each female may produce over 80 off-spring during her lifetime. The body louse produces more eggs during her lifetime than the pubic louse. Newly hatched lice mate with old, and hundreds of nits result every 2 weeks. The female body or head louse attaches herself to a hair and slides along it, laying eggs. If hair is not available, clothing fibers are used. Nits are firmly attached to one side of the hair. Crowded living conditions are most conducive to the spread of lice, which can be transmitted either by person-to-person contact or by fomites, such as hairbrushes, caps, scarves, coats, or carpets.[22] Sharing of clothing is a common source of transmission.

Treatment

The application of 1% gamma benzene hexachloride lotion to the affected skin area for 12–24 hours is effective in body-lice infestation.[2] For head-lice or crab-lice infestations, 1% gamma benzene hexachloride shampoo, 1% permethrin shampoo, or 0.3% pyrethrin shampoo applied for 10 minutes and then rinsed out results in an 80% cure rate. Malathion 0.5% lotion left on for 8–12 hours is also effective.[1,2] Resistance of head lice to permethrins, pyrethrins, and malathion has been reported.[22,23] Shampoo treatments will not, however, remove the gelatinous nits. The use of a warm damp towel for 30 minutes on the scalp will loosen the nits and allow their mechanical removal with a fine-toothed comb (nit comb). Most pediculicide shampoos are supplied with a nit comb. Retreatment in 7 days is recommended. Measuring the distance of the nit closest to the scalp surface will provide a baseline measurement to help determine adequacy of treatment on follow-up. The head lice is found on pillows in 4% of infested children.[24] Boiling of clothing, bedding, and other possible fomites is ovicidal and lousicidal, and it is necessary because nits may be attached to clothing. Sun drying and cold washing are ineffectiive.[24] The recent introduction of suffocation-based pediculicides (Nuvo Lotion) may provide a strategy that avoids resistance.[25] They are not rinsed out but allowed to dry-on overnight.

Patient Education

It is tempting for parents to use pediculicides repeatedly in children with lice infestations. The clinician should emphasize the hazards of central nervous system and other toxicities posed by such usage. All contacts should be identified and treated simultaneously. Students should be readmitted to school the morning after the first treatment.[26] 'No-nit' policies for return to school cannot be justified.[26] Cutting the child's hair short should be discouraged. Schoolmates should be examined by the school nurse to determine if other children are infested.[26] A firm diagnosis should be made as retained hair sheaths and external particulates may be mistaken for nits and induce considerable anxiety.[26] For a Patient Education Sheet on Head Lice, see CD-ROM.

Follow-up Visits

An office or visiting nurse follow-up to evaluate therapy 1 week after the initial visit is most helpful. If new eggs or nits are seen on the proximal hair shafts, as close or closer to the scalp than the original measurement, then retreatment is necessary. Nits will grow out with the hair shaft and by 7 days after suc-

cessful treatment should be at least 6–7 mm from the scalp margin.

PAPULAR URTICARIA

Clinical Features

Pruritic erythematous papules, with or without an erythematous, urticarial flare, are characteristically arranged in clusters in papular urticaria (Fig. 7.19).[27] Such clusters are usually seen over the shoulders, upper arms, and buttocks. Individual papules each have a tiny central punctum (Fig. 7.20). Papular urticaria occurs predominantly between the ages of 18 months and 7 years. In intense hypersensitivity, vesicles and bullae may be seen. Recurrent crops of these papules are the rule, with each crop lasting 2–10 days (Figs 7.21, 7.22). Occasionally, giant areas of erythema may occur (Fig. 7.23). Characteristically, the affected child is the only household member involved.

Fig. 7.19 Papular urticaria in a child. Grouped papules with surrounding urticarial flare due to cat fleas.

Fig. 7.20 Papular urticaria. New leson with central puncta.

Fig. 7.21 Papular urticaria. Grouped lesions on the lower neck where a puppy was carried by the child.

Fig. 7.22 Papular urticaria. Central papules with urticaria flare on arm of child.

Fig. 7.23 Papular urticaria. Giant red flare following insect exposure.

The problem may persist for 3–9 months and most often begins in spring or summer.

Differential Diagnosis

Insect bites, viral exanthems, photoeruptions, acute parapsoriasis, and the early stages of other papulosquamous diseases (see Ch. 9) may be confused with papular urticaria.

Pathogenesis

The lesions represent delayed hypersensitivity reactions to a variety of biting or stinging arthropods. Cat fleas are the usual offenders.[27] Less commonly, dog fleas, mosquitoes, lice, scabies, fowl mites, and grain or grass mites are responsible. Epicutaneous testing with homogenized arthropods has reproduced the urticarial papule within 4–8 hours. The pathologic fea-

tures of naturally occurring lesions are similar to those of a delayed-type (tuberculin) skin test with prominent eosinophilia.[28] Papular urticaria to bed bugs may be mediated by IgE to specific bed bug salivary proteins.[29]

Treatment

The logical therapy is to remove the offending insect.[27] Dogs or cats should be treated for fleas or mites by a veterinarian. Household fumigation may be necessary.[27] The child should be kept away from the pet. Protective clothing, such as long sleeves, may be useful. The prophylactic use of an oral antihistamine, such as cetirizine, may reduce the reactions. Use of insect repellents may make the child less attractive to the insect (see Table 7.1).[30,31] See CD-ROM for a Patient Education Sheet on Insect Repellents for Children. The most successful repellent for mosquitoes is Bite

Blocker, with DEET-containing insect repellents almost as efficaceous.[30] Caution should be exercised to not use DEET on large areas of skin or in concentrations greater than 10%.[30] DEET preparations that are 6.5 %, listed in Table 7.1, may be used cautiously on the child's skin. Fleas or mites living in carpets or furniture may be eliminated by treatment with a commercial insecticide. Window casings should be treated in the case of bird mites. Symptomatic relief may sometimes be obtained with topical midpotency glucocorticosteroid creams or ointments applied three times daily.

Patient Education

When only one member of the household is affected, it is difficult to convince some parents of the cause. The extreme sensitivity of the affected person to the offending arthropod should be explained. Often an obvious source is not evident from the initial history, and a thorough search should be made for the source, including inquiries into day care, preschool, and visits to neighbors, friends, and relatives. It is a great relief to both the parents and the child to learn that the sensitivity is limited to 3–6 months. For a Patient Education Sheet on Papular Urticaria, see CD-ROM.

Follow-up Visits

A visit within 2 weeks is most useful in reviewing the possible sources and evaluating the response to therapeutic measures. At the follow-up visit it is often easier to convince parents of the cause of the eruption.

HELMINTHS (PARASITIC WORMS)

Cutaneous Larva Migrans (Creeping Eruption)

Clinical features

Pruritic, serpiginous, erythematous, linear lesions of the skin that advance at the rate of 1 cm/day represent the classic pattern seen in cutaneous larva migrans (Fig. 7.24).[32] Lesions are usually on the feet (Fig. 7.25) and occasionally the arms or legs.[32,33] Vesicles and bullae may be present along the tract, and pulsatile edema within the erythematous, serpiginous tract may be observed. Some children complain of pain at the site, and edema of the area is noted in about 25% of cases. A history of a child having played along the shorelines of the southeastern or eastern United States is usually

Fig. 7.24 Creeping eruption. Serpiginous red track on the plantar surface of a child with A. braziliensis.

Fig. 7.25 Creeping eruption. Serpiginous tract accompanied by crusted and excoriated lesions from the child's scratching.

obtained. A second clinical form involves strictly the perianal area, buttocks, and thighs, with serpiginous tracts that spread 5–10 cm/hr. The child may have peripheral blood eosinophilia, with 10–35% eosinophils present.

Differential diagnosis

The annular erythemas, including ECM, urticaria, and even tinea infections, may be confused with cutaneous larva migrans. The rapid progression and advancement of the border in cutaneous larva migrans and the presence of pulsations within the serpiginous tract are useful differentiating features.

Pathogenesis

Two larvae are primarily responsible for the cutaneous lesions in cutaneous larva migrans found in North America. *Ancylostoma braziliensis* is the most common of these larvae and produces the clinical pattern involving the feet.[32,33] Children playing along the shore of the southern United States are at the greatest risk. *A. braziliensis* is the dog and cat hookworm, and ova of this organism are deposited in the soil or in the sandy beaches from dog and cat excretions and hatch into larvae that will penetrate bare skin. The larvae migrate 1–2 cm/day and produce the serpiginous lesions of the skin. Stools are negative for parasite eggs, and identification of the larvae within the tract is quite difficult because they are often found beyond the area of obvious inflammation. This parasite cannot complete its life cycle in humans, and the larvae disappear within 4–6 weeks of their onset.

The second form of cutaneous larva migrans is due to the larvae of *Strongyloides stercoralis*. These larvae usually penetrate the skin near the anus and spread onto the buttocks. They are able to leave the skin and may settle in the gastrointestinal tract, and a stool sample examined for ova and parasites will identify the *Strongyloides* larvae or eggs. Larvae from fish or squid nematodes may also produce a creeping eruption, particularly among travelers to the Caribbean.[1,20]

Treatment

Topical thiabendazole 15% cream, applied three times a day for 5–7 days, is the treatment of choice for creeping eruption caused by *A. braziliensis*.[34] Parents should be instructed to treat well beyond the area of obvious skin redness. Oral thiabendazole is also quite effective in a dose of 25 mg/kg two times a day for 2 days and should be used for creeping eruption caused by *S. stercoralis*. Oral albendazole, 400 mg/day for 7 days, and ivermectin, 200 μg/kg as a single dose, have also been shown to be efficacious.

Patient education

Parents should understand that these infestations may be acquired from sandy beaches or sandboxes, and only in certain regions of North America. Further, they should know that the lesions are not contagious to other children, and that usually one treatment protocol is curative.

Follow-up visits

A visit at 4–5 days after initiation of therapy is useful to evaluate the response.

Swimmer's Itch, Seabather's Eruption, and Jellyfish Stings

Clinical features

Pruritic papules appearing in areas not protected by the swimsuit are characteristic of swimmer's eruption, which has occurred in those who have swum in freshwater lakes of the upper Great Lakes region of North America.[35] The longer the water exposure, the more likely to develop swimmers' eruption. [35]

In seabather's eruption, the pruritic 2–5 mm papules occur under the swimsuit-covered areas after swimming in salt waters of the southern United States.[36] Jellyfish stings may be linear when the jellyfish tentacles strike the skin (Fig. 7.26).[37] The papules or linear lesions are persistent and may last for at least 2 weeks.

Fig. 7.26 Jellyfish eruption. Multiple linear erythematous areas where jellyfish tentacles contacted the skin.

Differential diagnosis

Papular urticaria, insect bite reactions, and infestations caused by scabies or other mites should be considered in the differential diagnosis. The strong historical and temporal association with swimming is a very useful differentiating point. Linear lesions of jellyfish stings may mimic phytophotodermatitis, in which plants such as tall grasses contact the skin and produce linear erythema or vesicles.

Pathogenesis

Parasitic flatworms have been implicated in swimmer's itch. Cercariae are released into the water from infected snails in freshwater lakes of the upper Great Lakes region. The parasites finish their cycle by penetrating the skin of warm-blooded hosts, but do not survive after penetration. The schistosomes usually come from the droppings of infested mammals and waterfowl and are then involved with the snail as intermediate host.

Seabather's eruption is due to cercariae of the *Linuche ungauiculata* jellyfish. When the seawater containing jellyfish larvae flows through the bathing suit, the larvae or adults contact the skin and discharge nematocysts.[37] Linear lesions of jellyfish stings are the direct result of contact with jellyfish tentacles.

Treatment

Because seabather's eruption is a self-limited disease, no specific anticercarial treatment need be introduced. Symptomatic treatment, such as the use of topical steroid preparations, oral antihistamines, or both, is usually recommended. In severe eruptions, oral prednisone for 5 days may be considered.

Patient education

Parents and patients should be given an explanation of the source of the itchy eruption and should know that it cannot be transmitted from the infested individual to other humans. They should also be told to recognize that this disease is self-limited and will disappear.

Seabather's eruption can be prevented or minimized by showering immediately after removal of swimwear.[38] A jellyfish sting inhibitor that also contains sunscreen (Nidara Technology LTD Jordan Valley, Israel) is effective when applied before swimming.[39] Immediate application of ice to a jellyfish sting will provide relief, as will topical papain-containing preparations.[38] Hyperpigmentation after jellyfish stings may require months to resolve.

Follow-up visits

Follow-up visits are usually unnecessary.

REFERENCES

1. Johnston G, Sladden M. Scabies: diagnosis and treatment. Brit Med J 2005; 331:619–622.
2. Report of the Committee on Infectious Diseases. 2003 Red book. Elk Grove Village, Ill: American Academy of Pediatrics; 2003.
3. Roberts LJ, Huffam SE Walton SF, et al. Crusted scabies: clinical and immunological findings in seventy-eight patients and a review of the literature. J Infect 2005; 50:375–381.
4. Ziemer M, Boer A. Eosinophilic pustulosis of infancy: not a distinctive inflammatory disease of the skin. Amer J Dermatopathol 2005; 27:443–455.
5. Burch JM, Krol A, Weston WL. *Sarcoptes scabiei* infestation misdiagnosed and treated as Langerhans cell histiocytosis. Pediatr Dermatol 2004; 21:58–62.
6. Gladstone HB, Darmstadt GL. Crusted scabies in an immunocompetent child: treatment with ivermectin. Pediatr Dermatol 2000; 17:144.
7. Usha V, Gopalakrishnan Nair TV. A comparative study of oral ivermectin and topical permethrin cream in the treatment of scabies. J Am Acad Dermatol 2000; 42:236.
8. Elgart ML. Cost benefit analysis of ivermectin, permethrin and benzyl benzoate in the management of infantile and childhood scabies. J Amer Acad Dermatol 2003; 4:1521–1524.
9. Centers for disease control and prevention (CDC). Unintentional topical lindane ingestion – United States 1998–2003. MMWR 2005; 54:533–535.
10. Sarwari AR Strickland T Pena C, et al. Tick exposure and Lyme disease at a summer camp in Maryland. WV Med J 2005; 101:126–130.
11. Li Z, Turner RP. Pediatric tick paralysis: discussion of two cases and literature review. Pediatr Neurol 2004; 31:304–307.
12. Hengge UR, Tannafel A, Tyring SK, et al. Lyme borreliosis. Lancet Infect Dis 2003; 3:489–500.
13. Nowakowski J, Nadelman RB, Sell R, et al. Long-term follow-up of patients with culture-confirmed Lyme Disease. Am J Med 2003; 11:91–96.
14. Committee on Infectious Diseases, American Academy of Pediatrics; Prevention of Lyme disease; Pediatrics 2000; 105:142.
15. Malouin R, Winch P, Leontsini E, et al. Longitudinal evaluation of and educational intervention for preventing tick bites in an area endemic for Lyme disease in Baltimore County. Am J Epidemiol 2003; 15:1039–1051.
16. Dumler JS, Walker DH. Rocky Mountain spotted fever – changing ecology and persisting virulence. N Eng J Med 2005; 353:551–553.
17. Fritz CL, Bronson LR, Smith CR, et al. Clinical, epidemiologic and environmental surveillance for ehrlichiosis and anaplasmosis in and endemic area of northern California. J Vector Ecol 2005; 30:4–10.

18. Oteo JB, Ibarra V, Blanco JR, et al. Dermacentor-borne necrosis, erythema and lymphadenopathy: clinical and epidemiological features of a new tick-borne disease. Clin Microbiol Infect 2004; 10:327–331.
19. Lui PC, Petersen D, Kimble RM, et al. Idiopathic necrotizing dermatitis: current management. J Paediatr Child Health 2005; 41:27–30.
20. Frundle TC. Management of spider bites. Air Med J 2004; 23:24–26.
21. Burgess I. Head lice. Clin Evid 2003; 10:1884–1889.
22. Hansen RC. Overview: the state of head lice management and control. Am J Manag Care 2004; 10(suppl):S260–S263.
23. Roberts RJ, Burgess IF. New head-lice treatments: hype or hope? Lancet 2005; 365:8–10.
24. Speare R, Cahill C, Thomas G. Head lice on pillows, and strategies to make a small risk even less. Int J Dermatol 2003; 42:626–629.
25. Pearlman D. A simple treatment for head lice: dry-on, suffocation-based pediculicide. Pediatrics 2004; 114:e275–e279.
26. Hansen RC, Ohaver J. Economic considerations associated with *Pediculus humanus capitis* infestation. Clin Pediatr 2004; 43:523–527.
27. Naimer SA, Cohen AD, Mumcuoglu KY, et al. Household papular urticaria. Isr Med Assoc J 2002; 4(suppl):911–913.
28. Garcia E, Halpern E, Rodriguez A, et al. Immune and histopathologic examination of flea bite-induced papular urticaria. Ann Allergy Asthma Immunol 2004; 92:446–452.
29. Leverkus M, Jocim RC, Schad S, et al. Bullous allergic hypersensitivity to bed bug bites mediated by IgE against salivary nitrophorin. J Invest Dermatol 2006; 126:91–96.
30. Fradin MG. Mosquitoes and mosquito repellents: a clinician's guide. Ann Int Med 1998; 128:931.
31. Committee to advise on tropical medicine and travel. Statement on personal protective measures to prevent arthropod bites. Can Commun Dis Rep 2005; 31:1–18.
32. Shinkar RM, Stocks R, Thomas E. Cutaneous larval migrans, creeping eruption sand worm. Arch Dis Child 2005; 90:998.
33. Hotez PJ, Brooker S, Bethony JM, et al. Hookworm infection. N Engl J Med 2004; 351:799–807.
34. Caumes E. Efficacy of albendazole ointment on cutaneous larval migrans in two young children. Clin Infect Dis 2004; 38:1647–1648.
35. Verbrugge LM, Rainey JJ, Reimink RL, et al. Prospective study of swimmer's itch incidence and severity. J Parasitol 2004; 90:697–704.
36. Kumar S, Hlady WG, Malecki JM. Risk factors for sea-bather's eruption: a prospective cohort. Pub Health Rep 1997; 112:59.
37. Segura-Puertas L, Ramos ME, Aramburo C, et al. One *Linuche* mystery solved: all three stages of the coronate scyphomedusa *Linuche unguiculata* cause seabather's eruption. J Amer Acad Dermatol 2001; 44:624–628.
38. Landow K. Best treatment of jellyfish stings? Postgrad Med 2000; 107:27.
39. Kimball AB, Arambula KZ, Stauffer AR, et al. Efficacy of a jellyfish sting inhibitor in preventing jellyfish stings in normal volunteers. Wilderness Environ Med. 2004; 15:102–108.

Chapter 8

Viral Infections

Viruses may involve the skin either by dissemination to skin during a systemic viral infection accompanied by viral replication in skin (viral exanthem) or by producing a virus-induced skin tumor. A number of viruses are epidermotropic and replicate within keratinocytes.

VIRAL EXANTHEMS

Any cutaneous eruption associated with an acute viral syndrome has been termed a *viral exanthem*. If mucosa is involved, it is termed an *enanthem*. The exact incidence of viral exanthems is unknown, but herpes simplex alone accounts for a yearly incidence of 5.1 children affected per 1000. Most clinicians who treat children report that viral exanthems are common. Enteroviral and adenoviral exanthems are the most frequently encountered in the United States and account for the majority of viral exanthems seen.[1] It should be emphasized that all viruses may cause an exanthem, including those that are rarely associated with one.[1]

Viral exanthems are seen frequently in general pediatric settings and are considered in the differential diagnosis of drug eruptions. Frequently, the clinician will see a child with a generalized eruption who received a medication for the illness. There is no current method to reliably distinguish a viral exanthem from a drug eruption. A variety of different patterns of viral exanthem are seen: a generalized maculopapular eruption that mimics measles (morbilliform), petechial eruptions, vesiculobullous eruptions, scarlet fever-like (scarlatiniform) eruptions, papulonodular eruptions, and oral erosions.[1] Morbilliform eruptions are the most common. It is important to recall that any viral exanthem, including morbilliform eruptions, may have a photodistribution or be exaggerated in areas of prior skin inflammation.[1-4] Some exanthems may also be photoactivated by ultraviolet injury.[4] Skin injury by factors other than ultraviolet light may also result in localization of the viral exanthem to the site of injury.[3] Exanthems may also be unilateral, as reported in the asymmetric periflexural exanthem (Fig. 8.1).[5,6]

VIRAL EXANTHEMS: THE MORBILLIFORM ERUPTIONS

Eruptions that mimic measles (morbilli) are called *morbilliform eruptions*.[1,7] They are seen as generalized, discrete, pink to red macules. The morbilliform eruptions include measles, rubella, enteroviral and adenoviral exanthems, roseola, the mononucleosis syndromes, and erythema infectiosum (EI).[1,7,8] Measles (morbilli) is the prototype and namesake of morbilliform eruptions and, although uncommon in highly immunized populations,[7] is considered first in this chapter. Other viruses may mimic measles. Parvovirus B19, enteroviruses, and adenoviruses are the most frequent causes of morbilliform eruptions in immunized children.[1,7-10] Rubella is still seen in the unimmunized and many other viruses may occasionally produce a morbilliform eruption (Box 8–1).[10]

Measles (Rubeola)

Clinical features

Classic measles: The features of classic measles include a severe prodrome followed by an exanthematous phase. During the entire course of the illness, the child appears quite ill. After an incubation period of 9–14 days, a prodrome of high fever, cough, rhinitis, and conjunctivitis appears.[1,7,11] The cough is described as barking, and a diagnosis of bronchitis or croup is

Fig. 8.1 Asymmetric periflexural exanthem. Annular erythema on the inner arm and adjacent axilla in an 8-year-old child.

Fig. 8.2 Koplik's spots. Bright erythema of buccal mucosa with pinpoint white macules in rubeola.

Box 8.1 Differential diagnosis of morbilliform eruptions caused by viruses

Measles (rubeola)

Rubella

Roseola

Boston exanthem

Erythema infectiosum

Infectious mononucleosis

Pityriasis rosea (presumed viral)

Hepatitis

Mumps

Echoviruses 1, 2, 4, 5, 7, 9, 13, 14, 22, 25, 30

Reoviruses 2, 3

Coxsackieviruses A1, 2, 3, 4, 5, 7

Respiratory syncytial virus

Cytomegalovirus

Adenoviruses 1, 2, 3, 4, 5, 7

Colorado tick fever

Dengue

Herpesvirus 6

Echovirus 16

Parvovirus B19

Epstein-Barr virus

---

papules. The eruption is preceded by intense erythema of the mucous membranes with focal 1 mm white areas, the so-called *Koplik's spots* (Fig. 8.2).[7,11–13] Bacterial otitis media, bacterial pneumonia, and encephalitis may complicate measles.[1,7,11–13] Their exact incidence in measles is unknown. Severe pneumonia and encephalitis are primary causes of death in measles and are more likely to complicate measles in young infants and the malnourished or immunodeficient child. Mortality related to measles in the United States is estimated at 1 per 1000.[1,7,11–13] Low vitamin A levels, in particular, have been implicated in the severity of measles.[7,14] Other complications of measles include myocarditis, pericarditis, thrombocytopenia, hepatitis, acute glomerulonephritis, and Stevens-Johnson syndrome.[7,11–13]

Atypical measles: In patients who have received killed measles vaccine, or in whom live measles vaccination has failed, a syndrome of high fever, abdominal pain, pulmonary consolidation, and an acral eruption consisting of vesicular, vesiculopustular, or purpuric lesions may occur (atypical measles) (Fig. 8.3).[15] This is rarely observed in North America.

Differential diagnosis

Classic measles: The severity of the prodrome, a high fever, and Koplik's spots in an acutely ill child are the most distinctive features differentiating measles from the other morbilliform eruptions (Boxes 8.1, 8.2). Viral isolation from mucosa, although difficult, will distinguish measles from other exanthems. Serologic tests for measles IgM obtained after 72 hours of rash or paired acute and convalescent sera, obtained 1 week

usually considered. The prodrome typically includes cervical lymphadenopathy and lasts 3–5 days.[7,11] The preauricular lymph nodes are enlarged. The prodrome is then followed by a cutaneous eruption.

The exanthem begins on the forehead as blotchy erythema and progresses to involve the face, trunk, and extremities, with multiple discrete macules and

Fig. 8.3 Petechiae and palpable purpura on the feet of an adolescent with atypical measles.

and 3 weeks after the onset of the illness and examined for measles IgG, will assist with a retrospective diagnosis.[14]

Atypical measles: Atypical measles may mimic meningococcemia and Rocky Mountain spotted fever, which are the main considerations in the differential diagnosis. Primarily acral petechiae may be the presenting symptom in echovirus 9 and other enterovirus infections. Other conditions to be considered in the differential diagnosis are listed in Box 8.3.

Pathogenesis

Despite the very active measles immunization program in the United States, outbreaks of measles continue to occur.[7,11,13] Measles has not been eradicated but is at the lowest incidence reported in the United States.[11] The cutaneous eruption is related to the presence of the measles virus within keratinocytes and endothelial cells of the superficial dermal vessels.[7,16] The clinical lesions are believed to be due to the host response to the virus within the skin. The measles virus, a paramyxovirus, replicates within keratinocytes and induces increased nuclear volume within the epidermal cells, producing multinucleated giant cells (Warthin-Finkeldy cells).[16]

Box 8.3 Differential diagnosis of the STAR* complex
Rubella
Human parvovirus B19
Hepatitis B
Adenovirus
Echoviruses
Coxsackieviruses
Epstein-Barr virus
STAR, sore throat, arthritis, rash.

The purpuric cutaneous eruption of atypical measles is thought to be the result of immune complex formation.[15]

Treatment

No specific treatment is available for classic or atypical measles. For children 1 year of age and older a single oral dose of 200 000 IU of vitamin A is recommended.[7] For children with evidence of vitamin A deficiency, the dose should be repeated in 1 day and at 4 weeks. Measles immune globulin may prevent or modify measles if given within 6 days of exposure.[7] The dose is 0.25 mL/kg given intramuscularly and, if the child is immune suppressed (including children with HIV infection) 0.5 mL/kg is given intramuscularly.[7] Symptoms should be treated and children should be closely monitored for complications. If secondary bacterial otitis media or bacterial pneumonia occurs, antibiotic therapy should be instituted.

Patient education

The high attack rate of measles should be emphasized, and the patient should be isolated during the contagious period (from the onset of respiratory symptoms through the third day of the cutaneous eruption).[7] Measles patients should be reported to local public health authorities.

Follow-up visits

Close contact should be maintained with the patient with measles to watch for bacterial superinfection, the development of severe pneumonia with pulmonary compromise, or encephalitis. A prompt revisit should be scheduled if fever recurs, headache or change in the level of consciousness is observed, or seizures or motor defects are noted. Frequent visits may be required during the course of the illness.

Rubella

Clinical features

Classic rubella: Classic rubella is a mild illness in most children.[3,7,10,17–20] Rubella acquired postnatally in infants and children usually is accompanied by few or no prodromal symptoms. Up to 50% of rubella infections may be entirely asymptomatic.[7,10,17–20] Mild lymphadenopathy may precede the cutaneous eruption by several days. The suboccipital and posterior auricular lymph nodes are usually prominently enlarged. A faint pink, macular eruption appears first on the face and spreads to the trunk and proximal

extremities. Within 48 hours, the face and trunk have cleared and the eruption involves the distal extremities. The child usually appears well. Rarely, petechiae or purpura may be seen. A monarthric arthritis may accompany the syndrome, particularly in adolescent girls.[17–20] It may present as the so-called STAR (*sore throat, arthritis, rash*) complex.[21] In the STAR complex, rubella and human parvovirus B19 are the most likely viruses responsible.[21] The arthritis may persist for several months. Fever is usually absent or low grade in young children with rubella, but may be present in older children and adolescents, particularly when arthritis is present.[3,7,17–19]

Congenital rubella: Rubella acquired during the first trimester of pregnancy may result in rubella embryopathy.[17–20] This may be manifested by neonatal purpura and petechiae caused by thrombocytopenia. Of cases of congenital thrombocytopenia, rubella is responsible for 10%.[17–20] Occasionally, jaundice caused by rubella hepatitis occurs. Accompanying features include deafness, congenital heart defects, cataract, retinopathy, glaucoma, growth retardation, behavioral disorders, meningoencephalitis, and psychomotor retardation.[17–20] Any or all of these features may accompany the typical rubella exanthem. Rubella embryopathy can develop during reinfection of the mother with rubella.[20] The exanthem may recur any time during the first 5 years. In infants with congenital rubella, rubella virus may be recovered from peripheral blood leukocytes, stool, or urine for months to years after birth.

Differential diagnosis

Classic rubella: In distinguishing classic rubella from measles, the absence of fever is helpful. Rubella may be difficult to distinguish from enteroviral exanthems, infectious mononucleosis syndromes, parvovirus B19 infections, or drug eruptions.[19] In the STAR complex, rubella may be indistinguishable from human parvovirus B19 infections or from other viral causes of the exanthem (see Box 8.3).[21] Culture of the virus from nasal mucosa will distinguish rubella from other exanthems and is more reliable than serology for rubella IgM.[7]

Congenital rubella: Other congenital infections may produce the thrombocytopenia and hepatitis seen with rubella.[18,20] These include toxoplasmosis, syphilis, cytomegalovirus (CMV), and herpes simplex virus (HSV). Rarely, neonatal lupus, Wiskott-Aldrich syndrome, and hereditary platelet disorders may mimic congenital rubella. The presence of cataracts and congenital heart defects should suggest congenital rubella. Viral cultures of urine and throat will distinguish rubella from other congenital infections.

Pathogenesis

Rubella virus, a rubrivirus, is a ribonucleic acid (RNA) virus that enters the bloodstream via the respiratory mucosa.[7] The mechanism of the exanthem is unknown but is believed to be the result of viral dissemination to skin. Rubella virus has been cultured from the synovia in rubella arthritis. Rubella embryopathy is still seen because young women are vaccine failures or have not received the vaccine. The exact mechanism of the embryopathy is unknown.[20]

Treatment

There is no specific treatment for rubella. If the patient is febrile, fever control measures will suffice. Nonsteroidal antiinflammatory agents may be required for the arthritis. The management of rubella embryopathy requires a multidisciplinary team to include ophthalmologists, cardiologists, neurologists, and developmental specialists.

Patient education

Exposure or potential exposure of susceptible women in the first trimester of pregnancy should be determined. If possible, the rubella patient should be kept isolated from pregnant women for 7 days after the rash has appeared.[7] In patients who acquire rubella postnatally, it is contagious from 2 days before the onset of the cutaneous eruption to 7 days after the onset. In congenital rubella, virus shedding usually ends by age 6 months but may continue up to 5 or 6 years.[7] The incubation period ranges from 14 to 21 days.[7]

When a pregnant woman is exposed to rubella, a serum specimen should be obtained and tested for rubella IgG antibody.[7] If antibody is present, the woman is probably immune and there is little risk of congenital infection.[7] If no rubella antibody is detectable, a second blood specimen should be obtained 2 or 3 weeks later. If antibody is present in the second specimen and not the first, infection is presumed to have occurred, and termination of pregnancy may be considered. If termination of pregnancy is not an option, immune serum globulin should be given, 0.55 mL/kg intramuscularly.[7]

Follow-up visits

Follow-up visits are usually unnecessary in postnatally acquired rubella. In congenital rubella a multidisciplinary approach, such as that offered by a birth defects clinic, is advisable.

Roseola (Exanthem Subitum, Human Herpesvirus 6 Infection)

Clinical features

Roseola occurs predominantly in infants under 2 years of age.[7,22,23] It is characterized by 2 or 3 days of sustained fever in an infant who otherwise appears well, following which the temperature falls (often to a subnormal level), and a pink, morbilliform, cutan-

Fig. 8.4 Roseola. Faint pink papules on the trunk of an infant with HHV-6 infection.

Fig. 8.5 Roseola. Pink macules on chest of infant with HHV-6 infection.

eous eruption appears transiently and fades within 24 hours (Fig. 8.4). Lesions are predominantly on the trunk (Fig. 8.5). A convulsion at the onset of fever is noted occasionally, but the exact incidence of febrile convulsions is unknown.[23] Mild edema of the eyelids and posterior cervical lymphadenopathy are occasionally seen. More frequently, human herpesviruses type 6 (HHV-6) and 7 (HHV-7) infection produces an illness with cough, fever, and otitis media or a febrile convulsion.[22–25] Febrile seizures are infrequent in HHV-6 or -7 infection, but HHV-6 or -7 should be considered in any febrile seizure, including status epilepticus attacks.[24,25] An infantile infectious mononucleosis syndrome has also been described.[22–24] HHV-6 or -7 infections are predominantly acute febrile illnesses in infants under 24 months of age.[7,22–24]

Differential diagnosis

Roseola can be distinguished from most other morbilliform eruptions (see Boxes 8.1, 8.2) by the distinctive history of 3 days of sustained fever in an infant followed by the appearance of a morbilliform eruption after the fever ends. It may be indistinguishable from echovirus 16 infections. Eruptions resulting from treatment with drugs may easily be confused with roseola in infants who received antibiotics for the febrile portion of the illness. The HHV-6 infections that cause otitis media may be difficult to distinguish from bacterial otitis media, and the infectious mononucleosis syndrome mimics illness induced by the Epstein-Barr virus (EBV) or CMV. The febrile convulsion may mimic bacterial or viral meningitis or epilepsy. HHV-6 or -7 can be identified by culture of peripheral blood leukocytes, by serodiagnosis, or from skin lesions by molecular diagnosis.[7,22–24]

Pathogenesis

HHV-6 or -7 infection is thought to be the major causative agent for roseola worldwide, whereas in North America, children with echovirus 16 infections probably account for some cases of roseola.[22,23] HHV-6 or -7 are herpes-group viruses that preferentially involve circulating leukocytes. They produce predominantly acute febrile illnesses in infants with elevated interleukin-6 levels,[25] and it may be associated with a few cases of infectious mononucleosis, leukemias, or histiocytic syndromes.[23]

Treatment

In roseola, fever can be controlled with wet dressings or tepid water sponge baths, supplemental fluids, and antipyretics. HHV-6 or -7 are insensitive to current antiviral agents, but in immunocompromised children with severe disease some authorities recommend treatment with ganciclovir.[7]

Patient education

Parents should be informed of the viral nature of this disorder and told that there is no necessity for antibiotics. If the child is seen during the febrile state, it is worthwhile to document the morbilliform eruption by personally observing it. Parents should be told that the virus responsible for roseola predominantly infects children under 24 months of age, and most older children and adults are immune.

Follow-up visits

To be certain to exclude other infections that may mimic roseola, a follow-up visit 2 days later is recommended to ascertain the course of the illness.

Human Parvovirus B19 Infection (Erythema Infectiosum)

Clinical features

The eruptions of EI (fifth disease) classically begin with an intense, confluent redness of both cheeks, the so-called *slapped-cheek appearance* (Fig. 8.6), seen in 75% of patients.[7,26] It may then spread to involve the arms (86%), legs (75%), chest (47%), and abdomen (45%), with a lacy, pink to dull-red macular eruption (Figs 8.7–8.9); 25% of patients will have only the lacy eruption on their extremities.[7,26] The original eruption lasts 3–5 days. Stimulation of cutaneous vasodilation, however, will cause the eruption to reappear up to 4 months later.[7,26] This may result from vigorous exercise, overheating of the skin, or sun exposure. Only 20% of affected children will have mild fever. Occasionally, morbilliform, vesicular, or purpuric skin eruptions are seen. A purpuric hand and foot eruption (purpuric gloves-and-socks syndrome) may develop (Figs 8.10, 8.11) and include facial lesions.[7,26,27] About 20% of infected children and adults are asymptomatic. During some outbreaks of EI, symmetric arthritis of hands, wrists, or knees will be observed.[7,21,26,28] The STAR complex is caused by parvovirus B19 as often as by rubella.[21] Joint symp-

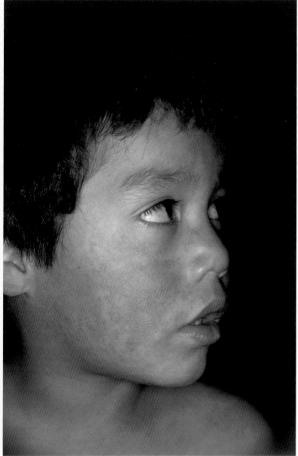

Fig. 8.6 Slapped-cheek appearance of a child with parvovirus B19 infection (erythema infectiosum).

Fig. 8.7 Lacy eruption on extensor arm of child with parvovirus B19 infection.

Fig. 8.8 Lacy pink eruption over the palms in erythema infectiosum.

Fig. 8.9 Lacy pink eruption on chest and upper abdomen.

toms usually resolve in 1–2 months. In patients with chronic hemolytic anemias, EI may be the cause of transient aplastic crises, and in immunosuppressed children it may be responsible for red-cell aplasia and severe anemia.[7,26,29] Immunosuppressed children may be susceptible to persistent infection.[7] Conjunctivitis

Fig. 8.10 Purpuric gloves-and-stockings syndrome. Glovelike purpura on hand of person with parvovirus B-19 infection. (Photograph courtesy of Joanna Burch MD.)

Fig. 8.11 Purpuric gloves-and-stockings syndrome. Stocking-like purpura on feet and ankles of person with parvovirus B-19 infection. (Photograph courtesy of Joanna Burch MD.)

may occasionally be a presenting symptom, and chronic infection has resulted in a picture of systemic necrotizing vasculitis.[7,26,29] Lupus-like illness and recurrent fever syndromes also are uncommon presentations of parvovirus B19 infections. EI in pregnant women may result in fetal death.[7,26,30]

Differential diagnosis

Drug eruptions and the other morbilliform eruptions may be considered in the differential diagnosis, but the lacy, mottled appearance of the EI eruption is characteristic. Occasionally, the more violaceous livedo reticularis pattern of skin mottling associated with collagen vascular disease (periarteritis nodosa or lupus erythematosus) may be confused with EI, especially if associated with arthropathy. The STAR complex can also be caused by rubella and other viruses (see Box 8.3).[21] The petechial or purpuric gloves-and-socks syndrome[27] should be differentiated from other petechial exanthems, such as enteroviral infections (Box 8.4) and noninfectious causes of purpura. Diagnosis can be confirmed by analysis of serum obtained within 30 days of the onset of illness for the presence of immunoglobulin M (IgM) B19 antibodies.[7,26,31] Parvovirus B19 DNA can be detected by PCR assays, but remain positive for 9 months so may not be indicative of recent infection.[7]

Pathogenesis

Human parvovirus B19 is the causative agent of EI.[7,26-29] The virus has been identified within EI skin lesions. The organism replicates in erythroid bone marrow cells, accounting for its role in red-cell aplasia of immunodeficiency and transient aplastic crises in children with chronic hemolytic anemias.[7,26] Suscept-

Box 8.4 Morbilliform viral exanthems with petechiae
Echovirus 9
EBV
Hepatitis
Atypical measles
Echoviruses 4, 7
Coxsackievirus A9
Respiratory syncytial virus
Rubella
Dengue
Parvovirus B19 (petechial gloves-and-socks syndrome)

ibility to infection has been linked to the presence of the erythrocyte P antigen, which serves as the receptor for parvovirus B19.[26,32] It is thought that hereditary lack of the receptor is protective against infection.[32] Among other viruses, parvovirus B19 has been implicated in the etiology of Kawasaki disease (see Ch. 11), although the association is controversial.[26]

Treatment

There is no specific treatment for EI, nor are there any specific control measures, although isolation of patients at risk for complications (pregnant women, immunosuppressed patients, patients with chronic hemolytic anemia) is recommended.[7] Administration of intravenous immunoglobulins may be effective in immunosuppressed children.[7] The disease may no longer be contagious once the skin eruption occurs.

Patient education

The patient or family should be informed of the dangers of parvovirus B19 virus to pregnant women, immunosuppressed patients, and patients with chronic hemolytic anemia (e.g. sickle cell disease). They should be advised to keep the infected child away from these individuals for 2 weeks, and good hand-washing techniques in the affected family should be emphasized. Pregnant women should be offered serologic testing for IgG antibody, and fetal ultrasonography may be useful. Children with EI may return to school or day care because they are no longer infectious.[7] They should also be told of the likely reappearance of the cutaneous eruption for up to 4 months. In children with the STAR complex, the likelihood of persistence of the arthritis should be emphasized.[21,26]

Follow-up visits

Follow-up visits are unnecessary for the child with normal immunity unless arthritis or exposure of persons at risk is involved.

Echovirus Exanthems

Clinical features

Echovirus exanthems result in morbilliform eruptions associated with two predominant clinical patterns: a morbilliform roseola-like pattern, and the petechial pattern (Figs 8.12, 8.13).[33-35] Infants and toddlers are

Fig. 8.12 Discrete red macules and a petechia in a child with echovirus infection.

Fig. 8.13 Enterovirus exanthem. Pink papules over the upper back.

more likely to have a viral rash with echovirus infections than are older children.[33,34] Echovirus 16 infection in children is usually seen in epidemic form and may mimic roseola in that the cutaneous eruption may appear after the end of 2 or 3 days of fever.[7,33] Since its first report, it has been known as the *Boston exanthem*, although it is found worldwide. The eruption is characteristically morbilliform, but vesicles or punched-out erosions have occasionally been described. The morbilliform eruption lasts 1–5 days. Cervical, suboccipital, and postauricular lymphadenopathy are seen. Aseptic meningitis may occasionally occur, but it is usually seen in children without the cutaneous eruption.

Echovirus 9 results in a morbilliform eruption with acral petechiae (see Fig. 8.9). Although a great number of viral infections may present with petechial eruptions (see Box 8.4), echovirus 9 accounts for most epidemics of petechial eruptions.[33,34] Echovirus 9 infects preschool children primarily, and they present with a syndrome of fever, sore throat, abdominal pain, and vomiting. Echoviruses 2, 4, 6, 11, 25, and 30 produce similar morbilliform exanthems, often without gastrointestinal symptoms (see Fig. 8.10). Aseptic meningitis is common.[7,33,34] The petechial eruption lasts 2–7 days.[33–35] Some coxsackieviruses produce similar clinical patterns.[33,34] Complete recovery follows.

Differential diagnosis

Roseola caused by HHV-6 or -7 should be considered in the differential diagnosis of echovirus morbilliform eruptions (see Boxes 8.1, 8.2). Roseola may mimic the Boston exanthem, but the fever and eruption in the latter often overlap. The identification of echovirus 16 in stools or throat washings helps to distinguish between these two disorders.[34,35] PCR analysis offers promise to distinguish enteroviral types.[36] Atypical measles, Rocky Mountain spotted fever, and meningococcemia are the major considerations of serious diseases in the differential diagnosis of echovirus 9 infections (see Box 8.4).[35] Other echoviruses, streptococcal infections, EBV, hepatitis, rubella, coxsackieviruses, dengue, and typhus may also be considered.

Pathogenesis

Echoviruses are small RNA viruses of the picornavirus group, which have been found worldwide.[7] There are 31 known types. The viruses are characteristically 'summer' viruses and produce epidemics, particularly in crowded living conditions. The incubation period is 3–5 days when the virus is spread by the enteric route.[7,35,36] The viruses use decay accelerating factor (CD55) as a receptor.[33,34] Despite enteric replication of the echovirus, gastrointestinal symptoms are uncommon, except for ECHO 9. It is not known whether the virus appears within the cutaneous eruption. The mechanism that produces the cutaneous eruption is also unknown.

Treatment

There is no specific treatment. Symptomatic fever control is useful.

Patient education

The contagious nature of the disease should be emphasized.

Follow-up visits

Follow-up visits are unnecessary.

Infectious Mononucleosis (Human Herpesvirus 4, 5, 6, and 7 Infections)

Clinical features

The annual incidence of infectious mononucleosis is estimated at 50 per 100 000 children, with the highest incidence found among adolescents and young adults.[7,37,38] As opposed to acute viral infections, the onset is often insidious. The usual presenting symptoms and signs are fatigue (100%), fever (in 85%), generalized lymphadenopathy (85%), sore throat with exudative tonsillitis (70%), headache (45%), and splenomegaly (45%).[7,37,38] Jaundice and hepatomegaly occur in up to 30% of patients. A pink, fleeting morbilliform eruption occurs in 15% of patients and may last 1–5 days.[7,37,38] Treatment of children with infectious mononucleosis with ampicillin, penicillin, or azithromycin for the sore throat results in an increase in incidence of morbilliform eruption in up to 80% of patients.[7,37,38] With antibiotic use, the eruption becomes bright red and more papular and may persist for 7–10 days (Fig. 8.14). The morbilliform eruption is the most characteristic seen with infectious mononucleosis, but occasionally other cutaneous eruptions may occur. Urticaria, and particularly cold urticaria, has been described as a prominent presenting feature,[39] and petechial eruptions associated with thrombocytopenia may be seen occasionally.[7,37,38] Palmar erythema has also been reported as a presenting symptom of infectious mononucleosis. Neurologic symptoms, such as spatial and visual distortion or signs of encephalitis, meningitis, neuritis, or Guillain-Barré syndrome, may accompany the cutaneous eruption.[7,37,38]

The acute phase with fever and sore throat lasts 2–3 weeks. Extreme fatigue and lethargy may persist

Fig. 8.14 Child with bright red morbilliform eruption of EBV-infectious mononucleosis plus ampicillin.

for 3 months, however.[7,37,38,40] Rare complications include splenic rupture, thrombocytopenia, agranulocytosis, hemolytic anemia, orchitis, and cardiac involvement.[37,38] Blood transfusions may occasionally precede the onset of mononucleosis because the viral agents are carried in leukocytes.[7,37,38] In children infected with the human immunodeficiency virus (HIV), EBV infections are commonly seen.[7,37,38]

Differential diagnosis

Laboratory studies are most useful in aiding with the diagnosis, with the detection of heterophil antibodies by Paul-Bunnell (heterophil) test as the most readily available.[7,38] In children under 4 years of age, it is often negative and EBV-IgM serology is preferred.[7,38] The laboratory findings most often encountered and their frequencies are shown in Table 8.1. During the early phase of infectious mononucleosis, the possibility of streptococcal pharyngitis is usually considered, as are other causes of pharyngitis. Infectious mononucleosis can be distinguished from the other morbilliform eruptions (see Boxes 8.1, 8.2) by its prolonged course, the prominent symptom of excessive fatigue, and the laboratory findings. If arthritis occurs, it must be differentiated from rubella or parvovirus B19 as causes of the STAR complex (see Box 8.3).[21] The petechial eruption must be differentiated from other causes of thrombocytopenic purpura in children, such as idiopathic thrombocytopenic purpura, lupus erythematosus, and malignancies. A similar syndrome may be produced by CMV, HHV-6 and HHV-7, rubella, and parvovirus B19, but exudative tonsillitis and heterophil antibodies are not present (see Table 8.1).[1,18,21,23,41] EBV mononucleosis is most pre-

valent in the adolescent, whereas CMV and others are more prevalent in infantile and childhood mononucleosis. CMV infectious mononucleosis may be accompanied by gastrointestinal symptoms such as colicky abdominal pain, vomiting, and diarrhea.[41] Tests of serum for IgM anti-EBV viral capsid antigen or isolation of EBV from oropharyngeal secretions will distinguish.[7,38,41]

Pathogenesis

It is now accepted that EBV (HHV-4) is responsible for most cases (85%) of infectious mononucleosis.[7,37,38] The incubation period is 4–8 weeks in adolescents but is usually shorter in prepubertal children. The period of communicability is uncertain because most patients with infectious mononucleosis excrete virus for at least 6 months after the onset of symptoms,[40] and there are asymptomatic carriers of EBV. In crowded conditions, intrafamilial spread of EBV is common, and infants may be infected. HHV-5 (CMV), HHV-6 and HHV-7, and parvovirus B19 may be responsible for the infectious mononucleosis syndrome, particularly in infants and toddlers.[3,37,38,41]

Treatment

In mild cases, no treatment is required. In hemolytic anemia, thrombocytopenic purpura, airway interference, neurologic involvement, or in selected patients with toxemia and prolonged fever, systemic glucocorticosteroids may be given. Prednisone, 2 or 3 mg/kg/day for 3 days, is recommended by many authorities for adolescents, although there is no demonstrable effect on fever, tonsillar swelling, or duration of illness.[42] Patients treated for 3 days with corticosteroids do not experience any adverse effects.[42] Ampicillin or penicillin should not be administered in routine cases because of the high frequency of drug rashes. Acyclovir has yet to be convincingly demonstrated to be efficacious in infectious mononucleosis, but the drug is active against EBV in vitro.[7]

Table 8.1 Frequency of laboratory findings in infectious mononucleosis	
Finding	**Patients (%)**
Epstein-Barr virus antibody IgG or IgM	85
Lymphocytosis	92
Atypical mononuclear cells in peripheral blood film	92
Liver enzyme abnormalities	80
Hypergammaglobulinemia	80
Heterophil antibodies	75
Indirect Coombs' test	50
Thrombocytopenia	50
Hyperbilirubinemia	40

Patient education

Concern that the spleen may rupture, which occurs in 0.5% of patients, should prompt avoidance of contact sports or other vigorous activity in which abdominal injury is likely.[7,37,38] Neurologic complications occur in 1.5% of cases, and patients should be warned about mental symptoms such as hallucinations and mood changes.[37,38] They should also be apprised of the prolonged convalescence from this disorder and of the need to increase activities in a stepwise fashion.

Follow-up visits

Weekly visits should be scheduled in patients with mild to moderate disease to ascertain the course of the disease and observe for complications. In severe disease, daily visits or hospitalization may be necessary.

Papular Acrodermatitis (Gianotti-Crosti Syndrome)

Clinical features

A distinct eruption called *papular acrodermatitis* (Gianotti-Crosti syndrome) is characterized by groups of large, flat-topped, nonpruritic papules that appear

in acral areas.[43] Involvement of the cheeks (Fig. 8.15), buttocks, and limbs is characteristic. Papules are particularly prominent over the hands, elbows, and knees (Figs 8.16–8.19), although with some outbreaks

Fig. 8.17 Gianotti-Crosti syndrome. Grouped papules around the elbow in child with EBV infection.

Fig. 8.15 Gianotti-Crosti syndrome. Multiple discrete papules on the cheek.

Fig. 8.18 Gianotti-Crosti syndrome. Grouped red papules on leg in child with EBV infection.

Fig. 8.16 Gianotti-Crosti syndrome. Skin-colored papules on back of the hand.

Fig. 8.19 Gianotti-Crosti syndrome. Grouped and linear papules around elbow in child with EBV infection.

Box 8.5 Viruses responsible for infectious mononucleosis

EBV

CMV

HHV-6

HHV-7

Rubella

Human parvovirus B19

the distribution is more widespread.[43,44] Focal facial involvement has been described in one outbreak.[44] The skin lesions may be preceded by low-grade fever and mild upper respiratory tract symptoms. Of children described as having this syndrome, 85% are less than 3 years of age, although it may occur in school-age children.[43] The eruption persists unchanged for 2–8 weeks and may be recurrent.[43] Generalized lymphadenopathy and hepatosplenomegaly develop in some children along with the cutaneous eruption. In such children, atypical lymphocytes are seen in peripheral blood films, and liver enzyme levels, especially serum aminotransferases, are elevated. EBV has been associated with outbreaks of papular acrodermatitis in North America,[45] and other viruses such as HHV-6, CMV and coxsackievirus A16 may be involved (Box 8.5).

In Europe, 30% of patients with papular acrodermatitis have mild viral hepatitis B; hepatitis B surface antigen (HBsAg) has been demonstrated in the lymph nodes in such children, with liver biopsy findings consistent with acute viral hepatitis.[43] Serologic tests for EBV-IgM will help distinguish.

Differential diagnosis

In irritant contact dermatitis, atopic dermatitis, licnenoid drug eruptions, and lichen planus, flat-topped acral papules that mimic papular acrodermatitis may be seen, but they are usually associated with severe pruritus and disruption of the skin surface.[45]

Box 8.6 Viruses responsible for papular acrodermatitis (Gianotti-Crosti syndrome)

EBV

CMV

Hepatitis B

Coxsackievirus A16

Pathogenesis

In infants with papular acrodermatitis in North America, EBV has been identified, but in a few infants HHV-6, CMV, or coxsackievirus A16 has been associated (Box 8.6).

Treatment

No treatment is needed for Gianotti-Crosti syndrome. Individual lesions are not responsive to topical steroids.

Patient education

The prolonged nature of the Gianotti-Crosti syndrome eruption should be emphasized. It should also be emphasized that several virus agents may be responsible for papular acrodermatitis, and its significance is the prolonged course.

Follow-up visits

Follow-up visits are unnecessary unless hepatosplenomegaly is present.

Hepatitis Viruses

Clinical features

Although viral hepatitis is usually not associated with exanthems, it is a disease that should not be overlooked when searching for the cause of a viral exanthem. Exanthems associated with hepatitis viruses A, B, C, and E are primarily morbilliform, but urticarial and scarlatiniform eruptions have been described.[7,46–50] Children infected with hepatitis A often have non-specific symptoms of low-grade fever, irritability, and upper respiratory tract symptoms without cutaneous involvement or mild jaundice.[7] Subclinical hepatitis is more likely to occur in a 10 to 1 ratio. The morbilliform eruption of hepatitis A, B, and E characteristically precedes the icteric stage by 1–10 days.[46,49,50] The entire disease may last 3–4 weeks. Both hepatitis A and E are primarily waterborne, enterically transmitted infections, with hepatitis A producing local outbreaks, whereas hepatitis E has produced large epidemics in the Indian subcontinent and Southeast Asia.[7] Urticarial eruptions may also be seen in the preicteric stages of hepatitis virus A infections.[7,47]

Differential diagnosis

The other viral exanthems, particularly rubella and parvovirus B19, should be considered during the prodromal phase of morbilliform and urticarial eruptions (see Boxes 8.1, 8.2). Urticaria resulting from other causes may be impossible to distinguish. The serum aminotransferase levels will be markedly elevated early in hepatitis, and will be an important distinguishing test. The eventual development of icterus, hepatic tenderness, and hepatic enlargement will allow a retrospective diagnosis of hepatitis. Pruritus may be severe during the icteric phase, particularly in hepatitis E. Diagnosis is usually made by the serologic test for IgM antihepatitis A or B or IgM antihepatitis E by enzyme-linked immunosorbent assay (ELISA) or radioimmunoassay.[7] Hepatitis C is detected by a recombinant immunoblot assay.[7]

Pathogenesis

Both hepatitis A and E are single-stranded RNA viruses that replicate in the liver but not the bowel. Virus shedding into the bowel occurs during the prodromal phase and may last throughout the remainder of the illness. A viremic phase that is believed to be responsible for the cutaneous eruptions may occur. The usual source of infection is human feces through contaminated water supplies and food, particularly shellfish.

Treatment

Only symptomatic treatment is usually given. Bed rest and adequate diet are supportive measures. For exposed individuals, human immune serum globulin, 0.02 mL/kg, is given as soon as possible after exposure.[50] For children under 2 years, hepatitis A vaccines given after exposure are preventive.[7]

Patient education

It should be emphasized that both hepatitis A and E are transmitted by the enteric route and possibly the oral route. Contaminated food or water sources should be sought. The importance of personal hygienic measures, such as hand washing, in preventing spread should be emphasized.[7,50] Vaccination for hepatitis A is recommended for children living in high-risk areas.[7,50]

Follow-up visits

Patients should be seen weekly until the jaundice has disappeared. Although the course is benign in 95% of children, hepatitis is variable and may progress to liver failure.

Fig. 8.20 Urticarial eruption of the leg in a child with preicteric hepatitis B.

Hepatitis B, C, and D Infections

Clinical features

Urticarial and serum-sickness-like eruptions are the most common skin eruptions seen with hepatitis B, and hepatitis-associated antigen may be detected in infected children 10 days after the eruption appears. Icterus usually does not develop.

If a child is infected with both hepatitis B and D, a fulminant picture of severe jaundice, with encephalopathy, bleeding, and fluid and electrolyte imbalance may ensue.

The urticarial or serum-sickness-like eruption of hepatitis B and C is characterized by joint swelling and fixed urticaria (Fig. 8.20) rather than a morbilliform exanthem.[48,49] It lasts 7–10 days and resolves with the onset of hepatic symptoms. Anaphylactoid purpura with purpuric papules on the distal extremities and a periarteritis nodosa pattern are rarely associated with hepatitis B infection.[7]

Differential diagnosis

A serum-sickness reaction resulting from drugs or serum products, or from rubella or parvovirus B19 infections, may mimic the prodrome of hepatitis. In hepatitis, however, the joint swelling is usually symmetric, in contrast to rubella, in which it is often monarthritic.

Pathogenesis

HBsAg antigenemia persists for 2 months in affected children and may last for several years. Hepatitis B virus has been identified as a double-stranded DNA virus that replicates via reverse transcriptase. It produces complete virus particles and capsids that circulate in the blood and can be detected ultrastructurally or by antibody testing.[7,50] Hepatitis C is a single-stranded RNA virus. Hepatitis D is a unique single-stranded RNA virus that cannot enter the hepatocytes unless accompanied by the hepatitis B virus. The morbilliform eruption is associated with HBsAg-positive hepatitis. Hepatitis antigen-antibody immune complexes have been identified in the sera and skin of patients with eruptions of the urticarial, anaphylactoid purpura, and periarteritis nodosa types.

Treatment

Exposed persons may be given doses of hepatitis B immunoglobulin (HBIG), 0.06 mL/kg, within 24 hours of exposure, and 1.0 mL of hepatitis B vaccine given intramuscularly within 7 days of exposure.[7,50] The vaccine should be repeated 1 and 6 months later. For perinatal exposure, 0.5 mL of HBIG should be administered within 12 hours of birth, with 0.5 mL of vaccine given within 7 days and at 1 and 6 months. The incubation period for hepatitis B and C is 6 weeks to 6 months.[50]

If children are hepatitis B positive, it is important to prevent them from donating blood or blood products and to protect laboratory personnel. Enteric transmission of hepatitis can occur, and contact with patients' blood should be avoided. Isolating the patients from contact with persons at risk for severe hepatitis may be important.

Patient education

The importance of evaluating contacts if hepatitis B is found should be emphasized.

Follow-up visits

A visit 2 weeks after the initial visit to determine whether the signs and symptoms of hepatitis B have developed is recommended. If the child is hepatitis B positive, sera should be retested for HBsAg and antibodies to HBsAg 3 months later to detect a possible chronic carrier.[7,50]

VIRAL EXANTHEMS: VESICULOBULLOUS ERUPTIONS

After dissemination to skin during a viremic phase, there may be productive viral infection of keratino-cytes, with ballooning degeneration of cells resulting in vesicle formation. This is particularly characteristic of the herpes group of viruses.

Herpes Simplex (Human Herpesvirus 1 and 2 Infections)

Clinical features

Grouped vesicles on an erythematous base are the characteristic lesions of herpes simplex in the skin, regardless of the location.[7,51,52] On mucous membranes, the blister roof is easily shed and the blister base (erosion) is seen. HHV infections may be primary or recurrent.[7,51,52] Recurrent infections represent reactivation of latent HSV. Sun-induced activation (photoactivation) is frequent in HSV infections.[53] In the immunosuppressed child the erythematous base may be lost, or large erosions may be seen. Several distinct clinical patterns are seen.

Primary infections

Gingivostomatitis: In infants and children, 60% of herpes simplex infections appear as a gingivostomatitis (Figs 8.21, 8.22) and are almost always caused by HSV type 1 (HSV-1).[7,51,52] It primarily appears in infants less than 6 months of age, with pain in the mouth and throat on attempted swallowing, accompanied by fever and irritability. Erosions are extensive throughout the oral cavity, with moist crusts and foul breath. The child often is unable to eat. It lasts 7–14 days. Many infants are asymptomatic or suffer a mild pharyngitis on their first encounter with HSV-1.

Recurrent herpes simplex virus infections: HSV after initial exposure may persist in nerve ganglia and be reactivated by a number of factors, including fever,

Fig. 8.21 Infant with primary herpes gingivostomatitis.

Fig. 8.22 Primary HSV-1 gingivostomatitis in an infant.

Fig. 8.23 Recurrent herpes lablialis on lip of pre-teen child.

ultraviolet light, trauma, and the menses.[7,51,52] The mechanisms of this reactivation of latent virus and its subsequent replication within epidermal cells are unknown. Nonetheless, once recurrent skin involvement appears, the disease is contagious and can be transmitted to other areas of skin or to other persons. This may be seen in wrestlers (herpes gladiatorum).[54]

Sites of involvement vary, but the most common are the lips (herpes labialis), eyes (herpes keratitis), nose, cheeks (herpes facialis), and fingers (herpetic whitlow).[7,51,52] When different skin locations are involved, the clinical appearance may vary, and all may be photoactivated.[53] In all forms, however, grouped vesicles on a red base are present. Regional lymphadenopathy may occur in all forms of herpes simplex.

Fig. 8.24 Recurrent herpes labialis of the lower lip and adjacent skin in a child.

Herpes labialis: Recurrent HSV infection of the lip occurs in 20% of all infants and children previously infected and accounts for the majority of all recurrent infections.[51,52] It appears as grouped vesicles on one portion of the lip, usually the lower lip, and typically follows an acute febrile illness or intense sun exposure (Figs 8.23, 8.24).[7,51-53] The period from the appearance of the vesicles until complete healing averages 8 days. HSV-1 can be recovered from the vesicles during the first 24 hours after onset. A prodrome of pain accompanies the lesions in 85% of patients.[51,52]

Herpes keratitis: Although the cornea is involved in only 8–10% of children infected with HSV-1, this is a serious infection, potentially leading to scarring and loss of vision.[7,51,55] Any HSV infection on the skin around the eye, whether accompanied by a red eye, should prompt a search for herpes keratitis (Fig. 8.25).

Fig. 8.25 Herpetic keratitis. Involvement of eyelid and conjunctiva in a child.

Dendritic ulceration of the cornea may be present and is an important characteristic.[55] Ophthalmologic consultation should be obtained.

Herpes facialis: Recurrent episodes of grouped vesicles on the cheek or forehead are less common than other forms of HSV of the head and neck, but frequently they are confused with impetigo (Fig. 8.26).[51,52]

Herpes hand and finger infections: HSV-1 infection of the hand and finger occurs in 10% of infants and children, with perhaps a predilection for thumb suckers (Figs 8.27, 8.28).[7,51,52]

Because it causes severe pain and erythema, it is often initially considered a pyoderma or cellulitis. A

Fig. 8.28 Herpetic whitlow on third finger of preschool child.

Fig. 8.26 Herpes facialis. Recurrent eruption of cheek in a child.

careful history will elicit the prodrome of pain, and careful examination will reveal thick-roofed blisters. Because the stratum corneum is thick on the palms and fingers, the vesicles appear deceptively deeper in the skin than in their epidermal location.[51,52]

Herpes progenitalis: Herpes progenitalis, predominantly caused by HSV type 2 (HSV-2) infection, occurs almost exclusively in adolescents and young adults.[7,51,56,57] Just as in HSV-1 gingivostomatitis, the symptoms may vary from none to severe widespread erosions, accompanied by fever, lymphadenopathy, severe pain, and lassitude. Recurrent herpes progenitalis characteristically presents with a prodrome of pain followed by the appearance of grouped vesicles on an erythematous base in a localized area of the genitalia. It is important to bear in mind that recurrent genital herpes is contagious and sexually transmitted.[7,56,57] It is a common venereal disease among adolescents and young adults.[57]

Neonatal herpes simplex: Neonatal herpes simplex may develop in approximately 10% of infants born of parents with active HSV-2 infection.[7,52,53] In natally acquired herpes simplex, 67% of cases are caused by HHV-2 and 33% by HHV-1.[7] Signs may be present at birth, but grouped vesicles on an erythematous base may appear up to 7 days after birth (Figs 8.29, 8.30). The disease may be mild, with primarily cutaneous manifestations, but central nervous system function may ultimately be impaired.[52,53] More usual is a systemic illness with jaundice, progressive hepatosplenomegaly, dyspnea, hypothermia, and central nervous system symptoms. A severe encephalitis ensues, and death occurs in 48–96 hours.[7,52]

Fig. 8.27 Herpetic whitlow of the thumb of baby who is a thumb sucker.

Fig. 8.29 Widespread blisters on the trunk in neonatal herpes.

Fig. 8.30 Perianal erosions in a newborn with HHV-2 infection.

Herpes simplex virus infections in immunodeficiency states: In infants or children with genetic immunodeficiency, those receiving immunosuppressive drugs,

Fig. 8.31 Discrete ulcers and hundreds of erosions associated with dermatitis in an infant with atopic dermatitis and widespread herpes simplex infection (Kaposi's varicelliform eruption, eczema herpeticum).

and those with severe protein-calorie malnutrition or cancer-associated immunodeficiency, atypical forms of HSV infection occur.[7,52] Grouped vesicles often become large bullae and may lack an erythematous border. Deep erosions may occur even in the absence of inflammation. Purpura or hemorrhage appears within the bullous lesions. After 24–48 hours of local skin involvement, generalized skin involvement and visceral involvement may ensue. Herpes encephalitis or pneumonia may result in death.

Kaposi's varicelliform eruption (eczema herpeticum): Infants and children with atopic dermatitis, burns, and other conditions that disrupt the epidermal barrier are susceptible to the development of generalized HSV infection characterized by high fever, lassitude, hundreds of skin vesicles, and sometimes death.[7,52] Severe infections may develop in these patients, even when their dermatitis is inactive (Fig. 8.31).

Differential diagnosis

A rapid clinical clue to HSV (or varicella-zoster virus [VZV]) infection is the finding of epidermal giant cells on a Tzanck preparation (Fig. 8.32; see Ch. 2 for technique).

Rapid diagnostic tests using fluorescent- or dye-labeled monoclonal antibodies are available to stain smears and are 90% or more reliable.[7,58] Isolation of HHV-1 or HHV-2 is the diagnostic gold standard but requires at least 24 hours. Molecular diagnosis using the polymerase chain reaction (PCR) techniques can

Fig. 8.32 Photomicrograph of smear of blister contents shows giant cells (transformed keratinocytes) in herpes simplex infection (Tzanck smear).

be done in less than 24 hours, but it is not widely available.[7]

Other virus infections to be considered in the differential diagnosis of herpes simplex are listed in Box 8.7.

Gingivostomatitis: Gingivostomatitis must be differentiated from aphthous ulcers, which are shallow, irregular, ragged, recurrent ulcerations on the oral mucosa. In erythema multiforme, in contrast to HSV gingivostomatitis, symmetric iris and target lesions are present on the skin. In herpangina, which is caused by enteroviruses, ulcers are limited to the anterior tonsillar pillars and have a linear arrangement; isolation of coxsackievirus A confirms the diagnosis.

Recurrent herpes simplex virus infection: Recurrent skin infection caused by HSV must be differentiated

---

Box 8.7 Vesiculobullous virus infections

Common
Herpes simplex
Varicella-zoster
Hand-foot-and-mouth disease (coxsackievirus A16)

Uncommon
Orf
Influenza
Coxsackieviruses A5, 9, 10
Echoviruses 4, 9, 11, 17, 25
Variola
Vaccinia (cowpox)

---

from herpes zoster. Because both infections demonstrate epidermal giant cells on Tzanck smear, antibody testing or viral culture is the preferred method for differentiating the two on first infection. The history of recurrent lesions in the same skin area suggests HSV rather than varicella-zoster virus. VZV infections often have three or more groups of vesicles; HSV infections have one or two.

Herpes labialis. Impetigo may mimic herpes labialis. Gram's stain and bacterial culture of the lesions will help distinguish the two.

Herpes keratitis: Herpes keratitis should be differentiated from bacterial conjunctivitis and epidemic adenovirus keratoconjunctivitis. The characteristic grouped vesicles on an erythematous base in periocular skin will help distinguish HSV from these infections. Furthermore, HSV is usually unilateral, whereas bacterial and adenovirus infections, although initially unilateral, often become bilateral.

Herpes hand and finger infections: HSV hand and finger infections are often confused with bacterial cellulitis. A Tzanck smear of the vesicle base is a rapid method of distinguishing HSV from bacterial infection. Candidal paronychia are not painful, in contrast to herpetic whitlow.

Herpes facialis: Impetigo may mimic facial herpes on the cheek or forehead. A Tzanck smear, HSV antibody test, or bacterial and viral culture will often distinguish the two.

Herpes progenitalis: Herpes progenitalis may mimic other venereal diseases. Also, it is not unusual to note more than one venereal disease simultaneously in the sexually active person.[7,57] A smear and culture for gonorrhea and a serologic test for syphilis are most helpful in such cases.

Neonatal herpes simplex: Other congenital infections (e.g. toxoplasmosis, other [congenital syphilis and viruses], rubella, CMV, and herpes simplex virus, the so-called *TORCH complex*) may mimic neonatal HSV. Vesicular skin lesions are not present in any of these, however. In neonatal bacterial sepsis, isolated vesicular or pustulovesicular lesions may occur. They are not grouped as in HSV infection, and Gram's stain and bacterial culture will distinguish them from herpes simplex.

Pathogenesis

HHV-1 and HHV-2 are complex DNA viruses with an incubation period of 2–12 days.[51] They are epidermotropic viruses, and productive viral infection occurs within keratinocytes. Active infection occurs despite high titers of specific antibody. This no doubt reflects the intracellular infection characteristic of these viruses in which antibody cannot interact with the active virus, which is transferred from cell to cell. There are two possible outcomes of epidermal cellular infection: productive and nonproductive infection. Productive infection is characterized by the biosynthesis of infectious progeny and epidermal cell death, producing the intraepidermal vesicle.[51] Nonproductive infection results in the perpetuation of all or part of the viral genome and survival of the epidermal cell, producing epidermal giant cells.[51] It is uncertain whether fusion of several epidermal cells or nuclear division without cytoplasmic division is responsible for the epidermal giant cells seen on Tzanck smear.

Treatment

Oral acyclovir, famciclovir, or valacyclovir are the specific therapy for localized cutaneous herpes simplex infections.[7,53,59] Oral acyclovir has been safe and effective in children. In severe primary HSV infections, such as herpes gingivostomatitis or Kaposi's varicelliform eruption, acyclovir may be very useful, especially if initiated within 72 hours of the onset, in doses of 20–40 mg/kg/day.[7] In localized forms of herpes simplex, such as those limited to a certain small area of skin, systemic therapy is usually not required. Neither topical nor systemic antiviral agents, however, will prevent recurrences of herpes simplex, although they may prevent transfection of the virus to adjacent skin sites or to family members or playmates if given prophylactically. In patients experiencing frequent, severe recurrences, 6 months of acyclovir prophylaxis (80mgm/kg/day in three doses) may be considered.[7]

In herpes keratitis, topical 5-iodo-2-deoxyuridine 0.1%, topical vidaribine 3%, or 1–2% trifluridine ophthalmic ointments are efficacious.[7,55] Before initiation of treatment, consultation with an ophthalmologist is recommended.

In neonatal HSV infections and in Kaposi's varicelliform eruption, intravenous acyclovir has proved effective.[7] Supportive measures, such as fever control, maintenance of fluid and electrolyte balance, and thermal regulation, are necessary. Infected patients shed virus and should be isolated.

Patient education

Patients with local cutaneous infection should be informed of the contagious nature of the disease. Avoidance of precipitating factors may be most useful (e.g. avoiding sun exposure or using sunscreens in sun-activated recurrent HSV, and discontinuing sexual activity in herpes progenitalis). In patients with atopic dermatitis or other skin diseases susceptible to disseminated HSV infections, optimal treatment of the underlying skin disease and consistency of care may be useful in preventing future episodes.

Follow-up visits

Careful ophthalmologic follow-up (every 1–2 days) is required in herpes keratitis. Disseminated infections often require hospitalization and intensive supportive therapy. Neonatal HSV requires careful developmental and neurologic examinations at 3-month intervals. Cutaneous herpes lesions may recur throughout childhood after neonatal HSV.

Chickenpox and Zoster (Human Herpesvirus 3 Infections)

Clinical features

Varicella (chickenpox): Varicella is characterized by the abrupt onset of crops of skin lesions.[7,60] Individual lesions begin as faint erythematous macules that progress to edematous papules and then to vesicles

Fig. 8.33 Varicella. Umbilicated vesicles on a red base.

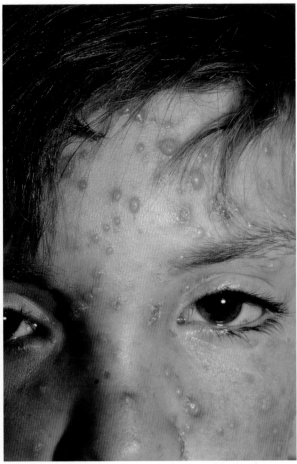

Fig. 8.34 Blisters, papules, and crusted lesion in a child with varicella.

Fig. 8.35 Large erosions (blister bases) in a child with bullous impetigo and varicella.

during 24–48 hours (Fig. 8.33). The vesicles then develop moist crusts that dry and are shed, leaving shallow erosions. Successive crops of lesions appear during the next 2–5 days, so that at any one time several stages of skin lesions can be observed concomitantly: macules, papules, vesicles, and crusted lesions (Fig. 8.34). Skin lesions may appear in sites of skin injury or be localized to areas of sun exposure. Lesions frequently involve mucous membranes, and isolated erosions may be seen in the conjunctiva, oral cavity, or nasal mucosa.[7,60] Fever is usually low grade, and associated symptoms are mild. In a single family, varicella lesions may vary from fewer than 10 in one child to hundreds in another. The total duration is 7–10 days, but frequently children stay home 14 days because of school or other contagion-restriction policy.[7] The disease is highly contagious from 1–2 days before the onset of the skin eruption to 5–6 days afterward.[7,60]

Secondary bacterial infection of one to three of the many varicella skin lesions is common (1–4%), producing the so-called *bullous varicella* (Fig. 8.35) Often, this is the result of *Staphylococcus aureus* infection, including MRSA. Pneumonia may complicate varicella in some children, and rarely, Reye's syndrome (encephalopathy and fatty infiltration of the liver) may ensue.[7] Severe generalized varicella infections may develop in immunosuppressed persons, with high fever, encephalitis, pneumonia, hepatitis, or disseminated intravascular coagulation.[7,60]

Herpes zoster: In children who have previously had varicella, recurrent infection results in herpes zoster.[7,61,62] Two to three groups of lesions appear within several adjacent dermatomes (Figs 8.36, 8.37). They begin as macules and edematous papules and progress to grouped vesicles on an erythematous base. Rarely, dermatomal pain may precede the eruption in

Fig. 8.36 Grouped blisters over several thoracic dermatomes in a child with herpes zoster.

Fig. 8.37 Many groups of blisters occurring over the arm in a child with herpes zoster.

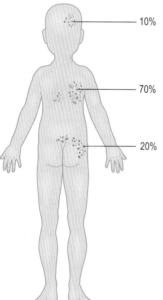

Fig. 8.38 Common distribution of herpes zoster in childhood: 10% cranial nerve involvement, 70% thoracic dermatome, 20% lumbosacral involvement.

Fig. 8.39 Involvement of the ear and adjacent skin associated with facial palsy in herpes zoster of geniculate ganglion (Ramsay Hunt syndrome).

Fig. 8.40 Grouped vesicles of cheek, mandible and ear in child with Ramsay Hunt syndrome.

children, and postzoster neuralgia may also occur, but rarely. Almost all children, however, have a mild illness lasting 7–10 days. Pruritus may be severe. The thoracic segments are involved in 70% of children with herpes zoster,[61] with the childhood distribution depicted in Figure 8.38. Infants may also develop zoster.[62] If the nose is involved, herpes zoster keratitis is likely to occur, and it may be as severe as HSV keratitis and may be recurrent.[61] Ophthalmic zoster is also more likely to be associated with severe pain than is zoster of other skin regions in children.[7,61] Herpes zoster involving skin around the eyes, nose,

and forehead requires a careful ophthalmologic examination. Reactivation of zoster may be manifest as acute peripheral facial paralysis in children.[63,64]

Herpes zoster may be the initial finding in acquired immune deficiency syndrome (AIDS), but it is rarely the presenting finding in childhood cancer. In immunosuppressed children, disseminated herpes zoster occurs 1–5 days after the dermatome infection begins. Even immunosuppressed children with disseminated herpes zoster recover without sequelae, but visceral involvement can occur. Involvement of the geniculate ganglion results in pain in the ear, vesicles on the pinnae, and facial palsy (Ramsay Hunt syndrome) (Figs 8.39, 8.40). Motor paralysis of other nerves may follow herpes zoster.

Differential diagnosis

Varicella: Typical varicella is seldom confused with other illnesses (see Box 8.7). In hand-foot-and-mouth disease, vesicles are limited to acral areas, and vesicular forms of insect-bite reactions (papular urticaria) usually have a typical history of bites. Acute pityriasis lichenoides may mimic varicella in that it produces crops of lesions in different stages. True vesicles are less common in pityriasis lichenoides, and papules with central purpura are more common. Rickettsialpox and dermatitis herpetiformis are rare in children, but may mimic varicella. A Tzanck smear of the vesicle base will differentiate varicella from these vesicular diseases. Occasionally, disseminated HSV infection will mimic varicella. Viral cultures or fluorescent antibody techniques may be necessary to distinguish between HSV and varicella.[7]

Herpes zoster: Local cutaneous HSV infections may also mimic herpes zoster in children. Usually, HSV involves one group of vesicles, and herpes zoster involves three to four clusters of grouped vesicles. Viral culture or fluorescent antibody tests may be required to distinguish the two.[7] Impetigo is sometimes confused with herpes zoster, but honey-colored crusts, Gram's stain of lesions, and bacterial cultures will help distinguish it from herpes zoster.

Pathogenesis

Human herpesvirus-3 (HHV-3) is a complex herpes-group DNA virus that infects in much the same way as herpes simplex (see Herpes Simplex, Pathogenesis, above). The incubation period ranges from 10 to 27 days and averages 14 days.[7,60] Productive infection occurs within keratinocytes, producing ballooning degeneration of cells and an intraepidermal blister.

Treatment

In the healthy child, varicella does not require specific therapy. Wet dressings, soothing baths, and oral antihistamines will give symptomatic relief of the pruritus in children.[7,60] Salicylates should not be administered.[7] Zoster immune globulin, if given within 72 hours after exposure of an immunosuppressed host (including newborns or hospitalized premature infants), may modify varicella.[7,61] Secondary bacterial infection of varicella lesions should be treated with antistaphylococcal drugs, such as dicloxacillin, 12.5–25.0 mg/kg/day in four divided oral doses for 7–10 days or if MRSA are isolated, with recommended regimens for MRSA.

Systemic antiviral agents, such as intravenous or oral acyclovir, valacyclovir, famciclovir, and foscarnet, have been used for childhood HHV-3 infections with success.[7,60,65] It is recommended that antivirals not be given to otherwise healthy children, but their use should be considered in those likely to have complications, such as adolescents and children with chronic pulmonary disease, especially if they are taking inhaled or systemic steroids, or children receiving chronic salicylate therapy. In immunosuppressed children, children with ophthalmic zoster, or children with Ramsay Hunt syndrome, acyclovir, 30 mg/kg/dose in four daily doses for 5 days, may be a valuable therapeutic strategy.[7,62] In acyclovir-resistant VZV, i.v. foscarnet 180 mg/kg/day in three doses for 14 days should be used. If administered within 72 hours of exposure, varicella vaccine is efficacious in preventing or attenuating varicella.[7,61,62]

Patient education

The highly contagious nature of varicella should be emphasized, and the child should be isolated until all lesions are crusted, which usually occurs 5–6 days after eruption of the lesions. Contact with the elderly, neonates, and immunocompromised children should be avoided.

Postvaricella scarring is always a concern for parents. What appear to be highly vascular purple-red scars return to normal skin color in 6–12 months and often leave little evidence of scarring. Patients should be advised to wait at least 1 year before seeking help for postvaricella scars.

Follow-up visits

A visit in 48 hours to assess the development of secondary bacterial infection is useful in children with varicella. Children with disseminated zoster, ophthalmic zoster, or Ramsay Hunt syndrome should be seen daily until symptoms improve.

Hand-Foot-and-Mouth Disease (Coxsackievirus Infection)

An abrupt onset of scattered papules that progress to oval or linear vesicles in an acral distribution should suggest hand-foot-and-mouth disease.[66] The individual lesions are seen on the palms, fingertips, interdigital webs, and soles of the feet, and are few in number (Figs 8.41, 8.42). Discrete oral lesions may also be seen (Fig. 8.43). Such children are not ill and characteristically are afebrile. During epidemics, incomplete forms may be seen.[66] In some epidemics, skin lesions may be more numerous and involve both proximal and distal extremities. Oral lesions appear as discrete, shallow, oval erosions. In recent years,

Fig. 8.43 Erosion of the tongue in a child with hand-foot-and-mouth syndrome.

fatal cases have been described that are predominantly caused by enterovirus 71.[66,67] Fatal cases often present with high fever.[66,67] Nail matrix arrest with shedding of nails may follow the acute infection.[68]

Differential diagnosis

In the early nonvesicular stage, rubella and the other morbilliform lesions must be considered (see Box 8.4), but the sparsity of lesions and the lack of truncal involvement make those diagnoses unlikely. In the vesicular stage, the disease may be confused with varicella, but the acral distribution of the lesions, the lack of pruritus, and the oval to linear nature of the individual vesicles will help differentiate hand-foot-and-mouth disease from varicella. Insect bites may also mimic hand-foot-and-mouth disease, particularly if they occur on exposed acral skin. Isolation of coxsackievirus or enterovirus 71 from throat washings or serologic evidence will distinguish.

Pathogenesis

Several coxsackievirus group A and B enteroviruses and enterovirus 71 have been found to be responsible for hand-foot-and-mouth disease.[7,66,67] The epidemic form is almost always caused by coxsackievirus A16 or enterovirus 71, but coxsackieviruses A2, A5, and A10 have also been associated. Molecular analysis reveals homology among coxsackievirus A16, A2, and enterovirus 71. The incubation period is 3–5 days, and the virus enters by the enteric route, with the eruption reflecting a viremic phase. The disease is contagious from 2 days before to 2 days after the

Fig. 8.41 Oval blisters of the palms in child with hand-foot-and-mouth disease (coxsackievirus A16 infection).

Fig. 8.42 Oval blisters on the feet of a child with hand-foot-and-mouth syndrome.

onset of the eruption, but virus excretion in feces may persist for 2 weeks.

Treatment

No treatment is necessary in mild cases. In severe illness with enterovirus 71 infection, immune globulin intravenous or the antiviral agent pleconaril may be effective.

Human Immunodeficiency Virus Infections

Clinical features

The cutaneous manifestations of HIV-1 disease in children are predominantly the result of bacterial, fungal, and viral infections.[7,69,70] Clinical findings of perinatally acquired HIV infection are usually noted at about 4 months of age, but may be first manifested as early as 3 months or as late as 21 months.[69,70] The initial features are usually lymphadenopathy, persistent diarrhea, hepatosplenomegaly, and failure to thrive. As HIV infection progresses to AIDS, more features of opportunistic infections appear. AIDS has many features that mimic hereditary immunodeficiency diseases, such as severe combined immunodeficiency (SCID). Often, the first sign of AIDS is persistent thrush, recalcitrant to antiyeast therapy. The failure to clear thrush should be distinguished from the infant who gets thrush, clears with therapy, and then has a recurrence after therapy. Infants with AIDS and thrush also will have failure to thrive, lymphadenopathy, hepatosplenomegaly, and esophageal involvement. Chronic cough, clubbing of the fingers, and hypoxemia are the features of *Pneumocystis carinii* pneumonia, the most common infection of children with AIDS.[69,70]

A dermatitis that mimics seborrheic dermatitis is observed in half of the children who have HIV infection. It is not specific. Severe herpes gingivostomatitis or zoster (Fig. 8.44) may be the presenting finding. Children with HIV infection may exhibit hundreds of molluscum contagiosum lesions, and giant molluscum lesions may be seen. Recurrent pyodermas caused by *S. aureus* are frequent, and cellulitis or septicemia may develop from cutaneous infections that otherwise should be well localized to the epidermis. Unusual dermatophyte infections in children, such as onychomycosis and widespread tinea faciei, may be found. Severe crusted scabies with hundreds of live mites, the so-called *Norwegian scabies*, may occur. Purpura is common and may be the result of thrombocytopenia or severe viral or bacterial infections. A

Fig. 8.44 Herpes zoster in a 12-year-old boy who is HIV positive.

persistent folliculitis called *eosinophilic folliculitis* may be seen.[69,70]

Drug eruptions are far more common than predicted, particularly morbilliform and toxic epidermal necrolysis reactions caused by trimethoprim-sulfamethoxazole.[69,70] A clinical syndrome that mimics acrodermatitis enteropathica may accompany the failure to thrive and result from nutritional zinc deficiency. Kaposi's sarcoma of skin has not been reported in children with HIV infection.

Differential diagnosis

Virtually every known skin infection will mimic some infection seen in the infant or child with AIDS. Severe malnutrition states and congenital immunodeficiencies may display the same findings. An HIV serology confirmed by Western immunoblotting techniques is the most sensitive tests utilized to distinguish HIV infection, and it should be done on every infant or child suspected of having HIV.[7] In HIV-1-exposed infants, it may be difficult using serologic tests alone to establish the diagnosis, and HIV DNA PCR may be required.[7]

Pathogenesis

The agent responsible for AIDS is HIV-1, a retrovirus that selectively infects T lymphocytes, including those that are epidermotropic.[7] It can be isolated from blood leukocytes and also found in small amounts in tears, semen, saliva, vaginal secretions, cerebrospinal fluid, and breast milk. Eighty percent of affected infants in the United States are infected by transplacental passage of HIV from the mother. Older children are infected by sexual contact and from blood products administered before 1985. In sexually active adolescents, seroprevalence is 0.2%. If the infant's mother was a prostitute or intravenous drug user, the likelihood of infant infection is quite high.[7] Once T lymphocytes are infected by HIV, it relentlessly destroys the child's cell-mediated immunity, leaving the child at the mercy of a huge variety of opportunistic infectious agents.

Treatment

Children with AIDS are best managed at large medical centers experienced in the care of AIDS patients. Infectious disease experts should be involved in their care. Treatment is directed at the specific opportunistic infection, and the antimicrobial selected is directed by culture and sensitivities. Combinations of antiretroviral drugs, including nucleoside analog reverse transcriptase inhibitors, protease inhibitors, and non-nucleoside reverse transcriptase inhibitors may effectively suppress the disease.[7,71] Assessment of the viral load by HIV RNA PCR will assist the evaluation of response to therapy.[70]

Patient education

Information about the transmission of HIV and support groups for AIDS families are essential. Preventive measures such as sex education for adolescents and treatment of HIV-positive mothers with antiretroviral agents may reduce the disease.[7,66] It should be emphasized that many unusual infections may be encountered, and vigilance for early signs and symptoms of infection must be encouraged. HIV vaccines show promise in infants and children.[72]

Follow-up visits

Frequent visits are required, and establishing a close relationship with an AIDS clinic is advisable.

VIRUS-INDUCED TUMORS

Certain viruses, such as human papillomaviruses and molluscum contagiosum viruses, do not destroy keratinocytes but induce keratinocyte proliferation, resulting in benign tumors of skin.

Warts (Human Papillomavirus Infection)

Clinical features

Human papillomavirus (HPV)-induced epithelial tumors produce a variety of clinical lesions known collectively as *warts*.[7,73–76] Different HPVs are associated with specific clinical patterns. Table 8.2 lists

Table 8.2 Clinical warts and associated human papillomavirus type

Clinical wart type	HPV type
Common wart	HPV-2a, b, c, d, e; some HPV-4
Plantar wart	HPV-1a, b, c; HPV-4, 60, 63, 65 (weight-bearing)
Flat warts	HPV-3a, b; HPV-10a, b
Condyloma acuminata	HPV-6a, b, c, d, e, f; HPV-11a, b; HPV-16

the clinical types of warts and the HPV type responsible.

Warts are very commonly seen in children. By age 11, 5% of children will have warts.[72,76]

The common wart *(verruca vulgaris)* appears as a solitary papule, with an irregular, rough surface (Figs 8.45–8.47). They are usually found on the extremities, but they may be found anywhere on skin, including the scalp and genitalia. *Periungual*

Fig. 8.45 Common wart on the hand.

Fig. 8.46 Traumatized common wart with focal hemorrhage.

warts occur around the cuticles of fingers or toes and are spread by trauma (Fig. 8.48). Mucosal warts are unusual but can appear on inner lip or tongue (Fig. 8.49). *Filiform* warts appear as spiny projections from the skin surface with a narrow stalk (Figs 8.50, 8.51). In children they are usually seen on the lips, nose, or eyelids. *Flat* warts have a flat-topped, smooth surface. They tend to be multiple and skin-colored to light tan (Fig. 8.52). They are grouped, will appear

Fig. 8.47 Common warts on a child's fingers.

Fig. 8.50 Filiform wart of posterior neck.

Fig. 8.48 Periungual warts.

Fig. 8.51 Filiform wart of eyebrow treated with cryotherapy by (tweezer-freeze) method.

Fig. 8.49 Mucosal warts of inner lip in child with Heck disease (HPV-13 infection).

Fig. 8.52 Multiple flat warts (verruca plana) of the cheek.

within sites of skin trauma, and are usually observed on the face or extremities. 'Fairy-ring' warts occur from injury resulting in partial removal of the wart (Fig. 8.53). *Plantar* (weight-bearing) warts appear as rough papules that disrupt the dermal ridges (Figs 8.51, 8.55). They are frequently painful when the child is walking. They may be grouped together to produce mosaic warts.

Fig. 8.53 'Fairy-ring' common wart incompletely removed by vesicant.

Fig. 8.56 Venereal warts (condyloma acuminata) of the foreskin in a male infant.

Fig. 8.54 Plantar (weight-bearing) wart.

Fig. 8.57 Condyloma of glans penis in preschool child.

Fig. 8.55 Plantar wart with secondary infection secondary to attempted self-removal with needle.

Fig. 8.58 Venereal warts in a female infant.

Fig. 8.59 Anal condyloma in female infant.

Venereal warts *(condylomata acuminata)* are multiple discrete or confluent papules with a rough surface that appear on the genital or oral mucosa, adjacent dry skin, or both (Figs 8.56–8.59).[73–75] Common warts also appear on genital or perigenital skin, particularly in toddlers.[73,75]

The natural history of warts is variable, and the incubation period is unknown, but transmission from child to child, adult to child, and mother to newborn is well documented.[73] Most warts spontaneously resolve in 12–24 months but may persist for longer periods in some children. Warts in the immunosuppressed child are very persistent. Most warts are asymptomatic, except weight-bearing warts, although large warts anywhere may develop painful fissures.

Differential diagnosis

Common warts and filiform warts are so characteristic that they present no diagnostic problem. Plantar warts must be differentiated from calluses, which have a smooth, rather than irregular, surface and preserve the dermal ridges. Condylomata acuminata must be distinguished from the moist, smooth papules of secondary syphilis (condylomata lata), which appear as moist papules in genital areas.[75] A serologic test for syphilis will readily distinguish the two. Flat warts are often overlooked and may be misdiagnosed as lichen planus, lichen nitidus, seborrheic keratosis, or birthmarks. The linear or grouped arrangement of flat warts is helpful in diagnosis, as is their occurrence along areas of skin trauma. Diagnosis can be established by biopsy and HPV molecular typing, but these procedures are rarely required, and warts remain a clinical diagnosis.

Pathogenesis

Immunity to warts is not well understood, but inducing inflammation around a single wart may result in regression of all others. The HPV is located within the epidermal cell nucleus, which may be an immunologically privileged site where viral antigen has little opportunity to interact with antibody or white blood cells and may encode receptors that prevent interferon release.[7,73] HPV induces vacuolated epidermal cells with eosinophilic inclusions. The HPV induces keratinocyte proliferation with relatively normal differentiation, giving rise to a benign epithelial tumor.

Treatment

There is no universally effective wart therapy. Wart therapy may be cytodestructive, immunologic, antiproliferative, or psychological.[72,76–79] Cytodestructive therapy is designed to destroy all of the epidermal cells within the wart tumor and, hopefully, all of the HPV as well. The recurrence rate for all wart treatment strategies is high, and it is unlikely the wart will resolve with a single treatment. Of cytodestructive therapies, cryotherapy usually has the lowest recurrence rate from a single treatment. Table 8.3 summarizes usual treatments for wart types.

Table 8.3 Treatment of viral warts

Type of wart	Treatment		Response rate (%)
	First choice	Alternative	
Common	Cryotherapy	Salicylic acid paint	60–90
Periungual	Imiquimod cream	Cantharidin	60
Flat	Retinoic acid	Imiquimod cream	50
Filiform	Surgery	Cryotherapy with forceps	50
Plantar	Salicylic acid plaster	Imiquimod cream	60
Venereal	Podophyllum or Condylox	Imiquimod cream	90

Cytodestructive therapies

Cryotherapy: A cryosurgery probe, spray unit, or copper bar cooled in liquid nitrogen may be used for cryotherapy, but a cotton swab with a loose, pointed tip is most commonly used. The cotton swab is dipped in a thermos containing liquid nitrogen ($-195°C$), and the saturated swab is applied to the center of the wart until a white ice ball extending 1–3 mm beyond the margin of the wart is formed. The freeze is maintained 10–30 seconds. Warts greater than 7 mm in diameter should not be frozen, because scarring is likely to result. In 1–2 days a blister, sometimes hemorrhagic, forms. Removing the blister roof in 1 week and refreezing may be necessary. Cryotherapy spray is best for common warts because it is the coldest but should not generally be used on periungual or plantar warts. Freezing a forceps with cotton wrapped around the ends in liquid nitrogen and grasping the narrow stalk of a filiform wart for 30–45 seconds (tweezer-freeze) is effective.

Salicyclic acid plasters: Cotton plasters impregnated with 40% salicylic acid can be used on plantar and periungual warts. The plaster is cut to size, the paper backing removed, and the gummed side placed against the wart. It should be secured by trainer's tape so the plaster does not move for 3–5 days. Sweating mobilizes the salicylic acid out of the plaster so that it may enter the skin. When the plaster is removed, the patient should soak the wart in water for 45 minutes, then rub off the dead, white skin of the wart. A new plaster is taped in place, and the process is repeated for two more changes.

Salicyclic acid paints: Nonprescription salicylic acid-containing solutions can be provided for home use. The solutions should be applied with a toothpick by microdrops. They should be applied once or twice a day for 4–6 weeks. This method will not work on warts over 5 mm. Redness around the base of the wart and itching may herald the onset of wart regression. These preparations should be used for periungual warts or small common warts.

Vascular selective lasers: The pulsed-dye laser will not scar and is equally effective as cryosurgery. Several treatment sessions may be required.

CO_2 *lasers, electrodesiccation, and X-rays*: CO_2 lasers, electrodesiccation, and X-ray therapies always result in scarring and other undesirable side effects, with high recurrence rates. They are not recommended.

Vesicants (cantharidin): Currently unavailable in the United States, the vesicant cantharidin can be quite effective in the treatment of periungual warts. If used on common warts, 'fairy-ring' warts may occur. It should be applied carefully with a toothpick to cover the size of the wart. It produces a tender blister beneath the wart 2 or 3 days after application, and the wart is eventually sloughed off. It is difficult to regulate the size of the blister, and the response may vary from application to application. Cantharidin should never be used in intertriginous areas.

Surgery: The recurrence rate after surgical excision of a wart approaches 100%, presumably because of transfection of HPV at the time of surgery. Removing a filiform wart by cutting its narrow base is one exception. Some authorities recommend the use of a sharp curette on the remaining plantar wart after 3 or 4 weeks of salicylic acid plasters.

Immunologic therapies

Interferon inducers: Imiquimod cream 5% applied daily for 1–2 months is a painless and effective treatment. The drug induces interferon production by keratinocytes. Instructions to discontinue when the warts become red will prevent crusting or oozing from excessive interferon release.

Alpha interferons: Alpha interferon preparations must be injected either intralesionally or subcutaneously twice weekly. The injection requirement limits their use in children.

Cimetidine: Some authorities have used 3 months of oral cimetidine, an H_2 blocking agent, at 30 mgm/kg/day in two doses to non-specifically improve immunity to HPV. This is usually used in conjunction with another strategy and should be reserved for resistant warts.

Vaccines: There are currently no effective wart vaccines.

Antiproliferative agents

Retinoic acid: Retinoic acid in a 0.025% cream or 0.05% cream may be used for flat warts and applied once or twice daily for 4–6 weeks. It is ineffective in common, plantar, or periungual warts.

Podophyllum: Podophyllum, a plant extract, is a microtubule inhibitor that blocks cell division. It can be effective against genital warts and common warts. It is applied by the healthcare provider in a 25% alcohol solution and applied with a toothpick to the warts. It should be washed off in 4 hours. It is an irritating substance, and application to perianal skin often induces defecation. A purified podophyllotoxin is now available for use by the patient (podofilox [Condylox]). It is applied carefully with a toothpick twice daily for 3 days, then 4 days later reapplied for 3 days if the warts remain. Podophyllum in excessive doses is a neurotoxin and can cause an areflexic coma.

Psychotherapy. Because warts regress without therapy, most studies demonstrate a placebo effect of 30%. Suggestion therapy such as 'buying the wart' from the child, or a variety of folk medicines, is expected to have a similar regression rate.

Patient education

It should be emphasized from the initial visit that one treatment is unlikely to cure the wart, and many treatments may be necessary (for the Patient Education Sheet on Warts, see CD-ROM). A careful explanation of the poor host immunity to the HPV is helpful.[76] For genital warts in infants and toddlers, the possibility of sexual abuse should be considered. However, it is well established that vertical transmission of genital warts from an infected mother can occur, and many genital warts are of common HPV types, with a parent, sibling, or caregiver having common warts of the same type.[75] This makes it impossible to diagnose sexual abuse by the presence of genital warts alone. The clinician should carefully examine the child for other forms of physical or sexual abuse, including examination of the oral cavity and genitalia. A history of unusual behavior in the child, such as withdrawal, sleep disturbances, phobias, or new onset of enuresis or encopresis, should be solicited. If suspicious history or physical findings other than the genital warts are obtained, reporting to the appropriate social agencies is recommended.[71]

Follow-up visits

A visit 2 weeks after initiating therapy is needed to ascertain the need for retreatment.

Molluscum Contagiosum

Clinical features

White or yellow-white 1–6 mm discrete papules with a central umbilication are seen in molluscum contagiosum (Figs 8.60, 8.61).[7,76,80–88] Lesions may extrude their contents through the central umbilication (Fig. 8.62). Occasionally, lesions as large as 15 mm will be found (Fig. 8.63). These 'giant' molluscum lesions can mimic orf (Fig. 8.64). A dermatitis often surrounds larger lesions (Figs 8.65, 8.66). Lesions larger than 6 mm may occasionally become red and purulent, healing with a slightly depressed scar. In infants and toddlers, lesions are usually observed around the eyes, axilla, and proximal extremities, but lesions can be found in other locations. In the child with atopic dermatitis, dozens to hundreds of lesions can be seen. Genital grouped lesions can be found in sexually active adolescents. Hundreds of lesions in

Fig. 8.60 Multiple molluscum umbilicated papules on an infant's face.

Fig. 8.61 Cluster of umbilicated molluscum papules in infant's scalp.

Fig. 8.62 Molluscum extruding their contents.

Fig. 8.63 'Giant' umbilicated, dome-shaped papule characteristic of molluscum contagiosum.

Fig. 8.64 Orf lesions mimicking molluscum on hand.

Fig. 8.65 Erythema and scaling surround resolving lesions of molluscum contagiosum (molluscum dermatitis) in antecubital fossa.

the older child or the presence of facial or perioral lesions should raise the suspicion of AIDS.[69,82]

Differential diagnosis

Warts, closed comedones, and tiny epidermal cysts may mimic molluscum contagiosum. Careful inspection, however, will reveal the central umbilication characteristic of molluscum contagiosum, and microscopic examination will differentiate the disease from other skin papules. At first glance, molluscum may appear to be blisters, but palpation and careful inspection will reveal their solid nature. Extrusion of the papule contents onto a glass slide and Wright's stain will reveal the characteristic viral inclusions. Serologic diagnosis is usually not required.[78]

Fig. 8.66 Large zone of dermatitis surrounding an umbilicated papule in molluscum dermatitis.

Lesions of molluscum dermatitis may mimic other forms of dermatitis, and pustular lesions may mimic bacterial folliculitis.

Pathogenesis

Molluscum contagiosum is caused by a poxvirus that induces epidermal cell proliferation.[7,76] Three types are recognized by restriction endonuclease analysis of viral DNA. Molluscum type 1 is believed to be responsible for common lesions on the extremities, head, and neck. Types 2 and 3 are most often associated with genital lesions in the adolescent or young adult. The incubation period is 2–7 weeks, and the child is contagious as long as active lesions are present.[83] The molluscum contagiosum viruses evade intracellular interferon production by encoding a faulty chemokine receptor.[80,84] Untreated molluscum may require 1–5 years to resolve.

Treatment

Removal of a papule is curative. In older children, the application of cantharidin covered for 4–6 hours with a Band-Aid, then soaked off in soapy water, is useful. The cantharidin should be applied as a microdrop with a wooden applicator. Excessive cantharidin may result in large and tender blisters. The use of a sharp dermal curette to remove the entire papule is considered the treatment of choice by some authorities although it can be quite painful, even if topical anesthetics are used beforehand.[88] Some clinicians prefer to empty the contents with a needle. In infants and young children this method is frightening and painful. In such children, daily or twice-daily application of imiquimod 5% cream is preferred.[86,87] Lesions are treated until they become red. Oral cimetidine has been reported to be successful by some.[85] Alternatives include application of a drop of potassium hydroxide, or podophyllum applied to the central umbilication with a wooden toothpick. This is less traumatic than curettage and may avoid scarring.[81,82] Recurrences are common because it is often difficult to detect the pinpoint early lesions of molluscum. Pustular molluscum lesions do not require antibiotics.

Patient education

The highly contagious nature of molluscum contagiosum should be emphasized. The lesions are benign, and patients should not be unduly concerned (for Patient Education Sheet on Molluscum Contagiosum, see CD-ROM).

Follow-up visits

A visit 1–2 weeks after initial therapy is advisable to determine the need for retreatment.

REFERENCES

1. Mancini AJ. Exanthems in childhood: an update. Pediatr Ann 1998; 27:398.
2. Norval M, El-Ghorr A, Garssen J. The effects of ultraviolet light irradiation on viral infections. Br J Dermatol 1994; 130:693.
3. Messner J, Miller JJ, James WD, et al. Accentuated viral exanthems in areas of inflammation. J Am Acad Dermatol 1999; 40:345.
4. Jones VF, Badgett JT, Marshall GS. Repeated photoreactivation of herpes simplex virus type I in an extrafacial dermatomal distribution. Pediatr Infect Dis J 1994; 13:238.
5. Coustou D, Leaute-Labreze P, Rioulac-Sage P, et al. Asymmetric periflexural exanthem of childhood: a clinical, pathologic, and epidemiologic prospective study. Arch Dermatol 1999; 135:799.
6. Gelmetti C, Grimalt R, Cambiaghi S. Asymmetric periflexural exanthem of childhood: report of two new cases. Pediatr Dermatol 1994; 11:42.
7. Report of the Committee on Infectious Diseases. Red book 2003. Elk Grove Village, Ill: American Academy of Pediatrics; 2000.
8. Weston WL, Morelli JG. Newly recognized infectious exanthems. Dermatol Nurs 1998; 10:191.
9. Kaplan SL: Newer pediatric pathogens. Adv Pediatr 1999; 46:189.
10. Davidkin I, Valle M, Peltola H, et al. Etiology of measles- and rubella-like illnesses in measles, mumps and rubella-vaccinated children. J Infect Dis 1998; 178:1567.
11. Duke T, Mgone SS. Measles: not just another viral exanthem. Lancet 2003; 361:763–773.
12. Koplik H: The diagnosis of the invasion of measles from a study of the exanthema as it appears on the buccal mucous membrane. Arch Pediatr 1896; 13:918.
13. Elliman D, Sengupta N. Measles. Curr Opin Infect Dis 2005; 18:229–234.
14. West CE. Vitamin A and measles. Nutr Rev 2000; 58:S46.
15. Fulginiti VA, Eller JJ, Downie AW. Altered reactivity to measles virus: atypical measles in children previously immunized with inactivated measles virus vaccine. JAMA 1967; 202:1075.
16. Schneider-Schaulies S, ter Meulen V. Pathogenic aspects of measles virus infections. Arch Virol 1999; 15:139.
17. Edlich RF, Winters KL, Long WB 3rd, et al. Rubella and congenital rubella (German measles). Long Term Eff Med Implants 2005; 15:319–328.
18. Weir E ,Sider D. A refresher on rubella. CMAJ 2005; 172:1680–1681.
19. Turner AJ. Surveillance of congenital rubella in Great Britain: rubella can be mistaken for parvovirus B19 infection. Br Med J 1999; 318:769.

20. Webster WS: Teratogen update: congenital rubella. Teratology 1998; 58:13.
21. Jundt JW, Creager AH. STAR complexes: febrile illness associated with sore throat, arthritis and rash. South Med J 1993; 86:521.
22. Zerr DM, Meier AS, Selke SS, et al. A population-based study of primary human herpesvirus 6 infection. N Eng J Med 2005; 352:768–776.
23. Stoeckle MY. The spectrum of human herpesvirus 6 infection: from roseola infantum to adult disease, Ann Rev Med 2000; 51:423.
24. Ward KN, Andrews NJ, Verity CM, et al. Human herpesviruses-6 and -7 each cause significant neurological morbidity in Britain and Ireland. Arch Dis Child 2005; 90:619–623.
25. Go T, Nakamura K. Frequent seizures with elevated interleukin-6 in the eruptive stage of exanthem subitum. Eur J Ped neurol 2002; 6:221–223.
26. Barton Rogers B. Parvovirus B19: twenty-five years in perspective. Pediatr Develop Pathol 1999; 2:296.
27. Harrel L, Strausberg I, Zeharia A, et al. Papular purpuric rash due to parvovirus B19 with distribution on the distal extremities and the face. Clin Infect Dis 2002; 35:1558–1561.
28. Drago F, Rampini E, Rebora A. Atypical exanthems: morphology and laboratory investigations may lead to an aetiological diagnosis in about 70% of cases. Br J Dermatol 2002; 147:255–260.
29. Barash J, Dushnitzky D, Sthoeger D, et al. Human parvovirus B19 infection in children: uncommon clinical presentations. Isr Med Assoc J 2002; 4:763–765.
30. Gilbert GL. Parvovirus B19 infection and its significance in pregnancy. Commun Dis Intell 2000; 24:69.
31. Chen MY, Lee KL, Hung CC. Immunoglobulin M and G immunoblots in the diagnosis of parvovirus B19 infection. J Formos Med Assoc 2000; 99:24.
32. Brown KE, Hibbs JR, Gallinella G. Resistance to parvovirus B19 infection due to a lack of virus receptor (erythrocyte p antigen). N Engl J Med 1994; 330:1192.
33. Sawyer MH. Enterovirus infections: diagnosis and treatment. Pediatr Infect Dis J 1999; 18:1033.
34. Zaoutis T, Klein JD. Enterovirus infections. Pediatr Rev 1998; 19:183.
35. Sukhai RN, Mumeke R. Enteroviral meningitis with a petechial rash in three children. Eur J Pediatr 2002; 161:226–227.
36. Takami T, Nakayama T, Kawashima H, et al. Determination of enterovirus serotype from sequence analysis of PCR products. J Clin Virol 2003; 26:763–773.
37. Godshall SE, Kirchner JT. Infectious mononucleosis: complexities of a common syndrome. Postgrad Med 2000; 107:175, 183.
38. Peter J, Ray CG. Infectious mononucleosis. Pediatr Rev 1998; 19:276.
39. Morais-Almeida M, Marinho S, Gaspar A, et al. Cold urticaria and infectious mononucleosis in children. Allergol Immunopathol 2004; 32:368–371.
40. Fafi-Kremer S, Morand P, Brion JP, et al. Long-term shedding of Epstein-Barr virus after infectious mononucleosis. J Infect Dis 2005; 191:985–989.
41. Meunier YA. Infectious mononucleosis-like syndrome and gastrointestinal disorders in acute aquired cytomegalovirus infection. Singapore Med J 2005; 46:421–423.
42. Thompson SK, Doerr TD, Henmgerer AS. Infectious mononucleosis and corticosteroids: management practices and outcomes. Arch Otolaryhol Head Neck Surg 131:900–904. 2005;
43. Caputo R, Gelmetti C, Ermacora E. Gianotti-Crosti syndrome: a retrospective analysis of 308 cases. J Am Acad Dermatol 1992; 26:207.
44. Yoshida M, Tsuda N, Morihata T, et al. Five patients with localized facial eruption associated with Gianotti-Crosti syndrome caused by primary Epstein-Barr virus infection. J Pediatr 2004; 145:843–844.
45. Tilly JJ, Drolet BA, Esterly NB. Lichenoid eruptions in children. J Am Acad Dermatol 2004; 51:606–624.
46. Tovo PA, Lazier L, Versace A. Hepatitis B virus and hepatitis C virus infections in children. Curr Opin Infect Dis 2005; 18:261–266.
47. Dollberg S, Berkun Y, Gross-Kieselstein E. Urticaria in patients with hepatitis A virus infection. Pediatr Infect Dis J 1991; 10:702.
48. Reichel M, Mauro TM. Urticaria and hepatitis C. Lancet 1990; 336:822.
49. Slowik MK, Jhaveri R. Hepatitis B and C viruses in infants and young children. Semin Pediatr Infect Dis 2005; 16:296–305.
50. Shepard CW, Finelli L, Fiore AE, et al. Epidemiology of hepatitis A and hepatitis B virus infection in United States children. Pediatr Infect Dis J 2005; 24:755–760.
51. Waggoner-Fountain LA, Grossmna LB. Herpes simplex virus. Pediatr Rev 2004; 25:86–93.
52. Kimberlin DW. Herpes simplex virus infections in neonates and early childhood. Semin Pediatr Infect Dis 200516:271–281.
53. Jones VF, Badgett JT, Marshall GS. Repeated photoreactivation of herpes simplex virus type 1 in an extrafacial dermatomal distribution. Pediatr Infect Dis J 1994; 13:238.
54. Anderson BJ. The epidemiology and clinical analysis of several outbreaks of herpes gladiatorum. Med Sci Sports Exerc 2003; 35:1809–1814.
55. Chong EM, Wilhemus KR, Matoba AY, et al. Herpes simplex virus keratitis in children. Am J Ophthalmol 2004; 138:474–475.
56. Brown ZA, Gardella C, Wald A, et al. Genital herpes complicating pregnancy. Obstet Gynecol 2005; 106:845–856.
57. Ramaswamy M, McDonald C, Sabin C, et al. The epidemiology of genital infection with herpes simplex virus types 1 and 2 in genitourinary medicine attendees in inner London. Sex Trasm Infect 2005; 81:306–308.
58. Goodyear HM. Rapid diagnosis of cutaneous herpes simplex infections using specific monoclonal antibodies. Clin Exper Dermatol 1994; 19:294.
59. Nikkels AF, Pierard GE. Treatment of mucocutaneous presentations of herpes simplex virus infections. Am J Clin Dermatol 2002; 3:475–487.
60. Hambleton S. Chickenpox. Curr Opin Infect Dis 2005; 18:235–240.
61. Takayama N, Takayama M, Takita J. Herpes zoster in healthy children immunized with varicella vaccine. Pediatr Infect Dis J 2000; 19:169.
62. Furuta Y, Ohtani F, Kawabata H, et al. High prevalence of varicella-zoster virus reactivation in herpes simplex-seronegative patients with acute peripheral nerve palsy. Clin Infect Dis 2000; 30:529.

63. Kurlan JG, Connelly BL, Lucky AW. Herpes zoster in the first year of life following postnatal exposure to varicella-zoster virus: four case reports and review of infantile herpes zoster. Arch Dermatol 2004; 140:1268–1272.

64. Furuta Y, Ohtani F, Aizawa H, et al. Varicella-zoster virus reactivation is an important cause of acute peripheral facial paralysis in children. Pediatr Infect Dis J 2005; 24:97–101.

65. Shafran SD, Tyring SK, Ashton R, et al. Once, twice or three times daily famciclovir compared with aciclovir for the oral treatment of herpes zoster in immunocompetent adults: a randomized, multicenter, double-blind clinical trial. J Clin Virol 2004; 29:248–253.

66. Frydenberg A, Starr M. Hand, foot and mouth disease. Aust Fam Physician 2003; 32:594–595.

67. Chang LY, Lin Ty, Huang YC. Comparison of enterovirus 71 and coxsackievirus A16 clinical illnesses during the Taiwan enterovirus epidemic, 1998. Pediatr Infect Dis J 1999; 18:1092.

68. Clementz GC, Mancini AJ. Nail matrix arrest following hand, foot and mouth disease: a report of five children. Pediatr Dermatol 2000; 17:7.

69. Mirchandani N, Hawit F, Silverberg NB. Cutaneous signs of neonatal and infantile immunodeficiency. Dermatol Ther 2005; 18:176–83.

70. Brady MT. Pediatric human immunodeficiency virus-1 infection. Adv Pedaitr 2005; 52:163–193.

71. Neely M, Kovacs A. Management of antiretroviral therapy in neonates, children and adolescents. Curr HIV/AIDS Rep 12004; :97–104.

72. Lambert JS. HIV vaccines in infants and children. Paediatr Drugs 2005; 7:267–276.

73. Silverberg NB. Human papillomavirus infections in children. Curr Opin Pediatr 2004; 16:402–409.

74. Leung AK, Kellner JD, Davies HD. Genital infection with human papillomavirus in adolescents. Adv Therapy 2005; 22:187–197.

75. Atabaki S, Paradise J. The medical evaluation of the sexually abused child: lessons from a decade of research. Pediatrics 1999; 104:178.

76. Silverberg NB. Warts and molluscum in children. Adv Dermatol 2004; 20:23–73.

77. Smolinski KN, Yan AC. How and when to treat molluscum contagiosum and warts in children. Pediatr Ann 2005; 34:211–221.

78. Harwood CA, Perrett CM, Brown VL, et al. Imiquimod cream 5% for recalcitrant cutaneous warts in immunosuppressed individuals. Br J Dermatol 2005; 152:122–129.

79. Orlow SJ, Paller A. Cimetidine therapy for multiple viral warts in children. J Am Acad Dermatol 1993; 28:794.

80. Tyring SK. Molluscum contagiosum: the importance of early diagnosis and treatment. Am J Obstet Gynecol 2003; 189:S12–S16.

81. Smith KJ, Yeager J, Skelton H. Molluscum contagiosum: its clinical, histopathologic and immunohistochemical spectrum. Int J Dermatol 1999; 38:664.

82. Kolokotronis A, Antonaides D, Katsoulides E, et al. Facial and perioral molluscum contagiosum as a manifestation of HIV infection. Aust Dent J 2000; 45:49.

83. Konya J, Thompson CH. Molluscum contagiosum virus: antibody responses in persons with clinical lesions and seroepidemiology in a representative Australian population. J Infect Dis 1999; 179:701.

84. Luttichau HR, et al. A highly selective CC chemokine receptor (CCR) 8 antagonist encoded by the poxvirus molluscum contagiosum. J Exp Med 2000; 191:171.

85. Yashar SS, Shamiri B. Oral cimetidine treatment of molluscum contagiosum. Pediatr Dermatol 1999; 16:493.

86. Bayeri C, Feller G, Goerdt S. Experience in treating molluscum contagiosum in children with imiquimod 5% cream. Br J Dermatol 2003; 149(suppl 66):25–29.

87. Ross GL, Orchard DC. Combination topical treatment of molluscum contagiosum with cantharidin and imiquimod 5% in children: a case series of 16 patients. Australs J Dermatol 2004; 45:100–102.

88. Weller R, O'Callaghan CJ, MacSween RM. Scarring in molluscum contagiosum: comparison of physical expression and phenol ablation. Br Med J 1999; 319:154.

Chapter 9 | Papulosquamous Disorders

Children affected with papulosquamous disorders have skin lesions characterized by red or violaceous macules that progress to papules and develop scales. The exact prevalence of this group of diseases is unknown.[1] However, psoriasis alone has a yearly prevalence of 3.1 per 1000 US children. Pityriasis rosea accounts for a further increase in the prevalence of papulosquamous eruptions in childhood. Thus, papulosquamous disorders are common in children and should be readily recognized by those caring for them. The clinician should recognize that this group of diseases is chronic, lasting months to years. It is important for the clinician to distinguish these diseases with raised lesions from flat, scaly conditions, such as the ichthyoses or the various forms of desquamation.

PSORIASIS

Clinical Features

Psoriasis is thought to be a hereditary disorder that requires an interplay of genetic and environmental factors for full clinical expression.[2] Childhood-onset psoriasis is more likely to demonstrate an affected family member than late-onset psoriasis.[3] Psoriasis is a clinical diagnosis based on the presence of thick, silvery scales on at least some lesions, the characteristic distribution, nail involvement, and the presence of the isomorphic phenomenon. The eruption consists of erythematous macular or papular lesions that develop a thick, silvery scale (Fig. 9.1).

Discrete scaly papules (guttate lesions) may be seen, or groups of papules may coalesce to form raised, sharply marginated, erythematous plaques. The sites of predilection for psoriasis (Fig. 9.2) include the scalp, ears, eyebrows, elbows, knees, gluteal crease, umbilicus, genitalia, and nails. Complete examination of the entire cutaneous surface is necessary because characteristic lesions with thick scale (Fig. 9.3) may be few in number. Scalp lesions commonly demonstrate thick scale (Figs 9.4; 9.5). The most common clinical picture of psoriasis (psoriasi vulgaris) in childhood is involvement of the ears (Figs 9.6; 9.7), elbows (Fig. 9.8), knees, and scalp by a few plaques.[3] Involvement of the anal crease is common (Fig. 9.9) and anal crease 'pinking' without scale may be an early sign of childhood psoriasis (Fig. 9.10). Genital involvement (e.g. perineal area, penis, inguinal folds, labia) occurs in 44% of children with psoriasis.[3] Gluteal cleft involvement is common (Fig. 9.11, 9.12), as is involvement of the penis.

Guttate psoriasis, the term given to the form of psoriasis with multiple discrete papules, begins on the trunk as multiple erythematous macules that mimic a viral exanthem (Figs 9.13, 9.14). Guttate psoriasis is more common in children than adults. As noted, the lesions progress to papules that develop a silvery scale (Fig. 9.15). These droplike papules (*guttata* is the Latin word for 'drop') are seen predominantly on the trunk and proximal extremities. Guttate psoriasis may follow a sore throat, particularly streptococcal pharyngitis, by 2–3 weeks.[3] Follicular accentuation of the skin lesions may be seen. Children with guttate psoriasis should be evaluated for pharyngeal[3] or rectal[3] streptococcal infection. Children with an episode of guttate psoriasis are likely to develop typical lesions of psoriasis vulgaris within 5 years.[1]

The isomorphic (Koebner) phenomenon, in which psoriatic lesions develop in sites of skin trauma several days after the traumatic event, is a useful diagnostic feature of psoriasis.[1] It occurs in a linear fashion along a scratch, but may also be precipitated by lacerations, abrasions, sunburn, insect bites, or pressure (Fig. 9.16). In some children it may appear in a nevoid distribution and mimic epidermal nevi.[4]

Fig. 9.1 Papules and plaques, some of which are covered with thick, silvery scales over the back of a child with psoriasis.

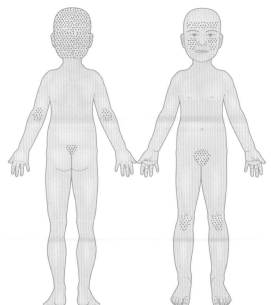

Fig. 9.2 The distribution of childhood psoriasis vulgaris.

Fig. 9.3 Plaque of psoriasis with silvery scale on the leg of a child.

Scalp involvement with psoriasis results in accumulation of thick scales throughout the scalp, with thickened scales along the frontal hairline and behind the ears (Fig. 9.17). The scalp is involved in the majority of children with psoriasis. Hair loss does not occur.

Involvement of the palms and soles is uncommon in children, but psoriasis may appear as fissured, painful, symmetric plaques (Figs 9.18, 9.19) or as multiple small, sterile pustules.[3,5] Pustular lesions on the palms and soles may be associated with common plaques of psoriasis elsewhere.[3,5] Children may also have involvement of the distal segment of one or more digits (Fig. 9.20).[6]

Nail signs in psoriasis (Box 9.1) include the following: multiple tiny pits on the surface of the nails (pitting) (Fig. 9.21); yellowing of the distal nail caused by separation of the nail plate from the nail bed (onycholysis); thickening of the distal nail (distal hyper-

Fig. 9.4 Scaly plaques of the scalp and face in psoriasis.

Fig. 9.5 Thick scale accumulations in scalp of child with psoriasis.

Fig. 9.7 Psoriatic scaly plaques in the ear canal in childhood psoriasis.

Fig. 9.8 Thick, scaly plaque above elbow in psoriasis.

Fig. 9.6 Scaly papules behind ear in childhood psoriasis.

Fig. 9.9 Scaly plaues in superior anal crease in a child.

Fig. 9.10 Pinking of superior anal crease without scale in childhood psoriasis.

Fig. 9.11 Scaly plaque on foreskin and red plaque on glans penis in child with psoriasis.

Fig. 9.12 Scaly plaque on foreskin in infantile psoriasis.

Fig. 9.13 Dozens of discrete, red papules scattered on the back of a child with acute guttate psoriasis after a streptococcal throat infection.

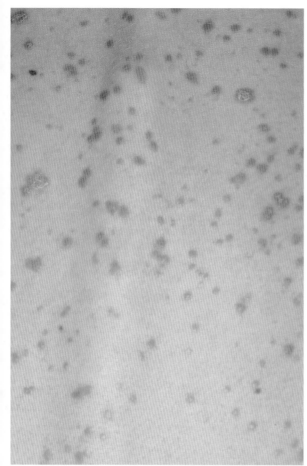

Fig. 9.14 Guttate psoriasis. Hundreds of small red papules.

Fig. 9.15 Guttate papules on the back of a child with streptococcal perianal cellulitis.

Fig. 9.16 Psoriasis appearing within the line of a previous scratch demonstrating the isomorphic (Koebner) phenomenon.

Fig. 9.17 Thick plaques without hair loss in a child with psoriasis.

Fig. 9.18 Scaly fissured psoriasis plaques on a child's palms.

Fig. 9.19 Scaly red plaque on child's thenar eminence.

Fig. 9.20 Red plaque of psoriasis with pustules involving child's distal thumb.

Fig. 9.21 Nail pitting in a child with psoriasis.

Fig. 9.22 Nail thickening and scaling in childhood psoriasis.

Box 9.1 Nail signs in psoriasis
Pitting of the nail surface
Distal onycholysis
Distal hyperkeratosis
Hyperkeratosis and crumbling of the entire nail

keratosis); or thickening, crumbling, and destruction of the entire nail (Fig. 9.22). All 20 nails may be involved and, rarely, nail changes may be the presenting feature of psoriasis in children. Nail changes are seen in 15% of children with psoriasis, but absence of nail involvement does not exclude the diagnosis of psoriasis.[3]

Erythroderma with thousands of pinpoint pustules, which eventuates in sheets of desquamation, is called *pustular psoriasis* and is quite rare in childhood but may result from treatment of psoriasis with systemic steroids (Figs 9.23–9.25).[3] Pustular psoriasis may rarely be accompanied by lytic bone lesions.[3,7]

Itching is a variable feature in psoriasis; most children do not complain of it. Scratching of lesions or picking off the scales may leave fine, bleeding points (Auspitz sign) (Fig. 9.26) and induce the isomorphic phenomenon and make individual lesions worse.

Arthritis is seldom seen. It develops in only 1% of children with psoriasis.[3,8] Arthritis may precede or follow psoriasis and usually begins as oligoarticular disease involving the metacarpophalangeal (MCP)

Fig. 9.23 Pinpoint pustules, erythema, and sheets of desquamation in a child with pustular psoriasis.

Fig. 9.24 Pinpoint pustules at border of childhood pustular psoriasis.

Fig. 9.25 Pinpoint pustules in psoriatic plaque on child's neck.

Fig. 9.26 Auspitz sign. Pinpoint bleeding areas where scale was lifted from psoriatic plaque.

Fig. 9.27 Childhood psoriatic arthritis. Erythema and swelling of the distal interphalangeal joints with total nail dystrophy.

Box 9.2 Differential diagnosis of papulosquamous disorders

Lichen planus

Lupus erythematosus

Lues (secondary syphilis)

Lichen striatus

Lichen nitidus

Psoriasis

Pityriasis rosea

Parapsoriasis

Pityriasis rubra pilaris

Dermatophyte infections

Dermatomyositis

Nummular eczema

joints, proximal interphalangeal (PIP) joints, or the axial skeleton (Fig. 9.27).[8,9]

Differential Diagnosis

Conditions to be considered in the differential diagnosis of papulosquamous disorders are listed in Box 9.2. Lichen planus with involvement of the elbows and knees can mimic psoriasis. However, the silvery scale and red color of psoriatic plaques distinguish them from the purple papules of lichen planus. Whitish plaques of the oral mucosa are seen in lichen planus, but not in psoriasis. The isomorphic phenomenon is also seen in lichen planus, but the papules are purple.

In contrast to psoriasis, linear epidermal nevi are present from birth. Flat warts occurring along a line of skin trauma do not have a scaly surface. Lichen striatus appears as a solitary lesion progressing down an extremity. Scaly macules on the elbows and knees seen in childhood dermatomyositis may be confused with psoriasis. The presence of a malar photo-eruption, muscle weakness and pain will help distinguish dermatomyositis. Hypertrophic cutaneous lupus lesions may mimic psoriasis, but the scale is thin, not thick, and central atrophy is present. Guttate psoriasis is most often confused with pityriasis rosea. The large 'herald patch' of pityriasis rosea is lacking in guttate psoriasis, and the overlying scale in pityriasis rosea is thin and central, rather than thick and diffuse, as in psoriasis. Early guttate lesions are not scaly and may be confused with a morbilliform viral exanthem, urticaria, drug eruption, or secondary syphilis.

Scaling in the scalp in psoriasis is nongreasy, in contrast to the seborrheic dermatitis of adolescents. Diffuse scaling of the scalp in African-Americans should make one consider tinea capitis. In atopic dermatitis of the scalp, the scales are mild, thin, and dry in contrast to the thick scales of psoriasis.

Nail pitting occurs in alopecia areata, but the pits are broader, more shallow, and fewer in number than in psoriasis. Onycholysis and hyperkeratosis of the nails occur in lichen planus, but synechiae from the cuticle to the fingertip and narrowing of the nail are seen. Fungal involvement of the nail is seen rarely in childhood, and usually only one or two nails are involved in contrast to psoriasis. Trachyonychia may be difficult to distinguish from psoriasis, although onycholysis and 'oil spots' found in psoriasis are usually not seen in trachyonychia. In the absence of classical psoriasis skin lesions elsewhere, it requires following the child over many months to finally distinguish the

two. All 20 nails are affected in ectodermal dysplasia and its variants, but alopecia, dental disorders, and other features are usually present to distinguish them from psoriasis.

Genital psoriasis must be differentiated from bacterial or candidal intertriginous infections by potassium hydroxide (KOH) examination and culture.

Pathogenesis

There are genetic factors involved in the development of psoriasis. The lack of complete concordance in monozygotic twins (67%) suggests a role for the combination of genetic and environmental factors.[2] Eight different psoriasis susceptibility genes (PSORS) have been identified.[2] The major psoriasis susceptibility gene (PSORS1) has been mapped to the major histocompatibility complex region of chromosome 6.

The classic pathologic features of psoriasis seen on skin biopsy denote inflammation associated with features of epidermal proliferation. The epidermis is thickened, with elongation of the rete ridges to the same level (regular acanthosis), increased epidermal mitosis, parakeratosis (nuclei retained in the stratum corneum), thinning of the granular layer, and microabscesses of neutrophils within the epidermis and stratum corneum. In the dermis the dermal papillae are clubbed, and there is vasodilation of dermal blood vessels with an infiltration of activated T lymphocytes.[10] T lymphocytes and the mediators they release are thought to be of primary importance in the development of a psoriatic lesion.[2] Increased numbers of epidermal cells enter the mitotic cellular pool; the epidermal turnover time in psoriasis is three to four times faster than that of normal skin.

The factors responsible for increased epidermal turnover are unknown. In many ways, the psoriatic epidermis mimics skin healing from a wound. In children the association with streptococcal infection is intriguing. Lymphocyte activation by streptococcal antigens has been implicated in the pathogenesis of guttate psoriasis.[11,12] Infection of the throat or perianal skin with streptococci may precipitate acute guttate psoriasis.[3]

Treatment

The treatment of psoriasis can be divided into three levels – topical, ultraviolet light, and systemic therapy – with the choice of treatment dependent on the severity of the disease. In most children, psoriasis can be controlled with topical therapy alone.[2,3,13,14]

Steroids are still the mainstay of topical therapy for children. Topical steroids improve psoriasis temporarily, with the most benefit obtained from moderate- to high-potency glucocorticosteroids. Low-potency topical steroids, such as 1% hydrocortisone, are ineffective in childhood psoriasis.[1] The maximal benefit is obtained with 2–4 weeks of daily therapy, and remissions are shorter than with phototherapy.

Topical calcipotriene (1,25-hydroxyvitamin D3 analog) may be equally effective as potent topical steroids in the management of childhood psoriasis, requiring 4 weeks to clearing.[15] The efficacy of topical calcipotriene is enhanced by alternating with potent topical steroids.[15] Topical calcipotriene is more irritating to the skin than topical steroids.[16]

Anthralin is a tricyclic hydrocarbon that is efficacious in the management of psoriasis by inhibiting epidermal proliferation through downregulation of the epidermal growth factor TGF-α and its receptor, the epidermal growth factor receptor.[17] The so-called 'short-contact' protocols are particularly useful. Anthralin 1% ointment is applied once daily to the psoriatic lesions for 20 minutes, then neutralized with a pH 7.0 soap, such as Dove soap, thoroughly washing off all of the anthralin. If not washed off, it produces considerable skin irritation. Anthralin also stains the skin and clothing brown. Most patients require 4–8 weeks of daily anthralin therapy to clear. There is no benefit from adding topical steroids to anthralin. Short-contact anthralin therapy is not quite as effective as topical calcipotriene.[17]

Tazarotene is a topically applied retinoid. It is similar in efficacy to midpotent topical steroids, but it is much more irritating.[10,18] It may also be used in combination with topical steroids.[18] Tazarotene is the best topical agent for treating psoriatic nail disease.

For the scalp, softening the scales with salicylic acid 3% in mineral oil or olive oil, or use of a phenol and saline scalp solution massaged in and left in overnight is useful. Then the scalp can be shampooed with a tar shampoo, and the scales can be gently mechanically removed with a comb and brush. This is repeated daily until the scales are gone. The tar shampoo may be drying, and conditioners applied after shampooing may be helpful. The use of steroid or calcipotriene lotions after shampooing may be necessary in resistant cases.[19,20]

Natural ultraviolet light (UVL) and artificial ultraviolet (UV) sources (phototherapy) are effective in the management of psoriasis. In general, psoriatic children have better therapeutic response to UVL if it is received in a structured phototherapy protocol rather than during sunbathing. Lubrication of the skin surface with mineral oil or petrolatum before UVL produces uniform penetration of UVL by reducing the reflection of light from the disrupted skin surface.[21] UVL therapy may be delivered as broad-band UVB (BB UVB, 290–320 nm) or narrow-band UVB (NB UVB, 311 nm) or photochemotherapy with methoxsalen and long-wave UVL (320–400 nm ultraviolet A [UVA]), so-called PUVA (psoralen ultraviolet A-range) therapy. NB UVB is more effective than BB UVB, but less effective than PUVA.[22] Because of potential mutagenicity, PUVA should be restricted to children over 12 years of age who have not responded to NB or BB UVB and it should be administered only by experienced dermatologists.[23] There is no evidence that BB or NB UVB treatment increase skin cancer risk in psoriasis patients.[24] Phototherapy may be used in combination with topical therapies or oral retinoids.[25–28]

Children with guttate psoriasis and evidence of streptococcal infection should be treated with antibiotics to eliminate the infection,[3] but there are no controlled trials proving its efficacy in improving psoriasis.[29]

Systemic steroids are contraindicated in childhood psoriasis because psoriatic erythroderma may follow withdrawal, resulting in fever, hypoalbuminuria, and other metabolic changes associated with generalized skin involvement.[5] Oral retinoids are efficacious in severe forms of childhood psoriasis, such as generalized pustular psoriasis and psoriatic erythroderma.[12] Retinoids should never be considered the drug of first choice in the management of childhood psoriasis. Methotrexate has been demonstrated to be efficacious in childhood psoriasis, but toxicity restricts its use to only the most recalcitrant cases.[30] The newer anti-TNF biologic agents are now being used in childhood psoriasis.[31,32] The use of systemic agents in the treatment of childhood psoriasis should always be managed by an experienced dermatologist.

Patient Education

Children with psoriasis have a chronic disease, and education is a crucial aspect of overall care. Patients and parents should understand that the disease is the result of both a genetic susceptibility and environmental factors (for Patient Education Sheets on

Psoriasis and Psoriasis Scalp Care, see CD-ROM). Childhood-onset psoriasis tends to increase in severity in adult life.[1,3] One should emphasize that good remission and good control of psoriasis can be achieved, but that sometimes childhood psoriasis is difficult to treat. One should explain that good treatments require 4–8 weeks to obtain significant improvement. It should also be stated that even if psoriasis clears, there is a hereditary susceptibility for psoriasis, and it can reappear in the future. Adolescents, in particular, need considerable emotional support. The occurrence of exacerbations at times of emotional stress is well recognized.

Patients should understand that trauma to the skin induces psoriasis, but severe restriction of activities is unwarranted. Not scratching psoriasis lesions should be stressed. In childhood guttate psoriasis, prompt administration of antibiotics with each sore throat or respiratory illness should be stressed, and children who have multiple episodes of poststreptococcal guttate psoriasis in a year might require prophylactic antibiotics.

Staphylococcus aureus can be cultured in large numbers from the skin surface in psoriasis. Occlusive dressings should be avoided because they enhance the overgrowth of skin bacteria. Hospitalized children with psoriasis will shed bacteria continually into the room air.

Follow-up Visits

Patients should be seen every 2 weeks during therapy to evaluate their response and to provide supportive care. Dermatology nurse specialists or psoriatic day-care centers are ideal for this type of specialized care. An advantage of phototherapy protocols is that emotional support for the patient can be provided with each treatment, and the parents and patient can develop a better understanding of the condition and the care required to successfully control psoriasis.

PITYRIASIS ROSEA

Clinical Features

Pityriasis rosea is most commonly seen in adolescents and children but has been described at all ages, including infancy.[33] It may be preceded by a prodrome of pharyngitis, lymphadenopathy, headache, and malaise, but in most children no history of constitutional symptoms is given. An annular, scaly, erythematous lesion (the herald patch) precedes the appearance of

Fig. 9.28 Pityriasis rosea. Herald patch, which is larger than other papules, is seen on child's chest.

the remainder of the lesions by 1–30 days (Fig. 9.28).[33] The herald patch is present in 12–94% of children.[34] It is usually on the trunk but may appear on the face or extremities. The herald patch, unlike the other lesions, shows central clearing and may mimic tinea corporis.[33]

Fig. 9.29 Lesions of pityriasis rosea following a 'Christmas tree' distribution.

The cutaneous lesions consist of multiple erythematous macules progressing to small, red papules that appear over the trunk (Fig. 9.29). The papules enlarge, becoming oval. The long axes of the oval lesions tend to be parallel to each other and follow the lines of skin stress (Fig. 9.30). A thin scale develops in the center of the oval lesions.[33] Individual lesions may be atypical in appearance, including vesicular, crusted, and purpuric types.[33] Asymptomatic oral lesions may be noted in 16% of cases.[33] In black skin, lesions over the proximal extremities, inguinal and axillary areas, and neck often predominate, with few lesions on the trunk (Fig. 9.31).[33] Despite the different distribution, the course is similar. The lesions last 4–8 weeks. Mild itching is common during the first week of the generalized eruption, but the lesions are asymptomatic thereafter.

Fig. 9.30 Inverse pityriasis rosea with lesions seen on the neck and face.

Fig. 9.31 Inverse pityriasis rosea with oval plaques with central scale on the neck of a black child.

Differential Diagnosis

The herald patch is often confused with tinea corporis before the appearance of the generalized eruption. If an antifungal agent is used, the development of the generalized papular eruption may be mistaken for a drug reaction to the antifungal. The herald patch may also be confused with a lesion of nummular eczema. Nummular eczema usually is crusted, in contrast to the dry, scaly herald patch. The generalized papular eruption may mimic urticaria, the viral exanthems, morbilliform drug eruptions, post-bone marrow transplantation eruption, or guttate psoriasis (see Box 9.2), but the presence of the herald patch is a useful distinguishing feature. As the lesions become more oval, secondary syphilis should be considered. Although secondary syphilis is usually characterized by lesions of the oral and genital mucosa and ham-colored macules on the palms and soles, the adolescent with 'pityriasis rosea' accompanied by oral, genital, and palmar lesions, fever, or lymphadenopathy should have a Venereal Disease Research Laboratories (VDRL) test to exclude secondary syphilis. The oval lesions may also be confused with pityriasis lichenoides chronica.

Pathogenesis

Because epidemics occur in a susceptible age group, pityriasis rosea has long been considered to be an infectious process. There is debate regarding the role of human herpesvirus (HHV)-7 as the causative agent.[34] Pathologic changes consist only of mild inflammation, with edema of the epidermis and dermis, and a mild perivascular accumulation of lymphocytes. Focal areas of parakeratosis are seen.

Treatment

Most children and adolescents require no therapy. A single dose of UVL, either natural sunlight exposure to redness or one minimal erythema dose of sunlamp exposure, will stop itching and hasten the disappearance of the lesions (Fig. 9.32).[33] Clearing of the rash following erythromycin 250 mg 4×/day for 2 weeks has been reported.[33] Oral antihistamines are rarely necessary. Topical steroids do not influence the lesions.

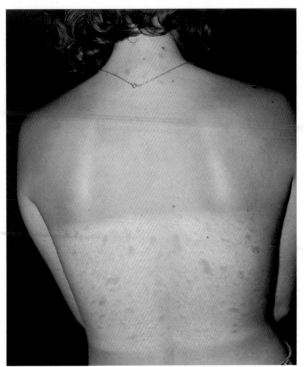

Fig. 9.32 The effect of sunlight on pityriasis rosea. Lesions present only in untanned areas of a child's back.

Patient Education

The long duration of the lesions should be explained, with assurance that they will disappear, leaving normal-appearing skin.

A repeat episode of pityriasis rosea may cause concern for the patient and parents, but multiple episodes occasionally occur and there is no need for concern.

Follow-up Visits

Follow-up visits are usually unnecessary except for follow-up on syphilis serology.

LUES (SECONDARY SYPHILIS)

Clinical Features

Secondary syphilis is characterized by discrete pink macules or pink papules with a fine scale distributed over the trunk and is associated with lymphadenopathy (see Ch. 5). Skin lesions erupt 4–8 weeks after the appearance of the chancre. Serologic tests for syphilis are always positive at the time of the secondary cutaneous eruption. A list of the cutaneous signs of secondary syphilis is presented in Box 9.3. The major

---

Box 9.3 Cutaneous signs of secondary syphilis

Major
Papular lesions
Condylomata lata
Mucous patches

Minor
Annular
Nodular
Pustular crusted lesions
Alopecia
Keratotic macules of palms and soles
Usually associated with generalized lymphadenopathy

---

signs include maculopapular lesions, condylomata lata, and mucous patches.[35]

Condylomata lata are moist, warty papules seen in the perineum and other intertriginous areas, such as under the breast and in the interdigital webs and axillae. The mucous patch is a papular lesion seen most often on the tongue as a red papule lacking tongue papillae. On the buccal mucosa, palate, tonsils, vaginal mucosa, glans penis, and coronal sulcus, it appears as a papule with a central erosion.

The maculopapular lesions, condylomata lata, and mucous patches contain hundreds of spirochetes and are infectious. Generalized lymphadenopathy accompanies these features in 85% of cases; low-grade fever, lethargy, and arthralgias accompany the eruptions in 50% of cases.

Minor variants of secondary syphilis include the following: annular lesions of the face, neck, and genitalia, most commonly seen in blacks; acral nodules that are few in number; sterile pustules and crusted lesions that mimic ecthyma; a 'moth-eaten' alopecia of the eyebrows and scalp hair; and keratotic, ham-colored macules of the palms and soles.

Untreated secondary syphilis may progress to nephrotic syndrome, cranial nerve palsies, meningismus, osteolytic lesions, syphilitic hepatitis, or neurosyphilis.

Differential Diagnosis

Syphilis is well known to mimic a wide variety of cutaneous conditions (see Box 9.2), most commonly pityriasis rosea.

The generalized eruptions may be differentiated from pityriasis rosea by the involvement of the palms and soles, lymphadenopathy, mucous patches, and a positive VDRL flocculation test.

Condylomata lata must be distinguished from venereal warts by the VDRL flocculation test or darkfield microscopic examination.

Mucous patches may be confused with geographic tongue, aphthous stomatitis, angular cheilitis, or other mucocutaneous syndromes.

For pathogenesis, treatment, patient education, follow-up visits, and references, see Chapter 5.

PITYRIASIS LICHENOIDES

Clinical Features

Pityriasis lichenoides, an uncommon disorder, may be seen in two distinct childhood forms: pityriasis lichenoides acuta (Mucha-Habermann disease) (pityriasis lichenoides et varioliformis acuta [PLEVA]) and pityriasis lichenoides chronica (PLC).[36] Both forms may occur in the same patient, or one form may progress to the other. Thus, they are considered two forms of the same disease.[36] The diseases usually have their onset between ages 3 and 15.[36] In pityriasis lichenoides acuta, the eruption consists of recurrent crops of red papules 2–4 mm in diameter (Fig. 9.33). The papules have central petechiae and progress to crusting (Figs 9.34, 9.35). Lesions in different stages are seen, particularly on the trunk. They heal with depressed scars. The eruption lasts approximately 9–12 months and is occasionally associated with low-grade fever. A very rare form of the condition includes acute high fever associated with ulcerative nodules.[37]

In pityriasis lichenoides chronica, salmon-colored, oval papules with central thin scales are seen primarily in the perineal area, thighs, and trunk (Figs 9.36, 9.37).[36] They are few in number, but may persist for 2–3 years.[36] Both forms may be seen simultaneously in the same child (Fig. 9.38). Both forms are seldom associated with itching.

Fig. 9.33 Acute pityriasis lichenoides. Crusted and petechial papules on trunk of child.

Fig. 9.34 Characteristic red papule with central crust in acute pityriasis lichenoides.

Fig. 9.35 Papules with central ulcer in acute pityriasis lichenoides.

Fig. 9.36 Chronic pityriasis lichenoides. Discrete, oval salmon-colored papules with a thin scale seen on a child's trunk.

Fig. 9.37 Chronic pityriasis lichenoides. Multiple scaly papules on child's leg.

Fig. 9.38 Both acute and chronic lesions mixed together on child with pityriasis lichenoides.

Differential Diagnosis

Pityriasis lichenoides acuta mimics varicella, and a child with 'prolonged varicella' should bring pityriasis lichenoides acuta to mind. Occasionally, insect bites or necrotizing vasculitis is confused with pityriasis lichenoides chronica. In pityriasis lichenoides acuta at least some lesions have a purpuric center, which is helpful to distinguish it from varicella or insect bites. The presence of lesions in many different stages is useful in separating pityriasis lichenoides acuta from vasculitis. Rarely, children will have lesions that appear similar to those of pityriasis lichenoides acuta, but upon histologic examination the infiltrating cells will demonstrate abnormal nuclear shapes and size. This condition is called *lymphomatoid papulosis*.[38] The exact incidence of lymphomatoid papulosis in children is unknown. Less than 10% of children with lymphomatoid papulosis will eventually develop a cutaneous T-cell lymphoma, mycosis fungoides.[39] A skin biopsy will distinguish.[38,39]

The chronic form mimics pityriasis rosea, and thus 'prolonged pityriasis rosea' should alert one to the diagnosis of pityriasis lichenoides chronica. Dry skin dermatitis, nummular eczema, secondary syphilis, guttate psoriasis, and tinea corporis sometimes confuse the diagnosis (see Box 9.2). The long duration and sparse number of lesions help distinguish.

Pathogenesis

Pityriasis lichenoides acuta is a vascular injury, with extravasation of erythrocytes, a superficial perivascular lymphohistiocytic infiltrate, and necrosis of the overlying epidermis. Focal parakeratosis is also seen. In contrast to necrotizing vasculitis, no fibrinoid necrosis of the vessel walls is seen, neutrophils are not present, and nuclear fragments are not found around vessels. The mechanism of the disease remains unknown.

The histologic findings in pityriasis lichenoides chronica are similar to those of pityriasis rosea. The mechanism of the disease is unknown.

Treatment

Treatment with oral erythromycin, 40 mg/kg/day for 1–2 months, may benefit some children.[40] For children who fail erythromycin therapy, a conservative approach is recommended. UVB phototherapy may control the disease and some authorities believe it is the treatment of choice for pityriasis lichenoides.[41] Topical steroids do not influence the disease, and claims for efficacy from high-dose tetracycline or low-dose methotrexate cannot be substantiated.

Patient Education

The prolonged course of these disorders should be emphasized.

Follow-up Visits

A visit in 1 month is useful to re-evaluate the child's disease state and determine response to therapy. In the child with lesions that persist for over 2 years, re-evaluation every 6–12 months is suggested, and additional biopsies should be considered because of the possibility of development of a cutaneous T-cell lymphoma.[38,39]

LICHEN PLANUS

Clinical Features

Lichen planus is a chronic papular skin disorder characterized by the appearance of purple, flat-topped papules.[42,43] The list in Box 9.4 is helpful in recalling the major features. The classic polygonal purple papules occur on the wrist and extensor surfaces of the forearm (Figs 9.39, 9.40). On the knees, feet, and lower legs, thick scaling is found over thickened, purple plaques (hypertrophic lichen planus) (Fig. 9.41). Bullae or erosions may be seen on the feet or head and neck.[44] The shaft of the penis is commonly involved (Fig. 9.42). Lichen planus may be inherited in an autosomal dominant manner.[42] The isomorphic phenomenon may be prominent (Fig. 9.43).

Oral lesions are rare and are seen most commonly on the buccal mucosa as white, thickened papules in a lacy pattern (Fig. 9.44).[45] Erosions or thickening of the tongue or gingivae may be seen.[45]

Box 9.4 The 'P's of lichen planus
Planar (flat-topped)
Pruritic (itchy)
Purple
Polygonal (angulated borders)
Papules
Penile

Fig. 9.39 Childhood lichen planus. Purple papules on wrist and forearm.

Fig. 9.40 Purple pruritic papules on wrist of girl with lichen planus.

In the scalp, a circumscribed area of hair loss with replacement of follicles by scarring rarely occurs.[42]

The nail changes of lichen planus are rare in children, but a roughening of the nail surface (trachyonychia) may be seen (Fig. 9.45).[46,47] Total destruction of all 20 nails with synechiae formation may precede, accompany, or follow the onset of skin lesions.[46,47] The nail is narrowed, with an overgrowth of fibrous tissue from the proximal nail fold across the nail plate

Fig. 9.41 Thick, scaly, purple plaques over the knee in a child with lichen planus.

Fig. 9.43 Isomorphic phenomenon in childhood lichen planus. Linear extension of lichen planus along the line of a scratch.

Fig. 9.42 Linear purple papules on the penis in a child with lichen planus.

Fig. 9.44 Lacy white thickening of the buccal mucosa in an adolescent demonstrating mucosal involvement in lichen planus.

to the tip of the digit. A few children with lichen planus will present with only nail involvement, which is often labeled trachyonychia until a nail biopsy is done or other mucocutaneous lesions of lichen planus develop.[47]

Fig. 9.45 Involvement in all 10 fingernails in childhood lichen planus

Fig. 9.46 Hundreds of discrete, pinpoint, white, flat-topped papules on a child with lichen nitidus.

Fig. 9.47 Isomorphic phenomenon in child with lichen nitidus.

Itching is severe in lichen planus, and the isomorphic phenomenon occurs commonly, with the appearance of lichen planus papules along an area of skin trauma.[43] Localized forms also occur in children. The natural history of lichen planus is to resolve in 9–18 months, leaving hyperpigmented areas in sites where lesions occurred.

A variant of lichen planus, called *lichen nitidus*, has histologic features identical to those of lichen planus but it is focal in nature.[48,49] It demonstrates tiny (1–2 mm), hypopigmented, flat-topped papules occurring in clusters, usually over the trunk or face (Fig. 9.46). Lesions may demonstrate the isomorphic phenomenon (Fig. 9.47).[48,49] They do not itch. Lesions of lichen nitidus have been found in 25% of children with lichen planus.

Differential Diagnosis

The characteristic purple color, with flat-topped papules with angulated borders, distinguishes lichen planus from other papulosquamous disorders (see Box 9.2). The hypertrophic lesions on the lower legs mimic psoriasis. Erosive lesions in the mouth mimic aphthous stomatitis and herpes simplex, and the white, lacy appearance of the buccal mucosa may be confused with premalignant leukoplakia or a white sponge nevus. A white sponge nevus is an autosomal dominant nevoid condition which presents as a thickened white plaque on the oral mucosa. A skin biopsy may be required to confirm the diagnosis of lichen planus.[43,45]

A variety of drugs can produce an eruption identical to lichen planus, including thiazide diuretics, quinacrine, chloroquine, quinine, quinidine, and gold, but these agents are rarely used in children.

Lichen nitidus may mimic keratosis pilaris, but the inspissated, dry, scaly, follicular plugs of keratosis pilaris are not seen, and lichen nitidus lesions are smooth-topped.[44,46]

Pathogenesis

Lichen planus results from an acute injury to the basal cells of the epidermis such that liquefaction degeneration of basal cells occurs and the dermal–epidermal junction is obscured. In bullous lichen planus the epidermis separates from the dermis. Amorphous colloid bodies representing degenerating basal cells combined with immunoreactants such as immunoglobulin A (IgA), immunoglobulin G (IgG), immunoglobulin M (IgM), complement, and fibrin are seen in the basal layer or just beneath it. The damaged basal cells have decreased ability to divide. Thus, there are features of prolonged retention of cells in the epidermis, with acanthosis, hyperkeratosis, and a thickened granular layer. The exact mechanism of the epidermal basal cell injury is unknown, but it is thought to be due to inflammatory injury by mononuclear cells that interact with the basement membrane. Hepatitis C has been associated with lichen planus.[50-52] The actual percentage of lichen planus patients with hepatitis C ranges from 3% to 60% and varies depending on geographic location.[50-52]

In lichen nitidus, the same pathologic changes occur, but they are limited to a single dermal papilla.

Treatment

Topical glucocorticosteroids are effective in controlling the itching and resolution of the lesions.[43] They are used twice daily, and 4–8 weeks of therapy are often required for remission. In children with severe generalized lichen planus, prompt relief from prednisone, 1–2 mg/kg/day in a single morning dose, can be expected in 2 weeks, although the lichen planus may return as the steroids are reduced. Oral lesions are usually asymptomatic, but when painful they will respond to topical steroid or topical isotretinoin gels applied to the mucosa. Lichen nitidus need not be treated.

Patient Education

Patients should be informed of the prolonged nature of lichen planus and the tendency for dyspigmentation to occur on healing. It should be emphasized that topical steroids are the most effective method to relieve the itching, but that the clearing of individual lesions will be slow.

Follow-up Visits

Follow-up visits every 2–4 weeks are needed to monitor the course of the disease and the response to therapy.

LUPUS ERYTHEMATOSUS

Clinical Features

In the pediatric age groups, lupus erythematosus (LE) occurs more often in females than in males.[53-55] The prevalence may be three times higher in black, Asian, or Hispanic children than in whites.[55] In approx-

imately 15% of all patients with LE, the onset is between the ages of 9 and 15 years, and the incidence is estimated at 1–6 per 100 000.[53-55]

A cutaneous eruption is present in 80% of adolescents with LE, and in 25% it is the presenting sign. The most frequent cutaneous sign is the erythematous maculopapular eruption over the cheeks and nose with a 'butterfly' distribution (Fig. 9.48).[53] It is covered by a fine scale and occurs in one-third to one-half of the patients. Next most common is the discoid lesion, a chronic, persistent skin change that progresses to scarring and pigmentary changes; in black patients, severe hypopigmentation may be seen (Fig. 9,49).[53,54-56] Discoid lesions are seen most frequently over the face, hands, ears, and scalp, where scarring hair loss results (Figs 9.50, 9.51).[57]

Fig. 9.48 Bright red, scaly plaques on cheeks of a girl with acute SLE.

Fig. 9.49 Atrophy, erythema, and scaling of preauricular skin of a child with DLE.

Fig. 9.50 Scaling and atrophy in ear canal of adolescent male with discoid lupus erythematosus.

Fig. 9.51 Scarring hair loss with redness and scaling of the underlying scalp in an 8-year-old girl with DLE.

Fig. 9.52 Subacute cutaneous lupus erythematosus. Annular, scaly patches on sun-exposed skin of adolescent girl.

Fig. 9.53 Acute phototoxic reaction with intense redness and skin detachment in SCLE.

More transient annular papulosquamous lesions limited to sun-exposed areas of skin are observed in subacute cutaneous lupus (Fig. 9.52).[58,59] Subacute cutaneous lupus erythematosus (SCLE) is more likely to occur in early childhood and be associated with genetic complement deficiencies[60] and the presence of anti-Ro and anti-La autoantibodies.[58–60] SCLE is the most photosensitive form of childhood lupus and phototoxic (Fig. 9.53) and bullous lesions (Fig.9.54) may occur after sun exposure.

Other kinds of skin involvement may occur in adolescents with LE, including telangiectatic erythema on the thenar and hypothenar eminences of the palms and the pulps of the fingers and diffuse erythema and telangiectasia of the cuticle, with erythematous, scaly macules occurring over the dorsa of the fingers between the knuckles (Fig. 9.55). A mottling of the extensor surface of the extremities, the

Fig. 9.54 Bullous SLE in child.

so-called *livedo reticularis*, occasionally occurs. Features of cutaneous vasculitis, such as subcutaneous nodules, splinter nail hemorrhages, purpuric acral infarcts, palpable purpura, and distal gangrene, may

Fig. 9.55 Classic hand findings in childhood SLE involving skin between knuckles. Contrast with involvement over the knuckles seen in childhood dermatomyositis demonstrated in Figures 9.61–9.63.

Fig. 9.57 Red-purple nodules on the upper arm of a girl with lupus profundus (panniculitis).

be seen (Fig. 9.56). Raynaud's phenomenon, a two-phase color change of the digit after cold exposure, with pallor and cyanosis, occurs in 35% of adolescents with systemic lupus erythematosus. Rarely, persistent, tender, red-purple nodules on the cheeks, proximal extremities, or trunk – which represent lupus panniculitic – will be seen in children (Fig. 9.57).[56] A distinct history of sun sensitivity may not be obtained in children with lupus, and careful questioning may be required to uncover photosensitivity.

Diagnosis depends on a constellation of clinical, pathologic, and serologic findings. Use of American Rheumatism Association (ARA) criteria for LE is recommended.[53,56]

The neonatal lupus syndrome (NLE) is characterized by congenital heart block or annular papulo-squamous skin lesions or both (Fig. 9.58).[61] Periorbital redness giving an 'owl-eye' appearance is characteristic (Fig.9.59).[62] Oval lesions that do not clear in the center are frequently seen (Fig. 9.60). Although affected infants do not meet ARA criteria for lupus, the association with maternal lupus or Sjögren's syndrome and the clinical skin lesions, skin pathology, and distinctive pattern of autoantibodies similar to those found in subacute cutaneous lupus permit the use of lupus in the diagnosis of this neonatal lupus syndrome. At delivery, 50% of the mothers of children with NLE will be asymptomatic. The skin lesions fade by 6–7 months of age, but the heart block will persist. Residual telangiectasia may persist for several years. In infants selected by cutaneous involvement, thrombocytopenia and hepatic disease were as frequent as cardiac disease and were more common in males with crusted skin lesions.[62]

Fig. 9.56 Vasculitis in childhood SLE. Note redness of thenar eminence and fingerpads with shallow erosions.

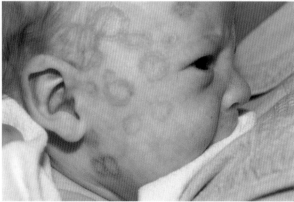

Fig. 9.58 Neonatal lupus syndrome. Five-week-old baby with annular papulosquamous lesions of the head and face.

Fig. 9.59 Charactistic 'owl-eye' periorbital involvement in NLE.

Fig. 9.60 Neonatal lupus syndrome. Four-week-old female with dozens of scaly, annular red macules on the forehead and cheeks and congenital heart block.

The most useful serologic test in the diagnosis of lupus is the fluorescent antinuclear antibody (ANA) test, which is positive in over 90% of children with LE.[56] Autoantibodies in LE are directed against a variety of nuclear components. The most specific is that directed against the nuclear acidic chromosomal proteins, such as the Sm antigen. It is very specific but is found in only 30% of patients. In addition to screening with a fluorescent ANA test, in some children in whom lupus is suspected an ANA profile in which immunodiffusion tests are done against soluble nuclear antigens may be performed. This is especially useful in detecting antibodies to Sjögren's syndrome A (SS-A) (Ro), which is a diagnostic marker for neonatal lupus syndrome and is found in 98% of reported babies.[61,62] A few babies will have autoantibodies to UI-RNP rather than anti-Ro.[61]

Depressed complement levels, especially the C4 level, are useful for detecting active vasculitis, particularly in the central nervous system and kidney. Direct immunofluorescence of skin biopsy specimens of involved skin is positive for granular deposits of IgG or C3 at the dermal–epidermal junction in 90% of patients. IgG deposits over basal keratinocytes are observed in subacute cutaneous lupus and neonatal lupus.[63]

The initial evaluation of patients with suspected LE should include the tests listed in Box 9.5.

In general, patients with discoid cutaneous lesions, subacute cutaneous lupus, or lupus panniculitis have a low incidence of disease in other organs, whereas those with the butterfly maculopapular eruption or vasculitis lesions are likely to have renal, central nervous system, or other vital organ involvement.[53]

Differential Diagnosis

Childhood dermatomyositis and lupus may present with similar cutaneous features. The photosensitive butterfly eruption may be seen in children with

---

Box 9.5 Initial laboratory evaluation of lupus erythematosus

Skin biopsy, formalin fixed for routine histologic study

Skin biopsy, frozen section, for immunofluorescence

Serum for antinuclear antibody and ANA profile

Serum for total hemolytic complement and complement components

Urinalysis

Complete blood cell count with differential and platelet count dermatomyositis or drug-induced photosensitivity, such as is seen with the phenothiazines, naproxen, or thiazide diuretics. A butterfly eruption may also be seen in polymorphous light eruption. Skin biopsy and immunofluorescence will be useful in distinguishing lupus erythematosus from these processes. The eruption may be scaly enough to consider psoriasis, lichen planus, or other papulosquamous disorders (see Box 9.2). Dermatophyte facial infection (tinea faciei) must be excluded by KOH examination of the scales.

Biopsy is necessary to differentiate discoid lesions of the face from psoriasis and lichen planus, and the discoid lesions of the scalp from other causes of circumscribed alopecia.

Drug-induced LE syndromes rarely cause cutaneous eruptions, but sometimes they may mimic LE. The drugs likely to produce LE syndromes are listed in Box 9.6. The livedo reticularis pattern is seen in dermatomyositis, scleroderma, and other collagen vascular diseases, as is Raynaud's phenomenon, palmar erythema, and cuticular telangiectasia.

Careful examination of the dorsa of the hands may help distinguish LE from dermatomyositis. In LE, scaly erythematous macules are seen between the knuckles on the dorsum of the hand, whereas in dermatomyositis, scaly macules or papules are seen over the knuckle pads. Compare Figure 9.55 with Figures 9.61–9.63.

The annular papulosquamous lesions of subacute cutaneous LE may mimic tinea corporis, erythema infectiosum, or pityriasis rosea, but a skin biopsy will distinguish.

The red-purple nodules of lupus panniculitis may be confused with vascular tumors or cutaneous lymphomas or leukemias.

Box 9.6 Drugs responsible for inducing lupus-like syndromes
High risk
Hydralazine
Procainamide
D-penicillamine
Practolol
Moderate risk
Isoniazid
Phenytoin
Ethosuximide
Propylthiouracil
Trimethadione

Fig. 9.61 Gottron's papules over the knuckles in juvenile dermatomyositis.

Fig. 9.62 Classic hand findings with involvement over knuckles in childhood dermatomyositis. Contrast with Figure 9.55 showing sparing of knuckles seen in childhood SLE.

Pathogenesis

Lupus erythematosus is associated with circulating immune complexes, which may account for many of the vasculitis features in the joints, kidneys, and central nervous system. In the skin there is an injury to epidermal basal cells with liquefaction degeneration, which may lead to dermal–epidermal separation.[63] A

Fig. 9.63 Hand findings in childhood dermatomyositis.

patchy accumulation of lymphocytes around dermal blood vessels and hair follicles is seen. These findings are found in acute, subacute, chronic (discoid), and neonatal skin lesions. In addition, discoid lupus shows epidermal atrophy and follicular plugs of scale.[63] Usually, no evidence of necrotizing vasculitis is found in the skin, although antigen-antibody complexes have been eluted from the skin. In lupus panniculitis, there is usually a dense lymphocytic infiltrate around subcutaneous vessels between fat lobules, without the superficial skin injury observed in other forms of cutaneous lupus.

The exact mechanism of skin injury and photosensitivity is unknown. A possible association with viruses or virus-induced tissue injury is suggested from animal models of LE-like diseases.

Treatment

It is beyond the scope of this book to discuss the treatment of systemic LE. The chronic cutaneous lesions respond to potent topical fluorinated glucocorticosteroids applied twice daily. In the discoid lupus form, response is slow, over many months. Hydroxychloroquine, 5 mg/kg/day, may be used if topical steroids alone are ineffective.[56] In children

treated with hydroxychloroquine, prior vision screening should be obtained by ophthalmologic consultation. Routine ophthalmologic and hematologic examination should be done throughout the treatment course.[56]

In children and adolescents with systemic involvement, skin lesions clear with immunosuppressive agents in the doses used to treat renal disease. Sometimes, skin lesions require additional topical therapy with potent or superpotent topical steroids for control.

Photoprotection should be a mainstay of therapy for cutaneous LE, even when photosensitivity is uncertain. Protective clothing and regular use of sunscreens are recommended.

Patient Education

Sun sensitivity should be discussed and the use of photoprotective agents strongly emphasized. Daily use of a sunscreen of at least SPF-30 is advised. In addition, it is advisable for the patient to avoid sun exposure between the hours of 10 a.m. and 4 p.m., during which time the majority of UVL reaches the earth's surface. The patient should be advised to wear a hat to protect the face from UV damage. Severe sunburn has resulted in systemic exacerbations of LE. Cosmetic coverings are helpful, both as sunscreens and for disguising unsightly skin lesions.

Follow-up Visits

After the initial visit, a visit in 2 weeks is useful for the evaluation of laboratory evidence, which may indicate potential systemic involvement. Often, adolescents presenting with acute symptoms such as fever, acute arthralgias, or renal disease must be hospitalized. It is important to remember that in 5–10% of those presenting with cutaneous lesions only, the disease may progress to involvement of internal organs. Thus, re-evaluation every 3 months is recommended.

DERMATOMYOSITIS
Clinical Features

The onset of most cases of childhood dermatomyositis is between 2 and 15 years.[64] The incidence is estimated as 0.5 per 100 000.[65,66] The most common presenting signs in childhood dermatomyositis are flat-topped red papules over the knuckles (Gottron's papules) (see Figs 9.61–9.63), a scaly rash over the elbows (Fig. 9.64) and knees, periungual erythema and telangiectasia (Fig. 9.65), periorbital edema with

Fig. 9.64 Dermatomyositis. Scaly, rosy-colored plaques over an elbow.

Fig. 9.65 Cuticular telangiectasia in dermatomyositis in adolescent male.

Fig. 9.66 Dermatomyositis. Purple-red discoloration of the eyelids.

Fig. 9.67 Dermatomyositis. Severe ulceration near the elbow with calcinosis cutis.

a violaceous hue of the eyelids (heliotrope) (Fig. 9.66), and malar erythema. A livedo reticularis pattern on the extremities may be prominent. The skin changes may precede, occur simultaneously with, or follow signs of muscle disease. Occasionally, the cutaneous features are present for months before muscle symptoms are noted.[64] Children with dermatomyositis appear ill, with low-grade fever, malaise, and anorexia noted.[66]

Weakness, with or without pain in the proximal muscles, is the most frequent symptom. Inability to run and climb stairs, easy fatigability during play, and inability to comb hair or reach upward may be presenting symptoms.[64,66] Difficulty swallowing secondary to pharyngeal muscle weakness may be seen.

As the disease slowly progresses, muscle weakness may be so profound as to make the child bedridden. Calcinosis of skin and muscle develops later in the course of the disease and becomes a major problem (Fig. 9.67).[66] Skin calcinosis is seen as crusted papules or plaques around joints or as nonhealing sores. Muscle calcification may result in contractures or severe muscular pain.

Differential Diagnosis

Lupus erythematosus is most often confused with dermatomyositis because of the facial photosensitive eruption. Examination of the dorsa of the hands (see the section on lupus, above) will help differentiate, as will muscle signs and symptoms. Muscle enzyme levels, particularly creatine phosphokinase (CPK), serum glutamate oxaloacetate transaminase (SGOT), and aldolase may be elevated and if dermatomyositis is expected they should be measured. Muscle biopsy, electromyography, ultrasonography, or magnetic resonance imaging may assist in the diagnosis.[66] Skin biopsy findings are not diagnostic but are consistent with a diagnosis of collagen vascular disease.

The scaly plaques on elbows and knees are often confused with psoriasis. In dermatomyositis the scale is thin, not thick, and there are associated muscle findings; the child appears ill in contrast to psoriasis.

The livedo reticularis pattern may also be found in periarteritis nodosa and lupus, and the cuticular telangiectasias are found in a number of collagen vascular diseases.

Pathogenesis

The mechanism of cutaneous injury is unknown.[66] Skin biopsies show edema of the upper dermis with a sparse perivascular mononuclear cell infiltrate, and immunofluorescent studies are usually non-specific. Children with dermatomyositis may have autoantibodies to aminoacyl t-rna such as Jo-1, and PM/SCL, or Mi-2 and have positive ANAs.[66]

Treatment

Systemic steroids, either high-dose intravenous pulsing or chronic oral therapy, and steroid-sparing drugs, such as intravenous immunoglobulin, azathioprine, methotrexate and mycophenil mofetil are the primary modes of therapy in dermatomyositis.[65,66] Aggressive early treatment of juvenile dermatomyositis decreases the incidence of calcinosis,[67,68] but once developed no single therapy has shown to be beneficial.[68] Skin lesions usually are controlled by systemic therapy, but occasionally potent or super-potent topical steroids will be required in addition. Hydroxychloroquine may also be helpful in treating resistant skin disease.[65]

Patient Education

It should be emphasized that a multidiscipline approach to care for children with dermatomyositis is required. Children should be treated in settings in which muscle disease specialists, dermatologists, and rheumatologists can coordinate the care, and physical therapy and nutritional support are available. Parents must recognize the serious and disabling nature of the condition, be prepared for long-term therapy, and be apprised of the potential complications of the disease and the long-term immunosuppressive therapy.

Follow-up Visits

If not hospitalized, the child should be seen weekly until good control of the disease is achieved.

Fig. 9.68 Lichen striatus. Linear, red, scaly papules extending down the flexor surface of a child.

Fig. 9.69 Lichen striatus lesions, which follow the lines of Blaschko.

Fig. 9.70 Pink linear plaque near thumb in early lichen striatus.

Fig. 9.71 Hypopigmented residual linear macules in healing lichen striatus.

Fig. 9.72 Lichen striatus extending down the digit.

Fig. 9.73 Lichen striatus on face of a girl.

LICHEN STRIATUS

Clinical Features

Lichen striatus is a disorder peculiar to childhood, characterized by linear, shiny, hypopigmented papules usually limited to one extremity (Fig. 9.68).[69] It does not follow vascular or neural structures, but tends to follow the lines of Blaschko (Fig. 9.69).[69] It is most common in ages 9 months to 6 years, with the majority of children being of preschool age.[69] Females are more commonly affected.[69] Although the lesions begin as pink or dull-red papules (Fig. 9.70), they quickly become hypopigmented (Fig. 9.71). Characteristically, the lesions begin on a buttock and spread down the leg, or begin on the shoulder and progress down the arm.[69] They may first be noticed distally, however. The lesion may extend down the digit (Fig. 9.72) and produce a linear nail dystrophy.[68] Occasionally, lesions will be noted on the face (Fig. 9.73). The lesions last 1 month to 3 years, with a mean of 6–12 months, and then spontaneously disappear.[69] Hypopigmented macules occur in 50% of cases and may persist for additional months.[69] Relapses of short duration have been noted after complete clearing.[69]

Differential Diagnosis

The linear lesions of lichen striatus are so characteristic that they are seldom confused with other lesions. The isomorphic phenomenon, seen in lichen planus, lichen nitidus, or psoriasis, may be confused with lichen striatus, but lesions will be present in other areas of the skin in these diseases. Epidermal birthmarks may also be confused for lichen striatus, but they are irregular on the surface rather than shiny and are present from birth, rather than being acquired later in life. Porokeratosis of Mibelli may be confused for lichen striatus, but it does not extend down an entire extremity. A skin biopsy will distinguish it from lichen striatus but is usually not required.

Pathogenesis

A chronic dermatitis is seen on histologic sections. It is thought to be an immune reaction to an aberrant skin clone secondary to somatic mutation.[69]

Treatment

Treatment is unnecessary. Topical steroids may be symptomatically helpful but do not influence the course of the disease.[69]

Patient Education

The benign nature and complete resolution of these lesions should be emphasized.

Follow-up Visits

A follow-up visit in 4 weeks is useful to examine for skin lesions in other areas to rule out other papulosquamous conditions.

Fig. 9.75 Porokeratosis of Mibelli on cheek of boy.

POROKERATOSIS OF MIBELLI
Clinical Features

Porokeratosis of Mibelli may appear as a segmental single lesion or as a group of lesions that may mimic lichen striatus or an epidermal nevus (Fig. 9.74).[70] The condition occurs more frequently in males and has a predilection for the face (Fig. 9.75), neck, forearms, and hands, although the knees (Fig. 9.76), buttocks, and feet may also occasionally be involved. Individual lesions appear as crater-like areas on the skin with a scaly, irregular, oval border.[70] The crateriform area may measure 5–50 mm in diameter, and several craters may be grouped together. The most important diagnostic feature of porokeratosis of Mibelli is the appearance of a scaly border in which a double row of scales surmounted by a furrow is observed. Diagnosis is by biopsy of the border of the lesion.

Fig. 9.74 Porokeratosis of Mibelli. Linear, scaly plaque with moatlike border in a 9-year-old child.

Fig. 9.76 Porokeratosis of the knee of a child.

Differential Diagnosis

Porokeratosis of Mibelli may be confused with lichen striatus or with epidermal nevi. However, in contrast to lichen striatus, lesions are often segmental and do not completely extend down an extremity. In contrast to epidermal nevi, they are never present at birth but develop later in childhood, and do not have as verrucous a surface. Biopsy is often useful in distinguishing among these possibilities.

Pathogenesis

The characteristic biopsy finding demonstrates focal areas of parakeratosis within the epidermis and, if proper sectioning of the double ridge has been obtained, a pair of focal parakeratotic columns with a normal or slightly thinned epidermis sandwiched between them.[70] Sparse or moderate inflammation may be seen beneath the parakeratotic columns. It is believed that this represents hyperplastic clones of keratinocytes, whose phenotypic expression is the result of activation by external trigger factors.[70] This would explain its generalized nature in immuno-suppressed patients or in patients with chronic sun damage.[70]

Treatment

The lesions of porokeratosis may produce some concern about cosmetic appearance in the parents, but no satisfactory therapy has been developed. Progressive growth may occur over 2–3 years, and some spontaneous resolutions have been reported. Case reports demonstrate successful treatment with cryo-surgery, 5-fluorouracil and salicylic acid, tretinoin and imiquimod,[71-74] but an adequate form of treatment for all cases remains elusive.[71]

Patient Education

The parents must be told that the cause is unknown. They must be warned against rushing into cosmetic surgery for improvement because the scarring after surgery may be worse than the lesion itself. The advantages of a conservative approach to such lesions should be emphasized. Malignant degeneration in porokeratosis may occur in less than 10% of patients, with the average time to development being 36 years.[75]

Follow-up Visits

Families should be instructed of the chronic nature of the disease and long-term risk for malignant degeneration.

JUVENILE PITYRIASIS RUBRA PILARIS
Clinical Features

Juvenile pityriasis rubra pilaris (JPRP) has its onset in the first or second decade of life.[76,77] The first sign is commonly salmon-colored diffuse thickening of the palms and soles (Figs 9.77, 9.78), with exaggerated scaling in the fissures (Fig. 9.79).[76,77] The involvement extends beyond the dorsopalmar and dorso-plantar junctions, often involving the knuckle pads (Figs 9.80, 9.81).

The condition may remain restricted to the palms and soles, but in the majority of children it will involve other areas of skin, such as circumscribed salmon-colored plaques of elbows and knees with a fine scale. The disease may also produce 2–6 mm red follicular papules, particularly over the distal extremities

Fig. 9.77 Salmon-colored scaly palms in childhood pityriasis rubra pilaris.

Fig. 9.78 Salmon-colored thickening of the sole in childhood pityriasis rubra pilaris.

Fig. 9.79 Scale and fissures on sole of child with JPRP.

Fig. 9.80 Involvement extending to the dorsa of the foot and toes in childhood pityriasis rubra pilaris.

Fig. 9.81 Preteen child with involvement of top of foot as well as soles in JPRP.

Fig. 9.82 Red follicular papules in childhood pityriasis rubra pilaris.

(Fig. 9.82). Widespread involvement of the trunk and progression to exfoliative erythroderma may rarely occur.[76] One feature frequently observed is the pre-sence of an area of uninvolved skin entrapped within a large plaque of involved skin (Fig. 9.83).[76] These so-called 'islands of sparing' were once considered a

Fig. 9.83 Red plaques on the trunk with 'island of sparing' in childhood pityriasis rubra pilaris.

diagnostic feature, but most now believe this can be seen in drug eruptions, psoriasis, and other conditions.[76] Despite widespread involvement, the child with JPRP usually has minimal to no itching. Scalp involvement has been reported, as has an asymptomatic white, lacy change of the oral mucosa. Most clinicians appreciate that a wide spectrum of disease may be observed, and as the condition evolves over many weeks, different skin sites may be affected.[76] The condition tends to be chronic, but most children clear spontaneously within 1 year.[76]

Differential Diagnosis

All of the papulosquamous eruptions may be considered in the differential diagnosis at some point (see Box 9.2). Psoriasis and guttate parapsoriasis are the most likely to be confused. Drug eruptions may mimic JPRP, and the involvement of the palms and soles may mimic poststreptococcal desquamation. However, the prolonged duration of JPRP and the characteristic salmon-colored thickenings should lead to a suspicion of JPRP. Skin biopsies are not diagnostic, but may suggest the diagnosis because of the 'moundlike' parakeratosis around follicular openings accompanied by hyperkeratosis and irregular acanthosis.[76]

Pathogenesis

The cause of the condition is unknown. A rare early onset form with an autosomal dominant pattern of inheritance has been reported.[76] Thickening of the epidermis, with increased keratinocyte proliferation and differentiation, is found.

Treatment

Childhood JPRP is quite difficult to treat. It is unresponsive to topical steroids and phototherapy.[76] Some children may respond to topical calcipotriene.[77] Oral retinoids, such as isotretinoin and etretinate have been successful.[75,76] Methotrexate has been used for refractory disease, but should be avoided in childhood because spontaneous remission is seen. Children unresponsive to topical calcipotriene or with extensive symptomatic disease should be treated with a 4–5 month trial of isotretinoin, 1 mg/kg/day. Management should be done by an experienced dermatologist.

Patient Education

Patients and parents should understand that this is a condition that can be quite persistent, and therapeutic responses are slow. One should state that the cause is unknown, and the therapy available treats the epidermal proliferation and not the triggering factors. The side effects of the systemic agent chosen should be carefully explained, and the risks and benefits of each therapy discussed.

Follow-up Visits

Follow-up visits should be at 2-week intervals until the response to therapy and side effects are determined. It is usually not necessary to treat until every skin area is cleared. If using retinoids, the clinician should provide a 'drug holiday' after 4 months of treatment.

REFERENCES

1. Krueger GG, Duvic M. Epidemiology of psoriasis: clinical issues. J Invest Dermatol 1994; 102:S14–S18.
2. Krueger G, Ellis CN. Psoriasis – recent advances in understanding its pathogenesis and treatment. J Am Acad Dermatol 2005; 53:S94–S100.
3. Rogers M. Childhood psoriasis. Curr Opin Pediatr 2002; 14:404–409.
4. Atherton DI, Kahana M, Russell-Jones R. Naevoid psoriasis. Br J Dermatol 1989; 120:837–841.
5. Matsuoka Y, Okada N, Yoshikawa K. Familial cases of psoriasis vulgaris and pustulosis palmaris et plantaris. Int J Dermatol 1993; 20:308–310.
6. Patrizi A, Bardozzi F, Neri I, et al. Psoriasiform acral dermatitis: a peculiar clinical presentation of psoriasis in children. Pediatr Dermatol 1999; 16:439–443.
7. Ivker RA, Grin-Jorgensen CM, Vega VK et al. Infantile generalized pustular psoriasis associated with lytic lesions of bone. Pediatr Dermatol 1993. 10:277–282.

8. Biondi-Oriente C, Scarpa R, Oriente P. Prevalence and clinical features of juvenile psoriatic arthritis in 425 psoriatic patients. Acta Derm Venereol Suppl (Stockh) 1994; 186:109–110.

9. Roberton DM, Abral DA, Malleson PN, et al. Juvenile psoriatic arthritis: follow-up and evaluation of diagnostic criteria. J Rheumatol 1996; 23:166–170.

10. Dando TM, Wellington K. Topical tazarotene: a review of its use in the treatment of plaque psoriasis. Am J Clin Dermatol 2005; 6:255–272.

11. Davison SC, Allen MH, Mallon E, et al. Contrasting patterns of streptococcal superantigen-induced T-cell proliferation in guttate vs. plaque psoriasis. Br J Dermatol 2001; 145:245–251.

12. Valdimarsson H, Sigmundsdottir H, Jonsdottir I. Is psoriasis induced by streptococcal superantigens and maintained by M-protein-specific T cells that cross-react with keratin? Clin Exp Immunol 1997; 107(suppl):21–24.

13. Leman J, Burden D. Psoriasis in children: a guide to its diagnosis and management. Paediatr Drugs 2001; 3:673–680.

14. Burden AD. Management of psoriasis in childhood. Clin Exp Dermatol 1999; 24:341–345.

15. Singh S, Reddy DC, Pandey SS. Topical therapy for psoriasis with the use of augmented betamethasone and calcitriene on alternate weeks. J Am Acad Dermatol 2000; 43:61–65.

16. Ashcroft DM, Po AL, Williams HC, et al. Systematic review of comparative efficacy and tolerability of calcipotriol in treating chronic plaque psoriasis. Br Med J 2000; 320:963–967.

17. Wall AR, Poyner TF, Menday AP. A comparison of treatment with dithranol and calcipotriol on the clinical severity and quality of life in patients with psoriasis. Br J Dermatol 1998; 139:1005–1011.

18. Tzung TY, Wu JC, Hsu NJ, et al. Comparison of tazarotene 0.1% gel plus petrolatum once daily versus calcipotriol 0.005% ointment twice daily in the treatment of plaque psoriasis. Acta Derm Venereol 2005; 85:236–239.

19. Reygagne P, Mrowietz U, Decroix J, et al. Clobetasol proprionate shampoo 0.05% and calcipotriol solution 0.005%: a randomized comparison of efficacy in subjects with scalp psoriasis. J Dermatolog Treat 2005; 16:31–36.

20. Duweb G, Alhaddar J, Abuhamid M. Calcipotriol solution in scalp psoriasis. Int J Tissue React 2006; 27:163–166.

21. Penven K, Leroy D, Verneuil L, et al. Evaluation of Vaseline oil applied prior to UVB TL01 phototherapy in the treatment of psoriasis. Photodermatol Photoimmunol Photodmed 2005; 21:138–141.

22. Bandow GD, Koo JY. Narrow-band ultraviolet B radiation: a review of the current literature. Int J Dermatol 2004; 43:555–561.

23. Nijsten TE, Stern RS. The increased risk of skin cancer is persistent after discontinuation of psoralen+ultraviolet A: a cohort study. J Invest Dermatol 2003; 121:ix–x.

24. Weischer M, Blum A, Eberhard F, et al. No evidence for increased skin cancer risk in psoriasis patients treated with broadband or narrowband UVB phototherapy: a first retrospective study. Acta Derm Venereol 2004; 84:370–374.

25. Lebwohl M, Drake L, Menter A, et al. Consensus conference: acitretin in combination with UVB or PUVA in the treatment of psoriasis. J Am Acad Dermatol 2001; 45:544–553.

26. Molin L. Topical calcipotriol combined with phototherapy for psoriasis. The results of two randomized trials and a review of the literature. Calcipotriol-UVB Study Group. Dermatology 1999; 198:375–381.

27. Carrozza P, Hausermann P, Nestle FO, et al. Clinical efficacy of narrow-band UVB (311 nm) combined with dithranol in psoriasis: an open pilot study. Dermatology 2000; 200:35–39.

28. Behrens S, Grundmann-Kallmann M, Schiener R, et al. Combination phototherapy of psoriasis with narrow-band UVB irradiation and topical tazarotene gel. J Am Acad Dermatol 2000; 42:493–495.

29. Owen CM, Chalmers RJ O'sullivan T, et al. A systematic review of antistreptococcal intervention for guttate and chronic plaque psoriasis. Br J Dermatol 2001; 145:886–890.

30. Dogra S, Handee S, Kanwar AJ. Methotrexate in severe childhood psoriasis. Pediatr Dermatol 2004; 21:283–286.

31. Papoutsaki M, Costanzo A, Mazzotta T, et al. Etanercept for the treatment of severe childhood psoriasis. Br J Dermatol 2006; 154:181–184.

32. Rich SJ, Bello-Quinter CE. Advancements in the treatment of psoriasis: role of biologic agents. J Manag Care Pharm 2004; 10:318–325.

33. Gonzalez LM, Allen R, Janniger CK, et al. Pityriasis rosea: an important papulosquamous disorder. Int J Dermatol 2005; 44:757–770.

34. Chuh AAT, Chan HHL, Zawar V. Is human herpesvirus 7 the causative agent of pityriasis rosea? A critical review. Int J Dermatol 2004; 43:870–876.

35. Baughn RE, Musher DM. Secondary syphilitic lesions. Clin Microbiol Rev 2005; 18:206–216.

36. Romani J, Puig L, Fernandez-Figueras MT, et al. Pityriasis lichenoides in children: clinicopathologic review of 22 patients. Pediatr Dermatol 1998; 15:1–6.

37. Miyamoto T, Takayama N, Kitada S, et al. Febrile uceronecrotic Mucha-Habermann disease: a case report and a review of the literature. J Clin Pathol 2003; 56:795–797.

38. Njisten T, Curiel-Lewandrowski C, Kadin ME. Lymphomatoid papulosis in children: a retrospective-cohort study of 35 cases. Arch Dermatol 2004; 140:306–312.

39. Fink-Puches R, Chott A, Ardigo M, et al. The spectrum of cutaneous lymphomas in patients less than 20 years of age. Pediatr Dermatol 2004; 21:525–533.

40. Truhan AP, Hebert AA, Esterly NB. Pityriasis lichenoides in children: therapeutic response to erythromycin. J Am Acad Dermatol 1986; 15:66–70.

41. Tay YK, Morelli JG, Weston WL. Experience with UVB phototherapy in children. Pediatr Dermatol 1996; 13:406–409.

42. Handa S, Sahoo B. Childhood lichen planus: a study of 87 cases. Int J Dermatol 2002; 41:423–427.

43. Sharma R, Maheshwari V; Childhood lichen planus: a report of fifty cases. Pediatr Dermatol 1998; 16:345–348.

44. Sanchez-Perez I, Rios Buceta L, Fraga J, et al. Lichen planus with lesions on the palms and/or soles: prevalence and clinicopathological study of 36 patients. Br J Dermatol 2000; 142:310–314.

45. Laeijendecker R, Van Joost T, Tank B, et al. Oral lichen planus in childhood. Pediatr Dermatol 2005; 22:299–304.

46. Joshi RK, Abanmi A, Ohman SG, et al. Lichen planus of the nails presenting as trachyonychia. Int J Dermatol 1993; 32:54–55.

47. Peluso AM, Tosti I, Piraccini BM, et al. Lichen planus limited to the nails in childhood: a case report and literature review. Pediatr Dermatol 1993; 10:36–39.

48. Tilly JJ, Drolet BA, Esterly NB. Lichenoid eruptions in children. J Am Acad Dermatol 2004; 51:606–624.

49. Soroush V, Gurevitch AW, Peng SK; Generalized lichen nitidus: a case report and literature review; Cutis 1999; 64:135–136.

50. Carrozzo M, Brancatello F, Dametto E, et al. Hepatitis C virus-associated oral lichen planus: is the geographical heterogeneity related to HLA-DR6. J Oral Pathol Med 2005; 34:204–208.

51. Nagao Y, Sata M. Hepatitis C virus and lichen planus. J Gastroenterol Hepatol 2004; 19:1101–1113.

52. Chuang TY, Stitle L, Brashear R, et al. Hepatitis C and lichen planus: a case control study of 340 patients. J Am Acad Dermatol 1999; 41:787–789.

53. Faller G Thomson PD, Kala UK, et al. Demographics and presenting clinical features of childhood systemic lupus erythematosus. S Afr Med J 2005; 95:424–427.

54. Bader-Meunier B, Armengaud JB, Haddad E, et al. Initial presentation of childhood-onset systemic lupus erythematosus: a French multicenter study. J Pediatr 2005; 146:648–653.

55. Klippel JH. Systemic lupus erythematosus: demographics, prognosis and outcome. J Rheumatol 1997; 48:67–71.

56. DeSilva TN, Kress DW. Management of collagen vascular diseases in childhood, Dermatol Clin 1998; 16:579–592.

57. Van Gysel D, de Waard-van der Spek FB, Oranje AP. Childhood discoid lupus erythematosus: a report of five new cases and review of the literature. J Eur Acad Dermatol 2002; 17:731–732.

58. Amato L, Coronella G, Berti S, et al. Subacute cutaneous lupus erythematosus in childhood. Pediatr Dermatol 2003; 20:31–34.

59. Parodi A, Caproni M, Cardinali C, et al.Clinical, histological and immunopathological features of 58 patients with subacute cutaneous lupus erythematosus: a review by the Italian group of immunodermatology. Dermatology 2000; 200:6–10.

60. Buckley D, Barnes L. Childhood subacute cutaneous lupus erythematosus associated with homozygous complement 2 deficiency. Pediatr Dermatol 1995; 12:327–336.

61. Lee LA. Neonatal lupus: clinical features and management. Paediatr Drugs 2004; 6:71–78.

62. Weston WL, Morelli JG, Lee LA. The clinical spectrum of anti-Ro-positive cutaneous neonatal lupus erythematosus. J Am Acad Dermatol 1999; 40:675–681.

63. David-Bajar KM, Bennion SD DeSpain JD, et al. Clinical, histologic and immunofluorescent distinctions between subacute cutaneous lupus erythematosus and discoid lupus erythematosus. J Invest Dermatol 1992; 99:251–257.

64. Peloro TM, Miller F III, Hahn TA, et al. Juvenile dermatomyositis: a retrospective review of a 30-year experience. J Am Acad Dermatol 2001; 45:28–34.

65. Callen JP. Collagen vascular diseases. J Am Acad Dermatol 2004; 51:427–439.

66. Dalakas MC, Hohlfeld R. Polymyositis and dermatomyositis. Lancet 2003; 362:971–982.

67. Fisler RE, Liang MG, Fuhlbrigge RC, et al. Aggressive management of juvenile dermatomyositis results in improved outcome and decreased incidence of calcinosis. J Am Acad Dermatol 2002; 47:505–511.

68. Boulman N, Slobodin G, Rozenbaum M, et al. Calcinosis in rheumatic diseases. Semin Arthritis Rheum 2005; 34:805–812.

69. Patrizi A, Neri I, Fiorentini C, et al. Lichen striatus: clinical and laboratory features of 115 children. Pediatr Dermatol 2004; 21:197–206.

70. Schamroth JM, Zlotogorski A, Gilead L. Porokeratosis of Mibelli: overview and review of the literature. Acta Dermato-venerealogica 1997; 77:207–213.

71. Dereli T, Ozyurt S, Ozturk G. Porokeratosis of Mibelli: successful treatment with cryosurgery. J Dermatol 2004; 31:223–227.

72. Danby W. Treatment of porokeratosis with fluorouracil and salicylic acid under occlusion. Dermatol Online J 2003; 9:33.

73. Agrawal SK, Gandhi V, Madan V, et al. Topical tretinoin in Indian male with zosteriform porokeratosis. Int J Dermatol 2003; 42:919–920.

74. Harrison S, Sinclair R. Porokeratosis of Mibelli: successful treatment with topical 5% imiquimod cream. Australas J Dermatol 2003; 44:281–283.

75. Maubec E, Duvillard P, Margulis A, et al. Common skin cancers in porokeratosis. Br J Dermatol 2005; 152:1389–1391.

76. Albert MR, Mackool BT. Pityriasis rubra pilaris. Int J Dermatol 1999; 38:1–11.

77. Thiers BH. The use of topical calcipotriene/calcipotriol in conditions other than plaque-type psoriasis. J Am Acad Dermatol 1997; 37:S69–S71.

Sun Sensitivity

Sun exposure in children may result in sunburn or sun-induced dermatoses in the skin. Abnormal reactions occur in the skin areas predominantly exposed to sunlight: the face, ears, back of the neck, 'V' of the neck, and extensor surfaces of the arms and hands. Sun sensitivity is suspected when the distribution of the cutaneous eruption is limited to these areas. The majority of children with sun sensitivity will have one of the idiopathic photodermatoses, erythropoietic protoporphyria (EPP), or lupus erythematosus (LE) (see Ch. 9). These conditions should be considered in every child with sun sensitivity.

SUNBURN

The acute result of excessive sun exposure is sunburn. Sunburn readily occurs in fair-skinned children, who have less melanin protection than darker-skinned children (Fig. 10.1) Intense sun exposure can produce sunburn in children with dark skin as well (Table 10.1). Any child who seeks medical assistance because of sunburn should be questioned about exposure to agents that make individuals sun sensitive.

Clinical Features

Erythema and skin tenderness begin 30 minutes to 4 hours after sun exposure, depending on the intensity of the exposure and the degree of the child's natural protection against the sun. They peak at 24 hours and may last up to 72 hours.[1] On the face, sunburn is usually most prominent on the nose and cheeks, with sun-protected areas under the nose, chin, and upper eyelids uninvolved (Fig. 10.2). On the extremities and trunk, protective clothing may produce sharp borders between burned and nonburned areas (Figs 10.3–10.6, see also Fig. 10.1). After intense sun exposure, edema and blistering occur (see Figs 10.2, 10.6). Some 2–7 days

after intense sun exposure, 5–10 cell layers of epidermis are shed in one piece as a white scale (desquamation). With acute sunburn, sleep is often disturbed because of the tenderness of the skin. Extensive sunburn causes a reduction in the sweating rate and may contribute to collapse from heatstroke, especially in infants under 6 months (Fig. 10.7). Sunburn over large areas of the body in a child may result in fever, headache, and fatigue.

Differential Diagnosis

It is occasionally difficult to determine in children what constitutes overexposure to sunlight (Box 10.1). In such a case one should consider the presence of a photosensitizing agent that would induce a sunburn reaction in an unusually short period (5–30 minutes of sun exposure). Agents that cause photosensitivity are listed in Chapter 18. Most have been associated with photosensitivity in adults, but they may also occur in children. Burning pain in the skin after 5 minutes of sun exposure should suggest EPP. In contrast, sunburn alone requires at least 30 minutes to produce symptoms. Rapid onset of sunburn and persistent sunburn reactions may be early clues to xeroderma pigmentosum (XP). In LE, the eruption occurs 1–7 days after sun exposure and is characterized by scaling and erythema, which is persistent for several weeks. Many viral exanthems appear primarily or are exacerbated in sun-exposed areas (see Ch. 8). The laboratory evaluation of photosensitivity, listed in Box 10.2, should be considered when determining the differential diagnosis of sun sensitivity.

Pathogenesis

The tanning or burning rays from the sun represent ultraviolet radiation. The exact cause of ultraviolet radiation damage to the skin is unknown, but it is thought to be a combination of direct effects on DNA,

Fig. 10.1 Sunburn in child with phototype I skin (always burns, never tans). Such children are often redheads with freckles.

Table 10.1 Skin photoypes and sun sensitivity

Skin Type	Description
I	Fair skin, always burns, never tans
II	Fair skin, usually burns, sometimes tans
III	Lightly pigmented, usually tans, sometimes burns
IV	Pigmented, always tans, never burns
V	Moderately pigmented, never burns
VI	Heavily pigmented (black) skin

generation of toxic oxygen species, the production of inflammatory mediators, and an inflammatory infiltrate of neutrophils and T lymphocytes.[1,2] Tanning is a protective response to ultraviolet radiation. Thus, tanning is always a sign of ultraviolet injury to the

Fig. 10.2 Acute sunburn of the face of the child. Note sparing of the upper eyelids, nasolabial folds, beneath the nose, and under the hair. Note the red papules of sweat duct obstruction.

Fig. 10.3 Acute sunburn with early vesiculation. Note sharp demarcation line at shoulder due to protective clothing.

Fig. 10.4 Acute sunburn on arm of child. Note the sharp demarcation due to protective clothing.

Fig. 10.5 Sunburn on back of adolescent. Note uninvolved skin protected by clothing.

Fig. 10.6 Sunburn with vesiculation on neck of adolescent.

Fig. 10.7 Sunburn in 1-month-old infant with heat exhaustion.

skin. Ultraviolet radiation effects are cumulative as well, with many types of cutaneous cells retaining the additive effects of years of radiation exposure.[3] Long-term effects are expressed as fine and deep wrinkling; scaly, red patches (actinic keratoses); and, ultimately, skin cancer formation.[3,4] Basal and squamous cell carcinomas of the skin are associated with chronic exposure to ultraviolet radiation, whereas malignant melanoma is more commonly seen in those patients with a history of multiple severe blistering sunburns.[5]

In acute ultraviolet injury the skin changes noted reflect immediate effects of radiation damage.[1,2] The first changes noted after prolonged sun exposure are vasodilation of the dermal blood vessels. There is evidence to implicate prostaglandin E_2 as a mediator of a portion of the pain and erythema of sunburn, but total inhibition of ultraviolet radiation-induced prostaglandin formation only inhibits sunburn by 30%.[2] Nitric oxide also plays a fundamental role in early

Box 10.1 Differential diagnosis of sun sensitivity

Sunburn

Idiopathic photodermatoses

Erythropoietic protoporphyria

Lupus erythematosus

Dermatomyositis

Photosensitizing drugs

Viral exanthems

Xeroderma pigmentosum

Box 10.2 Laboratory evaluation of photosensitivity

Red blood cell fluorescence

Red blood cell protoporphyrin levels

Antinuclear antibody and antinuclear antibody profile

Skin biopsy

sunburn.[1] Vitamins C and E given together orally for at least 1 week before ultraviolet radiation to the skin also decrease sunburn, presumably by acting as free radical scavengers.[6] Metabolic changes then occur within epidermal cells, and individual epidermal cells within the midepidermis, demonstrate clumping of tonofilaments and abnormalities of cytoplasmic and nuclear shape, producing the rounded, so-called *sunburn cell*.[7] Such cells lose their epidermal cell attachments; with increased sun exposure, a large number of these cells appear within the epidermis and produce an intraepidermal blister cavity.

Treatment

The pain and erythema of sunburn can be relieved by the use of wet dressings or cool compresses. Inhibitors of prostaglandin synthesis, such as aspirin or indometacin, may modify sunburn if given within 6 hours of exposure. There is no convincing evidence that vitamins C and E or systemic or topical glucocorticosteroids are beneficial in the treatment of established sunburn.[8] Topical anesthetics, such as benzocaine, are sensitizing and transient in their relief of pain and thus are not recommended. *Sunburn is 100% preventable, and prevention is by far superior to treatment.*

Patient Education

Depending on occupation, a majority of lifetime sun exposure is received before the age of 18 years. Thus, it is extremely important to protect infants, children,

Box 10.3 Sunscreen sun protection factor

$$SPF = \frac{\text{MED of sunscreened skin}}{\text{MED of unprotected skin}}$$

MED, minimal erythema dose, i.e. the minimal amount of UVB energy required to produce erythema to human skin.

Box 10.4 Recommendations for sunscreen use in children

Use a broad-spectrum sunscreen with UVB SPF of 30 or higher

Select a waterproof sunscreen preparation

Apply prior to sun exposure

Reapply every 1–2 hours

Box 10.5 Types of available sunscreens

UVB protection
PABA (*p*-aminobenzoic acid) and its derivatives

Cinnamates

Salicylates

Combinations of above ingredients

UVA protection
Dibenzoylmethane derivatives

UVB plus UVA protection
Benzophenones

Anthranilates

Physical agents that block light

and adolescents against sun exposure. Sun protection habits should be formed at an early age, because adolescents either do not realize or do not admit that they are sun sensitive, and they are likely to be non-compliant.[9] Also, many parents do not recognize the degree of sun sensitivity of their children. Infants younger than 6 months should not be subjected to sun exposure because of the decreased sweating rate and the likelihood of heatstroke.[10] For those older than 6 months, mid-day sun avoidance is still the best method of sun protection. If this cannot be done on a given day, clothing, natural shade, and umbrellas provide good sun protection. Special sun-protective clothing is also available, as are laundry additives which increase clothing sun protection levels.[11,12] Sunscreen agents with SPF (sun protection factor) of 30 or higher are recommended as an adjunct to other sun-protective measures (Boxes 10.3–10.5).[13] Because of the increasing evidence that ultraviolet A (UVA)

radiation is also damaging to the skin, many sunscreens now contain agents that block both ultraviolet B (UVB) and UVA (see Box 10.5).[14] Physical sun blocks, such as zinc oxide pastes and titanium dioxide, have become more cosmetically acceptable and are effective sun-protective agents. It must be remembered that sunburn is a gross sign of sun damage, and that cellular damage to the skin can occur even with the use of SPF-15 sunscreens or higher.[13,14] These creams and lotions should be applied to the skin prior to sun exposure. Sunscreens should be used throughout the spring, summer, and fall months and during the winter in sunny climates. Although local reactions to sunscreens are common, these reactions are mostly of the irritant type and not allergic; if allergic reactions occur, they are more frequently caused by the sunscreen vehicle and not the active ingredient.[15] Sun avoidance, such as planning outdoor activities before 10 a.m. and after 4 p.m., is preferable. Sunscreens should not be used to increase the amount of time spent in the mid-day sun. For a Patient Education Sheet on Sun Protection, see CD-ROM.

Follow-up Visits

Follow-up visits are unnecessary.

Box 10.6 Types of idiopathic photodermatoses

Papular polymorphous light eruption

Juvenile spring eruption (hydroa aestivale)

Actinic prurigo

Hydroa vacciniforme

Solar urticaria

Fig. 10.8 Erythematous papules and plaques in a 9-year-old male with papular polymorphic light eruption.

Fig. 10.9 Papular PMLE in a fair-skinned girl.

IDIOPATHIC PHOTODERMATOSES

Clinical Features

The idiopathic photodermatoses are a group of sun-sensitive conditions that may be separated by distinct clinical patterns. Five major types are reported (Box 10.6).

Papular polymorphous light eruption (PMLE) is the most common type.[16] The process begins in the spring and improves throughout the summer. In 75% of patients, onset of the disease is sudden, occurs within the first 3 decades of life, and affects predominantly females. New lesions appear within hours to days of sun exposure, remain 7–10 days, and usually heal without scarring. The clinical lesions are discrete erythematous papules and plaques (Figs 10.8, 10.9), occurring in sun-exposed areas. For unknown reasons, not all sun-exposed skin is affected. The majority of patients improve with age, and in some patients the disease may subside totally.[16]

Juvenile spring eruption (hydroa aestivale) is described in children of European descent, mainly boys aged 5–12 years.[17] Its prevalence in primary school-aged males in Dunedin, New Zealand is 12%.[18] It characteristically begins as 2–3 mm discrete papules or vesicles on the ears and cheeks of fair-skinned children. The episode lasts 1 week and reappears the next spring (Fig. 10.10). A small percentage (22%) of patients with juvenile spring eruption will at other times in their lives develop lesions more typical of plaque-type polymorphous light eruption, and some authorities consider it a localized variant of polymorphous light eruption.[17]

Actinic prurigo (Hutchinson's summer prurigo) is seen predominantly in Native Americans of the central plains of the United states and Canada and in Central and South America, although it has been described in other ethnicities.[19] Females predominate 2:1. It begins as a dermatitis predominantly occurring on the face and extensor surface of the forearms of school-age children. The lesions characteristically start in the early spring, when sufficient sunlight energy reaches the earth's surface. Lesions usually occur by age 5 years. The initial eruption consists of an itchy, acute facial or forearm dermatitis with edematous papules and vesicles (Figs 10.11, 10.12). As the spring progresses, the dermatitis becomes subacute, with crusting on the surface and epidermal thickening or lichenification (Fig. 10.13). Papular lesions may predominate on the face (Fig. 10.14). In the summer the eruption may spontaneously clear, to recur again the next spring. Some very sun-sensitive children will have the eruption throughout the year. It is characteristic that several patches of skin are involved, with uninvolved areas of skin in between. In Native

Fig. 10.10 Vesicles and crusts on the tops of the ears in a child with juvenile spring eruption.

Fig. 10.11 Actinic prurigo. Papules and lichenification of cheeks of Native American boy.

Fig. 10.12 Polymorphous light eruption. Photodermatitis of a Native American child, with vesicles and crusting of the face at springtime onset.

Fig. 10.13 Chronic polymorphous light eruption with lichenification by midsummer.

Fig. 10.14 Facial papules in girl with PMLE.

Fig. 10.15 Redness and chronic scaling of lower lip (actinic cheilitis) in Native American boy.

Americans a chronic cheilitis of the lower lip and conjunctivitis is common[19,20] (Fig. 10.15), and a family history of the disease is often obtained.

Hydroa vacciniforme is characterized by a few discrete, deep-seated vesicles on the cheeks, ears, or nose that heal with scarring (Fig. 10.16).[21] They are frequently persistent, lasting up to 4 weeks, and more episodes may occur with further sun exposure. Rarely, the eye may be affected with conjunctival injection, photophobia, lacrimation, and corneal ulceration.[22] This is the rarest of all forms of polymorphous light eruption. A severe hydroa vacciniforme-like eruption with systemic symptoms is associated with Epstein-Barr virus and lymphoid malignancies.[23]

Solar urticaria is an uncommon idiopathic photodermatosis and an uncommon cause of urticaria. Patients present with urticaria acutely after sun exposure (Fig. 10.17). The disease rarely presents before late adolescence.[24]

Fig. 10.16 Deep-seated vesicle on the ear of a child with hydroa vacciniforme.

Fig. 10.17 Solar urticaria. Wheal induced by sunlamp on back of hand of child.

Differential Diagnosis

Atopic dermatitis, in addition to other photosensitive states, may mimic idiopathic photodermatoses (see Box 10.1). During hot weather, sweating in children with atopic dermatitis may induce itching and dermatitis on the face and sun-exposed areas. A family history of atopic dermatitis, and the finding of flexural dermatitis in addition to photo-accentuated dermatitis, are useful differentiating features. Acute sensitivity to airborne substances may also lead to the appearance of a contact dermatitis predominantly on sun-exposed areas. In airborne contact dermatitis, the upper eyelids are usually involved, in contrast to polymorphous light eruption. LE, EPP, dermatophyte infections of the face, and sunburn are likely to be confused. Laboratory tests listed in Box 10.2 should be considered. Photodermatitis caused by drugs characteristically produces a diffuse involvement of sun-exposed areas, rather than the patchy areas of dermatitis seen with polymorphous light eruption. Solar urticaria must be differentiated from other causes of urticaria.

EPP and XP have an onset in early infancy rather than childhood, and they may have symptoms out of proportion to skin changes. They usually do not develop dermatitis-like changes.

Pathogenesis

The mechanism of any form of idiopathic photodermatosis is unknown, although actinic prurigo is most likely an autosomal dominant disorder.[25] Patients with idiopathic photodermatosis are generally more likely to be sensitive to both UVA and UVB, but may also be sensitive to either alone.[26] The biochemical changes responsible for initiating inflammation after sun exposure are unknown.

Treatment

Treatment of polymorphous light eruption involves the use of topical glucocorticosteroids in an ointment base applied twice daily for the dermatitis. In addition, wet dressings in the form of a face mask made of a damp washcloth, with eye, nose, and mouth holes, will serve to enhance the steroid effect on the face. This may be used for 2–3 days. Secondary bacterial infection is best treated with systemic antibiotics.

Sun avoidance is crucial in such patients and should be the mainstay of any treatment program. The child should restrict outdoor activities to the hours before 10 a.m. and after 4 p.m. Further photoprotection with a wide-brimmed hat, long-sleeved shirts, and sunscreens with UVB (SPF higher than 30) and UVA protection is necessary (see Box 10.5). A new topical preparation containing 0.25% alpha-glucosylrutin, 1% vitamin E, and a broad-spectrum highly UVA protective sunscreen appears to be highly effective in the prevention of the rash of PMLE.[27]

In cases of severe polymorphous light eruption, short treatment courses of broad-band UVB (290–320 nm), narrow-band UVB (311 nm) or psoralen and UVA may be considered.[16] Although it appears contradictory to treat a photosensitive disorder with a UVR, many studies have proven the efficacy of this approach.[16]

Thalidomide 100–200 mg/day initial dose is effective in the treatment of actinic prurigo. Once disease control has been achieved the dose is decreased with some patients requiring amounts as low as 25 mg/week[19] Recently, pentoxifylline 400 mg 2 or 3 times daily has been shown to be effective in the treatment of actinic prurigo.[28] Its side effect profile is much better than that of thalidomide. This study evaluated only 10 patients and larger trials will be necessary to confirm the results.

Patient Education

The concept of sun sensitivity must be understood by patients and their parents. Sun protection methods should be carefully explained and re-explained at each visit. Because of the delayed nature of the eruption, the relationship of the disease to sun exposure is difficult to comprehend. Many parents are reluctant to accept sun avoidance or to restrict their children's activities at school or play.

Follow-up Visits

A visit 1 week after initial therapy is useful to assess the therapeutic response. Visits at 4-week intervals thereafter are advised until the condition has cleared.

ERYTHROPOIETIC PROTOPORPHYRIA

Clinical Features

Erythropoietic protoporphyria (EPP)[29] is an autosomal dominant inherited disorder of porphyrin metabolism. The preschool child experiences burning, stinging, or itching sensations in the skin. Often, this occurs after a sun exposure of only 1–10 minutes. Despite the severe discomfort the child suffers, no skin lesions may be found. The child soon learns to

stay indoors. Intense sun exposure may result in facial edema, erythema, or urticaria, followed by petechiae, primarily on the face. Less often, vesiculation and crusting of the face appear (Figs 10.18, 10.19).

Fig. 10.18 Vesicles on nose of child with EPP.

Fig. 10.19 Crusting of the cheek and atrophic scarring in severe erythropoietic protoporphyria.

Fig. 10.20 Thickened papules over the dorsa of the left hand of a 12-year-old female with erythropoietic protoporphyria.

Fig. 10.21 Thickened papules over knuckles in child with EPP.

More commonly, however, acute skin changes do not occur, and chronic changes are apparent. Chronic changes usually do not appear until late childhood. Slightly thickened, skin-colored papules appear over the dorsa of the hands (Figs 10.20, 10.21), nose, and cheeks. Pitted scars on the face and perioral, linear, skin-colored papules may result from previous vesicular injury.

Skin biopsy specimens from sun-exposed skin show thickening of the small blood vessels of the papillary dermis, with a perivascular deposit of periodic acid-Schiff (PAS)-positive material. Direct immuno-fluorescence of such lesions demonstrates deposits of immunoglobulins, mostly immunoglobulin G (IgG), around superficial dermal blood vessels.

Children with EPP may suffer cholelithiasis, with porphyrin stones in the gallbladder, and 10% will have mild liver function abnormalities with 5% progressing to hepatic failure. A mild microcytic hypochromic anemia may also occur.

The diagnosis can be confirmed by quantitative red blood cell protoporphyrins.

Differential Diagnosis

Most other photosensitive states (see Box 10.1), such as polymorphous light eruption, LE, sunburn, and drug photosensitivity, can be excluded by the striking history of cutaneous burning seen in children with EPP, by a positive family history, and by laboratory studies. Occasionally, the family is unable to relate the symptoms to exposure to sunlight, and airborne allergens are suspected. This is particularly true if facial edema or urticaria is a major feature. A careful history, however, will reveal the role of sun exposure.

Pathogenesis

Abnormally elevated tissue levels of protoporphyrin IX, a normal precursor of heme, are found in EPP. The increased levels of protoporphyrin IX are due to a defect in the enzyme ferrochelatase. Permissive normal genes have been identified in EPP which, when co-inherited with the EPP gene, enable disease expression. Excessive protoporphyrin IX has been found in the circulating erythrocytes, plasma, liver, and bone marrow. Protoporphyrin IX absorbs light at 409 nm and becomes a molecule with an altered energy state. The molecule then transfers energy to molecular oxygen; toxic oxygen products are thought to be responsible for the injury to vascular membranes and perhaps to lysosomal membranes, with subsequent inflammation.

Light-producing 409 nm wavelengths are found in sunlight, reflected sunlight, sunlight traveling through window glass, and fluorescent lighting. Thus, a child could develop symptoms indoors or through window glass.

Treatment

Conventional sun protection methods have been uniformly unsuccessful because of the poor ability of sunscreen to protect in the 409 nm range and the small amount of light necessary to induce symptoms.

Oral administration of betacarotene is the treatment of choice. In children, a dosage of 40–120 mg/day will raise serum carotene levels to 600–800 µg/100 mL, the desired therapeutic range. The child becomes carotenemic, but sun tolerance is greatly increased. Children who previously refused to go outdoors may play for 3–4 hours outside without symptoms. Narrow-band UVB (311 nm) hardening similar to that used in PMLE is also effective. Other agents that quench reactive singlet oxygen have also been used. If an urticaria-like component is present, antihistamines are helpful.

Patient Education

The hereditary nature of the disease should be discussed with the patient and the parents, and all family members should be screened by protoporphyrin level determinations. Liver function tests may also be performed on family members. It must be emphasized that photosensitivity can occur with fluorescent lamps, such as those in overhead lighting in school.

Follow-up Visits

During the initiation of therapy, a visit every 2–3 weeks is useful to ascertain the response and to adjust the therapeutic dosage of betacarotene. After 4 weeks the serum carotene levels may be used to monitor for the correct dosage. After an effective therapeutic response is achieved, visits yearly to examine the patient for possible liver involvement and to obtain liver function tests are valuable.

PHYTOPHOTODERMATITIS

Clinical Features

Redness and blisters that occur in bizarre shapes, such as linear streaks, and that leave intense hyperpigmentation are characteristic of phytophotodermatitis

(Figs 10.22–10.24).[30] Exposure to plants in the spring and summer months from outdoor activities is the usual history. Some children present with only the hyperpigmented streaks, without a distinct history of erythema or blistering (Fig. 10.25). Exposure to limes or certain perfumes may also produce the syndrome.

Differential Diagnosis

The linear streaks of blisters may be confused with acute allergic contact dermatitis from plants such as poison ivy, whereas the hyperpigmented macules can be confused with incontinentia pigmenti because of the linear arrangement or irregular café-au-lait spots. The bizarre shapes and simultaneous, sudden onset of phytophotodermatitis lesions help differentiate from contact dermatitis.

Fig. 10.22 Phytophotodermatitis. Linear and bizarre shapes of hyperpigmentation in an 8-year-old boy from a fight with his brother; they were hitting each other with plants found along a lakeshore.

Fig. 10.23 Bizarre patterns of brown pigment on legs of boy with phytophotodermatitis.

Fig. 10.24 Hyperpigmentation of boy's hand from exposure to wild celery and sunlight.

Fig. 10.25 Linear hyperpigmentation secondary to contact with riverside grasses followed by sun exposure. No history of redness or vesiculation.

Pathogenesis

Plants that contain the furocoumarin psoralen are responsible. This includes the celery family and certain grasses and limes. The plants produce the psoralen transiently, usually after a rainy week. The child gets the psoralen onto the skin from the plant touching the skin (the epicutaneous application of a photosensitizer). The psoralen, when exposed to sunlight, produces a photodermatitis with blister formation, followed by intense stimulation of melanin production (see Fig. 10.24). The resultant hyperpigmentation may last for months.

Treatment

The acute dermatitis phase is treated as an acute allergic contact dermatitis with moderate-potency topical steroid ointments twice daily for 2 weeks. The hyperpigmentation is difficult to treat, but bleaching creams may be used if cosmetically important areas are involved.

Patient Education

Patients and parents should be advised that once hyperpigmentation occurs, it may persist for 6–12 months. They should be told of the nature of the photosensitizing chemical from plants and should avoid play in the area where the plants were contacted.

Follow-up Visits

A follow-up visit in 4 weeks to evaluate the progress of the condition is recommended.

XERODERMA PIGMENTOSUM
Clinical Features

Xeroderma pigmentosum (XP) is an autosomal recessive disorder of sun sensitivity of which eight different forms have been recognized.[31] Onset of skin lesions by 18 months of age is characteristic, with early sunburn reactions from minimal sun exposure and numerous freckles as the predominant findings. An important clue is that the sunburn may persist for several weeks rather than resolve within a week (Figs 10.26, 10.27). Telangiectasia of the sun-exposed areas and cutaneous atrophy develop within a few years of the other cutaneous findings. Actinic keratoses, which appear as persistent, red, scaly, rough macules in sun-exposed skin, are found next, and the child's skin appears prematurely aged (Fig. 10.28). In dark-skinned children these findings may be difficult to appreciate. Skin

Fig. 10.26 Xeroderma pigmentation. Redness of pre-teenager's hand from prolonged sunburn (three weeks after exposure).

Fig. 10.27 Xeroderma pigmentosum. Sunburn and telangiectasia of ear.

Fig. 10.28 Sun damage (actinic cheilitis) to lips and red, scaly macules (actinic keratosis) in adolescent with mild form of xeroderma pigmentosum.

cancers may develop by the age of 6–8 years, with basal and squamous cell carcinomas and malignant melanomas reported before puberty. Skin-colored or pigmented papules should be regarded as suspicious for skin cancers, and biopsy should be done promptly. The majority of precancerous and cancerous skin lesions occur on the head and neck. Early death from metastatic skin cancers is reported, with 10% of the patients dead before puberty. Ocular disease has a median age of onset of 4 years. Photophobia, eyelid atrophy, ectropion, corneal xerosis and scarring, and ocular neoplasms are seen. Up to 20% of affected patients have neurologic disease. Group A patients have severe early-onset neurologic disease. Groups D and G have milder adult-onset neurologic disease. Immunologic abnormalities, including defective natural killer cell function and a marked deficiency in cellular catalase, are seen. Diagnosis and classification of suspected XP are accomplished by examination of abnormal deoxyribonucleic acid (DNA) repair by the patient's cells after ultraviolet light exposure.

Differential Diagnosis

The early freckling should be differentiated from lentigines observed in multiple lentigines syndromes and the LEOPARD (lentigines, electrocardiogram [ECG] abnormalities, ocular hypertelorism, pulmonary stenosis, abnormalities of genitalia, retardation of growth, and deafness) and NAME (nevi, atrial myxoma, myxoid neurofibroma, ephelides) syndromes. Freckling is earlier in onset, macular, and tan, whereas lentigines are a darker brown. Ordinary freckles usually begin between the ages of 3 and 5 years, rather than before

2 years in children with XP, and are not accompanied by skin changes that make the child appear old. Actinic keratoses and skin cancers in prepubertal children may be seen in the basal cell nevus syndrome or in Bazex's syndrome, but not at an age as young as in children who have XP, nor do these children develop the other skin changes associated with XP. Diagnosis is suggested by skin biopsy showing severe actinic skin damage at an early age. Confirmation is made by culture of skin cells with evaluation of DNA repair.

Pathogenesis

Enzymes involved in several steps of DNA repair are abnormal.[31] Thus far, at least eight different defects in DNA repair can be found by the fusion of cultured cells from different patient groups with each other to determine if normal DNA repair is restored. Defects have been found in DNA damage recognition, DNA damage binding, DNA helicase and endonucleases. Failure to repair ultraviolet light damage results in carcinogenesis, and XP patients are an important model in the ultimate understanding of sun-induced cancers.

Treatment

Sun avoidance is essential to minimize skin damage and skin cancer formation. Children with XP should avoid sunlight, wear protective clothing, and use sunscreens with maximal SPF each day. Biopsy of any suspect skin lesion is necessary. Referral to a center with experience in management of this condition is recommended. Dermatologic, ophthalmologic, and neurologic consultations should be obtained.

Patient Education

The autosomal recessive inheritance of this disease should be emphasized. A great deal of effort stressing the critical role of sunlight in producing skin cancers is required. The need for frequent evaluations must be emphasized because many skin cancers are preventable or cured if detected early and treated.

Follow-up Visits

A cutaneous examination every 3 months is necessary, preferably at a center with experience in XP. At the follow-up visit, careful examination for skin cancers should be done, with biopsy of any suspect lesions.

An evaluation of the child's sun protection program should be performed at each visit.

REFERENCES

1. Terui T, Tagami H. Mediators of inflammation involved in UVB erythema. J Dermatol Sci 2000; 23:S1–S5.
2. Hruza LL, Pentland AP. Mechanisms of UV-induced inflammation, J Invest Dermatol 1993; 100:35S–41S.
3. Halladay GM. Inflammation, gene mutation and photoimmunosuppression in response to UVR-induced oxidative damage contributes to photocarcinogenesis. Mutat Res 2005; 571:107–120.
4. Matsumura Y, Ananthaswamy HN. Toxic effects of ultraviolet radiation on the skin. Toxicol Appl Pharmacol 2004; 15:298–308.
5. Oliveria SA, Saraiya M, Geller AC et al. Sun exposure and risk of melanoma. Arch Dis Child 2006; 91:131–138.
6. Placzek M, Gaube S, Kerkmann U, et al. Ultraviolet B-induced DNA damage in human epidermis is modified by the antioxidants ascorbic acid and D-alpha-tocopherol. J Invest Dermatol 2005; 124:304–307.
7. Claerhout S, Van Laethem A, Agostinis P, et al. Pathways involved in sunburn cell formation: deregulation in skin cancer. Photochem Photbiol Sci 2006; 5:199–207.
8. Han A, Maibach HI. Management of acute sunburn. Am J Clin Dermatol 2004; 5:39–47.
9. Benvenuto-Andrade C, Cestari TF, Mota A, et al. Photoprotection in adolescence. Skinmed 2005; 4:229–233.
10. American Academy of Pediatrics Committee on Environmental Health. Ultraviolet light: a hazard to children. Pediatrics 1999; 104:328–333.
11. Hatch KL, Osterwalder U. Garments as solar ultraviolet radiation screening materials. Dermatol Clinic 2006; 24:85–100.
12. Edlich RF, Cox MJ, Becker DG, et al. Revolutionary advances in sun-protective clothing – an essential step in eliminating skin cancer in our world. J Long Term Eff Med Implants 2004; 14:95–106.
13. Weinstock MA. Updated sunscreen advice: SPF 30. J Am Acad Dermatol 2000; 43:154.
14. Gasparro FP. Sunscreen, skin photobiology, and skin cancer: the need for UVA protection and evaluation. Environ Health Perspect 2000; 108:71–78.
15. Nixon RL, Frowen KE, Lewis AE. Skin reactions to sunscreens. Aust J Dermatol 1997; 38:S83–S85.
16. Stratigos AJ Antoniou C, Katsambas AD. Polymorphous light eruption. J Eur Acad Dermatol Venereol 2002; 16:193–206.
17. Beth-Jones J, Norris PG, Graham-Brown RA, et al. Juvenile spring eruption of the ears: a probable variant of polymorphic light eruption. Br J Dermatol 1991; 124:375–378.
18. Tan E, Eberhart-Phillips J, Sharples KL. Juvenile spring eruption: a prevalence study. NZ Med J 1996; 109:293–295.
19. Hojyo-Tomoka M-T, Vega-Memije M-E, Cortes-Franco R, et al. Diagnosis and treatment of actinic prurigo. Dermatol Ther 2003; 16:40–44.
20. Vega-Memije ME, Mosqueda-Taylor A, Irigoyen-Camacho ME, et al. Actinic prurigo cheilitis: clinicopathologic analysis and therapeutic results in 116 cases. Oral Surg Oral Med Oral Pathol Oral Radiol Endod 2002; 94:83–91.
21. Gupta J, Man I, Kemmett D. Hydroa vacciniforme: a clinical and follow-up study of 17 cases. J Am Acad Dermatol 2000; 42:208–213.
22. Jeng BH, Margolis TP, Chandra NS, et al. Ocular findings as a presenting sign of hydroa vacciniforme. Br J Ophthalmol 2004; 88:1478–1479.
23. Cho KH, Lee SH, Kim SW, et al. Epstein-Barr virus-associated lymphoproliferative lesions presenting as a hydroa vacciniform-like eruption: an analysis of six cases. Br J Dermatol 2004; 151:372–380.
24. Roelandts R. Diagnosis and treatment of solar urticaria. Dermatol Ther 2003; 16:52–56.
25. Schnell AH, Elston RC, Hull PR, et al. Major gene segregation of actinic prurigo among North American Indians in Saskatchewan. Am J Med Gen 2000; 92:212–219.
26. Schornagel IJ, Knol EF, van Weelden H, et al. Diagnostic phototesting in polymorphous light eruption: the optimal number of irradiations. Br J Dermatol 2005; 153:1234–1236.
27. Hadshiew IM, Treder-Conrad CV, Bulow R, et al. Polymorphous light eruption (PLE) and a new potent antioxidant and UVA-protective formulation as prophylaxis. Photodermatol Photoimmunol Photomed 2004; 20:200–204.
28. Torres-Alvarez B, Castenedo-Cazares JP, Moncada B. Pentoxifylline in the treatment of actinic prurigo. A preliminary report of 10 patients. Dermatology 2004; 208:198–201.
29. Murphy GM. Diagnosis and management of erythropoietic porphyrias. Dermatol Ther 2003; 16:57--64.
30. Bowers AG. Phytophotodermatitis. Am J Contact Derm 1999; 10:89–93.
31. Lehmann AR. DNA repair-deficient diseases, xeroderma pigmentosum, Cockayne syndrome, and trichothiodystrophy. Biochimie 2003; 85:1101–1111.

Chapter 11

Bullous Diseases and Mucocutaneous Syndromes

Blister formation in the skin of children usually brings to mind a viral infection (herpes simplex or zoster) or bullous impetigo. However, a large variety of non-infectious blistering skin diseases may be seen. These may be spontaneously occurring blisters, such as seen in acute allergic contact dermatitis, the immuno-bullous disorders, erythema multiforme (EM), masto-cytosis, the drug eruptions (Stevens-Johnson syndrome [SJS]), toxic epidermal necrolysis (TEN). Trauma-produced blisters are seen in the fragile skin of the hereditary mechanobullous disorders (epidermolysis bullosa). A history of trauma-induced blisters is important in distinguishing the hereditary mechano-bullous disorders from immunobullous disorders. In most of the hereditary mechanobullous disorders the onset of blisters is within the first 3 months of life.

Blisters in different skin regions may have quite different appearance. On the palms and soles blisters often have a thick roof of stratum corneum and appear deceptively deep in tissue when they are within the epidermis or at the dermal–epidermal junction. In contrast, blisters on mucous membranes shed their roofs quickly, so that only blister bases (erosions) are seen. Allergic contact dermatitis is discussed in detail in Chapter 4, infectious blisters in Chapters 5 (impetigo) and 8 (viral blisters), mastocytosis in Chapter 14, drug-induced blisters in Chapter 20, and mechanobullous diseases are discussed in Chapter 18.

SPONTANEOUS VESICULOBULLOUS ERUPTIONS

Viral blisters, bullous impetigo, chemical or thermal burns, papular urticaria, and acute dermatitis such as plant allergic contact dermatitis are the most common forms of blisters that appear spontaneously (Box 11.1). The injury in thermal burns is similar to that in sun-burn. EM is a recurrent blistering disease of the skin. SJS and TEN are uncommon but serious blistering mucocutaneous syndromes in children. Miliaria, aphthous ulcers, and geographic tongue are common, more benign forms of spontaneous vesiculobullous diseases, whereas the immunobullous diseases are quite uncommon to rare. All forms of mastocytosis may blister, especially the rare diffuse cutaneous masto-cytosis. Kawasaki disease is included in this chapter,

---

Box 11.1 Differential diagnosis of spontaneous vesiculobullous diseases

Commonly seen
Viral vesicles (HSV, varicella-zoster virus [VZV])

Bullous impetigo

Thermal or chemical burns

Friction blisters

Acute dermatitis

Miliaria

Uncommon disorders
Erythema multiforme

Stevens-Johnson syndrome

Toxic epidermal necrolysis

Autoimmune blistering disorders
Dermatitis herpetiformis, linear IgA dermatosis, pemphigus, pemphigoid

Mechanobullous diseases
Epidermolysis bullosa types, especially simplex

Mastocytosis

Bullous insect bite reactions

Lupus erythematosus

Lichen planus

Polymorphous light eruption

Incontinentia pigmenti

Bullous ichthyosis

although not truly a bullous disease, because it mimics the major mucocutaneous syndromes.

ERYTHEMA MULTIFORME

Clinical Features

Erythema multiforme (EM) is a syndrome characterized by the acute onset of oval or round, fixed, erythematous skin lesions appearing symmetrically on the skin.[1-3] Each lesion remains at the same site at least 7 days, and often for 2 or 3 weeks (Fig. 11.1). The lesions progress over several days to form concentric zones of color change in which the central zone of epidermal injury becomes dusky, blistered, or crusted. These lesions are called *target* or *iris* lesions (Fig. 11.2).[1-3] Prodromal symptoms in EM are conspicuously absent.[1-3] EM lesions are frequently recurrent and preceded by a lesion of herpes labialis (Fig. 11.3).[1-4] Skin lesions initially involve the dorsal surface of the hands and the extensor aspects of the extremities.[2-6] The palms and soles are frequently involved, with the flexor aspects of the extremities affected less frequently. The isomorphic (or Koebner) phenomenon has been reported in EM (Fig. 11.4). Systemic symptoms and signs are absent in EM. In 50% of children with EM there are no mucosal lesions, but when present, only the oral mucosa is involved and lesions are few (5 to 10) in contrast to hundreds on the skin (Fig. 11.5).[2,4,6] Target lesions may occur on the lips and be mistaken for SJS.[7] EM lasts an average of 3 weeks. It is most common in adolescents but may occur at all ages. Recurrences may occur yearly, but occasionally they happen every 1 or 2 months,

Fig. 11.2 'Target' or 'iris' lesions with characteristic central dusky necrotic zone in a child with erythema multiforme caused by herpes simplex virus.

Fig. 11.3 Herpes labialis crusted lesion present on child's lip at the onset of erythema multiforme.

Fig. 11.4 Isomorphic (Koebner) phenomenon in adolescent with erythema multiforme.

Fig. 11.1 Early fixed papules with a central dusky zone on the dorsum of the forearm of a child with erythema multiforme caused by herpes simplex virus.

particularly if the child has been treated with systemic steroids.[2] Recurrences may be induced by ultraviolet light and mimic polymorphic light eruption.[8]

Fig. 11.5 Oral involvement in erythema multiforme.

Fig. 11.6 Target lesions on the lip in a child with HSV-erythema multiforme.

There is no evidence that EM progresses to SJS or TEN.[1,2,5]

Differential Diagnosis

Acute urticaria is most often confused with EM.[4,5] This confusion results from the fact that urticaria may frequently have lesions with concentric color changes, with a pale edematous center and an erythematous border. In particular, giant urticaria, with large polycyclic lesions that are often accompanied by angioedema of the hands and feet, may be mistaken for EM. However, urticarial lesions are transient, usually lasting 24 hours or less, whereas EM lesions are fixed and stay at the same site for at least 7 days. Further, the first concentric zone of color change seen in EM minor is not pale in the center, as seen in urticaria, but rather demonstrates epidermal injury with crusting or blister formation.[5,6] Urticarial lesions will clear with subcutaneous epinephrine, and EM minor will not.[4,5] Skin biopsy will also distinguish EM from urticaria.[5,6]

Oral mucous lesions that are confused with EM include aphthous ulcers, herpes simplex infection, bullous pemphigoid, pemphigus, paraneoplastic pemphigus, and epidermolysis bullosa (see Box 11.1). Exfoliative cytologic study of the blister base will demonstrate epidermal giant cells of herpes simplex. Immunofluorescent examination of mucosal biopsies will distinguish the immunobullous diseases.

Pathogenesis

In the majority of affected children, EM is thought to be due to a herpes simplex virus (HSV)-specific host response to HSV antigens expressed on keratinocytes within the target lesion (Fig. 11.6).[2–6,9,10] There is compelling evidence to show that HSV antigens and deoxyribonucleic acid (DNA) are present within the skin lesions even when a distinctive preceding HSV episode is not observed.[3,4,9,10] Children with recurrent lesions may have recurrent HSV preceding most, but not all, EM episodes. HSV is carried to skin sites within CD34+ leukocytes.[10] HSV may reside within keratinocytes of previously involved skin and may reactivate at the same sites.[3,9,10] Children with EM may be unable to effectively clear HSV from keratinocytes. The central necrotic zone of a target lesion shows individual keratinocyte necrosis and inflammatory cells around superficial dermal blood vessels and up into the epidermis.[3] The outer red zone shows dilation of vessels and minimal inflammation. Sheets of necrotic epithelium, as observed in SJS or TEN, are conspicuously absent. In a few children, HSV may not be the precipitating agent. Epstein-Barr virus (EBV), cytomegalovirus (CMV), and other human herpesviruses have been implicated.

Treatment

For EM, symptomatic relief may be obtained from wet compresses or oral antihistamines. There is no evidence to support the use of systemic steroids in EM.[1,2] In children with recurrent episodes of EM, prophylaxis with oral acyclovir at 20 mg/kg/day may be considered.[11]

Patient Education

Patients should be informed of the role of HSV in EM, and children with recurrent episodes should attempt to reduce sun exposure or other factors that might precipitate the antecedent HSV infection.

Follow-up Visits

A visit in 24–48 hours is wise early in the disease to determine the progress of EM.

KAWASAKI DISEASE (MUCOCUTANEOUS LYMPH NODE SYNDROME)

Clinical Features

In Kawasaki disease the child presents with a high fever of abrupt onset that lasts longer than 5 days and is accompanied by conjunctival injection (Fig. 11.7).[12,13] One of three oral changes occurs: (1) erythema, fissures, redness, and dry crusting of the lips (Fig. 11.8); (2) diffuse erythema of the oropharynx; or (3) strawberry tongue.[12,13] One of four changes is seen in the extremities: (1) prominent edema and induration of the hands and feet (Fig. 11.9), (2) erythema of the palms and soles, (3) desquamation beginning at the tips of the digits and spreading proximally in transverse nail grooves [14] (Fig. 11.10), or (4) an erythematous eruption that is polymorphous in character at one point in time but mostly scarlatiniform and generalized.[12,13] The peeling of the fingertips may be recurrent after the acute phase of Kawasaki disease.[14] Lymph node masses larger than 1.5 cm, particularly in the cervical lymph nodes, may be noted. Kawasaki disease is a diagnosis of exclusion, so that other forms of acute febrile illnesses, including acute adenoviral infection, must be considered first.[12,13] Laboratory tests related to Kawasaki disease are non-specific, including an increased sedimentation rate of red blood

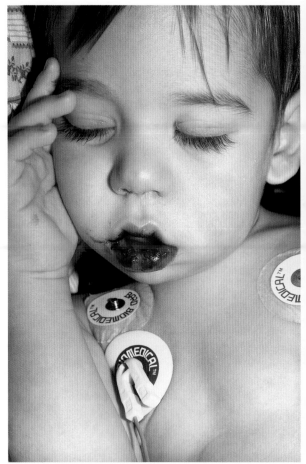

Fig. 11.8 Red, swollen, and dry, slightly crusted lips in a child with Kawasaki disease.

Fig. 11.9 Red, swollen fingers in an infant with Kawasaki disease

Fig. 11.7 Injected conjunctivae in a child with Kawasaki disease.

cells, elevated non-specific acute-phase reactants, mild anemia, and thrombocytosis that can be quite striking.[12,13]

Fig. 11.10 Peeling of fingertips from distal to proximal in Kawasaki disease.

Aneurysms of the coronary artery occur in 10–20% of patients with Kawasaki disease, and 2% will die from thrombosis of the aneurysms of coronary vessels.[12,13] Echocardiography may detect coronary aneurysms when present, but coronary angiography may be required. Although there is some evidence that coronary aneurysms may heal spontaneously, careful cardiac monitoring and involvement of a pediatric cardiologist are recommended. Other complications of vasculitis may occur, including gangrene of digits. Kawasaki disease was originally described in Japan, but cases have been reported from virtually all areas of the world.[12,13] It is recurrent in 4% of children.[12,13]

Differential Diagnosis

Many diseases with fever and mucocutaneous symptoms can be confused with Kawasaki disease. The most common conditions that mimic Kawasaki disease are acute adenovirus infections, SJS, measles, toxic shock syndrome, staphylococcal and streptococcal scarlet fever, and acute infections such as leptospirosis. By rigidly adhering to the United States Communicable Disease Center criteria for Kawasaki disease, one may be able to distinguish one condition from another.[12,13] A direct fluorescent test for adenovirus may distinguish it. Cultures can be very helpful in differentiating toxic shock syndrome (TSS) and staphylococcal scarlet fever from Kawasaki disease.

Pathogenesis

Kawasaki disease is a segmental vasculitis with major involvement of coronary vessels that mimics infantile periarteritis nodosa.[12,13] The pathogenesis is unknown, although the clustering of cases in winter and spring and close grouping have implicated an infectious agent. Although a number of infectious agents have been implicated, Kawasaki disease may represent a specific immune response pattern to different infectious agents. Coronary artery aneurysms develop during or after the acute inflammation.

Treatment

Intravenous gamma globulin (IVIG), if given within 10 days of the onset of fever along with low-dose salicylate therapy, has been recommended to prevent aneurysms.[12,13] IVIG is usually given in a single dose of 2 g/kg, although 400 mg/day for 4 days is also efficacious.[12,13] Children who present with a serum C reactive protein value of greater than 10 mg/mL, a lactic acid dehydrogenase value greater than 590 IU/mL, or a hemoglobin less than 10 g/dL may be nonresponsive to IVIG.[15,16] A polymorphism in plasma platelet-activating factor acetylhydrolase may predict resistance to IVIG[15] and one must remember that all IVIG batches are not the same.[15] Retreatment with IVIG may be required in patients with persistent fever. High-dose steroids are contraindicated and may increase the prevalence of heart disease in this syndrome.[12,13] Careful cardiac monitoring for arrhythmias is required. Involvement of a pediatric cardiologist is recommended.

Patient Education

Patients should be informed that Kawasaki disease is likely the result of a yet unknown infectious agent. They should be further advised of the seriousness of the heart disease, which may eventually prompt the need for careful monitoring of cardiac signs and symptoms. It should be encouraged that any restrictions of activities or long-term diagnostic tests be obtained under the care of a pediatric cardiologist.

Follow-up Visits

Frequently, the child with Kawasaki disease is hospitalized, and regular hospital follow-ups are performed. Management as an outpatient should be done only when good cardiac consultation and follow-up care are available. Long-term follow-up should follow the American Heart Association guidelines.[12,13]

APHTHOUS ULCERS

Clinical Features

Aphthous ulcers are common in childhood.[16,17] Recurrent, shallow erosions of the gums, tongue, palate, lips, and buccal mucosa are seen in aphthous ulcers (Figs 11.11, 11.12).[16–18] The erosions are 1–10 mm in diameter and have a gray-yellow base (see Fig. 11.12). Burning and tenderness may occur. Healing occurs in 7–10 days, without scarring. Recurrences are usually irregular, several months apart, and consist of two to four lesions (Fig. 11.13). In a more severe form, recurrences with numerous large (under 10 mm) lesions (Fig. 11.14) are so frequent, that the child is seldom free from discomfort.[18,19] Aphthae are usually limited to the mouth, but associated large ulcers on the mouth (Fig. 11.15) and the genitalia are seen in complex aphthosis,[19] and oral and genital aphthae

Fig. 11.12 Large aphthous ulcer with gray center.

Fig. 11.13 Aphthous ulcer on the lower lip of a child.

Fig. 11.14 Painful aphthous ulcer on side of tongue.

Fig. 11.11 Minor aphthous ulcer with red border in a child's mouth.

may be observed in association with iritis or uveitis, erythema nodosum, and central nervous system disease in the periodic fever syndromes associated with mouth ulcers (Fig. 11.16), including cyclic neutropenia, the FAPA (Fever, Aphthous ulcers, Pharyngitis,

Fig. 11.15 Large painful ulcer on side of tongue in child with complex aphthosis and vaginal lesions.

Fig. 11.16 Aphthous ulcer on tip of tongue of child with periodic fever (FAPA) syndrome.

Box 11.2 Differential diagnosis of recurrent or persistent oral ulcerations
Aphthous ulcers
Herpes simplex
Behçet's disease
Inflammatory bowel disease
Periodic fever syndromes
Pemphigus vulgaris
Stevens-Johnson syndrome
Paraneoplastic pemphigus

Adenitis) syndrome and in Behçet's syndrome.[18–22] Minor aphthae may be associated with inflammatory bowel disease or an upper respiratory tract illness.

Differential Diagnosis

Aphthous ulcers must be distinguished from herpes simplex and other viral oral ulcerations, autoimmune blistering diseases such as pemphigus, and EM (Box 11.2). Exfoliative cytologic study of the erosion will identify the epidermal giant cells of herpes simplex, and viral culture will distinguish the disorder from herpes simplex, coxsackieviruses A5, A10, and A16; and other enteroviruses. EM may present with oral erosions, but the symmetric target skin lesions will suggest the disorder. Erosions of the autoimmune blistering diseases will persist for many months, in contrast to days with aphthous ulcers. Evaluation of any child who has fever with aphthous ulcers should include Behçet's syndrome and the periodic fever syndromes, and other systemic manifestations should be sought.[18–22]

Pathogenesis

The mechanism of aphthous ulcers is unknown. Several studies have demonstrated lymphocytotoxic activity against oral epithelium, suggesting an autoimmune phenomenon. Biopsy shows ulceration of the epidermis and a mixed inflammatory infiltrate. Infectious agents have been implicated, and the cytotoxic response that produces the injury to oral epithelium may therefore be organism specific.

Treatment

Treatment is symptomatic. Mild attacks may respond to liquid antacids, oral cyanoacrylate dental adhesives, or daily rinsing with an enzyme solution containing amyloglucosidase and glucose oxidase.[23,24] Silver nitrate cautery will reduce pain without prolonging healing time[25] but cryotherapy will not.[26] Many mild episodes require no treatment. Severe lesions may require topical steroids, such as triamcinolone acetonide in a base that adheres to mucous surfaces. Oral prednisone, 1–2 mg/kg/day for 3–5 days, may be necessary for severe involvement that impairs eating.[23] Sucralfate suspension has been useful in some cases. If a periodic fever syndrome is diagnosed, some episodes can be aborted with 1 or 2 days of oral prednisone.[20–22]

Patient Education

The recurrent nature of this disorder and the lack of effective therapy should be emphasized. It should be clearly stated that the cause is unknown, and that therapy is therefore non-specific and aimed at symptomatic relief.

Follow-up Visits

Follow-up visits are necessary only when severe attacks occur.

GEOGRAPHIC TONGUE

Clinical Features

Children under 4 years of age are most commonly affected by geographic tongue, a benign inflammatory disorder.[16,17] Multiple annular, smooth patches that mimic blister bases on the tongue have a gray, slightly elevated border (Fig. 11.17).[27] There are usually no symptoms, but occasionally a child will complain of tenderness. The pattern of involvement changes from day to day, and spontaneous remissions occur.[27]

Differential Diagnosis

Diagnosis is usually easy because the migratory pattern occurs exclusively in geographic tongue. A dry tongue usually has fissures and is not migratory. Malnutrition usually produces diffuse redness and swelling of the entire tongue. Aphthous ulcers, EM, and viral ulcers do not migrate from day to day, and once established they remain fixed for at least 3–5 days.

Pathogenesis

Pathologic changes in the annular border of the lesion of the tongue are surprisingly similar to those in psoriasis. There are microabscesses in the epithelium and

Fig. 11.17 Geographic tongue.

epithelial thickening, but the pathogenesis is unknown. Although the smooth area looks like an erosion clinically, the epithelium is intact and there is no blister formation.

Treatment

Treatment is usually unnecessary because the lesions are asymptomatic. Oral liquid antacids taken before meals may help if pain occurs when eating.

Patient Education

The benign nature of this condition should be emphasized.

Follow-up Visits

Follow-up visits are unnecessary.

MILIARIA (HEAT RASH)

Clinical Features

There are two major forms of miliaria: miliaria crystallina and miliaria rubra.[28] Miliaria crystallina occurs in newborn infants or in areas of sunburn. Miliaria rubra (heat rash) occurs primarily in infants with induced sweating or heat retention. Airtight occlusion predisposes to miliaria. Miliaria crystallina is characterized by clear, thin-walled vesicles that are 1–2 mm in diameter, without erythema. The vesicles rupture within 24–48 hours and leave a white scale. They are seen on the head and neck and upper trunk in newborn infants and within areas of sunburn in other children.

The characteristic finding in miliaria rubra consists of 2–4 mm papules or papulovesicles surrounded by erythema (Fig. 11.18).[28–30] Lesions are seen in flexural areas, such as the neck, axilla, and groin, after excessive sweating. The face and upper chest may be involved. Miliaria rubra may occur in a localized skin area where airtight occlusion has occurred, for example, in an immobilized or comatose child lying on a plastic bed cover.

Both forms of miliaria may be secondarily infected by *Staphylococcus aureus*, producing pustules in the sweat pores (miliaria pustulosa), which is particularly troublesome in tropical or subtropical areas. If continued sweating occurs, repeated daily episodes of miliaria result. Allowing the skin to cool and dry produces mild desquamation and healing in a few days.

Fig. 11.18 Red pinpoint papules on chest of infant with miliaria rubra.

Fig. 11.19 Superficial sweat-duct obstruction in miliaria crystallina (left) does not result in inflammation, in contrast to midepidermal sweat-duct obstruction in miliaria rubra (right).

Differential Diagnosis

Box 11.1 presents the conditions to be considered in the differential diagnosis of miliaria crystallina and miliaria rubra. Miliaria crystallina can be distinguished from viral infections of skin or from acute dermatitis by the lack of erythema and the negative exfoliative cytologic findings. On smear of miliaria crystallina lesions, neither giant cells nor inflammatory cells are seen.

Miliaria rubra may be confused with neonatal acne, viral exanthems, candidiasis, or drug eruptions, but it is so characteristic that it is seldom misdiagnosed. The febrile child who receives an antibiotic may be mistakenly diagnosed as drug allergic when the eruption with fever was miliaria.

Pathogenesis

Occlusion of sweat ducts after sweating, with rupture of the sweat duct as it spirals through the epidermis, is seen in miliaria (Fig. 11.19). In miliaria crystallina the duct rupture is within the stratum corneum, whereas in miliaria rubra it occurs in the lower epidermis. Induction of sweating, overheating of the skin, and mechanical occlusion of the sweat pores are essential to the production of miliaria. The baby who is overclothed is particularly susceptible to miliaria.

Treatment

The treatment of choice consists of avoidance of further sweating and allowing the skin surface to dry and cool. If pustule formation occurs and secondary staphylococcal infection appears, systemic anti-staphylococcal antibiotics should be administered. Cooling lotions and other agents used for miliaria are not effective unless sweating is reduced. Avoidance of overclothing the baby will be preventive.

Patient Education

The role of overheating the skin and the ease of sweat-duct obstruction should be emphasized. The parent or caregiver who overdresses the infant or child should be duly informed. Avoidance of all airtight dressings, such as plastic occlusion, and the need for cooling the skin must be emphasized.

Follow-up Visits

Follow-up visits are unnecessary.

THE IMMUNOBULLOUS DISEASES

One should suspect an immunobullous disease in the circumstance of a persistent blistering condition, particularly if present for over a month.[31] Immunobullous diseases may present with intraepidermal blister formation, which results in a flaccid, easily eroded blister or a subepidermal blister that is tense (Box 11.3). All are chronic diseases and as a group are quite uncommon to rare.[31] All are characterized by the presence of autoantibodies; the immunobullous diseases are also called the *autoimmune blistering diseases*. In most diseases the autoantibodies are thought to play a role in the pathogenesis of the blister formation. In contrast to the hereditary mechanobullous diseases (see Ch. 18) in which there are gene mutations resulting in weakening of the epidermal structural proteins, in immunobullous diseases there are autoantibodies to these same structural proteins.[31] Treatment of immunobullous diseases requires long-term immunosuppressive therapy protocols, and the child should be managed by an experienced dermatologist.

Dermatitis Herpetiformis

Clinical features

The most common of this group of diseases is dermatitis herpetiformis (DH), characterized by severely pruritic vesicles or urticaria lesions (Figs 11.20, 11.21), which usually has its onset in adolescence.[31-34] In dermatitis herpetiformis, skin lesions are characteristically grouped. Involvement of elbows (Fig.11.22), knees, the upper trunk and buttocks is characteristic but lesions may occur anywhere including the hands (Fig.11.23) and feet, palms and soles, scalp and the mouth.[31,33]

Urticarial lesions are common and DH may present as chronic urticaria.[32] Itching is so severe that

Fig. 11.20 Blisters and excoriated papules on the back of an adolescent with dermatitis herpetiformis (DH).

Fig. 11.21 Numerous erosions with a few blisters involving entire back of child with DH. Note that central back is involved in contrast to neurotic excoriations.

Fig. 11.22 Grouped blisters and erosions around the elbow in child with DH.

Fig. 11.23 Grouped blisters on the dorsum of the hand in child with DH.

intact blisters are not seen but excoriations and erosions are seen instead. DH is associated with gluten sensitivity, but gastrointestinal symptoms are usually absent. The bowel pathology mimics gluten-sensitive enteropathy, but only involves focal bowel segments, so sufficient absorption can occur without diarrhea or weight loss.[31,33,34] DH is most prevalent in Northern European populations and may be associated with development of lymphomas in adult life.[35]

Differential diagnosis

There are frequent errors made in the diagnosis dermatitis herpetiformis, particularly if one relies on clinical features alone. It should be emphasized that the diagnosis of immunobullous diseases is based on a combination of clinical, histologic, and immunofluorescent findings. Immunofluorescence of a skin biopsy is frequently the diagnostic test for these dis-

eases, and one must select noninvolved skin adjacent to a blister for biopsy. One should never biopsy an old blister or a crusted lesion. Diagnosis is made by biopsy of blistered skin for routine histology and adjacent nonblistered skin for immunoflourescence.[31] On routine histology, dermal papillae are stuffed with neutrophils and a subepidermal separation is noted.[31] On direct immunofluorescence (IF) examination, granular IgA deposits are found in the tops of the dermal papillae.[31] These findings distinguish DH from the other immunobullous disorders (see Box 11.2) and other causes of clinical blisters and itchy skin diseases such as atopic dermatitis or scabies. If the IF is negative, it may have to be repeated.[31] In addition, like celiac disease, patients with DH may have serum anti-endomysial or IgA anti-gliadin antibodies.[34] It is never acceptable to diagnose DH based on the presence of an itchy skin disease.

Pathogenesis

Hereditary gluten sensitivity is involved in DH but exactly how it causes skin disease is unclear. IgA antibodies deposited in the dermal papillae may have anti-gliadin (gluten protein) activity but are bound to tissue transglutaminase in the cutaneous vessels of the dermal papillae.[31,36]

Treatment

The antineutrophil drug dapsone is the treatment of choice at 2 mgm/kg/day.[31,37] Before starting, a baseline complete blood count and a serum glucose-6-dehydrogenase (G6PD) level should be obtained, as children with G6PD deficiency may develop severe hemolysis with dapsone. Baseline liver function and renal function tests should also be obtained. Dapsone is only available in scored tablets of 25 mg or 100 mg. The half-life of dapsone is 24–30 hours, so once-daily dosing is preferred. Dapsone does not affect antibody deposition. The major side effects are hemolytic anemia and methhemoglobinemia. Methhemoglobinemia can be prevented by cimetidine at 30 mg/kg/day. For the first month, it is recommended to follow the blood counts weekly and liver and renal function tests monthly. As soon as a clinical response is obtained, dapsone can be administered every other day. A gluten-free diet can also reduce the dapsone requirement, but the child will need to follow the diet for at least 3 months. For children who do not respond to dapsone, sulfasalazine at 100 mg/kg/day may be considered, not to exceed 2 g per day. A pharmacist can make a suspension of 100 mg/5 mL if the child cannot take the 500 mg tablets.

Colchicine 0.2–0.5 mg/day has been recommended by some for dapsone failure and efficacy of infliximab has been demonstrated in gluten-sensitive enteropathy.[38]

Patient education

Parents should be provided information on a gluten-free diet.[33,34,37] There are many resources available. They should be advised of the side effects of dapsone, including the idiosyncratic hepatitis and foot drop neuropathy. They also should recognize that even if the child can reduce or eliminate dapsone requirements, the disease can recur.

Follow-up visits

While the child is taking dapsone, monthly visits to monitor blood counts and liver and renal function tests are recommended. As the child reduces dapsone or even tapers off dapsone, half-yearly evaluations may be useful.

Linear IgA Dermatosis

Clinical features

Tense blisters often grouped around the inguinal area are characteristic (Fig. 11.24).[39] Blisters can be seen anywhere on skin, however, and are characteristically sausage-shaped (Fig.11.25).

Multiple tense blisters can be seen with some hemorrhage (Fig.11.26) Usually, toddlers are affected but neonates[40] and older children have been reported.

Fig. 11.24 Numerous sausage-shaped tense bullae and crusted lesions in the pelvic area of a toddler with linear IgA dermatosis.

Fig. 11.25 Rosette of blisters on the leg of a child with linear IgA dermatosis.

Fig. 11.26 Tense blisters on the arm in a child with linear IgA dermatosis.

Most cases occur spontaneously, although some are drug-induced (vancomycin and phenytoins).[40] A few children have had disease induced by ultraviolet light exposure.

Differential diagnosis

Histology reveals a subepidermal blister and is indistinguishable from other subepidermal blisters. IF examination of adjacent unaffected skin reveals a linear deposition of IgA and, to a lesser extent, IgG along the basement membrane zone.[41,42] It is distinguished from the other immunobullous diseases including pemphigoid by the presence of IgA at the basement membrane zone.

Pathogenesis

Autoantibodies in linear IgA dermatosis disrupt adherence of the epidermis to the dermis, resulting in blister formation. The antibodies are primarily directed against the structural proteins linking the hemidesmosome of the epidermal basal cell to the collagens of the dermis.[42] The major antigen appears to be collagen 17. The mechanisms of drug-induced IgA autoantibodies are unclear.

Treatment

If drug-induced disease is suspected, then the drug should be stopped.[40] Like DH, linear IgA disease may respond promptly to dapsone and remit spontaneously within 2–3 months.[31,42,43] Linear IgA disease, whether drug induced or not, often does not recur, in contrast to DH. A few cases are refractory and may require the addition of another agent. Mycophenolate mofetil [41] and oral erythromycin[44] have been reported to be successful, but both take 2–3 months to demonstrate efficacy.

Patient education

Parents should be told that most children respond promptly to therapy and long-term therapy is rarely required.

Follow-up visits

Follow-up is determined by therapy. A first follow-up at 1–2 weeks is useful to determine effect of therapy and the possible requirement for additional treatments. As with treatment of DH, careful monitoring of dapsone is required and baseline blood counts, liver and renal function tests are required.

Pemphigus Foliaceous and Vulgaris

Clinical features

Pemphigus foliaceous, the most frequent form of childhood pemphigus, is characterized by moist crusts and flaccid blisters, usually on facial (Fig. 11.27) or upper trunk skin (Figs 11.28, 11.29).[31,45] The lesions, once they appear, are persistent. In the highlands of Brazil, an endemic form of pemphigus foliaceous (fogo selvaem) occurs.[45] Rarely, the child will present with a 'butterfly' facial rash that mimics lupus (pemphigus erythematosus).

In pemphigus vulgaris, oral erosions precede skin lesions by 3 months.[31,46,47] Large erosions of the lips (Fig. 11.30), tongue, and buccal mucosa are seen. Then, flaccid blisters and crusted lesions appear on

Fig. 11.27 Crusted erosion on temple of child with pemphigus foliaceous.

Fig. 11.28 Crusted lesions on arm of child with pemphigus foliaceous.

Fig. 11.29 Healing erosions on back of child with pemphigus foliaceous.

the body (Figs 11.31, 11.32). The oral lesions may be so painful as to interfere with eating and drinking, and weight loss may ensue. Other mucosal sites such as anus, vagina, and colon are sometimes involved.[47] A

Fig. 11.30 Completely eroded lips in adolescent with pemphigus vulgaris. His mouth was also severely eroded.

Fig. 11.31 Trauma-induced erosions in infant with pemphigus vulgaris.

Fig. 11.32 Bleeding erosions and healing lesions on back of toddler with pemphigus vulgaris.

Fig. 11.33 Red, oozing, eroded, verrucous plaques in axilla of child with pempigus vegetans variant of pemphigus vulgaris.

variant of pemphigus vulgaris, called pemphigus vegetans, in which exuberant, verrucous intertriginous lesions are found in axilla (Fig. 11.33) and groin.

Differential Diagnosis

Impetigo most mimics pemphigus foliaceous. The oral lesions of pemphigus vulgaris mimic major aphthous ulcers, herpes simplex stomatitis, and the oral lesions of Stevens-Johnson syndrome. The other immunobullous diseases [see Box 11.2] may also mimic. Diagnosis is based upon biopsy of adjacent normal skin for IF examination. In pemphigus foliaceous, IgG deposits between cells in the upper epidermis is seen; in pemphigus vulgaris, IgG deposits between cells of the entire epidermis is seen.

Pathogenesis

In pemphigus foliaceous, IgG autoantibodies to a structural protein expressed in the upper epidermis, desmoglein 1, is found.[31] Desmoglein 1 is important for cell–cell adherence in the upper epidermis and the autoantibodies disrupt the adherence, resulting in fragile outer epidermis that is separated by slight trauma or friction. In pemphigus vulgaris, the target antigen is desmoglein 3, which is found throughout the epidermis. The autoantibodies make the entire epidermis above the basal cells fragile.

Treatment

Pemphigus is most persistent, and long-term immunosuppressive treatment may be required.[31,48–50] The initial goal of therapy is to reduce inflammation in the skin, and the long-term goal is to suppress the auto-antibody production. Mild forms of pemphigus foliaceous with few lesions may be managed with topical superpotent corticosteroids such as clobetasol propionate applied twice daily.[31] However, more widespread pemphigus foliaceous and pemphigus vulgaris often require a two-drug treatment program: oral corticosteroids plus an additional immunosuppressive that will also act as a steroid-sparing agent. Prednisone at 2 mg/kg/day plus either cyclophosphamide at 1–3 mg/kg/day or mycophenolate mofetil at 50 mg/kg/day can be considered.[48,49] Prednisone should be kept at 2 mg/kg/day until lesions are almost clear, then reduced. To counter acid reflux disease induced by prednisone, a proton pump inhibitor or H_2 blocking agent should be administered as long as the child is on prednisone. Mycophenolate mofetil inhibits T- and B-lymphocyte purine synthesis and requires careful drug monitoring.[49] Mycophenolate mofetil is supplied as suspension of 200 mg/mL or 250 or 500 mg tablets. Cyclophosphamide also causes urinary bladder hemorrhage and the child should have good fluid intake while on the drug. Ideally, the child will be able to discontinue steroids after 3 months, but may continue long term on immunosuppressives for 3 years or more.[31,48] There are few convincing data to support the use of dapsone, IVIG, cyclosporine, or azathioprine in childhood pemphigus.

Fig. 11.34 Tense blisters on leg in childhood bullous pemphigoid.

Fig. 11.35 Vular blisters, erosions, and early scarring in preschool child with localized vulvar pemphigoid.

Patient education

Parents should be advised of the potentially life-threatening nature of pemphigus and the need for careful follow-up evaluations.

Follow-up

After obtaining baseline blood counts, liver function tests and glucose, weekly blood counts should be obtained during the first month at follow-up visits. Thereafter, monthly blood tests should be obtained.

Childhood Pemphigoid
Clinical features

Pemphigoid appears in two predominant clinical subtypes: infantile, and localized childhood vulvar.[31,51–55] Both types heal with scarring. The infantile form usually presents with blisters on acral areas (Fig. 11.34) including the palms and soles.[54] It can spread to

become more generalized after several months if untreated. The childood vulvar type presents as blisters and erosions on the vulvar skin (Fig. 11.35) or occasionally vaginal mucosal, and produces scarring.[51–53] The lesions are usually painful.

Differential diagnosis

Infantile pemphigoid may be mimicked by other immunobullous diseases [see Box 11.2], allergic

Box 11.4 Differential diagnosis of vulvar ulcers and erosions
Complex aphthosis
Behçet's disease
Lichen sclerosis et atrophicus
Inflammatory bowel disease
Epidermolysis bullosa

contact dermatitis or hand-foot-and-mouth disease. Vulvar pemphigoid can be mimicked by complex aphthosis, Behçet's disease and by other immuno-bullous diseases (Box 11.4). With scarring, forms of epidermolysis bullosa should be considered. Direct IF evaluation will distinguish, demonstrating linear IgG deposition along the basement membrane zone in pemphigoid.

Pathogenesis

Autoantibodies in pemphigoid are directed against hemidesmosome antigens, notably type 17 collagen that anchors the epidermal basal cell to the dermis. The autoantibodies disrupt attachment, allowing a subepidermal blister to occur.

Treatment

If detected early in the course of disease, pemphigoid lesions respond well to topical superpotent steroids (clobetasol propionate) twice daily for 3–4 weeks, or if widespread, to oral prednisone 2 mg/kg/day.[31,54]

Paraneoplastic Pemphigus

Clinical features

Paraneoplastic pemphigus (PNP) is characterized by the abrupt onset of severe and widespread lip and oral erosions (Fig. 11.36), target-like lesions on the skin (Fig. 11.37), and severe cuticle nail involvement (Fig. 11.38).[56–59] Oral lesions with severe mucositis interfere with eating and drinking, and weight loss ensues. Cough develops, which heralds severe pul-

Fig. 11.36 Hemorrhagic crusts on lips, eroded conjunctiva in boy with PNP. He had mediastinal Castleman's tumor.

Fig. 11.37 EM-like acral blisters in a child with PNP.

Fig. 11.38 Cuticular scarring and early fingernail loss in child with PNP.

monary involvement, and sloughing of airway mucosa (bronchiolitis obliterans) ensues. Mortality is 95%.

Differential diagnosis

Paraneoplastic pemphigus exactly mimics Stevens-Johnson syndrome at the outset (see Box 11.2). It can be distinguished by direct IF examination of skin with IgG deposits both within the epidermis, like pemphigus, and at the basement membrane zone, like pemphigoid. Both intraepidermal and subepidermal separations can be seen on histology.

Pathogenesis

Paraneoplastic pemphigus is often associated with a B-lymphocyte tumor of the mediastinum (Castleman's tumor).[56–59] The proliferating B lymphocytes produce a series of autoantibodies against epidermal and basement membrane antigens.[58] Autoantibodies against desmoplakin 1, envoplakin, periplakin, desmoplakin 2, and desmoglein 3 are found.[59] Additional autoantibodies against epidermal components are found less frequently.

Treatment

As soon as the diagnosis is established, administration of oral steroids plus mycophenolate mofetil is recommended.[59] Removal of the Castleman's tumor has occasionally been associated with remission.[56–59]

Patient education

The severe, life-threatening nature of the disease should be emphasized.

Follow-up visits

Prolonged hospitalization is usual and follow-ups are determined by response to therapy and complications of treatment.

REFERENCES

1. Leaute-Labreze C, Lamireau T, Chawki D, et al. Diagnosis, classification and management of erythema multiforme and Stevens-Johnson syndrome. Arch Dis Child 2000; 83:347–352.
2. Weston WL, Morelli JG. Herpes-associated erythema multiforme in prepubertal children. Arch Pediatr Adolesc Med 1997. 151:1014.
3. Weston WL. Herpes-associated erythema multiforme. J Invest Dermatol 2005; 124:xv–xvi.
4. Weston WL, Stockert SS, Jester JD. Herpes simplex virus in childhood erythema multiforme. Pediatrics 1992; 89:32.
5. Weston JA, Weston WL: The overdiagnosis of erythema multiforme. Pediatrics 1992; 89:802.
6. Weston WL. What is erythema multiforme? Pediatr Ann 1996; 25:106.
7. Weston WL, Morelli JG, Rogers M. Target lesions on the lips: childhood herpes simplex-associated erythema multiforme mimics Stevens-Johnson syndrome. J Am Acad Dermatol 1997; 37:848.
8. Wolf P, Soyer HP, Fink-Puches R, et al. Recurrent post-herpetic erythema multiforme mimicking polymorphic light and juvenile spring eruption: two cases in young boys. Br J Dermatol 1994; 131:364–367.
9. Brice SL, Leahy MA, Ong L. Examination of non-involved skin, previously involved skin and peripheral blood for herpes simplex virus DNA in patients with recurrent herpes-associated erythema multiforme. J Cutan Pathol 1994; 21:406.
10. Ono F, Sharma BK, Smith CC, et al. CD34+ cells in the peripheral blood transport herpes simplex virus DNA fragments to the skin of patients with erythema multiforme [HAEM]. J Invest Dermatol 2005; 124:1215–1224.
11. Tatnall FM, Schofield JK, Leigh IM. A double-blind, placebo-controlled trial of continuous acyclovir therapy in recurrent erythema multiforme. Br J Dermatol 1995; 132:267.
12. Wang CL, Wu YT, Liu CA, et al. Kawasaki disease: infection, immunity and genetics. Pediatr Infect Dis J 2005; 24:998–1004.
13. Barone SR, Pontrelli LR, Krilov LR. The differentiation of classic Kawasaki disease, atypical Kawasaki disease and acute adenoviral infection. Arch Pediatr Adolesc Med 2000; 154:453.
14. Michie C, Kinsler V, Tulloh R, et al. Recurrent skin peeling following Kawasaki disease, Arch Dis Child 2000; 83:353.
15. Minami T, Suzuki H, Takeuchi T, et sl. A polymorphism in plasma platelet-activating factor acetylhydrolase is involved in resistance to immunoglobulin treatment in Kawasaki disease. J Pediatr 2005; 14:78–83.
16. Stiehm ER. Lessons from Kawasaki disease: all brands of IVIG are not equal. J Pediatr 2006; 148:6–8.
17. Schulman JD. Prevalence of oral mucosal lesions in children and youths in the USA. Int J Paediatr Dent 2005; 15:89–97.
18. Rioboo-Crespo M del R, Planelis del Porzo P, Rioboo-Garcia H. Epidemiology of the most common oral mucosal diseases in children. Med Oral Patol Oral Cir Bucal 2005; 10:376–387.
19. Verpilleux MP, Bastujin-Garin S, Revuz J. Comparative analysis of severe aphthosis and Behçet's disease: 104 cases. Dermatology 1999; 198:247.
20. Marshall SE. Behçet's disease. Best Pract Res Clin Rheumatology 2004; 18:291–311.
21. Padeh S. Periodic fever syndromes. Pediatr Clin North Am 2005; 52:577–609.
22. Feder HM Jr. Periodic fever, aphthous stomatitis, pharyngitis, adenitis: a clinical review of a new syndrome. Curr Opin Pediatr 2000; 12:253.
23. Long SS. Periodic fever. Adv Exp Med Biol 2005; 568:101–115.
24. McBride DR. Management of aphthous ulcers. Am Fam Phys 2000; 62:149.

25. Fridh G, Koch G. Effect of a mouth rinse containing amylo-glucosidase and glucose oxidase on recurrent aphthous ulcers in children and adolescents. Swed Dental J 1999; 23:49.

26. Alidaee MR, Taheri A, Mansoori P, et al. Silver nitrate cautery in aphthous stomatitis: a randomized controlled trial. Br J Dermatol 2005; 153:521–525.

27. Arikan OK, Birol A, Tuncez F, et al. A prospective randomized conrolled trial to determine if cryotherapy can reduce the pain of patients with the minor form of recurrent aphthous stomatitis. Oral Surg Oral Med Oral Pathol Oral Radiol Endod 2006; 101:31–35.

28. Lacour JP, Perrin C. Eruptive familial lingual papillitis: a new clinical entity? Ped Dermatol 1997; 14:13.

29. Jainkittivong A, Langlais RP. Geographic tongue. Clinical characteristics of 188 cases. J Contemp Dent Pract 2005; 15:123–135.

30. Wenzel FG, Horn TD. Nonneoplastic disorders of the eccrine glands. J Am Acad Dermatol 1998; 38:1.

31. Weston WL, Morelli JG, Huff JC. Misdiagnosis, treatments, and outcomes in the immunobullous diseases in children. Pediatr Dermatol 1997; 14:264.

32. Powell GR, Bruckner SL, Weston WL. Dermatitis herpetiformis presenting as chronic urticaria. Pediatr Dermatol 2004; 21:564–567.

33. Zone JJ. Skin manifestations of coeliac disease. Gastroenterology 2005; 128:S87–S91.

34. Humbert P, Pelletier F, Dreno B, et al. Gluten intolerance and skin diseases. Eur J Dermatol 2006; 16:4–11.

35. Hervonen K, Vomanen M, Kautianen H, et al. Lymphoma in patients with dermatitis herpetiformis and their first-degree relatives. Brit J Dermatol 2005; 152:82–87.

36. Preiz K, Sardy M, Horvath A, et al. Immunoglobulin, complement and epidermal transglutaminase deposition in the cutaneous vessels in dermatitis herpetiformis. J Eur Acad Dermatol Venerol 2005; 19:74–79.

37. Chand NN, Mikas AA. Coeliac disease: current concepts in diagnosis and treatment. J Clin Gastroenterol 2006; 40:3–14.

38. Turner SM, Morghen M, Probert CS. Refractory coeliac disease: regression with infliximab and immunomodulators. Eur J Gastroenterol 2005; 17:667–669.

39. Kishida Y, Kameyama J, Nei M, et al. Linear IgA bullous dermatosis of neonatal onset: case report and review of the literature. Acta Paediatr 2004; 93:850–852.

40. Onodera H, Mihm MC Jr, Yoshida A, et al. Drug-induced linear IgA dermatosis. J Dermatol 2005; 32:759–764.

41. Allen J, Wojnarowska F. Linear IgA disease: the IgA and IgG response to dermal antigens demonstrates chiefly IgA response to LAD285 and a dermal 180 kDa protein. Br J Dermatol 2003; 149:1055–1058.

42. Sitaru C, Zillikens D. Mechanisms of blister induction by autoantibodies. Exp Dermatol 2005; 14:861–875.

43. Farley-Li J, Mancini AJ. Treatment of linear IgA bullous dermatosis of childhood with mycophenolate mofetil. Arch Dermatol 2003; 139:1121–1124.

44. Cooper SM Powell J, Wojnarowska F. Linear IgA disease: successful treatment with erythromycin. Clin Exp dermatol 2002; 27:677–679.

45. Ribeiro AM, Alvarez RR, Friedman H, et al. The profile of fogo selvagem (endemic pemphigus foliaceous) at the University Hospital of Brasilia-Brazil. Epidermiologic and clinical considerations. Int J Dermatol 2005; 44:293–298.

46. Ariyawardana A, Tilakaratne WM, Dissanayake M et al. Oral pemphigus vulgaris in children and adolescents: A review of the literature and case report. Int J Paediatr Dent 2005; 15:287–293.

47. Bruckner AL, Fitzpatrick JE, Hashimoto T, et al. Atypical IgA/IgG pemphigus involving the skin oral mucosa and colon. Pediatr Dermatol 2005; 22:321–327.

48. Minouni D, Nousar CH, Cummings DL, et al. Differences and similarities among expert opinion on the diagnosis and treatment of pemphigus vulgaris. J Amer Acad Dermatol 2004; 49:1059–1062.

49. Kawashita MY, Tsai K, Aoki V, et al. Mycophenolate mofetil as an adjuvant therapy for classical and endemic pemphigus foliaceous. J Dermatol 2005; 32:574–580.

50. Kong HH, Prose NS, Ware RE, et al. Successful treatment of childhood pemphigus vulgaris with anti-CD20 monoclonal antibody (rituximab). Pediatr Dermatol 2005; 22:461–464.

51. Fischer G, Rogers M. Vulvar disease in children: a clinical audit of 130 cases. Pediatr Dermatol 2000; 17:1.

52. Schoeffler A, Roth B, Causeret A, et al. Vulvar cicatricial pemphigoid of childhood. Pediatr Dermatol 2004; 21:52–3.

53. Edwards S, Wakelin SH, Wojnarowska F, et al. Bullous pemphigoid and epidermolysis bullosa acquisita: presentation, prognosis and immunopathology in eleven cases. Pediatr Dermatol 1998. 15:184–190.

54. Fisler RE, Saeb M, Liang MG, et al. Childhood bullous pemphigoid: a clinicopathologic study and review of the literature. Am J Dermatopathol 2003; 25:183–189.

55. Voltan F, Maeda JY, Muniz Silva MA, et al. Childhood bullous pemphigoid: report of three cases. J Dermatol 2005; 32:387–392.

56. Wang J, Zhu X, Li R, et al. Paraneoplastic pemphigus associated with Castleman tumor: a commonly reported subtype of paraneoplastic pemphigus in China. Arch Dermatol 2005; 141:1285–1293.

57. Lane JE, Woody C, Davis LS, et al. Paraneoplastic autoimmune multiorgan syndrome (paraneoplastic pemphigus) in a child: case report and review of the literature. Pediatrics 2004; 114:e513–e516.

58. Wang L, Bu D, Yang Y, et al. Castleman's tumours and production of autoantibody in paraneoplastic pemphigus. Lancet 2004; 363:525–531.

59. Mimouni D, Anhalt GJ, Lazarova Z, et al. Paraneoplastic pemphigus in children and adolescents. Br J Dermatol 2002; 147:725–732.

Skin Cysts and Nodules

Persistent masses in the skin often result in a child being brought in for medical examination. Often, parents are concerned that the skin lesion is cancer. Biopsy may be necessary to provide an accurate diagnosis in these conditions, which are rarely symptomatic except in weight-bearing areas. A large number of skin problems can produce nodules. When one observes a skin-colored nodule in an infant or child, an orderly list of possibilities does not easily come to mind. One should first remember that the most common palpable superficial nodule in infants and children is a lymph node. Some enlarged lymph nodes may appear in unusual locations. Occipital and cervical nodes are superficial and easily palpated, and sometimes may be mistaken for skin tumors or nodules.

The most common types of superficial skin nodules in infants and children are listed in Table 12.1.[1] An estimation of the approximate frequency of each skin nodule in infants and children is provided. Epithelial cysts and pilomatricomas together account for over two-thirds of such superficial nodules, and one should particularly remember these two major causes of skin nodules when making a diagnosis.[1] Overall, only 1% of such skin nodules turn out to be malignant growths. The main factors in suspecting whether one of these nodules is malignant are listed in Box 12.1. The most important factor is rapid, progressive growth. Hemangiomas can show rapid growth in infancy (see Ch. 13) and have a benign course. If a clinician is certain that a lesion is not a hemangioma and identifies a skin nodule with rapid, progressive growth, he or she should suspect malignancy and obtain a tissue sample for diagnosis.

SKIN CYSTS

Skin cysts are often solitary in children and produce skin-colored nodules that distort skin contours. They are the most common skin nodule, found predominantly on the lateral border of the eyebrow or under the scalp, in both infants and children (Figs 12.1–12.4).

Clinical Features

Epithelial cysts, dermoid cysts, branchial cleft cysts, and milia

Epithelial cysts are slow-growing, firm, round nodules that reach a maximum size of 1–15 cm (see Fig. 12.2). Epidermal cysts in the newborn period are found predominantly in the lateral border of the eyebrow or in the scalp.[1–3] They may also be seen on the palms and soles of newborns. They may not be recognized until childhood when the lesions grow larger. Whether these cysts contain follicular or other adnexal structures and are designated dermoid cysts does not vary their location or clinical features. The presence of midline pits or cysts on the nose poses a special problem related to possible intracranial connection.[4] Papules, cysts, or draining sinus tracts on the lateral aspect of the neck may be associated with branchial cleft cysts or sinus tracts (Fig. 12.5).[5] Midline cysts in perineum are called median raphe cysts (Fig. 12.6).

In adolescence, solitary cysts appear on the scalp, face, neck, and trunk in the region where acne vulgaris is seen (Fig, 12.7). They can be in unusual locations such as the plantar surface (Fig. 12.8). Multiple cysts in children or adolescents should suggest Gardner's syndrome which has associated multiple intestinal polyps which could become cancerous. Milia are tiny, superficial cysts seen on the faces of newborns and within the scar in scarring conditions such as epidermolysis bullosa (Fig. 12.9).

Table 12.1 Skin nodules and cysts in infants and children

Type	Approximate percentage of all nodules (%)
Epithelial cysts	59
Pilomatricomas	10
Fibromas	4
Neurofibromas	3
Lipomas	3
Lymphangiomas (lymphatic malformations)	3
Granuloma annulare	3
Juvenile xanthogranulomas	3
Mastocytomas	2
Miscellaneous lesions	9
Malignant tumors (usually sarcomas)	1

Box 12.1 Factors associated with likelihood of malignancy in superficial skin tumors in children*

Rapid, progressive growth

Ulceration

Fixed to deep fascia

Greater than 3 cm and firm

Occurs in first 30 days of life

* Listed in order of importance.

Steatocystoma multiplex

Steatocystoma multiplex appears as firm, skin-colored or yellowish nodules 1–3 cm in diameter in the axillae and on the neck, chest, and arms (Fig. 12.10). The condition is inherited as an autosomal dominant mutation of keratin 17. It can be associated with pachyonychia congenita type 2. It begins in late childhood or adolescence and is uncommon.[6,7]

Fig. 12.1 Dermoid cyst. Cystic nodule on lateral aspect of left eyebrow of newborn infant.

Fig. 12.2 Dermoid cyst on occipital scalp of infant.

Fig. 12.3 Persistence of dermoid cyst in 11-year-old girl.

Fig. 12.4 Inflamed dermoid cyst after family attempted to 'open it.'

Fig. 12.5 Branchial cleft cyst on the neck of a child.

Fig. 12.6 Median raphe cyst in perineum of infant.

Fig. 12.7 Inflamed epithelial cyst. This lesion may be inflamed secondary to infection or spontaneous rupture and foreign body reaction.

Fig. 12.8 Epidermal inclusion cyst on plantar surface of child's foot.

Fig. 12.9 Milia on the cheek of a child.

Fig. 12.10 Steatocystoma multiplex. Multiple oval 4–6 mm skin colored papules on 8-year-old's neck.

Eruptive vellus hair cysts

Eruptive vellus hair cysts commonly begin between ages 5 and 10 years as small, skin-colored papules appearing on the lower chest and upper abdomen, areas not usually involved with epithelial or dermoid cysts (Fig. 12.11).[8] Usually, five or more lesions are present.

Fig. 12.11 Eruptive vellus hair cyst. Superficial cystic lesions on the midportion of the chest and upper aspect of the abdomen.

Differential Diagnosis

For a list of skin nodules and cysts that should be included in the differential diagnosis, see Table 12.1. Epithelial and dermoid cysts are difficult to distinguish from one another without a biopsy. However, because both conditions are benign, a biopsy is usually not necessary. Midline nasal dermoid lesions are the exception. These appear as a midline pit, fistula, or swelling anywhere from the glabella to the nasal tip. These lesions may have intracranial extensions. Steatocystoma multiplex similarly has a different distribution, with locations around the axilla, neck, and onto the arms. Gardner's syndrome should be considered when multiple epithelial cysts are seen. Branchial cleft cysts are usually on the lateral aspect of the neck and may show inflammation.

Pathogenesis

Epithelial cysts and milia

Although epithelial cysts are commonly called *sebaceous cysts*, they contain neither sebum nor sebaceous glands. Epithelial cysts and milia are filled with keratin in laminated layers and lined by epithelium. When they are ruptured, foreign body reactions occur around the ruptured cyst wall.

Steatocystoma multiplex

Steatocystoma multiplex consists of intricately folded cyst walls of epithelial cells, with flattened sebaceous gland lobules within or close to the cyst wall.

Dermoid cysts

Dermoid cysts represent sequestration of skin along lines of embryonic closure and contain an epithelial lining plus either mature sebaceous glands, eccrine sweat glands, or mature hair.

Branchial cleft cysts

Branchial cleft cysts are defects of embryological closure. They may drain into the pharynx or onto the skin.[9]

Eruptive vellus hair cysts

Most authorities consider eruptive vellus hair cysts a developmental anomaly of body hair follicles. Obstruction at the neck of the follicular channel results in cystic dilation of the follicle, retention of vellus hairs, and atrophy of the hair bulbs.

Treatment

Most cysts require no treatment and may be best left alone. If cosmetic improvement can be obtained, surgical excision is the treatment of choice. Midline nasal dermoid cysts require meticulous surgical excision in an effort to prevent intracranial extension and complications. Before surgery, neuroimaging studies may help to predict intracranial involvement.[4] Branchial cleft cysts and sinus tracts require complete surgical excision to avoid recurrence. No effective therapy for vellus hair cysts is available.

Patient Education

Patients should be aware of the benign nature of these growths despite their prominent size. In children with multiple epithelial cysts, bowel examination for signs of Gardner's syndrome is indicated.

Follow-up Visits

A visit 1 week after surgery to explain the pathologic findings is beneficial.

ADNEXAL TUMORS

A variety of benign growths arises from epithelial adnexal structures (e.g. sebaceous glands, hair follicles, sweat glands) and produce skin nodules or tumors. Some, such as the sebaceous nevus and epidermal nevus, appear at birth and are discussed in the section on birthmarks (see Ch. 21). Most adnexal tumors do not appear until adult life, but four types – pilomatricomas, syringomas, trichoepitheliomas, and basal cell carcinoma – may be seen in childhood or adolescence.

Clinical Features

Pilomatricoma

Pilomatricomas (calcifying epitheliomas) appear as solitary, hard, multilobular, 2–5 mm papules covered by normal skin on the face or extremities (Figs 12.12–12.14).[10] They may have a blue color. Pilomatricomas often begin in infancy or during early school years, but they are not hereditary. Pilomatricomas account for up to 10% of all skin nodules and

Fig. 12.13 Inflamed pilomatricoma on child's cheek.

Fig. 12.14 Multilobulated pilomatricoma on adolescent's thigh.

Fig. 12.12 Pilomatricoma. Firm blue papule on the face of a child.

tumors in children.[1] They may be present in newborns. They are a result of a mutation in hair matrix cells.[11]

Fig. 12.15 Syringomas. Multiple skin-colored papules on the face and lower eyelid.

Fig. 12.17 Trichoepithelioma on child's nose.

Syringomas

Syringomas appear at puberty as small (1–2 mm), skin-colored to yellowish, soft papules (Fig. 12.15). They occur on the eyelids, cheeks, axillae, abdomen, and vulva. They are more common in girls than boys. Most often, lesions are limited to the eyelids.[12]

Trichoepitheliomas

Trichoepitheliomas appear as numerous, round, skin-colored nodules primarily on the midface area of children and adolescents (Figs 12.16, 12.17). The nodules are 2–8 mm in diameter and also may be seen on the upper trunk, neck, and scalp. A few fine telangiectasias may be observed over the lesions. Multiple lesions are inherited as an autosomal dominant trait, whereas solitary lesions may appear spontaneously without a family history.[13] Tumors of deep sweat glands (syringocystadenoma papilliferum) may arise within a nevus sebaceous at adolescence (Fig. 12.18).

Fig. 12.18 Syringocystadenoma papilliferum arising within a linear nevus sebaceous.

Basal cell carcinoma

Basal cell carcinoma is uncommon in school-age children and adolescents.[14] These lesions appear on the face or upper trunk as a solitary nodule with overlying telangiectasia. They may be seen in otherwise unaffected children, but their presence should suggest three syndromes: the basal cell nevus syndrome associated with a defect in the PTCH gene,[15] xeroderma pigmentosum, and the Bazex's syndrome (Table 12.2). The basal cell carcinoma may progress to ulceration and local invasion of the dermis and deeper tissues. It does not metastasize.

Differential Diagnosis

Pilomatricomas and basal cell carcinoma are characteristically solitary and firm, in contrast to syringomas and trichoepitheliomas. Trichoepitheliomas and syringomas may be confused with acne vulgaris or the

Fig. 12.16 Multiple trichoepitheliomas on the nose of a child.

Table 12.2 Syndromes associated with basal cell carcinoma in children

Clinical feature	Basal cell nevus syndrome	Bazex's syndrome	Xeroderma pigmentosum
Inheritance	Autosomal dominant	Autosomal dominant	Autosomal recessive
Palmar pits	Present	Present	Absent
Multiple freckles	Absent	Absent	Present
Prominent dilated pores on arms and dorsa of hands	Absent	Present	Absent
Jaw cysts	Present	Absent	Absent
Defective teeth	Present	Absent	Present

multiple angiofibromas of tuberous sclerosis because they occur on the face. The latter are red rather than skin colored, however. An ultrasound may be beneficial in diagnosing pilomatricoma.[16] A skin biopsy will distinguish between the lesions of tuberous sclerosis, trichoepithelioma, or syringoma. Confirmatory diagnosis of all four adnexal tumors is made by skin biopsy.[17,18]

Pathogenesis

Pilomatricoma

Pilomatricoma is considered a benign hyperplasia of the cells of the hair matrix. It is a tumor located in the deep dermis and is composed of islands of basophilic cells and nuclear 'shadow' cells. Calcium deposits appear throughout the tumor.

Syringoma

Syringoma is a benign hyperplasia of the cells of the eccrine sweat ducts. Numerous small ducts are located in the mid to upper dermis with 'tennis racquet' shapes and surrounding fibrosis.

Trichoepitheliomas

Trichoepitheliomas consist of multiple horn cysts and basophilic tumor islands in the mid-dermis. They are believed to be derived from the cells of the hair follicle.

Basal cell carcinoma

Basal cell carcinomas are composed of solid masses of cells that contain a large nucleus and little cytoplasm and extend down from the epidermis. Separation from the surrounding fibrous tissue by a clear space is commonly observed. In xeroderma pigmentosum, ultraviolet light-induced DNA damage cannot be repaired because of autosomal recessive inheritance of various enzyme deficiencies.[19] The pathogenesis of basal cell epitheliomas in the basal cell nevus syndrome is associated with mutations in the hedgehog signaling pathway.[15] The cause of the Bazex's syndrome is currently unknown.

Treatment

Excision is the treatment of choice for pilomatricomas and basal cell carcinoma. Multiple syringomas and trichoepitheliomas are difficult to treat, and treatment of multiple lesions often has poor cosmetic results. A recent study suggested beneficial therapy of trichoepithelioma with topical imiquimod three times a week.[20]

Patient Education

The benign nature and origin of pilomatricoma, syringoma, and trichoepithelioma should be discussed. Basal cell epitheliomas should be considered to be slowly progressing malignant tumors. In the hereditary syndromes, careful evaluation of family members is necessary.

Follow-up Visits

Children with basal cell carcinoma should be examined every 6 months for the appearance of further skin tumors. The importance of avoiding exposure to the sun and using sunscreens should be emphasized at each visit.

220 | Textbook of Pediatric Dermatology

SKIN NODULES

Fibromas

Clinical features

Dermatofibroma: The presenting symptom of dermatofibroma is a small, firm, well-defined, often pigmented nodule on the leg or trunk of children, adolescents, or adults (Figs 12.19, 12.20). Dermatofibroma may follow minor skin trauma or may appear spontaneously. Multiple lesions can also occur. Lateral pressure on the lesion will produce dimpling of its surface. The lesions may become as large as 1–2 cm in diameter, and they persist indefinitely.

Hypertrophic scars: A hypertrophic scar is an overgrowth of fibrous tissue that remains at the site of the original injury (Fig. 12.21). These lesions usually enlarge for several months after the injury along the area of the injury. Eventually, the hypertrophic scar will stabilize for several months before regressing in size.

Fig. 12.21 Hypertrophic scar. Site of previous chickenpox lesions.

Keloids: Keloids are firm, progressively enlarging nodules with a shiny, hairless surface. They may be painful or itch. They may occur on the extremities but are predominantly located on the earlobes (Fig. 12.22),

Fig. 12.19 Dermatofibroma on arm of 2-year-old child. Firm pink plaque with exaggerated dermal ridges.

Fig. 12.20 Dermatofibroma. Firm, well-defined brownish-red nodule on the leg of an adolescent.

Fig. 12.22 Keloid nodule on ear lobe from piercing.

Fig. 12.23 Keloid and epithelial cyst. Superior lesion is an epithelial cyst, and lower lesion is a keloid that formed in an excision scar of a previously excised epithelial cyst.

presternal area, neck (Fig. 12.23), and face after skin trauma. They often have stellate shapes. The tendency to form keloids may be inherited.[21] Keloids are associated with increased TGF-β upregulations.[22] They may progressively enlarge for 20–40 years and form lobulated or pedunculated masses.

Digital fibrous tumor of childhood: Digital fibrous tumor of childhood is a firm nodule occurring around the fingernail or toenail.[23] The lesion may be present at birth or will usually arise before 1 year of age. Because excision often results in rapid recurrence, the lesion is also called recurrent digital fibrous tumor. The lesion may initially grow rapidly and require a skin biopsy to confirm that it is not a sarcoma. It will usually spontaneously involute within several years.

Differential diagnosis

Dermatofibromas: Dermatofibromas may be pigmented and mimic melanoma. They are more likely to be confused with other skin nodules, however (see Table 12.1).

Keloids and hypertrophic scars: Keloids are seldom misdiagnosed, but early keloids mimic ordinary scars. The keloid will extend beyond the bounds of the original injury, whereas the hypertrophic scar will remain within the area of injury.

Digital fibrous tumor of childhood: Digital fibrous tumors may mimic the fibrous thickening overlying a

subungual exostosis, a callus, or a corn. A radiograph of the digit should be obtained before biopsy.

Pathogenesis

Dermatofibromas: Dermatofibromas contain numerous fibroblasts with excessive deposition of collagen and proliferation of the overlying epidermis. They are believed to be a reactive proliferation of fibroblasts in response to trauma.

Keloids and hypertrophic scars: Keloids produce nodular patterns of collagen fibers associated with the new blood vessel formation, as expected in healing. However, as the vessels regress, collagen deposition continues and fails to thin as expected. Hypertrophic scars may be a similar process to a lesser degree.

Digital fibrous tumor of childhood: Digital fibrous tumors show proliferating fibroblasts that contain eosinophilic cytoplasmic inclusions thought to represent myofilaments.

Treatment

Dermatofibromas, if symptomatic or worrisome, may be excised. Keloids can be treated by injections of intralesional glucocorticosteroids, which results in softening and flattening of the keloid. Often, triamcinolone acetonide, 5–10 mg/mL in saline solution, is injected. Surgery alone will result in rapid reappearance of the keloid, but surgery followed by frequent intralesional injections of glucocorticosteroids may be effective therapy for large keloids. Steroid injections may result in hypopigmentation surrounding the lesion. Applications of silicone occlusive sheeting may or may not benefit keloids or scars.[24] Months of application may be required. Recurring digital fibrous tumors should be allowed to involute spontaneously if possible because surgical excision may be followed by recurrence.[25]

Patient education

The benign nature of these disorders should be emphasized.

Follow-up visits

Keloids may be injected with steroids at 4–6 week intervals.

Fig. 12.24 Neurofibroma. Soft, skin-colored papule on midplantar skin of child.

Neurofibromas

Neurofibromas may be present at birth or develop later in life. The neurofibroma is a soft, easily inverted, skin-colored to brown papule or nodule that may occur anywhere on the skin (Fig. 12.24). Occasionally, a large clustering of neurofibromas will form a plexiform neurofibroma. Neurofibroma may occur as solitary lesions or may be associated with neurofibromatosis. Neurofibromatosis is discussed in Chapter 17. Solitary lesions may precede the other features of neurofibromatosis.

Differential diagnosis

The differential diagnoses of neurofibromas are listed in Box 12.2. A biopsy may be necessary to confirm the diagnosis.

Pathogenesis

Neurofibromas are benign tumors of nerve sheath cells.

Box 12.2 Differential diagnosis of neurofibromas
Angiolipoma
Hemangioma
Lipoma
Lymphangioma
Mucous cyst
Melanocytic nevus

Patient education

The nature of neurofibromas and their association with multiple neurofibromatosis should be carefully explained to the family, and a complete family history and evaluation of family members should be done.

Follow-up visits

Children with a solitary neurofibroma should be followed every 6–12 months and examined for the appearance of café-au-lait spots or other signs and symptoms of neurofibromatosis.

Lipomas
Clinical features

Lipomas are soft, subcutaneous nodules unattached to overlying skin (Fig. 12.25). They are usually solitary, begin in adolescence, and are most commonly found on the neck, upper aspect of the chest, and arms. Angiolipomas, variants of lipomas, may present as painful subcutaneous nodules, usually on the upper arms of adolescent females.

Differential diagnosis

Epithelial cysts, neurofibromas, and other skin nodules may mimic lipomas, but the ability to easily slide the overlying skin over the lesion helps to confirm the deep subcutaneous location of lipomas.

Pathogenesis

A lipoma is composed of nodules of normal-appearing fat cells. Capillary proliferation is seen in angiolipoma in addition to an excess of normal fat cells.

Fig. 12.25 Lipoma. Soft subcutaneous nodule unattached to overlying skin.

Treatment

Lipomas are usually asymptomatic. Angiolipomas may be painful and may require excision for pain relief.

Patient education

The benign nature of these nodules should be emphasized.

Follow-up visits

Follow-up visits are unnecessary.

Lymphangiomas (Lymphatic Malformation)

Lymphangiomas (lymphatic malformations) are often present at birth and are discussed in detail in the section on vascular malformations (see Ch. 13). They may, however, be overlooked until later in infancy and childhood, and their presenting symptom is solitary, soft swellings of the face, neck, trunk, or extremities that show progressive growth.

Granuloma Annulare

Clinical features

Small, firm papules or nodules that form a circle or semicircle are characteristic of granuloma annulare.[26] They may be skin colored, but more often a dusky, violaceous hue is seen. Stretching the skin reveals the ring of papules or nodules. The lesions occur predominantly in acral areas, on the digits, ankles, and wrists (Figs 12.26–12.32); 50% of affected children have a single ring of lesions. Occasionally, large, firm, subcutaneous nodules may be seen, or multiple small papules are found. Lesions are usually asymptomatic but occasionally can be painful.[27]

Fig. 12.26 Granuloma annulare. Unilateral oval lesion on dorsum of foot.

Fig. 12.27 Granuloma annulare. Large and small annular plaques on ventral surface of arm. Central resolution can be seen in larger lesions.

Fig. 12.28 Granuloma annulare. Grouping of firm papules on palm of hand.

Fig. 12.29 Granuloma annulare. Annular papules distorting skin over proximal interphalangeal joint of fourth digit.

Fig. 12.30 Granuloma annulare. Typical annular lesion on one wrist; solitary nodule of GA on the other wrist.

Fig. 12.31 Granuloma annulare. Annular pink papules with dusky purple center.

Fig. 12.32 Early granuloma annulare. Multiple pink annular patches on child's arm. Subtle elevated borders could be appreciated only by palpation.

Differential diagnosis

Small granuloma annulare lesions are often mistaken for dermatophyte infections. The lack of epidermal change or scaling and the deep palpable portion help distinguish granuloma annulare from tinea corporis. Large nodules of granuloma annulare may mimic rheumatoid nodules, and subcutaneous granuloma annulare may be histologically and clinically indistinguishable from rheumatoid nodules. In granuloma annulare, no systemic symptoms are noted. Occasionally, other annular lesions (e.g. lichen planus, sarcoidosis, syphilis, necrobiosis lipoidica diabeticorum) are confused with granuloma annulare. A biopsy may be necessary to confirm the diagnosis.

Pathogenesis

Focal areas of collagen degeneration surrounded by lymphocytes and epithelioid cells are seen in the mid-dermis and reticular dermis in granuloma annulare. The mechanism of the disease is unknown.

Treatment

Because lesions are asymptomatic, only reassurance is necessary. Although it is tempting to treat such conditions, spontaneous remission in several years is the rule.[26] No effective therapy is available.

Patient education

The benign nature of this disorder and its natural history should be stressed. Its distinct separation from rheumatoid disease states should be explained.

Follow-up visits

Follow-up visits are unnecessary.

Rheumatoid Nodules

Clinical features

True rheumatoid nodules are uncommon in children. They are seen in rheumatoid arthritis, rheumatic fever, and systemic lupus erythematosus as 1–4 cm subcutaneous nodules not attached to overlying skin. They develop over bony structures such as a joint and are usually associated with severe rheumatoid disease with positive rheumatoid factor. The overlying skin has a normal color.

Differential diagnosis

Rheumatoid nodules are most often confused with granuloma annulare (see Table 12.1). However, epithelial cysts, adnexal tumors, lipomas, and other skin nodules may also be confused with rheumatoid nodules.

Pathogenesis

Foci of collagen degeneration surrounded by macrophages are seen in the deep dermis and subcutaneous fat. The mechanism of production of rheumatoid nodules is unknown, but most investigators regard this condition as a form of immune complex disease.

Treatment

If the nodules are symptomatic, excision is the treatment of choice. Therapy used to control other rheumatic symptoms rarely influences rheumatoid nodules.

Patient education

Information about the nature of the associated disease should be given to the patient and family members.

Follow-up visits

The timing of follow-up visits should be based on the severity of the associated systemic illness.

Necrobiosis Lipoidica Diabeticorum

The lesions of necrobiosis lipoidica diabeticorum are irregularly shaped, yellow-red plaques on the lower leg (Fig. 12.33). The lesions may show central atrophy or sclerosis. Often, the lesions are bilateral and symmetric. A skin biopsy specimen of a lesion may have the histologic appearance of granuloma annulare. Children with necrobiosis lipoidica diabeticorum may have associated diabetes mellitus and should be evaluated with a fasting serum glucose test.

Fig. 12.33 Necrobiosis lipoidica diabeticorum. Large plaque on lower leg of female adolescent. Note elevated border and yellow-red coloration.

Fig. 12.34 Juvenile xanthogranuloma. Yellow-orange lesion on the scalp.

Fig. 12.35 Yellow-orange nodule of JXG in infant's scalp.

Fig. 12.36 Juvenile xanthogranuloma. Lesion on the abdomen has more of a brown-orange color.

Fig. 12.37 Juvenile xanthogranuloma. Grouping of lesions on lower aspect of trunk and on thigh.

Fig. 12.38 Juvenile xanthogranuloma. Orange-brown coloration is seen on close inspection.

Juvenile Xanthogranulomas

Clinical features

Juvenile xanthogranulomas (JXG) are orange to yellow-brown soft nodules that appear on the skin of infants and children (Figs 12.34–12.36). The nodules are often multiple, numbering five to ten (Figs 12.37, 12.38). They may be present at birth and often involute spontaneously over several years.[28] Lesions are seen in the iris and may be mistaken for retinoblastoma, or they may cause vision loss.[29] Although involvement is primarily in the skin, nodules have been described in the testes, lung, liver, spleen, and pericardium.[30]

Differential diagnosis

Xanthomas, spindle and epithelioid melanocytic nevi, histiocytosis, and mastocytomas all may appear as orange or yellow-brown nodules at first presentation (Box 12.3). Skin biopsy may be necessary to distinguish juvenile xanthogranuloma from these conditions. Stroking the skin surface covering, a mastocytoma will produce urticaria within the nodule (Darier's sign).

Box 12.3 Differential diagnosis of orange or yellow-brown nodules

Benign cephalic histiocytosis
Langerhans cell histiocytosis
Juvenile xanthogranuloma
Mastocytoma
Spindle and epithelioid cell melanocytic nevus
Xanthoma

Pathogenesis

Within the dermis, large accumulations of macrophages appear. Their cytoplasm gradually fills with lipid, creating a particular type of giant cell called the *Touton giant cell*. Regressing lesions show fibroblastic proliferation. There is no apparent relationship between juvenile xanthogranuloma and either abnormalities of lipid metabolism or malignant histiocytosis.

Treatment

Treatment of the individual lesions is usually not necessary. Examination by an ophthalmologist may be necessary to evaluate and possibly treat eye lesions if they occur. Eye lesions are rare and appear to be more likely associated with multiple cutaneous lesions in children younger than 2 years of age.[31] Patients with juvenile xanthogranulomas and multiple café-au-lait spots may have an increased risk of granulocytic leukemia.[32,33]

Patient education

The natural history of this lesion and the need for careful observation for eye involvement in high-risk patients should be emphasized.

Follow-up visits

Ophthalmologic follow-up may need to be done to monitor for eye changes. Examination and quantitation of skin lesions can be completed during routine examinations.

Mastocytomas

Mastocytomas are usually present at birth and are discussed in detail in Chapter 14. They may not become apparent until 1–2 months of age and appear as macular red or red-brown lesions, usually on the trunk.[34]

Pyogenic Granulomas

Clinical features

Pyogenic granulomas are most common in acral areas, such as the hands and fingers, and on the face (Fig. 12.39). They appear as solitary, dull red, firm nodules that are 5–6 mm in diameter. The surface may be smooth and glistening, but often it is ulcerated and crusted. The lesion bleeds easily when traumatized. Surgical excision has resulted in the appearance of multiple satellite lesions in a few instances. Pyogenic granuloma may occur at any age, but in childhood it is most common in the first 5 years of life. The majority of patients have no history of a predisposing factor.[35]

Differential diagnoses

Pyogenic granuloma is often misdiagnosed as a hemangioma, glomus tumor, melanocytic nevus, wart, molluscum contagiosum, or malignant melanoma.[36] All of these lesions can ulcerate and crust if traumatized. It is important to obtain tissue for pathology in order to distinguish pyogenic granuloma from the other lesions, which may have serious medical consequences.

Pathogenesis

Proliferation of capillaries within a circumscribed area with flattened or ulcerated epidermis on top and epidermal proliferation at the sides, producing a 'collarette' of epidermis, is seen. Pyogenic granuloma may be caused by increased expression of vascular endothelial growth factor (VEGF).[37]

Treatment

Shave biopsy followed by curettage and electrocautery is the treatment of choice.[38] The removed tissue should be sent for pathological examination. Pulse dye laser treatment may be effective for smaller lesions but repeated treatments may be necessary.[39]

Patient education

The clinician should explain to the patient and parents that this growth is not malignant, will not disappear without treatment, and represents an abnormal healing response.

Follow-up visits

A visit 1 week after removal of the lesion is useful to inform the patient of the pathologic diagnosis and evaluate healing.

Smooth-Muscle Hamartoma

Smooth-muscle hamartomas are present a birth, but they may not be noted until later in infancy or childhood. The lesions may have excess hair and may be hyperpigmented when compared with normal skin. On palpation, the lesional hairs may become erect as a result of the excess smooth muscle within the lesion. Biopsy of the lesion will show abundant smooth-muscle bundles within the dermis.[40]

Calcified Nodules

Cutaneous calcinosis results from precipitation of insoluble calcium salts within cutaneous tissues. This can occur in congenital or acquired lesions. Solitary or multiple lesions can be present that are firm or rock hard. They are usually asymptomatic but can be painful and discharge chalky material through the skin. Underlying metabolic disease, connective tissue disease, or malignancy may be associated, or the lesion can be idiopathic. In newborn infants, a solitary calcified nodule of the ear may form (Figs 12.40, 12.41), whereas in children with dermatomyositis or other collagen vascular diseases, multiple nodules

Fig. 12.39 Pyogenic granuloma. Smooth, glistening surface on an erythematous papule.

Fig. 12.40 Calcified nodule. Lesion on ear of infant.

Fig. 12.41 Calcified nodule of ear in preteen.

may form on the extensor surfaces of hands and elbows. Biopsy confirmation is necessary before a comprehensive systemic evaluation is begun.

Piezogenic Pedal Papules

Piezogenic pedal papules are common, sometimes painful papules that may occur on the feet (Fig. 12.42) and wrist.[41] The lesions represent herniations of fatty subcutaneous tissue into connective tissue. The herniations are seen when pressure is applied to the heel or wrist. Painful lesions can be excised or treated with orthopedic padding.[41]

Knuckle Pads

Knuckle pads are thickening of the skin overlying digital joints (Fig. 12.43). The lesions grow slowly and

are asymptomatic.[42] The lesions are sporadic and idiopathic. They are rarely associated with trauma. The lesions can persist indefinitely. Treatment is usually unsuccessful and unnecessary because the lesions are asymptomatic.

Panniculitis

Inflammation in the subcutaneous fat may be first seen as painful lesions that feel as if they are deep beneath the skin. Biopsy will identify the inflammation within the fat. The cause of panniculitis may not be found, or it can be associated with infection, trauma, metabolic, or systemic disease.[43] Biopsy confirmation may be necessary before a comprehensive systemic evaluation is begun. One type of panniculitis, subcutaneous fat necrosis of the newborn infant, is described in Chapter 21.

Fig. 12.42 Piezogenic pedal papules. Lesions on the foot are seen as multiple soft, compressible papules that appear when pressure is placed on the heel.

Fig. 12.43 Knuckle pads over the proximal interphalangeal joints of both hands.

Sarcoidosis

Sarcoidosis is a systemic disease associated with granulomas. Skin lesions can occur with or without systemic symptoms. The skin lesions may appear as indurated papules or plaques. Skin biopsy showing the granulomas of sarcoid should prompt a systemic evaluation for sarcoidosis.[44]

Corns and Calluses

Clinical features

Corns and calluses are areas of thickened skin that appear on sites of prolonged pressure or friction. Patients who have these lesions often believe they are warts. Corns are more circumscribed (2–5 mm), may be painful and are better demarcated than calluses (Fig. 12.44). Paring the surface off the lesions will reveal a central core in a corn. Corns are found primarily on the feet and are the result of poorly fitting shoes. Calluses are diffuse areas of thickened skin, 5–20 mm in diameter, on the palmar surfaces of hands or fingers or the weight-bearing areas of the feet. Paring the surfaces of these lesions will reveal normal skin grooves.

Differential diagnosis

Plantar warts are most often confused with corns and calluses. Shaving off the skin surface with a razor blade will reveal interrupted skin ridges with a central area containing black dots in a wart, interrupted skin ridges with a central core of keratin in a corn, and normal skin ridges in a callus. Patients with unexplained focal or diffuse thickening of the palms or soles may have a variety of palmoplantar kerato-

Fig. 12.44 Corn. Circumscribed epidermal thickening with central core.

derma. These conditions may be associated with metabolic or structural abnormalities and may require intensive investigation.

Pathogenesis

Prolonged pressure or friction from ill-fitting shoes produces corns and calluses on the feet. Playing a musical instrument, using playground equipment, or working with tools produces corns and calluses on the hands. The thickening is due to epidermal proliferation and an increase in the number of cells in the stratum corneum.

Treatment

Reducing the lesion with a razor blade by shaving off the excess stratum corneum and then covering the lesion with a salicylic acid 40% plaster for 1–7 days will relieve the discomfort of corns and calluses. Changing shoes may also benefit the patient.

Patient education

The patient should be told that the lesion is not a wart and that prolonged pressure and friction are responsible for the genesis of the lesion.

Follow-up visits

Follow-up visits are unnecessary.

Histiocytosis

Clinical features

The histiocytoses include a group of benign and fatal disorders which are characterized by proliferation of histiocytes.[45] Lesions may be present at birth or appear during infancy or childhood (Figs 12.45–12.50). The cutaneous lesions of Langerhans cell histiocytosis (LCH) may consist of discrete red, orange, and/or yellow-brown papules or nodules. The presenting symptom may be a crusted, scaling dermatitis of the scalp, postauricular, perineal, and axillary areas. The presence of red-brown purpuric papules and nodules within or peripheral to areas of dermatitis should alert the clinician to a diagnosis of LCH.

Congenital self-healing reticulohistiocytosis consists of papules and nodular lesions present at birth that can look like the lesions of LCH or a pyogenic granuloma (Figs 12.51, 12.52).[46,47] Larger lesions

Fig. 12.45 Langerhans cell histiocytosis. Crusted purpuric papules on lower abdomen with underlying lymphadenopathy.

Fig. 12.46 Langerhans cell histiocytosis. Diaper dermatitis similar to Figure 4.21.

Fig. 12.47 Langerhans cell histiocytosis. More severe dermatitis in diaper area unresponsive to conventional therapy.

Fig. 12.48 Langerhans cell histiocytosis. Erosions in both inguinal areas in this infant.

Fig. 12.49 Langerhans cell histiocytosis. Scaly and crusted papules in infant's scalp.

Fig. 12.50 Langerhans cell histiocytosis. Petechial papules and scaly plaques on infant's trunk.

Fig.12.51 Congenital self-healing reticulohistiocytosis. At birth, this lesion looks similar to a pyogenic granuloma.

Fig.12.52 Congenital self-healing reticulohistiocytosis. Nodule present at birth with crateriform central erosion.

can demonstrate a crateriform central erosion (see Fig. 12.52).

Benign cephalic histiocytosis consists of 2–5 mm, yellow-red to tan papules that develop on the face and upper part of the body (Figs 12.53, 12.54).[48] The lesions usually begin between 6 and 12 months of age. They consist of non-Langerhans cell histiocytes.

Differential diagnosis

Histiocytosis lesions include the differential diagnosis of juvenile xanthogranulomas, eczema, seborrheic dermatitis, diaper dermatitis, and scabies.[49] The presence of petechiae or purpura within or peripheral to areas of dermatitis suggests LCH.

Pathogenesis

The Langerhans cell is a specific monocyte-macrophage that expresses CD1, a glycoprotein, and contains Birbeck granules.[50] Langerhans cells are found within the epidermis of skin, regional lymph nodes, thymic epithelium, and bronchial mucosa. The histiocyte is a monocyte-macrophage. The associated histiocytic syndromes represent infiltrations with histiocytic cells that may or may not be Langerhans cells.

LCH is an umbrella term that includes the diseases previously called *histiocytosis X*. The diagnostic feature of LCH is the presence of lesional histiocytes, at least some of which are phenotypically like normal Langerhans cells.[50] The lesions may contain varying proportions of LCH cells, macrophages, lymphocytes, eosinophils, neutrophils, and plasma cells. Skin, bone, spleen, liver, lungs, and lymph nodes may

Fig. 12.53 Benign cephalic histiocytosis. Multiple tan flat-topped papules on face.

Fig. 12.54 Benign cephalic histiocytosis. Multiple red-tan papules on face.

Benign cephalic histiocytosis usually requires no therapy and should resolve during childhood. A patient has been documented with diabetes insipidus and benign cephalic histiocytosis.[51] Congenital self-healing reticulohistiocytosis requires close clinical observation to confirm a benign course. LCH survival and therapy are dependent on the number of organs involved and the severity of the involvement.[45] Therapy for LCH may also involve surgical removal of lesions, chemotherapy, or observation. Chemotherapy may include corticosteroids, alkylating agents, cytokines, or immunoglobulin. Before therapy, a systemic evaluation is required to identify the extent and severity of disease.

Patient education

A thorough evaluation is necessary to identify the type and extent of histiocytic syndromes. Parents should be informed of the unusual nature of LCH and should be given information on the benign or malignant course that their child can expect.

Follow-up visits

Diagnosis and treatment of these conditions requires coordination with a pathologist, radiologist, pediatric oncologist, and primary care physician. Follow-up visits should be arranged to inform the patient and the patient's family of the severity and extent of disease and possible therapies directed by the pediatric oncologist.

be affected. Great clinical heterogeneity of LCH exists despite more uniform pathologic features. LCH may be localized to bone or skin, may be associated with diabetes insipidus and/or exophthalmos, or may have lethal multiorgan involvement. Studies have considered a relationship between human herpesvirus 6 and LCH.[45]

Benign cephalic histiocytosis lesions consists of non-Langerhans cell histiocytes.

Treatment

Treatment of these disorders depends on the specific diagnosis and extent of disease. A biopsy is usually necessary to confirm the diagnosis. Additional biopsies may be needed for electron microscopic examination and immunohistochemistry to confirm the specific type of histiocytosis.

Fig. 12.55 Embryonal rhabdomyosarcoma on the face of an infant.

Rhabdomyosarcomas

Clinical features

Rhabdomyosarcomas are the most common malignant soft-tissue tumors in childhood.[52] They are far more common than melanomas in prepubertal children. The head (Fig. 12.55) and neck and urogenital tract are the usual sites of involvement. Two peaks of age in childhood have a higher incidence of rhabdomyosarcoma: ages 1–5, and during adolescence. The tumor usually appears as a mass lesion of the neck, face, or extremity, or is seen as a subcutaneous and/or intradermal nodule that has normal-appearing skin. Occasionally, the surface of the skin covering the tumor becomes reddened. The lesion may produce local signs of destruction depending on the location. For example, in the orbit, it may produce exophthalmos or ptosis; in the ear canal, a bloody discharge with a polypoid ear mass; and in the nasal passages, obstruction of one of the airways and bleeding. In the genitourinary tract, it may appear as urinary obstruction. Grapelike masses of tumor protruding from the vagina are another presentation of rhabdomyosarcoma.

Rhabdomyosarcomas may spread either by local extension or by hematogenous or lymphatic metastases. Approximately 75% of the metastases will become apparent within 6 months of the appearance of the original lesion. The most frequent sites involved with metastases are the regional lymph nodes, lungs, liver, bone marrow, bone, and brain. Head and neck tumors have been reported to extend directly into the brain, and may occur as frequently as in one-third of all cases.

Differential diagnosis

The feature of rapid, progressive growth will help distinguish rhabdomyosarcoma from the other skin nodules and cysts of infants and children listed in Table 12.1. Ulceration is not an early sign of rhabdomyosarcoma, but the tumor is fixed to deep fascia, is often greater than 3 cm, and is firm in consistency.

Pathogenesis

Rhabdomyosarcoma is a malignant tumor of striated muscles. There is no hereditary pattern and there are no known precipitating factors. They are separated into the two common histological types of either embryonal or alveolar rhabdomyosarcoma.[52]

Treatment

Therapy has included radiation and combination chemotherapy in the initial stages of disease after wide surgical excision. Debulking the tumor with wide surgical excision is the first treatment of choice. New therapeutic protocols are currently being evaluated.[52]

Patient education

Prognosis should be discussed with the family, keeping in mind that a number of factors are important in the survival rate. The prognosis is better for the embryonal type than the alveolar type of rhabdomyosarcoma.[52] The location of the original lesion is an important factor, with the best prognosis occurring in orbital lesions, the next best with bladder, and the worst with lesions beginning on the head and neck. Referral to a pediatric oncology facility as soon as the diagnosis is suspected is indicated.

Follow-up visits

Follow-up visits should be arranged for family support, but a pediatric oncologist should be involved in determining frequency of visits.

Neuroblastoma, Leukemia, and Lymphoma

Lymphoma, leukemia (Fig. 12.56), and neuroblastoma (Fig. 12.57) can present as inflamed cutaneous papules or nodules.[53–55] Neuroblastomas may blanch when stroked.[56] The lesions may appear as the primary manifestation of disease or as a metastases of known disease. Cutaneous T-cell lymphoma is also

Fig. 12.56 Leukemia. Firm purple nodules on the back of an infant with congenital leukemia.

Fig. 12.57 Cutaneous neuroblastoma as blue nodule was the first sign of this infant's disease.

Fig. 12.58 Hypopigmented patch as early sign of cutaneous T-cell lymphoma in 6-year-old.

Fig. 12.59 Persistent eczematous patches and plaques in 8-year-old with cutaneous T-cell lymphoma.

Fig. 12.60 Eroded nodule on child's arm with Ki+ T-cell lymphoma.

atrophy (Fig. 12.58). The diagnosis may require several skin biopsies as well as special stains of the biopsies for immunological markers.[57] Unknown nodules or lesions that demonstrate rapid progressive growth (see Box 12.1), should be biopsied for specific diagnosis (Figs 12.59, 12.60). Therapy will need to be directed by a pediatric oncologist.

REFERENCES

1. Knight PJ, Reiner CB. Superficial lumps in children: what, when, and why? Pediatrics 1983; 72(2):147153.
2. Hsu HC, Lin HF. Eyelid tumors in children: a clinicopathologic study of a 10-year review in southern Taiwan. Ophthalmologica 2004; 218(4):274–277.
3. Pryor SG, Lewis JE, Weaver AL, et al. Pediatric dermoid cysts of the head and neck. Otolaryngol Head Neck Surg 2005; 132(6):938–942.
4. Paller AS, Pensler JM, Tomita T. Nasal midline masses in infants and children. Dermoids, encephaloceles, and gliomas. Arch Dermatol 1991; 127(3):362–366.

called mycosis fungoides. It can present in children with hypopigmented patches and possibly hypopigmented plaques that may demonstrate cutaneous

5. Todd NW. Common congenital anomalies of the neck. Embryology and surgical anatomy. Surg Clin North Am 1993; 73(4):599–610.

6. Covello SP, Smith FJ, Sillevis Smitt JH, et al. Keratin 17 mutations cause either steatocystoma multiplex or pachyonychia congenita type 2. Br J Dermatol 1998139(3):475–480.

7. Rugg EL, Leigh IM. The keratins and their disorders. Am J Med Genet C Semin Med Genet 2004 Nov 15;131C(1):4-11.

8. Grimalt R, Gelmetti C. Eruptive vellus hair cysts: case report and review of the literature. Pediatr Dermatol 1992; 9(2):98–102.

9. Davenport M. ABC of general surgery in children. Lumps and swellings of the head and neck. Br Med J 1996; 312(7027):368–371.

10. Julian CG, Bowers PW. A clinical review of 209 pilomatricomas. J Am Acad Dermatol 1998; 39(2 Pt 1):191–195.

11. Xia J, Urabe K, Moroi Y, et al. Beta-catenin mutation and its nuclear localization are confirmed to be frequent causes of Wnt signaling pathway activation in pilomatricomas. J Dermatol Sci 2006; 41(1):67–75.

12. Pruzan DL, Esterly NB, Prose NS. Eruptive syringoma. Arch Dermatol. 1989; 125(8):1119–1120.

13. Lee DA, Grossman ME, Schneiderman P, et al. Genetics of skin appendage neoplasms and related syndromes. J Med Genet 2005; 42(11):811–819.

14. Price MA, Goldberg LH, Levy ML. Juvenile basal cell carcinoma. Pediatr Dermatol 1994; 11(2):176–177.

15. High A, Zedan W. Basal cell nevus syndrome. Curr Opin Oncol 2005; 17(2):160–166.

16. Hwang JY, Lee SW, Lee SM. The common ultrasonographic features of pilomatricoma. J Ultrasound Med 2005; 24(10):1397–1402.

17. Kirchmann TT, Prieto VG, Smoller BR. CD34 staining pattern distinguishes basal cell carcinoma from trichoepithelioma. Arch Dermatol 1994; 130(5):589–592.

18. Marrogi AJ, Wick MR, Dehner LP. Benign cutaneous adnexal tumors in childhood and young adults, excluding pilomatrixoma: review of 28 cases and literature. J Cutan Pathol 1991; 18(1):20–27.

19. Cleaver JE. Cancer in xeroderma pigmentosum and related disorders of DNA repair. Nat Rev Cancer 2005; 5(7):564–573.

20. Urquhart JL, Weston WL. Treatment of multiple trichoepitheliomas with topical imiquimod and tretinoin. Pediatr Dermatol. 2005; 22(1):67–70.

21. Bayat A, Walter JM, Bock O, et al. Genetic susceptibility to keloid disease: mutation screening of the TGFbeta3 gene. Br J Plast Surg 2005; 58(7):914–921.

22. Campaner AB, Ferreira LM, Gragnani A, et al. Upregulation of TGF-beta1 expression may be necessary but is not sufficient for excessive scarring. J Invest Dermatol 2006; 126(5):1168–1176.

23. Beckett JH, Jacobs AH. Recurring digital fibrous tumors of childhood: a review. Pediatrics 1977; 59(3):401–406.

24. O'Brien L, Pandit A. Silicon gel sheeting for preventing and treating hypertrophic and keloid scars. Cochrane Database Syst Rev. 2006(1):CD003826.

25. Albertini JG, Welsch MJ, Conger LA, et al. Infantile digital fibroma treated with Mohs micrographic surgery. Dermatol Surg 2002; 28(10):959–961.

26. Smith MD, Downie JB, DiCostanzo D. Granuloma annulare. Int J Dermatol 1997; 36(5):326–333.

27. Brey NV, Malone J, Callen JP. Acute-onset, painful acral granuloma annulare: a report of four cases and a discussion of the clinical and histologic spectrum of the disease. Arch Dermatol 2006; 142(1):49–54.

28. Janssen D, Harms D. Juvenile xanthogranuloma in childhood and adolescence: a clinicopathologic study of 129 patients from the Kiel pediatric tumor registry. Am J Surg Pathol 2005; 29(1):21–28.

29. Hildebrand GD, Timms C, Thompson DA, et al. Juvenile xanthogranuloma with presumed involvement of the optic disc and retina. Arch Ophthalmol 2004; 122(10):1551–1555.

30. Freyer DR, Kennedy R, Bostrom BC, et al. Juvenile xanthogranuloma: forms of systemic disease and their clinical implications. J Pediatr 1996; 129(2):227–237.

31. Chang MW, Frieden IJ, Good W. The risk of intraocular juvenile xanthogranuloma: survey of current practices and assessment of risk. J Am Acad Dermatol 1996; 34(3):445–449.

32. Cambiaghi S, Restano L, Caputo R. Juvenile xanthogranuloma associated with neurofibromatosis 1: 14 patients without evidence of hematologic malignancies. Pediatr Dermatol 2004; 21(2):97–101.

33. Shin HT, Harris MB, Orlow SJ. Juvenile myelomonocytic leukemia presenting with features of hemophagocytic lymphohistiocytosis in association with neurofibromatosis and juvenile xanthogranulomas. J Pediatr Hematol Oncol 2004; 26(9):591–595.

34. Ben-Amitai D, Metzker A, Cohen HA. Pediatric cutaneous mastocytosis: a review of 180 patients. Isr Med Assoc J. 2005; 7(5):320–322.

35. Patrice SJ, Wiss K, Mulliken JB. Pyogenic granuloma (lobular capillary hemangioma): a clinicopathologic study of 178 cases. Pediatr Dermatol 1991; 8(4):267–276.

36. Frieden IJ, Esterly NB. Pyogenic granulomas of infancy masquerading as strawberry hemangiomas. Pediatrics 1992; 90(6):989–991.

37. Bragado R, Bello E, Requena L, et al. Increased expression of vascular endothelial growth factor in pyogenic granulomas. Acta Derm Venereol 1999; 79(6):422–425.

38. Ghodsi SZ, Raziei M, Taheri A, et al. Comparison of cryotherapy and curettage for the treatment of pyogenic granuloma: a randomized trial. Br J Dermatol 2006; 154(4):671–675.

39. Tay YK, Weston WL, Morelli JG. Treatment of pyogenic granuloma in children with the flashlamp-pumped pulsed dye laser. Pediatrics 1997; 99(3):368–370.

40. Gagne EJ, Su WP. Congenital smooth muscle hamartoma of the skin. Pediatr Dermatol 1993; 10(2):142–145.

41. Redbord KP, Adams BB. Piezogenic pedal papules in a marathon runner. Clin J Sport Med 2006; 16(1):81–83.

42. Peterson CM, Barnes CJ, Davis LS. Knuckle pads: does knuckle cracking play an etiologic role? Pediatr Dermatol 2000; 17(6):450–452.

43. Schuval SJ, Frances A, Valderrama E, et al. Panniculitis and fever in children. J Pediatr 1993; 122(3):372–378.

44. English JC 3rd, Patel PJ, Greer KE. Sarcoidosis. J Am Acad Dermatol 2001; 44(5):725–743; quiz 744–746.

45. McClain KL, Natkunam Y, Swerdlow SH. Atypical cellular disorders. Hematology (Am Soc Hematol Educ Program) 2004:283–296.

46. Ricart J, Jimenez A, Marquina A, et al. Congenital self-healing reticulohistiocytosis: report of a case and review of the literature. Acta Paediatr 2004;93(3):426–429.

47. Berger TG, Lane AT, Headington JT, et al. A solitary variant of congenital self-healing reticulohistiocytosis: solitary Hashimoto-Pritzker disease. Pediatr Dermatol 1986; 3(3):230–236.

48. Jih DM, Salcedo SL, Jaworsky C. Benign cephalic histiocytosis: a case report and review. J Am Acad Dermatol 2002; 47(6):908–913.

49. Talanin NY, Smith SS, Shelley ED, et al. Cutaneous histiocytosis with Langerhans cell features induced by scabies: a case report. Pediatr Dermatol 1994; 11(4):327–330.

50. Geissmann F, Lepelletier Y, Fraitag S, et al. Differentiation of Langerhans cells in Langerhans cell histiocytosis. Blood 2001 1; 97(5):1241–1248.

51. Weston WL, Travers SH, Mierau GW, et al. Benign cephalic histiocytosis with diabetes insipidus. Pediatr Dermatol 2000; 17(4):296–298.

52. Breitfeld PP, Meyer WH. Rhabdomyosarcoma: new windows of opportunity. Oncologist 2005; 10(7):518–527.

53. Harms D. New entities, concepts, and questions in childhood tumor pathology. Gen Diagn Pathol 1995; 141(1):1–14.

54. de la Luz Orozco-Covarrubias M, Tamayo-Sanchez L, Duran-McKinster C, et al. Malignant cutaneous tumors in children. Twenty years of experience at a large pediatric hospital. J Am Acad Dermatol 1994; 30(2 Pt 1):243–249.

55. Young G, Toretsky JA, Campbell AB, et al. Recognition of common childhood malignancies. Am Fam Physician 2000; 61(7):2144–2154.

56. Maris JM, Matthay KK. Molecular biology of neuroblastoma. J Clin Oncol 1999; 17(7):2264–2279.

57. Wain EM, Orchard GE, Mayou S, et al. Mycosis fungoides with a CD56+ immunophenotype. J Am Acad Dermatol 2005; 53(1):158–163.

Chapter 13 | Vascular Lesions

VASCULAR TUMORS AND MALFORMATIONS

Vascular birthmarks are one of the most common forms of birth defects. The classification of vascular birthmarks has in the past been confusing. We prefer the classification of Mulliken and Glowacki (Box 13.1), which divides vascular birthmarks into vascular tumors and vascular malformations.[1,2] Although they may occasionally appear similar at birth, the natural history of these lesions is quite distinct, and within a few months of age they can usually be differentiated (Table 13.1).

Vascular Tumors

Clinical features[3]

Infantile hemangiomas: Although generally classified as vascular birthmarks, only 20% of infantile hemangiomas are present at birth. The other 80% arise between 2 and 4 weeks of age. Hemangiomas are common and by 1 year of age, 10–12% of children born at full term will have developed an infantile hemangioma. Twenty percent of preterm babies weighing less than 1000 g will develop an infantile hemangioma. Females are affected at least twice as often as males.

There are three major types of infantile hemangioma presentations (Box 13.2). The most common is a pale white to gray-blue macule (Figs 13.1, 13.2). The other types are the telangiectatic (Figs 13.3, 13.4) and the papular (Fig. 13.5) forms. At the time of presentation it is impossible to predict what form the infantile hemangioma will eventually take or its final size. Because all infantile hemangiomas are derived from the same cell type, and all have the same natural history, the terms *strawberry* and *cavernous* should

not be used to describe infantile hemangiomas. These terms should be replaced by describing the location of the infantile hemangioma within the skin (see Box 13.1). Bright-red, papular infantile hemangiomas should be referred to as *superficial infantile hemangiomas* (Fig. 13.6), whereas blue, nodular infantile hemangiomas should be referred to as *deep infantile hemangiomas* (Fig. 13.7). The majority of infantile hemangiomas contain both a superficial and a deep component (Figs 13.8, 13.9) and should be labeled as *mixed infantile hemangiomas* (see Box 13.1).

At 4–8 weeks of age, infantile hemangiomas undergo a rapid growth phase that continues until the infant is 6–9 months of age. During this time the rate of growth of the infantile hemangioma is much greater than the growth rate of the infant. This rapid growth phase is a characteristic feature of infantile hemangiomas. After the rapid growth phase, the infantile hemangioma growth slows and approximates the growth rate of the infant. As they grow, most infantile hemangiomas will feel soft and be easily compressible. The growth phase is eventually followed by regression of the infantile hemangioma. This begins sometime in the second year of life. The regression phase begins with paling of the infantile hemangioma (Fig. 13.10), followed by flattening of the tumor. This phase slowly continues, and by 5 years of age 50% of infantile hemangiomas have reached maximal regression. By 9 years of age 90% of infantile hemangiomas will have reached maximal regression. Maximal regression of the infantile hemangioma does not define a return to normal skin. Residual postinfantile hemangioma regression includes hypopigmentation, telangiectasia (Fig. 13.11), fibrofatty deposits, and scarring if the infantile hemangioma has previously ulcerated.

Although infantile hemangiomas are usually benign lesions, they can be associated with certain local and

Box 13.1 Classification of infantile hemangiomas and vascular malformations

Infantile hemangiomas
Superficial

Mixed

Deep

Vascular malformations
Capillary (port-wine stain)

Telangiectatic

Hypertrophic capillary (angiokeratoma)

Venous

Arteriovenous

Lymphatic

Cutis marmorata telangiectatica congenita

Mixed

Table 13.1 Differential diagnosis of infantile hemangiomas and vascular malformations

Infantile hemangiomas	Vascular malformations
Tumor of endothelial cells	Developmental abnormality
Only 20% present at birth	Always present at birth
Undergo rapid growth	Stable growth
Always undergo regression	Never regress

Box 13.2 Clinical presentation of infantile hemangiomas

Blue-gray macule

Telangiectatic

Papular

Fig. 13.1 Macular pale white presentation of an infantile hemangioma.

Fig. 13.2 Macular pale precursor of an infantile hemangioma.

Fig. 13.3 Telangiectatic presentation of an infantile hemangioma.

systemic complications (Box 13.3). Ulceration and subsequent infection are the most common forms of complications of infantile hemangiomas. Ulcerations (Fig. 13.12) occur during the rapid growth phase of infantile hemangiomas primarily located in the diaper area.[4] Infection is usually with *Staphylococcus aureus*, but *Pseudomonas aeruginosa* may also be seen. Infants with periorbital infantile hemangiomas should always be referred for ophthalmologic evaluation for amblyopia and/or astigmatism. Superficial cervicofacial infantile hemangiomas in a 'beard distribution' are associated with upper airway infantile hemangiomas.[5] Large lumbosacral infantile hemangiomas spanning the midline may be associated with underlying anomalies of the spine and spinal cord.[6] Large facial infantile hemangiomas may be associated with central nervous system malformations (most commonly Dandy-Walker posterior fossa malformations), abnormal central nervous system arteries, cardiac and

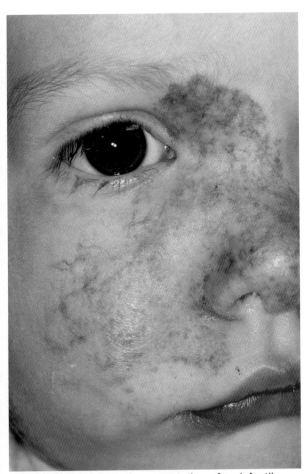

Fig. 13.4 Telangiectatic presentation of an infantile hemangioma.

Fig. 13.5 Papular presentation of an infantile hemangioma.

Fig. 13.6 Superficial infantile hemangioma.

Fig. 13.7 Deep infantile hemangioma.

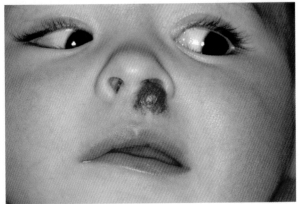

Fig. 13.8 Mixed superficial and deep infantile hemangioma that obstructs breathing.

large vessel defects, and ophthalmologic abnormalities (PHACE syndrome [*p*osterior fossa malformation, infantile *h*emangiomas, *a*rterial anomalies, *c*oarctation of the aorta and other cardiac defects, and *e*ye abnormalities]).[7]

Magnetic resonance imaging (MRI) of the lower spine should be obtained on children with large lumbosacral infantile hemangiomas. Brain and cardiac imaging should be performed if one is considering the

Fig. 13.9 Mixed superficial and deep infantile hemangioma.

Fig. 13.10 Paling of a mixed superficial and deep infantile hemangioma in an 18-month-old female. This is often the initial sign of regression of the infantile hemangioma.

Fig. 13.11 Residual hypopigmentation and telangiectasia postregression of an infantile hemangioma in a 17-year-old female.

Fig. 13.12 Ulceration of an infantile hemangioma on the buttock of a 3-month-old infant.

Box 13.3 Complications of infantile hemangiomas
Local
Obstruction of vital function
Ulceration
Infection
Systemic
High-output cardiac failure

possibility of the PHACE syndrome (Fig.13.13). Obstruction of a vital function (e.g. vision, Figs 13.13–13.15), breathing (Fig.13.16), eating, urination, or defecation and high-output cardiac failure may also be seen. A solitary cutaneous infantile hemangioma

Fig. 13.13 Widespread facial infantile hemangiomas in PHACE syndrome.

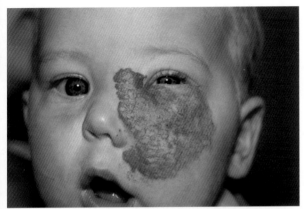

Fig. 13.14 Mixed superficial and deep infantile hemangioma in a 4-month-old male, leading to partial visual obstruction.

Fig. 13.15 Deep infantile hemangioma obstructing vision.

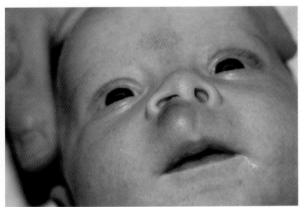

Fig. 13.16 Deep infantile hemangioma obstructing breathing.

Fig. 13.17 Sudden change of a kaposiform superficial hemangioendothelioma to deep purple as part of the Kasabach-Merritt syndrome.

causing high-output cardiac failure is an exceedingly rare event. Although historically described in infantile hemangiomas, platelet trapping with consumption coagulopathy (Kasabach-Merritt syndrome) is rarely if ever seen with these tumors, but it is seen most commonly in association with kaposiform hemangioendothelioma or tufted angioma.[8]

Kaposiform hemangioendothelioma: Kaposiform hemangioendotheliomas are rare vascular tumors that often are present at birth and are usually seen before 2 years of age.[9] They occur equally in males and females. Mature lesions have a nodular and infiltrative growth pattern and a characteristic purple color. Lesions are usually solitary. They may be seen in the retroperitoneum and the skin, but hepatic kaposiform hemangioendothelioma has not been reported. These are very aggressive local tumors, and although not

metastatic they can be fatal. As opposed to infantile hemangiomas, kaposiform hemangioendotheliomas do not regress spontaneously.

Platelet trapping with consumption coagulopathy may occur. A large, rapidly growing, soft, compressible vascular tumor is noted to suddenly become firm and to become dark purple (Fig. 13.17).

Laboratory evaluation will show a decreased platelet count and abnormal blood clotting consistent with a consumption coagulopathy. Although quite rare, it is a medical emergency.

Histologically, the tumor consists of a combination of plump and spindle-shaped endothelial cells. The areas containing the spindle cells are slitlike vascular spaces resembling Kaposi's sarcoma. The cells are locally aggressive and form irregular lobules and sheets of cells that infiltrate the dermis and subcutaneous tissue.

Fig. 13.18 Plaque-type tufted angioma on the neck of a 4-year-old girl.

Fig. 13.19 Satellite lesions of tufted angioma on the neck of the same girl in Figure 13.12.

Fig. 13.21 Nodular-type tufted angioma on the thigh of a 2-week-old boy.

Fig. 13.20 Solitary tufted angioma on leg.

Tufted angiomas: Tufted angiomas present as two distinct clinical patterns.[10,11] The most common of these are slowly expanding, dusky, reddish-blue vas-cular plaques. More than 50% occur on the head, neck, upper trunk, and upper arms (Fig. 13.18). Satellite lesions may be seen (Fig. 13.19). The majority arise within the first two decades of life. Regression in this type of tufted angioma is not expected. Kasabach-Merritt syndrome may also be seen with this tumor.

The less common form presents as a solitary vascular tumor on a lower extremity (Figs 13.20, 13.21). This type of tumor does not exhibit the slow expansion seen in the other clinical type of tufted angioma, and satellite lesions are not seen. Regression of this type of tufted angioma has been reported.[12]

Histologically, the blood vessels in tufted angiomas occur in discrete tufts (hence the name) described as 'cannonball-like.' The tufts consist of endothelial cells closely packed together.

Congenital infantile hemangiomas

Congenital infantile hemangiomas[13,14] are fully developed at birth and do not exhibit the rapid growth phase seen in infantile hemangiomas. There are two types of congenital infantile hemangiomas: rapidly involuting congenital infantile hemangioma (RICH), and noninvoluting congenital infantile hemangioma (NICH).

There are three presentations of RICH: a red-purple tumor with coarse telangiectasia present on the surface; a flat infiltrative tumor with violaceous overlying skin; and a raised grayish tumor with multiple tiny telangiectasias surrounded by a pale halo (Fig. 13.22). They are most commonly seen on the head, neck, or limbs. The natural history of RICH is to involute rapidly within the first 6–14 months of life, leaving abnormal atrophic baggy skin as a residue. Occasionally, RICH will not involute completely and will subsequently resemble NICH. Histologically, RICH have large lobules of capillaries surrounded by fibrous tissue. Hemosiderin, thrombosis, and focal calcification may be seen.

NICH are also seen predominantly on the head, neck, and limbs. They present as plaquelike tumors with a pink to purple color and coarse superficial telangiectasia. NICH grow proportionately with the child without signs of regression. Histologically, NICH contain lobular collections of small, thin-walled vessels with dilated dysplastic veins interlobularly.

Differential diagnosis

The differential diagnosis of an infantile hemangioma depends on the time of presentation to the physician.

Fig. 13.22 Dull red plaque with surrounding halo in rapidly involuting congenital hemangiona [RICH] at age 2 months.

A mature infantile hemangioma that has undergone a rapid growth phase followed by the initiation of regression is difficult to confuse with anything else.[3] The greatest difficulty in the differential diagnosis of infantile hemangiomas occurs with those present at birth. The telangiectatic presentation of infantile hemangiomas can easily be confused with a telangiectatic vascular malformation.[15] Only observation over time will differentiate between these two types of birthmarks. Deep infantile hemangiomas can be mistaken for lymphatic malformations, and again time will simplify the differential. Kaposiform hemangioendothelioma can be differentiated by the color and infiltrative growth pattern. Classic tufted angiomas are more plaquelike and are usually located from the chest up. The nodular type of tufted angioma may be difficult to differentiate from certain types of venous malformations, RICH, or NICH. RICH and NICH may be separated by either their rapid involution or lack of involution. Subcutaneous sarcomas are rare but should be considered when an infant presents with a firm, rather than rubbery-feeling, rapidly growing mass.

Firm rapidly growing lesions which are fixed to the deep tissue may require biopsy and MRI to obtain the correct diagnosis.

Pathogenesis

Infantile hemangiomas are benign tumors of capillary endothelium.[16] Proliferating infantile hemangiomas are associated with an overabundance of mast cells, and as the tumor regresses, the mast cell number also decreases. It is not unusual for mast cells to be associated with blood-vessel growth, and it is unknown whether this is a primary or secondary event. Endothelial cell proliferation is enhanced by certain angiogenic factors, such basic fibroblast growth factor, vascular endothelial growth factor, insulin-like growth factor 2, and angiogenin.[16] Infantile hemangiomas can be identified histologically by the presence of glucose transporter protein (GLUT-1) and Lewis antigen (LeY).[16] Regression in infantile hemangiomas is asynchronous, with parts of the tumor regressing while other portions continue to grow. As with the beginning of growth of the tumor, the mechanism of initiation of regression remains unknown, although it is likely to be secondary to endothelial cell apoptosis. Kaposiform hemangioendotheliomas are aggressive tumors of endothelial cells. Tufted angiomas are also comprised of endothelial cells, but the mechanism of tuft formation is unknown. The pathogenesis of RICH and NICH is unknown, although NICH behave more as a vascular malformation rather than a true tumor. Kaposiform hemangioendothelioma, tufted angiomas, RICH, and NICH do not stain with GLUT-1 or LeY.

Treatment

The first question that arises regarding treatment of infantile hemangiomas is which ones should be treated (Box 13.4).[3] Certainly, all infantile hemangiomas with the potential to interfere with a vital function should be treated. Periorbital infantile hemangiomas may cause pressure on the eye, leading to astigmatism, or they may partially or totally obstruct vision, causing amblyopia. High-output cardiac failure, although rare, is a medical emergency and requires immediate referral to a cardiologist. Infantile hemangiomas in the diaper area frequently ulcerate.[6] Ulcerated infantile hemangiomas are severely painful and at risk for superinfection. Facial infantile hemangiomas can be disfiguring, and early treatment minimizes the extent of infantile hemangioma growth and the eventual residua. Other infantile hemangiomas should be observed and treated only if complications arise.

For years, the mainstay of treatment for infantile hemangiomas has been oral glucocorticosteroids (Box 13.5).[3] From 30% to 60% of infantile hemangiomas are reported to be responsive to glucocorticosteroid therapy. Treatment should be started at 2 mg/kg and adjusted depending on the response of the tumor. Some authors advocate using higher doses of glucocorticosteroids. Responsive infantile hemangiomas

will demonstrate an effect from treatment within 7 to 10 days, manifested as softening of the tumor, lightening in color, or a noticeable decrease in growth rate. Systemic glucocorticosteroids should be used as the first line of treatment for high-output cardiac failure and those rapidly growing infantile hemangiomas that threaten to interfere with a vital function. Systemic glucocorticosteroid therapy is not without side effects, and treatment should be maintained for as short a time as possible. The use of intralesional steroids has also been advocated for the treatment of infantile hemangiomas, but we believe that this procedure should be done only by those with experience.

Interferon alpha-2a has been demonstrated to be effective for infantile hemangiomas that are unresponsive to glucocorticosteroids.[3] Treatment is initiated daily by subcutaneous injection at a dose of 3 million U/m^2 and continued until the infantile hemangioma is fully in a regressive state. On average, treatments have been continued for 9–12 months. Treatment with interferon alpha-2a is expensive and potentially toxic. Fever and myalgias occur in almost every case, as do reversible elevation of liver function tests, neutropenia, and anemia. The most worrisome side effect of interferon alpha-2a is spastic diplegia, which may persist after cessation of therapy. Therefore, use of interferon alpha-2a should be restricted to truly endangering or life-threatening infantile hemangiomas unresponsive to glucocorticosteroids.[3]

The vascular-specific pulsed dye laser has added another option for the treatment of infantile hemangiomas.[4,17] This form of therapy is excellent for the treatment of ulcerated infantile hemangiomas, leading to a rapid decrease in the pain associated with

Box 13.4 Indications for treatment of infantile hemangiomas
High-output cardiac failure
Obstruction of vital function
Ulceration
Infection
Facial location
Diaper area location

Box 13.5 Treatment options for infantile hemangiomas
Oral glucocorticosteroids
Vascular-specific pulsed dye laser
Interferon alpha-2a

Fig. 13.23 Ulceration of an infantile hemangioma on the buttock of a 5-month-old infant.

Fig. 13.24 Same infantile hemangioma 4 weeks later after one pulsed dye laser treatment.

the ulceration and complete healing of 75% of the ulcerations within 2 weeks and 90% after two laser treatments (Figs 13.23, 13.24).[4,17] Superficial papular infantile hemangiomas treated before or early in the rapid growth phase also respond well to treatment. The treatment is simple and fast, and side effects are nearly nonexistent. The limitation of vascular pulsed dye lasers in the treatment of infantile hemangiomas is their minimal depth of penetration into the skin. Vascular pulsed dye laser treatment minimally alters the long-term outcome of mixed or deep infantile hemangiomas. Non-specific laser therapy, such as the carbon dioxide or the neodymium:yttrium, aluminum, garnet (Nd:YAG) laser, although effective in destroying hemangiomas, often leads to scarring and a worse outcome than natural regression.

The response of kaposiform hemangioendotheliomas to treatment is unpredictable.[9] Multiple therapies have been used, including surgery, glucocorticosteroids, vincristine, interferon, antiplatelet aggregating agents, embolization, and radiotherapy. Heparin is contraindicated for the treatment of disseminated intravascular coagulopathy associated with kaposiform hemangioendotheliomas because it has been shown to increase the growth rate of the tumor and worsen the clinical situation. Patients should be referred for comprehensive multispecialty care.

The response of tufted angiomas to treatment is also variable, but treatment with either vascular pulsed dye laser or interferon alpha-2a has been reported to be succesful.[12] Fortunately, this tumor is not as aggressive as kaposiform hemangioendothelioma and does not always require treatment.

Systemic glucocorticosteroids should be used as the first line of treatment for Kasabach-Merritt syndrome. Heparin and fresh frozen plasma may also be needed to control bleeding. Heparin is contraindicated in Kasabach-Merritt secondary to kaposiform hemangioendothelioma. Combination chemotherapy may be beneficial.[8]

Surgical excision is indicated for NICH and the residua post RICH regression.

Patient education

The natural history and potential complications of infantile hemangiomas should be discussed with the patient's family. They should be aware of the difficulty of predicting the eventual size and type of the infantile hemangioma, the final outcome, and the need for treatment. The need for frequent follow-up visits, until the infantile hemangioma growth and complication pattern is evident, should be emphasized. Parents should be told of the aggressive nature of kaposiform hemangioendotheliomas and the need for prompt treatment. The chronic nature of tufted angiomas and poor response to most treatments should be discussed. Parents should be told that congenital nonprogressive infantile hemangioma may or may not involute and that time will separate the two.

Follow-up visits

Infantile hemangiomas need to be followed closely during the rapid growth phase. Initially, visits should be every 2 weeks, and if no complications occur and the infantile hemangioma growth has stabilized the time between visits can be lengthened.

Children with periorbital infantile hemangiomas should be referred for ophthalmologic evaluation and management. For mostly deep periorbital infantile hemangiomas, one may consider MRI to evaluate the extent and relationship to the eye of the deep component. Once regression has begun and no complications have been noted, follow-up should be on a yearly basis.

Patients with hemangioendotheliomas will need to be treated aggressively until the tumor is under control.

The follow-up of tufted infantile hemangiomas will depend on their location, rate of growth, and response to chosen treatment.

Congenital nonprogressive infantile hemangiomas should be followed every 6 months for the first 18 months of life to determine if rapid involution will occur.

Vascular Malformations

Clinical features

Vascular malformations are developmental errors of blood and/or lymphatic vessel formation. By definition, vascular malformations are always present at birth.[1] They do not undergo a rapid growth phase, but rather grow proportionally with the child. Vascular malformations should be classified according to the predominant vessel type within the birthmark (see Box 13.1).[1]

Capillary malformations (port-wine stains) are the most common type of vascular malformation. Eyelid, occipital, and nuchal vascular birthmarks are very common in light-skinned newborns. Small lesions over the eyelids often fade, but the occipital and nuchal lesions will remain. Excluding these, port-wine stains occur in 3 per 1000 births. The name *port wine stain*

derives from the dark red color that is common in mature capillary malformations (Fig. 13.25). However, most port-wine stains present as light pink macules (Fig. 13.26). The dark red color (port-wine) slowly develops as the patient ages. Along with the darkening in color, maturing port-wine stains develop progressive nodularity and blebbing, and may lead to overgrowth of the underlying soft tissue and bone.[18,19] The rate of progression of any individual port-wine stain cannot be predicted, but approximately 67% of patients with facial port-wine stains will develop these changes by the fifth decade.[18,19]

In patients with facial port-wine stains, the possibility of the Sturge-Weber syndrome should be considered. The Sturge-Weber syndrome is the association of a facial port-wine stain with central nervous system (seizures, mental retardation, hemiplegia) and ophthalmologic (glaucoma) abnormalities. The overall

Fig. 13.25 Dark red port-wine stain with central blebbing in a 14-year-old female.

Fig. 13.26 Typical light-pink port-wine stain in a 3-year-old male.

Fig. 13.27 Bilateral port-wine stain in a 2-year-old female with the Sturge-Weber syndrome.

Fig. 13.28 Hypertrophy of the left arm and hand in a 6-year-old male with the Klippel-Trenaunay syndrome.

Fig. 13.29 Massive overgrowth of leg in Klippel-Trenaunay-Weber syndrome.

Fig. 13.30 Angiokeratomas overlying vascular malformation.

Fig. 13.31 Angiokeratoma circumscriptum in a 6-month-old female demonstrating thickened epidermis overlying a capillary malformation.

risk of a facial port-wine stain having the associated abnormalities of the Sturge-Weber syndrome is 8%, but the chances increase with increasing size of the facial port-wine stain (Fig. 13.27). Infants with bilateral facial port-wine stains are at the highest risk (33%).[20] Patients with a port-wine stain, venous malformation or mixed capillary–venous malformation covering an extremity are at risk for the development of overgrowth of that extremity (Klippel-Trenaunay syndrome) (Figs 13.28, 13.29). As the child gets older the overgrowth can become enormous and can be associated with severe varicosities, venous stasis, ulceration, and recurrent infection, leading to a state of chronic lymphedema.[21] Occasionally, port-wine stains are extensive and cover large areas of skin.

Telangiectatic vascular malformations are capillary malformations in which individual rather than confluent telangiectasias are the presenting feature.[15]

They should be considered a variant of port-wine stains. The risk of development of Sturge-Weber and Klippel-Trenaunay syndromes in association with telangiectatic malformations is unknown.

Hyperkeratotic capillary malformations (angiokeratomas) are distinguished by their acanthotic, hyperkeratotic epidermis overlying a capillary malformation (Fig. 13.30). Five separate conditions are classified as angiokeratomas, but only angiokeratoma circumscriptum is congenital.[22] Angiokeratomas should be considered a mixed developmental abnormality of vessels and epidermis. They are most commonly seen on an extremity as unilateral bands or as plaques composed of blue-black papules or nodules with a warty, hyperkeratotic surface (Fig. 13.31).

Venous malformations are developmental errors in vein formation.[21,23,24] These malformations may contain any size of vessel from venules to large drain-

Fig. 13.32 Distinct blue venous pattern of a venous malformation in an 11-year-old female.

Fig. 13.34 Superficial lymphatic malformation. Grouping of gelatinous skin-colored papules on the abdomen.

Fig. 13.33 Venous malformation with a large nodule in a 9-year-old male.

Fig. 13.35 Superficial lymphatic malformation. After minor trauma, lesions may darken, the result of bleeding into the lesion.

ing veins. Their distinct venous pattern is often obvious at presentation (Fig. 13.32). Occasionally, large nodules will develop within these lesions (Fig. 13.33).

Arteriovenous malformations (fistulae) are direct connections between an artery and the venous system, bypassing the capillary bed.[24] They are often initially trivial-appearing lesions but with time may expand rapidly. They are high-flow lesions and may have a notable pulsation and/or thrills and bruits. Localized pain, hyperhidrosis, hypertrichosis, and hyperthermia of a relatively banal-looking vascular lesion should raise the suspicion of an arteriovenous malformation. Arteriovenous malformations are the rarest type of vascular malformation.

Lymphatic malformations are in general referred to as *lymphangiomas* – a misnomer because the lesions are developmental errors in the formation of lymphatic vessels and not tumors as the suffix *-oma* designates.

There are two clinical types of lymphatic malformations: superficial and deep. Superficial lymphatic malformations consist of multiple clusters of small vesicles covering limited skin areas, usually less than 10 cm in diameter (Figs 13.34, 13.35). Deep lymphatic malformations present as dermal or subcutaneous, squishy nodules. They vary in size from a few centimeters to large, ill-defined, grotesque, rubbery, skin-colored, subcutaneous nodules that may underlie areas of more superficial lymphatic malformations.[25] They are usually solitary and involve the face, trunk, and extremities. Histologically, they may consist of either small or large (cystic hygroma) lymphatic vessels.

In cutis marmorata telangiectatica congenita, two clinical presentations may be seen. The first is a mottled pattern of blue or dusky-red erythema present at birth (Fig. 13.36). In the second form there is

Fig. 13.36 Permanent mottled appearance of cutis marmorata telangiectatica congenita.

Fig. 13.37 Venous pattern of cutis marmorata telangiectatica congenita (congenital phlebectasia).

atrophy of the skin and larger, depressed, blue venous malformations (congenital phlebectasia) (Fig. 13.37). Both types may be seen in the same patient. Often, a single extremity is involved, but the lesions may occur bilaterally on the extremities or on the trunk. A gradual increase in the size of the lesions is expected as the child grows, but the lesions become less noticeable within the first few years of life.[26] Associations with musculoskeletal or other vascular malformations may occur.

Occasionally, vascular malformations will contain a mixture of many different types of vascular components. They present as a composite of the presentation of each individual component.

Differential diagnosis

In older children, port-wine stains and telangiectatic malformations are rather characteristic and are sel-dom confused with other lesions. At birth, port-wine stains and telangiectatic vascular malformations must be differentiated from the macular and telangiectatic presentations of infantile hemangiomas.[3,15] These lesions will eventually be distinguished by the presence or absence of a rapid growth phase.

Congenital solitary angiokeratomas and angiokeratoma circumscriptum must be differentiated histor-ically from the acquired forms of angiokeratoma. Although quite rare, the development of numerous angiokeratomas at a young age should alert the clin-ician to the possibility of either Fabry's disease or α-fucosidosis.

As with the capillary malformations, venous and arteriovenous malformations are usually quite char-acteristic. Nodular malformations of venules may be confused with tufted angiomas, RICH, and NICH. Rarely, these lesions are disfiguring and can be mis-taken for vascular malignancies such as Kaposi's sarcoma and angiosarcomas.

Superficial lymphatic malformations may be mistaken for a disorder with grouped vesicles, such as herpes simplex, herpes zoster, or dermatitis herpetiformis. There is no erythematous base in circumscribed lymphangioma, however, and the lesions appear gelatinous, not fluid-filled. As noted, hemorrhage into such lesions results in darkening, which may be confused with melanoma.

Deep lymphatic malformations may be confused with lipomas, plexiform neurofibromas, and other soft subcutaneous masses.

In contrast to cutis marmorata telangiectatica con-genita, mottling of newborn skin is a transient vasodilatation and is relieved by rewarming the skin. The livedo reticularis pattern of collagen vascular dis-ease is flat, is not depressed over the discolored areas, is always bilateral, and is associated with systemic signs and symptoms.

Pathogenesis

All vascular malformations should be considered developmental errors in vessel formation. Most are sporadic and are likely caused by genetic mosaicism.

Treatment

The vascular-specific pulsed dye laser is recognized as the treatment of choice for capillary and telangiec-tatic vascular malformations.[27] Standard therapy was with a wavelength of 585 nm and a pulsed duration of

0.5 milliseconds. Vascular-specific pulsed dye lasers capable of emitting longer wavelengths and longer pulse duration are now available. Theoretically, they have the advantage of deeper depth of penetration into the dermis and the ability to destroy larger-caliber vessels. Comparative studies of different wavelengths and pulse duration are few, with only a small number of patients enrolled.[28,29] Response of these lesions to treatment depends on the age of the patients at the beginning of treatment and the size of the lesion.[27,29] The younger the child at the beginning of treatment and the smaller the lesion, the more increased the likelihood of complete removal (Figs 13.38, 13.39). Treatments can safely be started as early as 2 weeks of age. Large lesions are improved by treatment, but total removal is less likely. Response to treatment is slow, and even small lesions in very young infants will frequently take 1–3 years for complete removal. Vascular-specific pulsed dye lasers are very safe, and side effects are minimal. Treatment has been greatly improved by the introduction of topical anesthetic creams, which significantly decrease the pain associated with the procedure.

Unlike port-wine stains, telangiectatic vascular malformations have a much smaller vessel load to destroy to return the skin to normal. Most of these lesions will be completely removed in three to six treatments (Figs 13.40–13.43).[15]

Treatment of all other types of vascular malformations, including the Klippel-Trenaunay syndrome, is difficult and must be handled on an individual basis.[21,25,30] Referral to a multidiscipline specialty clinic with specific expertise in dealing with these types of birth defects is optimal.

Patient education

Parents of babies with capillary and telangiectatic malformations should be told about the possibility of treatment with vascular-specific pulsed dye lasers. They should be referred to the nearest treatment center as soon as possible.

If a large facial port-wine stain is present, the possibility of the Sturge-Weber syndrome should be discussed, and the patient should be referred for neurologic and ophthalmologic consultation.

For other types of vascular malformations, the difficulty of treatment should be discussed, and, if possible, the child should be referred to a specialty clinic with expertise in managing the specific types of lesions.

Follow-up visits

The frequency of follow-up visits is determined by the degree of complications associated with a given malformation.

ACQUIRED VASCULAR LESIONS

Pyogenic Granuloma

Clinical features

Pyogenic granulomas are most common in acral areas, such as the hands and fingers, and on the face (Fig. 13.44).[31] They appear as solitary, dull-red, firm nodules that are 5–6 mm in diameter. The surface may be smooth and glistening, but often it is ulcerated and crusted. The lesion bleeds easily when traumatized. Removal by surgical excision followed by

Fig. 13.38 Before laser treatment of port-wine stain in an 8-year-old female.

Fig. 13.39 Same patient shown in Figure 13.38, 2 years later, after 10 laser treatments.

Fig. 13.40 Telangiectatic malformation in a 4-month-old female.

Fig. 13.41 Same patient shown in Figure 13.40, 2 months after initial laser treatment.

Fig. 13.42 Same patient shown in Figure 13.40, after second laser treatment.

Fig. 13.43 Same patient shown in Figure 13.40, 10 months after initial laser treatment. Only three laser treatments were required to achieve almost total clearing of the telangiectatic malformation.

suturing has resulted in the appearance of multiple satellite lesions in a few instances. Pyogenic granuloma may occur at any age, but in childhood it is most common in the first 5 years of life. The majority of patients have no history of a predisposing factor.

Differential diagnosis

Pyogenic granuloma is often misdiagnosed as a hemangioma, glomus tumor, Spitz nevus, juvenile xanthogranuloma, wart, molluscum contagiosum, or malignant melanoma. All of these lesions can ulcerate and crust if traumatized. Pathologic study distinguishes pyogenic granuloma from these other lesions.

Pathogenesis

Proliferation of capillaries within a circumscribed area, with flattened or ulcerated epidermis on top and epidermal proliferation at the sides, producing a 'col-

Fig. 13.44 Pyogenic granuloma. Smooth, glistening surface of the erythematous papule.

larette' of epidermis, is seen. Pyogenic granuloma is believed to be caused by an abnormal healing response.

Treatment

Excision by curettage with electrocautery to the base is the treatment of choice. Pulse dye laser treatment is effective for lesions 0.5 cm and smaller.[32]

Patient education

It should be explained to the patient and family that this growth is not malignant but will not disappear without treatment and represents an abnormal healing response.

Follow-up visits

A visit 1 week after removal of the lesion is useful to inform the patient and family of the pathologic diagnosis and evaluate healing.

Spider Telangiectasia

Clinical features

A spider telangiectasia is a small lesion consisting of a central arteriole from which superficial blood vessels radiate peripherally (Figs 13.45–13.47). They usually appear between ages 2 and 6 years and are located in sun-exposed areas, usually on the cheeks, nose, dorsa of the hands, and forearms. Sometimes, the central arteriole is raised and prominent and it may be pulsatile on diascopy. Approximately 40% of light-skinned children will have these lesions.

Differential diagnosis

Spider telangiectasia must be differentiated from the telangiectatic mats of the autosomal dominant Osler-Weber-Rendu syndrome, in which confluent telangiectasia compose each lesion and multiple lesions are

Fig. 13.45 Vascular spider with prominent central feeding vessel on the cheek of a child.

Fig. 13.46 Vascular spider (nevus araneus).

Fig. 13.47 Vascular spider on face of child.

Fig. 13.48 Vascular telangiectasias on lips of child with hereditary hemorrhagic telangiectasia (HHT, Osler-Weber-Rendu syndrome).

seen over the dorsum of the hands, lips, and face (Figs 13.48, 13.49). Associated epistaxis, peptic ulcer-like symptoms, or both may be important systemic symptoms to help differentiate the two conditions. Spider telangiectasia may be confused with the telangiectatic mats seen in collagen vascular diseases such as scleroderma and lupus erythematosus.

Pathogenesis

The cause of these lesions is unknown, but sun exposure may be a factor.

Treatment

If the cosmetic appearance is a concern to the child, lesions may be removed without scarring using the pulsed dye laser at 585 nm. A single treatment is over 90% effective.[29]

Patient education

The common and nonserious nature of these lesions should be emphasized.

Follow-up visits

Follow-up visits are unnecessary.

Cherry Angiomas and Diffuse Angiokeratomas

Clinical features

True cherry angiomas are rare in childhood and usually appear as 1–3 mm solid-red, dome-shaped, blanching papules (Fig. 13.50).[33] The appearance of multiple cherry angiomas around the umbilicus and scrotum, which increase progressively with age, should bring to mind two diagnoses: Fabry's disease and α-fucosidosis. In Fabry's disease, attacks of pain, numbness, and tingling of the hands and feet often accompany the eruption.[34] The usual onset of the eruption is between 4 and 12 years of age. In α-fucosidosis, severe mental retardation and neuromuscular spasticity accompany the disorder.[35]

Differential diagnosis

Cherry angiomas and angiokeratomas must be differentiated from small pyogenic granulomas and small superficial infantile hemangiomas. Usually, the differentiation is quite simple. Cherry angiomas are small (2–5 mm) and dome-shaped with a normal epithelium over them. Pyogenic granulomas have a friable, often crusted surface and bleed easily. When they first appear, angiokeratomas have a smooth surface but later will develop a rough, scaly surface.

Pathogenesis

Fabry's disease is an X-linked recessive disorder in which activity of a specific lysosomal hydrolase, α-galactosidase A, is deficient. The glycosphingolipid, ceramide trihexoside, accumulates within endothelial cells and produces the cutaneous vascular lesions. Rearrangements or point mutations in the gene encoding α-galactosidase have been found. On electron microscopy, the endothelial cells of the affected vessels are shown to contain multiple laminated inclusions diagnostic of the disease. In α-fucosidosis the lysosomes of the endothelial cells are widely dilated, but the material is washed out during tissue fixation so

Fig. 13.49 Telangiectasias on hand of child with HHT.

Fig. 13.50 Cherry angioma on the trunk of a child.

the cells appear empty. Fibroblast culture and analysis of α-galactosidase A activity may be performed to confirm the diagnosis of Fabry's disease. In α-fucosidosis, an autosomal recessive trait, fibroblast cultures may also be useful in confirming the diagnosis.

Treatment

The future treatment for Fabry's disease or α-fucosidosis will be either enzyme replacement or bone marrow transplant.[36,37] Cherry angiomas may be easily treated with the pulsed dye laser at 585 nm, if desired.

Patient education

The patient and family should be informed about the seriousness of each of these conditions and referred for genetic counseling. They should be advised that prenatal diagnosis is possible for future pregnancies, and that molecular probes are available to screen carrier females. Enzyme replacement or gene therapy should be considered.

Follow-up visits

Follow-up visits should be arranged with the appropriate pediatric care specialists.

REFERENCES

1. Spring MA, Bentz ML. Cutaneous vascular lesions. Clin Plast Surg 2005; 32:171–186.
2. Enjolras O, Mulliken JB. Vascular tumors and vascular malformations (new issues). Adv Dermatol 1997; 13:375,
3. Miller T, Frieden IJ. Hemangiomas: new insights and classification. Pediatr Ann 2005; 34:179–187.
4. Morelli JG, Tan OT, Yohn JJ, et al. Treatment of ulcerated infantile hemangiomas in infancy. Arch Pediatr Adol Med 1994; 148:1104.
5. Orlow SJ, Isakoff M, Blei F. Increased risk of symptomatic infantile hemangiomas of the airway in association with cutaneous hemangioma in a 'beard' distribution. J Pediatr 1997; 131:643.
6. Albright AL, Gartner JC, Weiner GS. Lumbar cutaneous hemangiomas as indicators of tethered spinal cords. Pediatrics 1989; 83:977.
7. Metry DW. Potential complications of segmental hemangiomas. Semin Cutan Med Surg 2004; 23:107–115.
8. Maguiness S, Guenther L. Kasaback-Merritt syndrome. J Cutan Med Surg 2002; 6:335–339.
9. Cooper JG, Edwards SL, Holmes JD. Kaposiform hemangioendothelioma: case report and review of the literature. Br J Plast Surg 2002; 55:163–165.
10. Jones EW, Orkin M. Tufted angioma (angioblastoma): a benign progressive angioma, not to be confused with

Kaposi's sarcoma or low-grade angiosarcoma. J Am Acad Dermatol 1989; 20:214.
11. Ishikawa K, Hatano Y, Ichikawa H, et al. The spontaneous regression of tufted angioma. A case report of regression after two recurrences and a review of 27 reported cases in the literature. Dermatology 2005; 210:346–348.
12. Okada E, Tamura A, Ishikawa O, et al. Tufted angioma (angioblastoma): case report and review of 41 cases in the Japanese literature. Clin Exp Dermatol 2000; 25:627–630.
13. Krol A, MacArthur CJ. Congenital hemangiomas: Rapidly involuting and noninvoluting congenital hemangiomas. Arch Facial Plast Surg 2005; 7:307–311.
14. North PE, Waner M, James CA, et al. Congenital nonprogressive hemangioma: a distinct clinicopathologic entity unlike infantile hemangioma. Arch Dermatol 2001; 137:1607–1620.
15. Morelli JG, Huff JC, Weston WL. The treatment of congenital telangiectatic vascular malformations with the vascular specific pulsed dye laser. Pediatrics 1993; 92:603.
16. Phung TL, Hochman M, Mihm MC. Current knowledge of the pathogenesis of infantile hemangiomas. Arch Facial Plast Surg 2005; 7:319–321.
17. David LR, Malek MM, Argenta LC. Efficacy of pulse dye laser therapy for the treatment of ulcerated hemangiomas: a review of 78 patients. Br J Plast Surg 2003; 56:317–327.
18. Geronemus RG, Ashinoff R. The medical necessity of evaluation and treatment of port wine stains. J Dermatol Surg Oncol 1991; 117:76.
19. Klapman MH, Yao JF. Thickening and nodules in port-wine stains, J Am Acad Dermatol 2001; 44:300.
20. Tallman B, Tan OT, Morelli JG, et al. Location of port wine stains and the likelihood of ophthalmic and/or CNS complications. Pediatrics 1991; 87:323.
21. Enjolras O, Chapot R, Merland JJ. Vascular anomalies and the growth of limbs: a review. J Pediatr Orthop B 2004; 13:349–357.
22. Schiller PI, Itin PH. Angiokeratomas: an update. Dermatology 1996; 193:275.
23. Enjolras O, Ciabrini D, Mazoyer E, et al. Extensive pure venous malformation in the upper or lower limb: a review of 27 cases. J Am Acad Dermatol 1997; 36:219.
24. Upton J, Coombs CJ, Mulliken JB, et al. Vascular malformations of the upper limb: a review of 270 patients. J Hand Surg 1999; 24:1019.
25. Marler JJ, Mulliken JB. Current management of hemangiomas and vascular malformation. Clin Plast Surg 2005; 32:99–116.
26. Garzon MC, Schwieger E. Cutis marmorata telangiectasia congenita. Semin Cutan Med Surg 2004; 23:99–106.
27. Kelly KM, Choi B, McFarlane S, et al. Description and analysis of treatments for port wine stain birthmarks. Arch Facial Plast Surg 2005; 7:287–294.
28. Yung A, Sheehan-Dare R. A comparative study of a 595-nm with a 585-nm pulsed dye laser in refractory port wine stains. Br J Dermatol 2005; 53:601–606.
29. Smit JM, Bauland CG, Wijnberg DS, et al. Pulsed dye laser treatment, a review of indications and outcome based on published trials. Br J Plast Surg 2005; 58:981–987.
30. Lee A, Driscoll D, Gloviczki P, et al. Evaluation and management of pain in patients with Klippel-Trenaunay syndrome: a review. Pediatrics 2005; 115:744–749.
31. Lin RL, Janniger CK. Pyogenic granuloma. Cutis 2004; 74:229–231.

32. Tay Y-K, Weston WL, Morelli JG. Treatment of pyogenic granulomas in children with the flashlamp-pumped pulsed dye laser. Pediatrics 1997; 99:368.

33. Luba M, Bangs SA, Mohler AM, et al. Common benign skin tumors. Am Fam Physician 2003; 67:729–738.

34. Mohrschlager M, Braun-Falco M, Ring J, et al. Fabry disease: recognition and management of cutaneous manifestations. Am J Clin Dermatol 2003; 4:189–196.

35. Kanitakis J, Allombert C, Doebelin B, et al. Fucosidosis with angiokeratomas. Immunhistochemical and electronmicroscopic study of a new case and literature review. J Cutan Pathol 2005; 32:506–511.

36. Mignani R, Cagnoli L. Enzyme replacement therapy in Fabry's disease: recent advances and clinical applications. J Nephrol 2004; 17:354–363.

37. Miano M, Lanino E, Gatti R, et al. Four-year follow-up of a case of fucosidosis treated with unrelated donor bone marrow transplant. Bone Marrow Transplant 2001; 27:747–751.

Chapter 14

Vascular Reactions: Urticaria, Erythemas, and Purpuras

Urticaria, erythemas, and purpuras are considered together in a single chapter because they represent a spectrum of disease characterized by progressive signs of injury to cutaneous blood vessels. All are accompanied by vasodilation (erythema) and leakage of fluid from blood vessels (edema). Leakage of red blood cells also occurs in the purpuras as a further sign of vascular insult. Included in this chapter is pyoderma gangrenosum, a rare but life-threatening dermatosis.

URTICARIA

Urticarial states are common in infancy and childhood, although the exact incidence is not known. Several large studies indicate that 3% of preschool children and about 2% of older children suffer from urticaria.[4–8] Children who have atopic dermatitis in infancy have an increased incidence of urticaria.[5] The high incidence of urticaria in healthy children undoubtedly includes children with a single episode of short-lived urticaria rather than persistent urticaria.[6–8] Interestingly, of all children with urticaria, only 3–5% have what can be documented as immunoglobulin E (IgE)-mediated allergic urticaria.[6–8] In contrast, approximately 15% of children with urticaria have a physical urticaria, with the bulk of these diagnoses classified as 'idiopathic.'[7,8] Rarely, children with persistent idiopathic urticaria may have urticarial vasculitis. For purposes of presenting a clinical approach to urticaria, transient urticaria and persistent urticaria are discussed separately.

Transient Urticaria and Angioedema
Clinical features

Transient urticaria in children often follows infection,[7,8] ingestion of certain foods,[9,10] encounters with stinging or biting insects,[11] ingestion of medications[7,8,12,13] (see Ch. 22) or rarely occurs with inflammatory systemic diseases such as collagen vascular disease or thyroiditis (Box 14.1).[7,8] The eruption is sudden in onset and pruritic, with erythematous raised wheals scattered over the body.[1,2,6] The wheals are usually 2–15 mm in diameter, flat-topped, and have tense edema (Fig. 14.1). The edema can be appreciated by stretching the skin slightly to demonstrate whitish centers. The erythematous borders with pale centers can be quite large and mistaken for target lesions of erythema multiforme.[14] Occasionally, giant urticarial lesions up to 30 cm in diameter with polycyclic borders will appear (Figs 14.2, 14.3). Such wheals commonly last from 20 minutes to 3 hours, disappear, then reappear in other areas. The entire episode of transient urticaria often lasts 24–48 hours; rarely, it lasts as long as 3 weeks. Transient urticaria, as it resolves, may leave flat, dusky areas lasting several days that mimic bruises (Fig. 14.4).[1,6,12,14] More typical are pink wheals scattered on the skin (Figs 14.5, 14.6).

Subcutaneous extension of lesions, called *angioedema*, may occur.[5,8,12] These lesions appear as large, deep swellings with indistinct borders around the eyelids and lips. They may also appear on the face, trunk, genitalia (Fig. 14.7), and extremities. The face, hands, and feet are involved in 85% of patients, and other areas are involved in 15%.[4,5] Up to half of children with transient urticaria may have angioedema, with swelling of the hands and feet commonly seen. When examined within the first 4 weeks of illness, all of the persistent urticarias may be indistinguishable from transient urticaria.

Hereditary angioedema accounts for only 0.4% of cases of urticaria, but its specific diagnostic tests and high mortality deserve special mention. It is an auto-

Box 14.1 Transient urticaria

Infectious associations
Streptococcus
Infectious mononucleosis (Epstein-Barr virus)
Hepatitis
Adenovirus
Enterovirus
Parasites

Bites and stings
Bees
Wasps
Scorpions
Spiders
Jellyfish

Drugs
Penicillin
Cephalosporins
Salicylates
Morphine, codeine, and other opiates
Nonsteroidal antiinflammatory drugs
Barbiturates
Amphetamines
Atropine
Hydralazine
Insulin

Blood and blood products

Foods
Peanuts
Nuts
Eggs
Shellfish
Strawberries
Tomatoes

Systemic diseases
Collagen vascular diseases
Lupus erythematosus
Juvenile rheumatoid arthritis
Polyarteritis nodosa
Dermatomyositis
Neonatal lupus syndrome
Sjögren's syndrome
Rheumatic fever
Inflammatory bowel diseases
Crohn's disease
Ulcerative colitis

Miscellaneous
Aphthous stomatitis
Behçet's disease
Thyroiditis

Fig. 14.1 Central wheal with red border in acute urticaria.

Fig. 14.2 Multiple polycyclic red wheals of different sizes in a child with urticaria. Commonly mistaken for erythema multiforme.

Fig. 14.3 Multiple shapes of urticarial lesions in a child.

somal dominant condition with repeated attacks of swelling of the extremities, face, and throat, accompanied by abdominal pain.[15,16] The onset usually follows trauma, such as surgery, dental manipulation, or accidents. It presents as a diffuse, brawny swelling of the extremities in 75% of patients, abdominal pain in 52%, and swelling of the face and throat in 30%.[15,16] Its onset is usually in adolescence, with the more severe symptoms associated with the menses. Abdominal pain eventually becomes a major complaint in

Fig. 14.4 Dusky centers with red borders in resolving childhood urticaria.

Fig. 14.5 Typical pink wheals of urticaria.

Fig. 14.6 Pink wheals on the leg of a child with urticaria.

Fig. 14.7 Angioedema of the scrotum and foreskin in an infant.

93% of patients. They do not have typical urticarial wheals, but 26% have lesions resembling erythema multiforme. Severe airway edema accounts for the mortality of almost 30% in untreated patients. Only

25% of patients give a positive family history. The diagnosis should be suspected if the serum C4 level is persistently low. It is confirmed by functional assay of the C1 esterase inhibitor. In some children hereditary

Box 14.2 Differential diagnosis of urticaria
Erythema multiforme
Mastocytosis
Flushing
Reactive erythemas
Juvenile rheumatoid arthritis
Vasculitis
Guttate psoriasis
Pityriasis rosea (early lesions)

Box 14.3 Differential diagnosis of angioedema
Cellulitis and erysipelas
Lymphedema
Acute contact dermatitis
Idiopathic scrotal edema of children
Melkersson-Rosenthal syndrome

angioedema is associated with lupus erythematosus or other collagen vascular diseases.[15,16]

Differential diagnosis

The conditions to be considered in the differential diagnosis of urticaria are listed in Box 14.2. A skin biopsy is recommended in atypical forms of urticaria.[17] Urticaria, especially giant urticaria, is frequently confused with erythema multiforme.[14] Urticarial lesions may blanch in the center, showing a red border and thus concentric zones of color change, as is seen in erythema multiforme. However, it should be remembered that individual urticarial lesions are transient, usually lasting less than 3 hours, whereas erythema multiforme lesions are fixed and stay in place at least 7–14 days.[14] Also, the target lesions of erythema multiforme reveal disruption of the epidermis in the center, with blisters, crusts, or scabs. Frequently, when polycyclic urticarial wheals of different sizes and shapes accompany edema of the hands and feet, erythema multiforme is incorrectly diagnosed.[14] Urticarial lesions often clear with the administration of subcutaneous epinephrine; erythema multiforme does not.[14] A skin biopsy will also distinguish the two. Urticaria can be differentiated from mastocytosis by a skin biopsy because increased numbers of mast cells are seen in mastocytosis. Flushing states are flat rather than elevated. In juvenile rheumatoid arthritis, faint erythematous macules with a clear center are present and are associated with a spiking fever. Vasculitis lesions have nonblanching purpuric centers, whereas psoriasis and pityriasis rosea demonstrate scaling overlying the erythematous papules.

Angioedema (deep hives) (Box 14.3) should be differentiated from cellulitis and erysipelas, which are tender, warm, red lesions. Chronic thickening of tissues occurs in lymphedema, in contrast to the acute stretching of tissue seen in angioedema. Angioedema of the hands and feet, which accompanies urticaria, may be confused with erythema multiforme.[14] A skin biopsy will distinguish. Persistent angioedema of the face or lip should bring to mind lupus erythematosus or other collagen vascular diseases. Considerable deep edema can develop in acute contact dermatitis, but vesiculation of the overlying epidermis and epidermal papules will help distinguish it from angioedema. Idiopathic scrotal edema of children and the Melkersson-Rosenthal syndrome are rare and can be distinguished from angioedema by the furrowed tongue and cranial nerve palsies of Melkersson-Rosenthal syndrome and the limitation of angioedema to the scrotum in idiopathic scrotal edema.

Pathogenesis

Histamine is undoubtedly the major chemical mediator of transient urticaria, and the mast cell is central in all forms of transient urticaria and angioedema.[1,2] Histamine may be directly released from cutaneous mast cells in the case of certain foods or opiate drugs. Specific IgE antibodies bound to mast cell surfaces that 'recognize' certain antigens, such as penicillin and other drugs, foods, and venom of certain stinging insects, result in the release of histamine after combination with antigen. In some, autoantibodies to the epsilon receptor on skin mast cells may be responsible.[1–3] Rechallenge studies are few, and in suspected urticarial reactions to drugs only 4% could be reproduced.[13]

Complement fragments, activated by immune complexes, may activate mast cells to release histamine or exert vasoactive effects of their own on cutaneous blood vessels. The latter mechanism is most often associated with infection, but careful documentation of the mechanism of histamine release involved with each inciting substance is not available. Eicosanoids may induce mast cell mediator release and have been implicated in exacerbations of urticaria,[1,2] and other cytokines have been implicated in urticaria.

In hereditary angioedema, a deficiency of the C1 esterase inhibitor permits unregulated cleavage of complement proteins once the complement system is activated, with particular consumption of C4. A C2 kinin activates the clotting system via the Hageman factor in hereditary angioedema.[15,16] Complement cleavage products may be responsible for the edema and erythema.

Treatment

Oral antihistamines are valuable in symptomatic control of urticaria. Hydroxyzine hydrochloride, 1–2 mg/kg/day in a single dose, or diphenhydramine hydrochloride, 5 mg/kg/day in four divided doses, is the most prescribed.[5,8] If urticaria at night is the problem, administration of hydroxyzine 1 hour before bedtime may allow a single treatment per day. Combinations of H$_1$ blocking agents such as cetirizine in the morning and hydroxyzine at bedtime may be effective. Nonsedating antihistamines are less effective in controlling urticaria. In angioedema not controlled by antihistamines, the addition of pseudoephedrine, 4 mg/kg/day in four divided doses, is useful but nightmares and sleep disturbances and sympathomimetic side effects limit its use to older children. The same drugs may be used to treat chronic angioedema. In acute angioedema of the airway, epinephrine 1:1000, 0.01 mL/kg/dose to a maximum dose of 0.5 mL, or albuterol inhalers may be used.[4,5] There is no evidence to support the use of systemic glucocorticosteroids in urticaria or angioedema. The addition of H$_2$ blocking drugs to H$_1$ antihistamines is of little additional benefit, and H$_2$ blockers are ineffective when used alone. Cromolyn sodium preparations, which may be efficacious in treatment of airway or bowel reactions, have not been particularly useful in skin. Leukotriene antagonists, such as zafirlukast or montelukast, may be useful in treating exacerbations that result from nonsteroidal antiinflammatory usage.[12] Allergen avoidance is an important strategy if the allergen can be identified. Virtually any drug may produce urticaria, but certain drugs are more frequently implicated. Drugs such as penicillin and aspirin account for most drug-induced urticaria, and their use should be specifically questioned in review of the patient's history. Cephalosporins produce an urticarial serum-sickness-like reaction. Foods suspected of causing the urticaria could be avoided if nutrition is not compromised. Restriction diets are of little value if a suspected food factor has not been identified.

In hereditary angioedema, acute attacks are managed by intravenous fluid replacement and airway maintenance.[17] Administration of danazol or stanozolol (synthetic attenuated testosterones), increases C1q esterase inhibitor levels and prevents the attacks of angioedema. Fresh-frozen plasma or ε-aminocaproic acid may be useful before surgical procedures.[17]

Patient education

It should be explained that cause-and-effect relationships often cannot be found in transient urticaria and angioedema, but that lesions can be expected to resolve by 1 month in most instances. One should emphasize that control of symptoms is possible with the use of antihistamines. An extensive and expensive allergy work-up is not indicated in children who have had urticaria less than 6 weeks, and work-up of chronic urticaria should be guided by history.

Patients with angioedema should have an adrenergic agent available for airway attacks, and patients with hereditary angioedema should be advised of the high mortality rate and the need to continue taking prophylactic drugs.[5]

Follow-up visits

In transient urticaria and angioedema a visit 1 week after the initial evaluation is useful for monitoring the course of the disease. In chronic urticaria it is useful to reevaluate precipitating factors periodically if a factor has not been identified. Patients with hereditary angioedema should be seen after 1 month of therapy to remeasure the C1 esterase inhibitor and adjust the drug dosage.

Persistent Urticaria

The physical urticarias

Urticaria that persists for over 4 weeks may be simply prolonged common urticaria or may be caused by one of the physical urticarias, urticarial vasculitis, or mastocytosis. The physical urticarias, which account for 15% of this group, consist of dermatographism, heat- and exercise-induced urticaria, delayed-pressure urticaria, cold urticaria, and familial cold urticaria.[1,7,8,18–28]

Clinical features

Dermatographism: Dermatographism occurs in 1% of adolescents and is characterized by wheal and erythema after minor stroking of or pressure on the skin

Fig. 14.8 Dermatographism. Light stroking of the skin evokes intense wheal and flare reaction.

Fig. 14.10 Heat- and exercise-induced urticaria. Pinpoint central wheal surrounded by large, blotchy erythema.

Fig. 14.9 Dermatographism in child with chronic urticaria.

Fig. 14.11 Heat and exercise urticaria. Blotchy pink macules on neck of adolescent.

(Figs 14.8, 14.9),[1,7,8] often results in mild itching. The wheal reaches maximal size in 6–7 minutes and persists for 10–15 minutes. Wheals are commonly found around the belt area and may follow widespread insect bites and transient episodes of urticaria. The wheal is seen in comatose children (e.g. in encephalitis, meningitis, drug overdose) and has been termed *tache cérébrale*. Dermatographism is also seen in about half of children with mastocytosis. Dermatographism may persist for years, but most patients can expect spontaneous regression within 2 years.

Heat- and exercise-induced urticaria: Heat- and exercise-induced urticaria (cholinergic urticaria) is characterized by a large (10–20 mm), blotchy erythema surrounding tiny (1–3 mm) central wheals (Figs 14.10, 14.11).[1,7,8] It occurs in up to 3% of adolescents. Heating of the skin or exercise sufficient to raise the body temperature 0.5°C will induce attacks of multiple wheals with itching. Hot or spicy foods, febrile illnesses, and hot baths may also initiate attacks. The onset is characteristically in adolescence, but the condition tends to persist into the young adult years.

Delayed pressure urticaria: Delayed pressure urticaria, which occurs primarily in adolescents, appears after prolonged pressure with a heavy weight.[1,7,8] A 7 kg weight suspended from an extremity by a strap for 15 minutes will reproduce the disease. Painful, deep swellings begin 4–6 hours after pressure and last up to 24 hours. Spontaneous remissions have been reported, but the natural history is unknown.

Cold urticaria: Cold urticaria appears in three forms: it may be associated with cryoglobulins and immune complex disease, it may appear as an acquired form not associated with cryoproteins, or it may occur as autosomal dominant familial cold urticaria.[1,19–21] In the form associated with cryoglobulins, infectious associations are the most common, particularly infectious mononucleosis.[19] In a few children with cryoproteins, the signs and symptoms of collagen vascular disease are often present. This disease is quite uncommon in children. The acquired form occurs after rewarming an area of skin exposed to cold. Wheals appear, and itching is severe.[20] Cooling the entire body may result in widespread wheals and fainting. To test for acquired cold urticaria, an ice cube is applied to the patient's skin for 2–10 minutes, and the skin is allowed to rewarm. The wheal appears during the rewarming. There may be a spontaneous remission, but the natural history is not known.

Familial cold urticaria: Familial cold urticaria is an autosomal dominant condition beginning shortly after birth.[20] The gene has been localized to chromosome 1q and C1AS1 gene mutations have been found that encode the protein cryopyrin.[21] Familial cold urticaria is genetically similar to the Muckle-Wells syndrome and chronic infantile neurologic cutaneous and articular syndrome, all inherited autoinflammatory recurrent fever syndromes.[21] Erythematous macules appear in exposed areas 30 minutes after exposure to a cold wind, but not after ingestion of iced drinks or ice. Older children complain of burning in the skin. Fever and chills, arthralgias, and headaches appear and last up to 48 hours.[21] A leukocytosis occurs during the attacks. The patient tends to suffer these attacks throughout life.

Differential diagnosis. The physical urticarias are often confused with other forms of urticaria (see Box 14.2).[1,7] The role of light pressure in dermatographism and deep pressure in delayed-pressure urticaria should help distinguish these disorders from the other forms of urticaria. Heat- and exercise-induced urticarias may be distinguished from other types of urticaria by the characteristic tiny central wheal with a large rim of erythema. The cold urticarias may be distinguished by the history of cold exposure, and in the familial form by the systemic symptoms accompanying the skin lesions.[21] Box 14.4 lists the conditions to be considered in the differential diagnosis of cold urticaria.

Pathogenesis. The physical urticarias differ from other urticarial states in that histamine does not appear to be the chemical mediator of the disease.[1] Histamine skin levels are normal in dermatographism, heat- and exercise-induced urticaria, cold urticaria with cryoglobulins, urticarial states, and familial cold urticaria. Histamine has been implicated in acquired cold urticaria and delayed-pressure urticaria.[2,6,18] In dermatographism and heat- and exercise-induced urticaria, mediation through cholinergic fibers of the

Box 14.4 Differential diagnosis of cold urticaria
Cryoglobulinemia and immune complex diseases
Systemic lupus erythematosus and other collagen vascular diseases
Macroglobulinemia
Mycoplasma infections (cold hemagglutinins)
Syphilis
Familial cold urticaria
Acquired cold urticaria

autonomic nervous system has been implicated. The vasoactive split products of the complement system may be involved in the cryoglobulinemic and familial cold urticarial forms. In familial cold urticaria, functional dysregulation of leukocyte cryopyrin is related to the inflammatory skin, joint, and febrile responses.[21]

Treatment. Many patients with physical urticaria require no therapy. If symptoms are severe enough to require therapy, H_1 blocking antihistamines such as hydroxyzine hydrochloride, 1–2 mg/kg/day in a single evening dose, or cetirizine, 2.5–5.0 mg once daily, may reduce the symptoms in dermatographism and heat- and exercise-induced urticaria.[2,18] This is surprising because histamine is not involved in the pathogenesis. There is little additional benefit from adding an H_2 blocking agent. Delayed-pressure urticaria does not respond to antihistamines but may respond to prednisone, 1 mg/kg/day for 4–5 days, but prednisone is generally not required.[2] There is no satisfactory treatment for cold urticaria other than cold avoidance, although cyproheptadine, 2–4 mg three times a day, and desloratidine 5mg in older children, has been reported to provide relief.[20,22]

Patient education. Patients with the physical urticarias must be instructed to reduce their exposure to the precipitating factors. Patients with dermatographism and delayed-pressure urticaria should not wear backpacks or carry other heavy weights and should avoid tight-fitting clothing and excessive friction or pressure on the skin. Patients with heat- and exercise-induced urticaria need to avoid excessive heating of the skin, vigorous exercise, hot baths, and other factors resulting in increased body heat. Patients with cold urticaria should avoid ice-cold food or drinks, dress warmly in cold weather, and avoid swimming in cold water.

Follow-up visits. A visit 2 weeks after the initial evaluation will be useful to monitor the progress of the disease and the therapeutic response.

Urticarial vasculitis

Clinical features. Urticarial vasculitis is characterized by fixed wheals distributed symmetrically over the extremities.[23,24] It is rare in childhood and may be associated with systemic symptoms.[30] Lesions remain fixed in the same area for 24–72 hours and may be accompanied by mild arthralgias or malaise

Fig. 14.12 Urticarial vasculitis. Fixed urticaria on foot and toes in adolescent boy.

(Fig. 14.12). Most patients have an elevated erythrocyte sedimentation rate and depressed serum complement levels.[24] Urticarial vasculitis may be associated with systemic lupus erythematosus or juvenile rheumatoid arthritis.[23] The natural history is not known. Although the findings are similar to those in necrotizing vasculitis with palpable purpura, most patients do not progress to palpable purpura.

Differential diagnosis. Urticarial vasculitis may be distinguished from other conditions (see Box 14.2) by the elevated erythrocyte sedimentation rate, depressed serum complement levels, the finding of small-vessel vasculitis on skin biopsy, and the associated systemic symptoms.[24]

Pathogenesis. Urticarial vasculitis has been associated with circulating immune complexes, resulting in injury to postcapillary venules in the upper dermis.[24] Immunofluorescence has demonstrated immunoglobulins and complement split products around inflamed venules. Neutrophils and degenerating neutrophil nuclei are seen around the venules on skin biopsy, with swelling of the venule wall and fibrin deposition.[24] The inflammatory events are most probably mediated through the interaction of immune complexes with the complement and clotting systems.

Treatment. If a cause for immune complex disease, such as streptococcal infection, can be determined, it can be eliminated, but such associations are difficult to document. There is no known effective treatment. Antihistamines, indometacin, dapsone, colchicine, and low-dose prednisone therapy have been utilized, with variable success.[24]

Patient education. Patients should be advised of the difference between urticarial vasculitis and other urticarias.

Follow-up visits. Monthly visits are advisable to determine whether the disorder has progressed to involve vessels of other organs. Urinalysis, erythrocyte sedimentation rate, and complement levels may be used to follow the course of the disease.

Mastocytosis (including urticaria pigmentosa)

Clinical features. There are four distinct forms of mastocytosis observed in childhood.[25] The most common are the solitary mastocytoma (discussed in Ch. 12) (Figs 14.13–14.15) and urticaria pigmentosa.[25,26] The uncommon forms are diffuse cutaneous mastocytosis (bullous mastocytosis) and the rare telangiectasia macularis eruptiva perstans.[27–29] There appears

Fig. 14.15 Soliatry mastocytoma with bulla on hand of infant.

to be both a hereditary and nonhereditary form of urticaria pigmentosa. In the far more common nonhereditary form, the blotchy macular and nodular pigmented lesions of appear in the first 8 months of life

Fig. 14.13 Mastocytoma. Pink plaque on the skin of an infant. Note tan borders.

Fig. 14.14 Solitary mastocytoma. Typical brown macules on chest of infant.

Fig. 14.16 Urticaria pigmentosa. Scattered brown blotchy macules and papules on trunk of infant.

Fig. 14.17 Urticaria pigmentosa. Infant progressed to develop dozens of brown macules and papules on trunk.

Fig. 14.18 Large blotchy tan macules and plaques in child with urticaria pigmentosa.

Fig. 14.19 Tense edema and redness within macule of urticaria pigmentosa after stroking (Darier's sign).

Box 14.5 Drugs producing histamine release in mastocytosis

Opiates (codeine, meperidine [Demerol], morphine)

Polymyxin B

Acetylsalicylic acid

(Fig. 14.16). One or two lesions are noted initially, but numerous lesions accumulate during the next few months (Fig. 14.17). The majority of lesions appear on the trunk (Fig. 14.18), although some may appear on the face and extremities. Individual lesions are often red at first and may easily become blistered.[22,23] The characteristic blotchy, brown pigmentation may not appear until 6 months after the onset of the lesions. Stroking the pigmented lesion will result in tense edema within the lesion and an erythematous flare surrounding the area (Darier's sign) (Fig. 14.19). Half of patients with mastocytosis will demonstrate dermatographism in uninvolved skin. Skin biopsy will confirm the diagnosis.[25,26] Spontaneous clearing by age 6 or 7 years is usual.

The hereditary form, seen in less than 2% of childhood urticaria pigmentosa, often has it's onset after 12 months of age, initially with only a few lesions.

More lesions accumulate slowly with age, and lesions do not spontaneously resolve. Systemic symptoms develop with time.

Spontaneous bulla formation within mastocytosis lesions may occur or be induced by a variety of drugs (Box 14.5). These drugs, or rubbing of the skin, may induce enough histamine release to produce systemic symptoms, such as flushing, tachycardia, hypotension with fainting, diarrhea, and vomiting.[25,26] As the child ages, it becomes more difficult to urticate the lesions, or to induce blisters, or both. Often, by age 5 these lesions are asymptomatic, and by adolescence only residual flat pigmentation remains.

Enlargement of the liver and spleen, systemic flushing episodes, and peptic ulcer symptoms should suggest systemic mastocytosis. Systemic mastocytosis occurs in up to 2% of infants with urticaria pigmentosa, with the hereditary subtype.[25,26] Bony involvement can be documented by radiologic examination, and bone-marrow examination will reveal increased numbers of mast cells. Extreme infiltration of the liver sufficient to produce cirrhosis may occur. In the infant who has urticaria pigmentosa without systemic symptoms, routine skeletal surveys and bone marrow examinations are not warranted.

Diffuse cutaneous mastocytosis (bullous mastocytosis) presents as blisters (Fig. 14.20) in the neonatal

Fig. 14.20 Diffuse cutaneous mastocytosis. Linear blisters from stoking the infant's skin.

Fig. 14.21 Diffuse cutaneous mastocytois. Thickened, leathery yellowish skin with prominent urticaria wheals develops with time.

period, often accompanied by flushing episodes.[25,26] The blisters are often large and they peel, leaving large, eroded bases. After a severe blistering episode, 5–10 days may be required to regranulate mast cells, and the baby experiences recurrent episodes. When the baby is evaluated, marked dermatographism is present. A leathery thickening with yellow-tan skin usually does not appear until 3–8 months of age (Fig. 14.21).[25,26] Severe syncopal episodes and death from prolonged hypotension have been reported. Gastrointestinal symptoms are seen as the child becomes older, including chronic diarrhea states and recurrent episodes of vomiting associated with abdominal pain.[28] Gastrointestinal stromal tumors may appear in adults. In addition to gastrointestinal involvement, bone marrow involvement is more likely. It is an autosomal dominant disorder, often associated with *c-kit* mutations.[28]

Differential diagnosis. Mastocytosis can be differentiated from other conditions by skin biopsy (see Box 14.1). The bullous lesions must be differentiated from other bullous diseases of infancy. Diffuse cutaneous mastocytosis has been confused with staphylococcal scalded skin syndrome, especially recurrent scalded skin syndrome, and with epidermolysis bullosa. Systemic mastocytosis may mimic histiocytosis or vasculitis.[29] Systemic mastocytosis has been associated with elevated serum tryptase levels.[30]

Pathogenesis. Excessive numbers of mast cells accumulate with the dermis in mastocytosis.[25,26] It is believed that hereditary mastocytosis represents reactive mast cell hyperplasia caused by activating mutations in the *c-kit* receptor in response to stem cell factor.[28] Excessive histamine release from these mast cells results in whealing or blister formation. The blister is subepidermal and may bleed. Histamine is undoubtedly responsible for the local and systemic effects. Flushing and syncopal episodes are due to prostaglandin D_2 release, and bleeding is caused by heparin release by cutaneous mast cells.[25,26] Increased bone marrow apoptosis and cluster formation is observed in *c-kit* mutations as it is in other myelodysplastic disorders.[28] It has been appreciated that children with systemic mastocytosis demonstrate chromosomal abnormalities in the bone marrow cells demonstrating genetic instability of hematopoietic cells.[28]

Treatment. Most infants with solitary mastocytomas or urticaria pigmentosa require no treatment.[25,26] Flushing episodes or other systemic symptoms may be controlled by the use of hydroxyzine hydrochloride, 2–4 mg/kg/day divided into four doses. Solitary mastocytomas may be treated with 2 weeks of superpotent topical steroids.[31] Oral cromolyn sodium has been reported to be valuable in infants with gastrointestinal involvement. Diffuse cutaneous mastocytosis may respond to psoralen ultraviolet A-range (PUVA) therapy or narrow-band UVB phototherapy.[32]

Patient education. It is essential that the child with mastocytosis not be given cough syrups with codeine or other medications with opiates. Parents should be provided the list in Box 14.5 of medications to be avoided. If surgery is contemplated, preoperative medications should be carefully selected. Substitution of other antipyretics for aspirin is also advised. The natural course should be emphasized. Genetic counseling is valuable for diffuse cutaneous mastocytosis.

Follow-up visits. A follow-up visit in 2 weeks is useful in determining the presence or absence of systemic symptoms. If treatment is given, monthly visits are advisable.

ERYTHEMAS

Erythemas of the skin without wheal production are uncommon in infants and children. Often called the *reactive erythemas*, they include the annular erythemas (including erythema chronicum migrans, erythema marginatum, and erythema annulare), erythema multiforme, and erythema nodosum. Erythema multiforme is covered in detail in Chapter 11 and erythema chronicum migrans in Chapter 5.

Annular Erythemas

Clinical features

Annular, polycyclic, and partially marginated lesions are called annular erythemas. One should remember that giant urticaria can assume annular shapes.

Erythema annulare. In erythema annulare the lesions have erythematous borders, a trailing scale, and a dusky center (Fig. 14.22). These lesions may occur anywhere on the skin.[33–36] Multiple lesions are usually present, and they slowly enlarge. They last for several months and tend to recur. In infants the lesions may be associated with a maternal collagen vascular disorder, particularly with Sjögren's syndrome and auto-

Fig. 14.23 Erythema marginatum. Fleeting, semiannular erythema on the face of an infant with acute rheumatic fever.

immune thyroiditis.[34] A distinct annular erythema is *erythema annulare centrifugum*, which has a fine, white scale just inside the red zone ('trailing scale') and may be associated with hidden infection such as urinary tract infections.[35] Annular red plaques has been reported as a presenting finding of childhood cutaneous T-cell lymphoma.[36]

Erythema marginatum: Erythema marginatum is a transient eruption consisting of curvilinear, migrating areas of erythema that form incomplete circles (Fig. 14.23). The marginated lesions may move rapidly over the skin within several hours and disappear.[37,38] Inducing cutaneous vasodilation may make the lesions more visible. It is found in only 3% of children with acute rheumatic fever,[37] despite being one of the Jones criteria for diagnosis, and is associated with the fever and well-established carditis. A thorough eva-

Fig. 14.22 Erythema annulare. Concentric zones of red and dusky skin.

Box 14.6 Differential diagnosis of annular erythemas

Erythema annulare

Erythema annulare centrifugum

Erythema chronicum migrans

Erythema marginatum

Tinea corporis

Pityriasis rosea

Subacute cutaneous lupus erythematosus

Neonatal lupus syndrome

Sarcoidosis

Syphilis

Juvenile rheumatoid arthritis

luation for acute rheumatic fever is indicated. It may also be seen after streptococcal infections without evidence of acute rheumatic fever and has been described in children with hereditary angioedema.[38]

Differential diagnosis

Conditions to be considered in the differential diagnosis of annular erythemas are listed in Box 14.6. Dermatophyte lesions have a scaly border and may be diagnosed by potassium hydroxide (KOH) examination and fungal cultures. Granuloma annulare lesions have a distinct nodular and papular border without epidermal change. The lesions of pityriasis rosea may be annular on occasion and have central clearing. Lupus erythematosus, sarcoidosis, and syphilis may also present with annular lesions. The transient urticarial lesions of juvenile rheumatoid arthritis tend to be limited to the abdomen, and clear slightly in the center.

Pathogenesis

Two of the erythemas demonstrate infectious agents within the skin lesions, with an attendant host response. In erythema chronicum migrans, *Borrelia burgdorferi* is found (see Ch. 5); in erythema multiforme, herpes simplex virus is noted (see Ch. 11). In erythema annulare and in erythema marginatum, the mechanism of disease is unknown. In erythema marginatum associated with hereditary angioedema, bradykinin has been implicated.[38] Dense accumulation of lymphocytes that surround superficial dermal blood vessels is seen on skin biopsy, which helps distinguish annular erythemas from urticaria.[38] Skin biopsy is useful in erythema annulare associated with T-cell lymphomas as characteristic T-cell infiltrates and epidermal abscess containing atypical lymphocytes are seen.[36]

Treatment

No treatment is useful for erythema annulare. Children with erythema marginatum are treated with penicillin for associated rheumatic fever or streptococcal infections and with hereditary angioedema, with anabolic steroids. Children with cutaneous T-cell lymphoma may be treated with a variety of protocols.[36]

Patient education

Clinicians should emphasize to the patient and family that these eruptions are skin reactions that do not require treatment but serve as a clue to a systemic disorder.

Follow-up visits

A visit 1 week after the initial evaluation is useful to discuss the results of laboratory evaluation for systemic disorders. The need for follow-up care is determined by the nature of the associated systemic disorder.

Erythema Nodosum

Clinical features

Erythema nodosum is characterized by the abrupt onset of symmetric, very tender, erythematous nodules on the extensor surface of the extremities (Fig. 14.24).[39–41] Occasionally, lesions will involve other areas of skin, such as the soles of the feet, eyelids, hands, or trunk. Widespread involvement is more characteristic of infants (Fig. 14.25). The nodules have indistinct borders (Fig. 14.26). Occasionally, it will be unilateral at presentation. The lesions may be so painful that the patient will limp. A prodrome of cough, sore throat, and fever will occur in about 25% of children.[39] It occurs most commonly in adolescents and is uncommon before age 2 years. Females predominate at a ratio of 1.7:1. Lesions last 2–6 weeks. Recurrences are reported in 4% of children. Lesions resolve as a bruise, with a color change to purple, then yellow-brown. Infectious causes, such as β-hemolytic streptococcal infections, tuberculosis, sarcoidosis, histoplasmosis, tularemia, Epstein-Barr virus (EBV), hepatitis B, Yersinia, and coccidioidomycosis, are the most

Fig. 14.24 Tender red nodules with indistinct borders in a teenage girl with erythema nodosum.

Fig. 14.25 Atypical location of erythema nodosum in an infant.

Fig. 14.26 Erythema nodosum on anterior leg of teenage girl.

common associations.[39-42] Streptococcal infections account for 30% of cases.[39,40] A careful history should be obtained for preceding infections.

Inflammatory bowel disease, Behçet's disease, the hereditary period fever syndromes, and Hodgkin's disease are uncommon associations.[40-44] Drugs may uncommonly produce erythema nodosum, particularly oral contraceptives in adolescent females.

Differential diagnosis

Erythema nodosum may be confused with many other processes involving the subcutaneous fat. In contrast to erythema nodosum, thrombophlebitis usually occurs on the lateral or flexor surface of the lower legs and heals with fibrosis. The nodose lesions of polyarteritis nodosa are associated with an exaggerated dusky, mottling pattern called *livedo reticularis* that is seen on the overlying skin. Giant insect-bite reactions may be confused with erythema nodosum, but a central punctum will help differentiate. Panniculitis can be distinguished on biopsy of skin to include subcutaneous fat. Vasculitis and eosinophilic cellulitis may also mimic erythema nodosum. The lesions of erythema nodosum are usually so characteristic that they are seldom confused with those of other disorders.

Pathogenesis

Erythema nodosum is a chronic injury of the blood vessels of the lower dermis and subcutaneous fat. Initially, the perivascular inflammation is neutrophilic, then lymphocytic, then granulomatous as the lesions age. There is increasing evidence to implicate circulating immune complexes in the pathogenesis of erythema nodosum as a part of the host immune response to an infectious agent. Fat cell destruction usually does not occur in erythema nodosum, so it is not a true panniculitis.

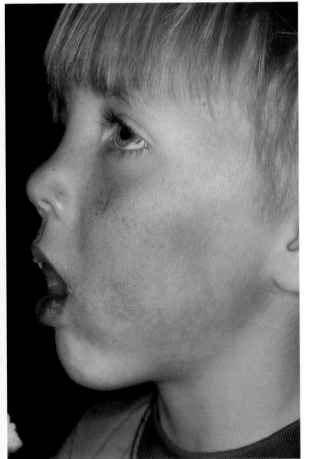

Fig. 14.27 Gustatory flushing (Frey's syndrome). Redness to cheek minutes after eating.

Treatment

Symptomatic treatment with acetylsalicylic acid or antihistamines may suffice because in many cases the erythema nodosum resolves within 3 weeks. In patients with acutely tender lesions that interfere with walking, nonsteroidal antiinflammatory agents, such as indometacin, may be tried.[45] Although some relief can be obtained with prednisone, oral steroids are not generally recommended and should not be used chronically. Thalidomide, effective in erythema nodosum associated with leprosy, has been used successfully in erythema nodosum of other causes.[45] The restricted availability of thalidomide in the United States limits its use.

Patient education

It should be emphasized that erythema nodosum is a response to infection or to certain inflammatory diseases. A search for such associations should be guided by the history and should not involve expensive laboratory tests. Parents should be reassured that most children recover within 3 weeks.

Follow-up visits

A return visit in 1 week is useful to ascertain the need for, or response to, therapy.

Gustatory Flushing

Clinical features

Gustatory flushing usually develops in early infancy and may first present when solid foods are introduced. An erythematous flush of one cheek occurs during or just after eating, lasting from 5 to 60 minutes (Fig. 14.27).[46–48] Sweating may develop within the flushed area, and tearing of the adjacent eye may occur.[47] Frequently, the infant is misdiagnosed as having a food allergy. Spontaneous remission has been reported after several years.

Differential diagnosis

Urticaria and food allergy are often considered in the diagnosis. However, gustatory flushing always occurs in the same site and does not move from skin area to skin area as urticaria would. Food allergy reactions should occur with specific foods and be widespread and not localized. Gustatory flushing occurs with any foods that stimulate the taste buds. Herpes facialis may be considered, but it presents with persistent erythema that lasts for at least 3 days and usually evolves to vesicle formation. Contact dermatitis also produces a persistent erythema on the cheek.

Pathogenesis

Gustatory flushing is caused by cross-linking of the parasympathetic nerve fibers innervating the parotid gland to the sympathetic fibers supplying the sweat glands and cutaneous vessels along the distribution of the auriculotemporal nerve. Foods that would ordinarily stimulate salivation instead produce flushing and sweating.[46,47] In infancy, cases are believed to be due to a congenital malformation resulting in cross-linking of nerve fibers. It may result from nerve regeneration after parotid surgery or injury in older children.

Treatment

There is no known effective treatment. Topical antiperspirants will control the sweating. If antiperspirants fail, injections of botulinum toxin have been effective.[48]

Patient education

Clinicians should emphasize that the condition does not represent allergy, and that spontaneous remission can be expected in most infants. Allergy evaluation should be discouraged.

Follow-up visits

Routine follow-up visits are unnecessary.

PURPURAS

Purpuric lesions always prompt investigation into bleeding states. They may involve small areas (e.g. petechiae) or large areas (e.g. ecchymoses). Palpable purpura (purpuric papules), dissecting purpura, and chronic pigmented purpura are presented in this section. Neonatal purpura (Box 14.7), acral petechiae and purpura (Box 14.8), and flat generalized petechiae and purpura (including thrombocytopenic purpuras,[49] vaccine purpuras,[50] and purpura seen after application of EMLA cream[51]) (Box 14.9) are not discussed, but are presented to aid the reader in making a differential diagnosis of these lesions.

Box 14.7 Differential diagnosis of neonatal purpura

Congenital infection
Toxoplasma
Enterovirus
Rubella
Cytomegalovirus
Herpes simplex
Syphilis
Coagulation defects
Autoimmune disorders (systemic lupus erythematosus and erythroblastosis fetalis)
Vascular tumors with platelet trapping syndrome (Kasabach-Merritt)

Box 14.8 Differential diagnosis of flat acral purpura

Rocky Mountain spotted fever
Meningococcemia
Atypical measles
Coagulation disorders
Progressive pigmentary purpura

Box 14.9 Differential diagnosis of flat generalized purpura

Thrombocytopenic states (idiopathic thrombocytopenic purpura, leukemia)
Coagulation disorders
Trauma (including child abuse)

Palpable Purpura (Purpuric Papules)

Clinical features

Discrete 1–5-mm papules with petechial centers or those that are completely purpuric characterize palpable purpura (Fig. 14.28).[52–55] They are usually found on the lower extremities and are symmetric and numerous (Fig. 14.29). Palpable purpura should immediately bring to mind vasculitis or septicemia. The vasculitis that occurs is called *cutaneous necrotizing venulitis* and can be associated with IgG or IgA (anaphylactoid purpura, Henoch-Schönlein purpura [HSP]) and may be associated with vasculitis of renal, gastrointestinal, joint, or cerebral vessels.[52–56] The lesions may begin as discrete urticarial wheals,[23,24,25] then progress to papular purpura and pustular purpura (Fig. 14.30). Eventually, cutaneous infarcts, purpuric bullae,[52] and gangrene with subsequent ulceration

Fig. 14.28 Numerous purpuric macules and papules on the buttocks of a child with necrotizing venulitis.

Fig. 14.29 Papules with purpuric centers on the leg of a child with necrotizing venulitis (Henoch-Schönlein purpura).

Fig. 14.30 Purpuric papules, pustules and bullae on leg of child with necrotizing venulitis.

Fig. 14.31 Acute hemorrhagic edma of infancy. Large purpuric macules on infant's arm.

and scarring will occur. In infants, large 10 cm or greater purpuric plaques with associated edema may be found. (Figs 14.31, 14.32). These are frequently seen on the genitalia or buttocks. This is termed acute hemorrhagic edema of infancy.[6,56] The course and associated findings are similar to that in children who experience typical palpable purpura of the legs (Fig. 14.33).[6,56] Arthralgia or arthritis of the knees and ankles is found in 80% of all children with HSP.[52–56] Cramping abdominal pain, vomiting, hematemesis, and melena signal gastrointestinal involvement. Abdominal pain is common but in most children lasts less than 24 hours. The kidney is involved in 70% of children.[54] Most have asymptomatic microscopic hematuria, but only 25% on the first visit. Some children may present with a nephrotic syndrome. Up to 10% of children may progress to chronic renal fail-

ure. Rarely, with involvement of the central nervous system vessels, seizures, paresis, or coma occur.

Most episodes of necrotizing venulitis have skin changes that last 4–6 weeks and then resolve.[52–54] In addition to necrotizing vasculitis, septicemic states also present with palpable purpura, which may evolve to pustules. Lesions are acral, symmetric, and few in number. Palpable purpura is seen in chronic meningococcemia, gonococcemia, and subacute bacterial endocarditis and is frequently associated with arthritis or arthralgias of the large joints. Blood cultures or genital cultures will confirm the diagnosis. It is difficult to culture organisms from lesions, but they may be identified by specific immunofluorescence from smears of lesions. Rarely, *Pseudomonas*, staphylococcal, deep fungal, or Gram-negative septicemia is responsible. Palpable purpura is also seen in collagen

Fig. 14.32 Acute hemorrhagic edema of infancy.

Fig. 14.33 Acute hemorrhagic edema of infancy. Nonblancing large macules on leg. Biopsy (stitches on leg) showed necrotizing venulitis.

Box 14.10 Differential diagnosis of palpable purpura
Necrotizing venulitis, IgA type (anaphylactoid [Henoch-Schönlein] purpura) or IgG type
Meningococcemia
Gonococcemia
Staphylococcal sepsis
Pseudomonas sepsis
Subacute bacterial endocarditis

vascular diseases of childhood, especially juvenile rheumatoid arthritis and lupus erythematosus.[23,24] It occurs in long-standing disease, often years after the diagnosis was confirmed. It is also seen in the periodic fevers.[44]

Differential diagnosis

Biopsy plus bacterial and fungal culture will distinguish infectious causes of palpable purpura from one another (Box 14.10). Immunofluorescent examination of a skin biopsy will reveal immunoglobulin A (IgA) deposits surrounding superficial cutaneous blood vessels in typical HSP[52,53] and IgG deposits in a few children. Antineutrophil cytoplasmic antibodies (ANCAs) may help in the diagnosis to exclude periarteritis nodosa.[54,55] Associated collagen vascular disease is usually already established, and diagnostic serologies are not routinely required.

Pathogenesis

In necrotizing venulitis and in septicemic states, circulating immune complexes have been implicated in the production of lesions through their interaction with the complement and clotting systems. The prodrome of upper respiratory tract infection, and sometimes positive streptococcal throat cultures, has implicated infectious agents as likely triggers of immune complex formation in HSP. An association with parvovirus B19, hepatitis B and C and vaccination against hepatitis B, pneumococci, and influenza in childhood HSP may also be found.[49,50,52,53]

Drugs such as propylthiouracil, hydralazine, and zafirlukast have been associated with necrotizing venulitis.

Fibrinoid necrosis of venule walls in the upper dermis, with perivascular accumulation of neutrophils, nuclear fragments, and extravasation of red blood cells, is seen on skin biopsy. Organisms may also be detected with Grams stains of skin biopsies in the septicemic states.

Treatment

In necrotizing venulitis with skin involvement only, no treatment is required. The skin lesions are unlikely to respond to corticosteroids.[52,53] Prednisone, 2 mg/kg/day, may be indicated with internal organ involvement, particularly bowel disease. The administration of systemic antibiotics, with the choice of agent based on appropriate cultures, is indicated for septicemic states. In severe prolonged necrotizing venulitis, pulse therapy with intravenous methylprednisolone and plasmapheresis or cyclophosphamide orally or pulsed intravenously may be useful.[52] Azathioprine has been successfully used for maintenance therapy.

Patient education

The serious nature of vasculitis of internal organs and septicemic states should be emphasized. Future upper respiratory tract illnesses should be brought to the physicians attention promptly, and appropriate cultures should be obtained. Early treatment of an associated streptococcal infection may be required.

Follow-up visits

In necrotizing venulitis, weekly follow-up visits are recommended for the first 4 weeks to monitor internal involvement, particularly of the kidney. Microscopic examination of the urinary sediment and protein determination are required. Thereafter, evaluations of renal function every 3 months are valuable to identify the children at risk of renal failure.

Nodular Purpura with Livedo: Polyarteritis Nodosa (Periarteritis Nodosa)

Clinical features

There are four polyarteritis syndromes in childhood: infantile polyarteritis nodosa, Kawasaki disease, nodular vasculitis, and chronic cutaneous polyarteritis nodosa.[57-60] The infantile form may represent Kawasaki disease without cutaneous findings and is considered with Kawasaki disease in Chapter 11.

Nodular vasculitis may demonstrate solitary red, tender nodules that mimic individual lesions of erythema nodosum (Fig. 14.34).[57] The cutaneous findings of livedo reticularis (Fig. 14.35) plus palpable, tender, linear, purple nodules (Fig. 14.36) are found in children with chronic cutaneous polyarteritis nodosa (Figs 14.37, 14.38).[57-60] Typically, older children rather than toddlers are affected. Fever, myalgias, arthralgias, and gastrointestinal symptoms are observed in 70%.[58,59] Hypertension, renal disease, pulmonary involvement, and localized neuropathy (mononeuritis

Fig. 14.34 Nodular vasculitis. Red nodule with ulcerations on one leg of adolescent girl.

Fig. 14.35 Livedo pattern in adolescent boy with periarteritis nodosa.

Fig. 14.36 Linear red nodules on leg of child with periarteritis nodosa.

Fig. 14.37 Periarteritis nodosa on leg of child.

Fig. 14.38 Linear tender red nodules and livedo reticularis in childhood polyarteritis nodosa.

multiplex) may be observed. The skin lesions are usually located symmetrically on the proximal extremities and persist for weeks, with recurrent crops of new nodules appearing. Exacerbations may occur on cold exposure. Focal areas of skin infarction and ulceration may accompany the nodules.[57–59] The course is quite chronic and may last for years.[57–59] Newborns of mothers with long-standing polyarteritis nodosa may develop a transient polyarteritis nodosa with lesions lasting 3 months. ANCAs may be present, and the affected child may have a positive antinuclear antibody test. The erythrocyte sedimentation rate is virtually always elevated.

Differential diagnosis

Livedo patterns must be distinguished from mottling, which may be seen transiently with cold exposure. Mottling disappears on rewarming and livedo patterns do not. Cutis marmorata telangiectasia congenita has a livedo pattern but is present from birth, not acquired. Careful palpation of the skin within the livedo area may be required to detect the linear nodules of periarteritis nodosa. Selection of a site for skin biopsy is critical. A biopsy specimen must include a linear nodule, with subcutaneous fat, to detect the characteristic pathology because artery involvement is segmental. Biopsy of the livedo area or a shallow biopsy may miss the pathology.

Pathogenesis

Polyarteritis nodosa is an inflammatory segmental disease of the walls of cutaneous arteries. Neutrophilic infiltration of the arterial wall and adjacent periarterial tissue is seen.[59] Thrombosis of vessels may be found. In children there is an association with parvovirus B19, hepatitis B and C, and with streptococcal infection. Mixed cryoglobulinemia may be found.[59]

Treatment

Most children respond well to low-dose oral steroids (0.5 mg/kg prednisone).[58] In children who require high-dose oral steroids, low-dose once-weekly methotrexate, pulsed intravenous cyclophosphamide, oral azathioprine and tumor necrosis factor alpha blockade have been used successfully.[58,60]

Patient education

Avoiding cold exposure is advisable. The child and the family should be informed about the chronic and persistent nature of this condition and advised of potential systemic complications and the need for monitoring of renal, gastrointestinal, and pulmonary involvement.

Follow-up visits

Initially follow-up visits should be every 2 weeks until disease control is established. After the disease is stabilized, evaluation of renal status and other systemic complications should be performed every 4–6 weeks.

Nodular Purpura: Pernio

Clinical features

Pernio is characterized by asymptomatic purple to purple-red nodules, several days to weeks after exposure to wetness and cold.[61,62] The nodules are usually on the digits and may be accompanied by a livedo pattern of the adjacent skin (Fig. 14.39). Other acral areas, such as the ears, may also be involved (Fig. 14.40). The livedo pattern slowly fades and the nodules remain for weeks. Occasionally, the nodules will ulcerate and are then quite painful. Ulcerated pernio lesions are usually on the toes and are called kibes.[61] The cold exposure may seem trivial rather than severe, and associated wetness is required.[61,62] Pernio has been associated with anorexia nervosa in adolescent girls.

Differential diagnosis

The nodules of pernio must be differentiated from lymphoma or leukemia states, which also produce red-purple nodules. Pernio lesions have an insidious onset rather than the abrupt onset of lymphomas and, once established, do not grow but remain stable. Poly-arteritis nodosa nodules are linear rather than oval and tender rather than nontender. A skin biopsy will distinguish the two conditions.

Pathogenesis

The exact mechanism of the response to cold injury is not known. Some children may have cryoproteins.[61] Pathology shows mid-dermal inflammation, including a lymphohistiocytic infiltrate around blood vessels, but is not specific.

Treatment

In most circumstances no treatment is required.

Patient education

Protection against cold and wetness is critical.

Fig. 14.40 Purple nodule on the ear of toddler with pernio.

Fig. 14.39 Purple, oval, nontender nodules on the toes in a child with pernio.

Follow-up visits

A follow-up visit in 2 weeks may be useful to ascertain the course of the condition and to reinforce the cold and wetness avoidance.

Dissecting Purpura (Disseminated Intravascular Coagulation)

Clinical features

Dissecting purpura, or disseminated intravascular coagulation, has an acute onset, with high fever and extensive, large, dissecting purpuric areas on the extremities.[63] The purpuric 'lakes' are large and are not associated with petechiae (Fig. 14.41). The condition has been associated with overwhelming infections, such as meningococcemia, *Escherichia coli* septicemia, and Rocky Mountain spotted fever, or it may follow common childhood infections, such as streptococcal pharyngitis or varicella, by 5–10 days.[63] Vascular collapse is common, and mortality is high in untreated patients. Even in those who survive, large areas of infarcted skin require long-term management. Survivors often will have impaired thyroid function.[64]

Differential diagnosis

The large purpuric lakes are so characteristic that they are not confused with other purpuric diseases.

Pathogenesis

The syndrome is triggered by the massive release of tissue thromboplastin with widespread fibrin deposition in the blood vessels of skin, lungs, and kidneys;

Fig. 14.41 Purpuric lakes with hemorrhagic blisters in a child with disseminated intravascular coagulation.

fibrinolysis; and consumption of coagulation factors, leading to secondary bleeding.[63] Proteins C and S are particularly consumed by the infections as well. Protein C is a vitamin K-dependent plasma serine protease that acts as an anticoagulant by inactivating clotting factors Va and VIIIa after clotting is initiated. Protein S acts as a cofactor for protein C in the inactivation of clotting factor Va. When protein C or protein S is deficient, intravascular hypercoagulability results, with widespread thrombosis.[63]

Treatment

Replacement of consumable clotting factors with fresh plasma, protein C concentrate, or platelet concentrates is the treatment of choice.[63] Most children require hospitalization. With persistent disseminated intravascular coagulation, heparin, 100 U/kg intravenously every 4–6 hours, may be given. Antibiotic treatment of the triggering bacterial infection is necessary. With extensive areas of skin necrosis, admission to a burn unit with appropriate debridement, prevention of secondary infection, and biologic dressings may be useful.[63]

Patient education

Advice to the patient and family depends on the nature of the triggering disease. Counseling regarding the grave prognosis and need for long-term care should be provided.

Follow-up visits

While the child is hospitalized, daily follow-up visits are useful to evaluate response to therapy.

Chronic Pigmented Purpura

Clinical features

Chronic pigmented purpura is characterized by an insidious onset and slow progression of grouped non-palpable petechiae over the extremities, trunk, or neck (Fig. 14.42) in adolescents.[65–67] Individual lesions show fresh and old petechiae intermixed and an interplay of red, brown, and yellow spots. Lesions are usually flat (Fig. 14.43), but a lichenified epidermis may overlie the lesions (Fig.14.44). The grouped petechiae are oval and may begin unilaterally[67] but progress to become symmetric. The lower extremities are most commonly involved, with more lesions

Fig. 14.42 Golden-brown and cayenne-pepper macules on the neck of a child with progressive pigmentary purpura.

Fig. 14.43 Pigmented macule in progressive pigmentary purpura.

Fig. 14.44 Lichenified brown plaque in child with progressive pigmented purpura.

Fig. 14.45 Annular pigmented macules in progressive pigmentary purpura (purpura annularis telangiectoides of Majocchi).

in dependent areas.[65–67] Lesions may progress to involve the entire trunk and upper extremities. Annular lesions may occur (Fig. 14.45). Itching is usually mild or absent, and no systemic symptoms are associated with chronic pigmented purpura. Spontaneous remission occurs within 1–2 years, but the natural course of the disease is not well documented.

Differential diagnosis

The lesions of grouped petechiae of multiple ages are so characteristic that this type of purpura is seldom confused with other disorders. Occasionally, trauma (e.g. child abuse) or a mild bleeding disorder is suspected.

Pathogenesis

A mild capillaritis is seen in these disorders, with extravasation of red blood cells, hemosiderin deposits, and a mild perivascular lymphocytic infiltration of superficial dermal blood vessels.[52] The vascular injury is mild, and its cause is unknown.

Treatment

There is no specific therapy. Reduction of venous stasis may be helpful.

Patient education

The expected remission and the mild nature of this disorder should be emphasized.

Follow-up visits

Follow-up visits are unnecessary.

Pyoderma Gangrenosum

Clinical features

Pyoderma gangrenosum begins as a 3–8 mm red papule that progresses within hours to a pustule, then to an ulceration surrounded by edematous, lilac-colored loosely attached epidermis (Figs 14.46, 14.47).[68–71] The ulceration rapidly and relentlessly enlarges to greater than 2 cm or more. Often, a history of preceding trauma is obtained.[68–71] Ulcers can appear anywhere, but the legs are most common and are seen in 80% of cases (Fig. 14.48).[68–71] Skin ulceration at sites of trauma (pathergy) such as venipuncture sites or attempts at surgical debridement may be seen (Fig. 14.49). A history of an associated

Fig. 14.48 Ulcer on thigh of child with pyoderma gangrenosum.

Fig. 14.46 Pyoderma gangrenosum. Ulceration with characteristic loosely attached epidermis and purple border.

Fig. 14.47 Loose, undermined purple border to ulcer in pyoderma gangrenosum.

Fig. 14.49 Multiple ulcerated lesions following attempted surgical debridement of pyoderma gangrenosum lesion (pathergy).

disease, such as inflammatory bowel disease, rheumatoid arthritis, or myelodysplastic disease may be obtained.[68–71] The mortality rate is 10%.

Differential diagnosis

Spider or other insect bites are often misdiagnosed.[71] Infections such as herpes simplex virus (HSV) or ecthyma gangrenosum are often mistaken for pyoderma gangrenosum. The presence of the characteristic lilac, loosely-attached, epidermal edges to the ulcer distinguishes pyoderma gangrenosum. A skin biopsy to include the loosely attached epidermal edge demonstrating an undermined epidermis with neutrophils replacing the upper dermis will distinguish.[71]

Pathogenesis

Pyoderma gangrenosum is considered one of the neutrophilic dermatoses because sheets of neutrophils replacing the reticular dermis and undermining the adjacent epidermis are found. Activated neutrophils are believed responsible for the tissue damage.[71] The association with other disorders with activated neutrophils, such as inflammatory bowel disease, rheumatoid arthritis, and myelodysplasia, reinforces the concept. Recently, one associated form of pyoderma gangrenosum has been mapped to chromosome 15q.[55]

Treatment

Immunosuppressive drugs, such as ciclosporin and tacrolimus, are the most effective in controlling the disease.[71] The condition is often responsive to high-dose glucocorticosteroids, but steroid side effects from long-term usage limit their usefulness. Antineutrophil drugs, such as dapsone and colchicine, may be useful in combination. Good response to infliximab have been reported.[72] Topical tacrolimus may be a useful adjunct. Many cytotoxic agents have been used, but no rigorous evaluation is avaliable.[71]

Patient education

The clinician should explain to the patient and family the life-threatening nature of the disease and the requirement of days to weeks to accomplish a remission. It should also be emphasized that an endoscopic examination for inflammatory bowel disease, a bone marrow examination for myelodysplasia, and an arthritis consultation are required, and that long-term immunosuppressive therapy will be required.

Follow-up visits

Weekly visits are required until remission is accomplished, after which monthly visits are necessary. Frequent monitoring of side effects of the immunosuppressive agents is required.

REFERENCES

1. Doutre M. Physiopathology of urticaria. Eur J Dermatol 1999; 9:601.
2. Staumont-Salle D, Dombrowicz D, Capron M, et al. Eosinophils and urticaria. Clin Rev Allergy Immunol 2006; 30:13–18.
3. Blank M, Gisondi P, Mimouni D, et al. New insights into the autoantibody-mediated mechanisms of autoimmune bullous diseases and urticaria. Clin Exp Rheumatol 2006; 24:S20–S25.
4. Smit de V, Cameron PA, Rainer TH. Anaphylaxis presentations to an emergency department in Hong Kong: incidence and predictors of biphasic reactions. J Emerg Med 2005; 28:381–388.
5. Wiener ES, Bajaj L. Diagnosis and emergent management of anaphylaxis in children. Adv Pediatr 2005; 52:195–206.
6. Carder KR. Hypersensitivity reactions in neonates and infants. Dermatol Ther 2005; 160–175.
7. Sackesen C, Sekerel BE, Orhan F, et al. The etiology of different forms of urticaria in childhood. Pediatr Dermatol 2004; 21:102–108.
8. Kozel MM, Sabroe RA. Chronic urticaria: aetiology, management and current and future treatment options. Drugs 2004; 64:2515–2536.
9. Di Lorenzo G, Pacor ML, Mansueto P, et al. Food-additive urticaria: a survey of 838 patients with recurrent chronic idiopathic urticaria. Int Arch Allergy Immunol 2005; 138:235–42.
10. Colver AF, Nevantaus H, Macdougall CF, et al. Severe food-allergic reactions across the UK and Ireland, 1998–2000. Acta Paediatr 2005; 94:689–695.
11. Ellis AK, Day JH. Clinical reactivity to insect stings. Curr Opin Allergy Clin Immunol 2005; 5:349–354.
12. Kidon MI, Kang LW, Chin CW, et al. Early presentation with angioedema and urticaria in cross-reactive hypersensitivity to nonsteroidal antiinflammatory drugs amoung young Asian, atopic children. Pediatrics 2005; 116:e675–e680.
13. Lammintausta K, Kortekangas-Savolainen O. Oral challenge in patients with suspected cutaneous adverse drug reactions: findings in 784 patients during a 25-year period. Acta Derm Venereol 2005; 85:491–496.
14. Weston WL. What is erythema multiforme? Pediatr Ann 1996; 25:106–108.
15. Gompels MM, Lock RJ, Abinum M, et al. C1 inhibitor deficiency: consensus document. Clin Exp Immunol 2005; 141:189–190.
16. Bork K, Meng G, Staubach P, et al. Hereditary angioedema: new findings concerning symptoms, affected organs and course. Am J Med 2006; 119:267–274.
17. Boyle RJ, Nikpour M, Tang ML. Hereditary angio-oedema in children: a management guideline. Pediatr Allergy Immunol 2005; 16:288–294.
18. Stone KD. Adavances in pediatric allergy. Curr Opin Pediatr 2004; 16:571–578.

19. Morais-Almeida M, Marinho S, Gaspar A, et al. Cold urticaria and infectious mononucleosis in children. Allergol Immunopathol 2004; 32:368–371.

20. Alangari AA, Twarog FJ, Shih MC, et al. Clinical features and anaphylaxis in children with cold urticaria. Pediatrics 2004; 113:e313–e317.

21. Pradalier A, Cauvain A, Oukachbi Z. Inherited auto-inflammatory recurrent fevers. Allerg Immunol 20064; 38:5–9.

22. Juhlin L. Inhibition of cold urticaria by desloratidine. J Dermatol Treat 2004; 15:51–59.

23. DeAmicis T, Mofid MZ, Cohen B, et al. Hypocomplementemic urticarial vasculitis: report of a 12-year-old girl with systemic lupus erythematosus. J Amer Acad Dermatol 2002; 47:S273–S274.

24. Black AK. Urticarial vasculitis. Clin Dermatol 1999; 17:565–569.

25. Ben-Amitai D, Metzker A, Cohen HA. Pediatric cutaneous mastocytosis: a review of 180 patients. Isr Med Assoc J 2005; 7:320–322.

26. Kiszewski AE, Duran-McKinster C, Oroozco-Covarrubias L, et al. Cutaneous mastocytosis in children: a clinical analysis of 71 cases. J Eur Acad Dermatol Venereol 2004; 18:285–290.

27. Gibbs NF, Friedlander SF, Harpster EF. Telangiectasia macularis eruptiva perstans. Pediatr Dermatol 2000; 17:194–196.

28. Yanagahori H, Oyama N, Nakamura K, et al. *c-kit* mutations in patients with childhood-onset mastocytosis and genotype–phenotype correlations. J Mol Diag 2005; 7:252–257.

29. Dunst KM, Huemer GM, Zelger BG, et al. A new variant of mastocytosis: report of three cases clinicopathologically mimicking histiocytic and vasculitic disorders. Br J Dermatol 2005; 153:642–646.

30. Klion AD, Noel P, Akin C, et al. Elevated serum tryptase levels identify a subset of patients with a myeloproliferative variant of idiopathic hypereosinophilic syndrome associated with tissue fibrosis, poor prognosis and imatinib responsiveness. Blood 2003; 101:4660–4666.

31. Burkhart IA. Solitary mastocytosis successfully treated with a moderate potency topical steroid. J Drugs Dermatol 2004; 3:309–310.

32. Smith ML, Orton PW, Chu H, et al. Photochemotherapy of dominant diffuse cutaneous mastocytosis. Pediatric Dermatol 1990; 7:251–254.

33. Helm TN, Bass J, Chang LW. Persistent annular erythema of infancy. Pediatr Dermatol 1993; 10:46–48.

34. Miyagawa S, Tanaka M, Okamoto S, et al. Autoimmune thyroid disease in anti-Ro/SSA-positive children with annular erythema: report of two cases. Br J Dermatol 2004; 150:1005–1008.

35. Weyers W, Diaz-Cascajo C, Weyers I. Erythema annulare centrifugum: results of a clinicopathologic study of 73 patients. Am J Dermatopathol 2003; 25:451–462.

36. Cogrel O, Boralevi F, Lereux S, et al. Lymphomatoid annular erythema: a new form of juvenile mycosis fungoides. Br J Dermatol 2005; 152:565–566.

37. Zomorrodi A, Wald ER. Sydenham's chorea in western Pennsylvania. Pediatrics 2006; 117:e675–e679.

38. Starr JC, Brasher GW, Rao A, et al. Erythema marginatum and hereditary angioedema. South Med J 2004; 97:948–950.

39. Kakourou T, Drosatou P, Psychou F, et al. Erythema nodosum in children: a prospective study. J Am Acad Dermatol 2001; 44:17–21.

40. Mert A, Ozaras R, Tabak F, et al. Erythema nodosum: an experience of ten years. Scand J Infect Dis 2004; 36:424–427.

41. Weinstein M, Turner D, Avitzur Y. Erythema nodosum as a presentation of inflammatory bowel disease. CMAJ 2005; 173:145–146.

42. Fauroux B, Clement A. Paediatric sarcoidosis. Paediatr Resp Rev 2005; 6:128–133.

43. Al-Otaibi LM, Porter SR, Poate TW. Behçet's disease: a review. J Dent Res 2005; 84:209–222.

44. Fietta P. Autoinflammatory diseases: the hereditary periodic fever syndromes. Acta Biomed Ateneo Parmense 2004; 75:92–99.

45. Winter HS. Treatment of pyoderma gangrenosum, erythema nodosum and aphthous ulcerations. Inflamm Bowel Dis 1998; 4:71–74.

46. Cliff S, Lever R, Moss AL, et al. Frey's syndrome without hyperhidrosis. J Roy Soc Med 1998; 91:388–389.

47. Ott H, Brost H, Poblete-Gutierrez P, et al. Auriculotemporal syndrome in childhood. Acta Derm Venereol 2004; 84:160–161.

48. Eckardt A, Kuettner C. Treatment of gustatory sweating (Frey's syndrome) with botulinum toxin. Head Neck 2003; 25:624–628.

49. Tancabelic J, Stout LA, Wetering J. Acute immune thrombocytopenic purpura in children and adolescents in South Dakota, 1998–2004. SDJ Med 2005; 58:465–468.

50. Demichelli V, Jefferson T, Rivetti A, et al. Vaccines for measles, mumps and rubella in children. Cochrane Database Syst Rev 19:CD004407, 2005.

51. Neri J, Savoia F, Guareschi E, et al. Purpura after application of EMLA cream in two children. Pediatr Dermatol 2005; 22:566–568.

52. Ishii Y, Takizawa T, Arakawa H, et al. Hemorrhagic bullous lesions in Henoch-Schöenlein purpura. Pediatr Int 47: 2005; 694–697.

53. Motoyama O, Iitaka K. Familial cases of Henoch-Schöenlein purpura in eight families. Pediatr Int 2005; 47:612–615.

54. Trapani S, Micheli A, Grisolia F, et al. Henoch-Schöenlein purpura in childhood: Analysis of 150 cases over a 5-year period and review of the literature. Semin Arthritis Rheum 2005; 35:135–137.

55. Cadnapaphornchai MA, Saulsbury FT, Norwood VF. Hypocomplementemic urticarial vasculitis: report of a pediatric case. Pediatr Nephrol 2000; 14:328–329.

56. McDougall CM, Ismail SK, Ormerod A. Acute hemorrhagic edema of infancy. Arch Dis Child 2005; 90:316.

57. Quintana G, Matteson EL, Fernandez A, et al. Localized nodular vasculitis: a new variant of localized cutaneous polyarteritis nodosa? Clin Exp Rheumatol 2004; 22:S31–S34.

58. Ozen S, Anton J, Arisov N, et al. Juvenile polyarteritis: results of a multicenter survey of 110 children. J Pediatr 2004; 145:517–522.

59. Agard C, Mouthon L, Mahr A, et al. Microscopic polyangiitis and polyarteritis nodosa: how and when do they start? Arthritis Rheum 2003; 49:709–715,

60. Feinstein J, Arroyo R. Successful treatment of childhood onset refractory polyarteritis nodosa with tumor necrosis factor alpha blockade. J Clin Rheumatol 2005; 11:219–222.

61. Weston WL, Morelli JG. Childhood pernio and cryoproteins. Pediatr Dermatol 2000; 17:97–101.

62. Simon TD, Soep JB, Hollister JR. Pernio in pediatrics. Pediatrics 2005; 116.e472–e475.

63. Gurgey A, Aytac S, Kanra G, et al. Outcome in children with purpura fulminans: report on 16 patients. Am J Hematol 2005; 80:20–25.

64. den Brinker M, Dumas B, Visser TJ, et al. Thyroid function and outcome in children who survived meningococcal septic shock. Intensive Care Med 2005; 31:970–976.

65. Torrelo A, Requena C, Medeiro IG, et al. Schamberg's purpura in children: a review of thirteen cases. J Am Acad Dermatol 2003; 48:31–33.

66. Tristani-Firouzi P, Meadows KP, Vanderhooft S. Pigmented purpuric eruptions of childhood: a series of cases and review of the literature. Pediatr Dermatol 2001; 18:299–304.

67. Mar A, Fergin P, Hogan P. Unilateral pigmented purpuric eruption. Australas J Dermatol 1999; 40:211–214.

68. Gailbraith SS, Drolet BA, Kugathasan S, et al. Asymptomatic inflammatory bowel disease presenting with mucocutaneous findings. Pediatrics 2005; 116:e39–e44.

69. Yayli S, Bahadir S, Alpay K, et al. Pyoderma gangrenosum in association with juvenile rheumatoid arthritis. J Dermatol 2005; 32:827–830.

70. Bakhshi S, Sethuraman G, Singh MK, et al. Atypical pyoderma gangrenosum as a manifestation of childhood acute lymphoblastic leukemia. Pediatr Dermatol 2005; 22:543–545.

71. Bhat RM, Shetty SS, Kamath GH. Pyoderma gangrenosum in childhood. Int J Dermatol 2004; 43:205–207.

72. Kaur MR, Lewis HM. Severe recalcitrant pyoderma gangrenosum treated with infliximab. Br J Dermatol 2005; 153:689–691.

Chapter 15 | Hair Disorders

Hair loss is far more common in children than is excessive hair. This chapter is divided into two sections: hair loss and excessive hair.

COMMON FORMS OF HAIR LOSS

When evaluating hair loss in children, one should determine whether it is congenital or acquired, circumscribed or diffuse. This results in four diagnostic categories of hair loss (Box 15.1). Hair loss, or *alopecia*, accounts for approximately 3% of children's visits to a dermatologist. It causes the parents and the child considerable anxiety and the health team considerable frustration. Among the numerous causes of hair loss in children, three types account for the great majority of visits to the clinician: alopecia areata, tinea capitis (see Ch. 6), and traumatic alopecia. All three are forms of acquired, circumscribed hair loss (Box 15.2). These three conditions should always be considered in the differential diagnosis of hair loss.

Alopecia Areata

Clinical features

Alopecia areata is characterized by complete or almost complete hair loss in circumscribed areas (Fig. 15.1). Usually, from one to three areas are involved.[1,2] Almost all patients present with loss of scalp hair, but body hair, sexual hair, eyelashes, and eyebrows may be involved.[1,2] The appearance of a circumscribed area that is completely devoid of hair without any scalp change is a constant feature. Scalp erythema or scaling may occur in alopecia areata after sunburn. A positive family history for alopecia areata is found in 10–42% of the patients.[1,2,3]

Nail disease occurs in 10–66% of children with alopecia areata.[1-3] Nail pitting is the most common

change and appears as shallow, wide (1–2 mm) depressions in the nail plate. The pits are wider than those seen in psoriasis (Fig. 15.2).

The prognosis for most children is excellent. Complete regrowth of the hair occurs within a year in the majority of children with alopecia areata.[2,3] Spontaneous remission is the rule. Approximately 30% will have a future episode of alopecia areata with 7–10% having chronic disease.[3]

Ophiasis, an unusual subtype involving less than 5% of all patients with alopecia areata, begins in the occiput or along the frontal scalp and spreads, with many patches of alopecia along the hair margins (Fig. 15.3). Ophiasis is likely to eventuate in loss of all of the scalp hair (alopecia totalis) (Figs 15.4, 15.5), or all of the scalp and body hair (alopecia universalis). When this occurs, the prognosis for regrowth is extremely poor.[3]

Differential diagnosis

Hair pulling or other forms of traction alopecia may mimic alopecia areata. Broken-off hairs, scalp petechiae, and a history of trauma are features that help distinguish these conditions. Tinea capitis, particularly the black-dot form, may be confused with alopecia areata. Careful examination of the scalp will reveal broken-off hairs within the follicle, and microscopic examination of these hairs in potassium hydroxide (KOH) 10% will reveal hyphae within the hair shaft. A fungal culture will help confirm the diagnosis. Although a scalp biopsy may be helpful in difficult cases, it is rarely necessary.

The scarring alopecias may present as circumscribed areas of hair loss, but a history of inflammation or injury and scalp thickening and color change seen in these conditions will help distinguish them from alopecia areata.

Fig. 15.1 Alopecia areata. Circumscribed patch of completely bald scalp.

Fig. 15.2 Nail pitting in a child with alopecia areata.

Fig. 15.3 Ophiasis pattern of alopecia areata, with hair loss starting in occiput.

Fig. 15.4 Alopecia totalis. Almost complete loss of scalp hair.

Circumscribed alopecia may be congenital. It is characteristic of certain birthmarks in the scalp, particularly sebaceous nevus and aplasia cutis congenita. These alopecias are usually not difficult to differentiate from alopecia areata. The history of onset at birth, and the yellow plaques or scarred areas in the scalp, will differentiate congenital circumscribed alopecias from alopecia areata.

Pathogenesis

The hair follicle is an immune privileged site that does not normally express major histocompatibility complex (MHC) class I or II antigens. In alopecia areata these antigens are expressed on the follicular epithelium. This is regarded as loss of immune privilege and allows for recognition by the immune system. Alopecia areata is thought to be an auto-

Fig. 15.5 Alopecia totalis. Ophiasis progressing to a completely bald scalp.

immune disease in which activated T lymphocytes attack the growing hair.[4,5] This is seen histologically as a dense perifollicular T-lymphocytic infiltrate.[6] Alopecia areata is a polygenic disorder with multiple susceptibility genes interacting with environmental factors.[4,5]

The injury to the growing hair results in premature conversion of growing hairs to resting hairs that are shed. Evaluation of clinically normal scalp hairs to determine the anagen (growing) to telogen (resting) ratio can be used to predict the likelihood of short-term hair regrowth.[7] Eighty percent of patients with a normal trichogram at the margin of a lesion with alopecia areata and 85% of patients with a normal trichogram in an unaffected area of the scalp will have complete hair regrowth within 1 year.[7]

Treatment

There is no specific treatment for alopecia areata. Because spontaneous regrowth occurs in 90% of cases, the prognosis is good in most patients. Many forms of local therapy, including intralesional or superpotent topical steroids, anthralin, minoxidil, contact sensitizers, and combinations of the above, have demonstrated short-term hair regrowth, but they do not alter the long-term course of alopecia areata.[1-4] Some authorities recommend the short-term administration of systemic glucocorticosteroids. This will induce hair growth in most cases. This therapy should be reserved for patients with ophiasis or alopecia totalis who have not responded to topical therapies. However, the suppression of inflammation and hair regrowth is temporary and variable. Withdrawal of steroids may result in prompt loss of the hair that has grown back. The risks of side effects of chronic systemic glucocorticosteroids outweigh the benefits.

In complete hair loss, referral to a dermatologist may be useful, and prompt attention should be given to obtaining a wig for the child. Excellent children's wigs are manufactured, and a physician's prescription may allow the family to obtain a wig at reduced prices. A support group, the National Alopecia Areata Foundation, has a number of North American chapters that provide excellent psychological support and the latest treatment information for persons with alopecia areata.

Patient education

Parents should be informed that there is no specific treatment regimen for alopecia areata. However, in children with the usual type of alopecia areata, with one to three circumscribed patches of complete scalp hair loss, it is important to emphasize the excellent prognosis even without treatment. Explaining the proposed mechanism of the disease and the excellent chances for spontaneous recovery will greatly aid understanding of the problem. Ophiasis patients should be told of the poor prognosis. Considerable effort should be devoted at the first visit to answering questions for the child and the family. The risks and benefits of all current therapy should be explained in detail, and the psychological benefits of wearing a wig should be discussed.

The clinician should provide the patient and family with information about the National Alopecia Areata Foundation, which can be contacted by mail at PO Box 150760, San Rafael, CA 94915-0760; by email at www.alopeciaareata.com; or by phone at 415-472-0760.

Follow-up visits

In the usual type of alopecia areata, a visit every 3 months is useful to check on progress and the chances for spontaneous regression. In the alopecia totalis, a visit in 2 weeks to re-explain the illness and encourage the use of a wig is most helpful. Frequent visits may be necessary to establish the proper physician–patient relationship.

Tinea Capitis

Tinea capitis is a major cause of acquired, circumscribed hair loss in children. It is covered in detail in Chapter 6.

Traumatic Alopecia

Traumatic alopecia results from hair injury produced by traction, friction, chemical, or other injury to hair. The common types seen in childhood include trichotillomania, hair pulling and the traction alopecia seen with various popular hairstyles.

Hair pulling

Clinical features. Circumscribed areas of hair loss with irregular borders and hairs broken off at different lengths are seen in hair pulling. Frequently, scalp excoriations and perifollicular petechiae are present (Fig. 15.6). Commonly, only one area of the scalp is involved (Fig. 15.7), with the frontoparietal and frontotemporal scalp being the most usual sites. Rarely, the eyebrows or eyelashes may be plucked (Fig. 15.8).[8] Hair pulling in children should be divided into three categories: acute hair pulling asso-

Fig. 15.8 Trichotillomania of the eyelashes.

ciated with stress, trichotillomania, and hair pulling associated with other psychiatric conditions. Children who outgrow the habit of hair pulling without any major intervention do not have true trichotillomania. The estimated lifetime prevalence of trichotillomania is 0.5–1% or higher, with the majority of patients exhibiting onset of trichotillomania before the age of 18 years.[9,10] The mean age of onset is 8 years for males and 12 years for females.[10] The condition is more common in females.[10]

Differential diagnosis. The diseases considered in the differential diagnosis of hair pulling are the same as those for alopecia areata and tinea capitis (see Box 15.2). One should also consider the possibility that someone other than the affected child, such as a sibling, playmate, parent, or baby-sitter, is doing the hair pulling. Self-haircutting (which is associated with other artifactual skin diseases) must be differentiated from hair pulling.

Fig. 15.6 Trichotillomania. Hair broken at many different lengths associated with scalp excoriations.

Pathogenesis. Traumatic events, such as the death of a family member or close friend, separation or divorce of parents, or difficulties in school, may precipitate acute hair pulling. Trichotillomania is an impulse control disorder leading to chronic hair pulling.[9,10] Hair pulling may be associated with a large variety of psychiatric diagnoses and symptoms.[9,10] Parents often vehemently deny such hair pulling because they have not personally observed it.

Fig. 15.7 Trichotillomania. Characteristic crown pattern with hairs broken at different lengths.

Treatment. The search for antecedent traumatic events is helpful. In children in whom a precipitating event can be identified, relief of stress will result in ending the nervous habit. Application of oils to the hair makes it more difficult to pull. Psychodynamic therapy, chemical treatments with antidepressants, and behavior modification have all been used to treat trichotillomania. However, it is difficult to evaluate which therapy is most effective and which patients will benefit most from whatever form of therapy is chosen. Some children persist with trichotillomania into adult life. In severe forms that are associated with other signs of emotional stress, psychiatric referral may be indicated.

Patient education. A careful search for a precipitating event, and an explanation of the complex nature of the process, are crucial to patient and parent education. The clinicians and others should avoid blaming the child or one or more family member. If a precipitating event can be identified, the clinician should suggest that remedying the circumstances surrounding that event will likely lead to cessation of the hair pulling. If no precipitating event can be demonstrated, the clinician should explain that this may be a difficult problem to treat. It should also be emphasized that hair pulling may just be a reaction to acute stress or a nervous habit; however, it may be a sign of significant chronic stress or other emotional problems, and if the child is having other psychosocial difficulties, counseling may be useful.

Follow-up visits. A follow-up visit in 1–2 months is useful in evaluating progress. Continued reassurance should be given. If the problem persists, referral to a child psychologist or psychiatrist is indicated.

Traction alopecia

Clinical features. Thinning of hair in particular areas of the scalp may result from constant traction or friction. Very few fractured hairs are found in the involved areas, although the hairs may be smaller in diameter than those found in adjacent areas (Fig. 15.9). The thinning is often patchy, depending on the nature of the trauma. The history of methods of hair care and types of hairstyle is crucial for the diagnosis.[11]

Differential diagnosis. The differential diagnosis is the same as for alopecia areata and tinea capitis (see Box 15.2).

Pathogenesis. Several different sources of traction or friction have been identified as responsible for traction alopecia.[11] The hairstyle, chemical or thermal

Fig. 15.9 Traction alopecia. Hair loss caused by tight braiding.

treatment, or friction produces incomplete and complete fractures of hair. One should always consider child abuse (e.g. pulling the child by the hair). Neonatal occipital alopecia is physiologic hair loss exacerbated by the rubbing of the baby's head on the sheet or mattress. Massage alopecia may occur from vigorous scalp massage and frequent shampooing. Marginal alopecia (alopecia at the edge of normal scalp hair) is seen with hair straightening or tight hair curlers. Cornrow alopecia, ponytail alopecia, and braid alopecia are all related to tight hairstyles. Hot-comb alopecia occurs on the vertex of the scalp and may involve scarring. It is the result of use of a hot comb to straighten or style hair. Marginal alopecia is sometimes seen in hot-comb alopecia.

Treatment. Discontinuation of the trauma to the hair is the obvious treatment of choice. The use of mild shampoos and wide-toothed combs with rounded ends, infrequent shampooing, and gentle brushing are all important components of therapy. Recovery may take 3–6 months.

Patient education. The susceptibility of certain hair types to such trauma should be explained and the benefits of being gentle with the hair emphasized.

Follow-up visits. A follow-up visit in 3–6 months is useful to assess hair regrowth.

UNCOMMON FORMS OF HAIR LOSS

The remaining types of hair loss are uncommon or rare. No attempt is made to consider these numerous conditions in detail, but an orderly approach to them is presented. The clinician should first determine whether the hair loss is circumscribed or diffuse, then determine whether it has been present from birth or acquired later in life. This results in four diagnostic categories: congenital circumscribed alopecia, acquired circumscribed alopecia, congenital diffuse alopecia, and acquired diffuse alopecia (see Box 15.1). In congenital diffuse alopecia, a further diagnostic step, the hair mount examination, is necessary. Only the general clinical features of each group and the differential diagnoses are given. Telogen effluvium is discussed in more detail later in this chapter.

The mechanisms of hair loss in most of these unusual forms of alopecia have not been uncovered. However, certain associations are of therapeutic importance. An extraordinary number of clinical conditions are associated with hair loss, and hair loss should be characterized into one of the preceding four types to permit proper diagnosis and therapy.

Congenital Circumscribed Alopecia

Clinical features

Localized areas of scalp hair loss present from birth usually overlie a birthmark, such as a sebaceous or epidermal nevus.[12] The scalp surface is smooth, particularly in newborns or infants with circumscribed hair loss, and yellow to tan (Fig. 15.10). As the child gets older, a plaque is noted. A congenital circumscribed alopecia may also occur in aplasia cutis congenita (Fig. 15.11). Aplasia cutis congenita occurs most commonly as an isolated defect, but it may be associated with other malformations or genetic syndromes.[13,14]

Fig. 15.10 Nevus sebaceus. Absence of hair in the area of yellow-orange plaque of a birthmark.

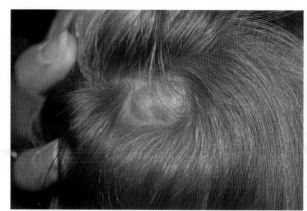

Fig. 15.11 Localized scarring of the scalp in aplasia cutis congenita.

Differential diagnosis

Nevus sebaceus is identified by its characteristic yellow color. Epidermal nevi are flesh-colored and have a rough, warty surface. Aplasia cutis congenita demonstrates scarring of the scalp in a circumscribed area and represents failure of formation of one or more layers of the scalp. In the other rare forms, circumscribed patches of hair loss without scalp changes are present. The differential diagnosis of this type of alopecia is given in Box 15.3.

Treatment

Treatment of sebaceous nevi, epidermal nevi, and aplasia cutis congenita is surgical excision. Following hormonal stimulation at puberty, sebaceous nevi become thickened and verrucous. They may also develop basal cell carcinomas and other adnexal tumors. Tumor development in sebaceous nevi is rare prior to the age of 16 years.[15]

Acquired Circumscribed Alopecia: Scarring Forms

Clinical features

Circumscribed hair loss acquired during childhood, other than alopecia areata, tinea capitis, and traction

Box 15.3 Differential diagnosis of congenital circumscribed hair loss
Sebaceous nevus
Aplasia cutis congenita (scarlike)
Epidermal nevus
Hair follicle hamartomas
Triangular alopecia of the frontal scalp

Fig. 15.12 Acquired circumscribed inflammatory scarring alopecia.

alopecia, is usually scarring in nature (Fig. 15.12). That is, the hair follicles are replaced by fibrous tissue following injury to the hair follicles after infection, trauma, or inflammatory skin disease.

Differential diagnosis

Box 15.4 presents the conditions to be considered in the differential diagnosis.

Congenital Diffuse Alopecia
Clinical features

Diffuse scalp hair loss present from birth usually results in the complaint that the child's hair simply will not grow. Such children never require haircuts. Included in this group are hair shaft defects in which the failure of hair growth is the result of structural defects that causes weakening and the breaking off of hairs

Box 15.4 Differential diagnosis of acquired, scarring, circumscribed hair loss

Postinfectious

Kerion caused by tinea capitis

Pyoderma

Varicella

Postinflammatory

Lichen planus

Lupus erythematosus

Postinjury

Physical trauma (e.g. abrasion, cuts)

Chemical or thermal burns

Radiation injury

(Figs 15.13–15.20).[16,17] The child has short, broken hairs of equal length. In many forms of ectodermal dysplasia, reduced numbers or absence of hair follicles produce the clinical picture of congenital dif-

Fig. 15.13 Three-year-old male with congenital trichorrhexis nodosa.

Fig. 15.14 Severe tichorrexis nodosa with hairs breaking just above follicular orifice.

Fig. 15.15 Photomicrograph of hair mount demonstrates broomstick fracture of trichorrhexis nodosa.

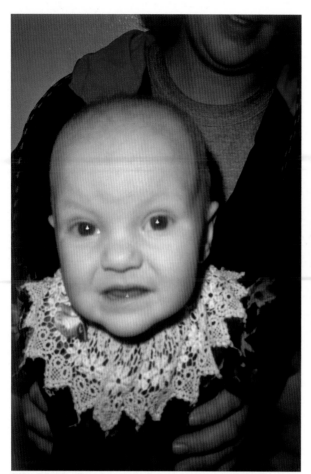

Fig. 15.16 Two-year-old female with monilethrix.

Fig. 15.17 Photomicrograph of hair mount demonstrates beading of the hair in monilethrix.

Fig. 15.18 Child suffering from trichorrhexis invaginata in Netherton's syndrome.

Fig. 15.19 Photomicrograph of hair mount demonstrates bamboo hair in trichorrhexis nodosa.

fuse alopecia. Children with genetic diseases associated with photosensitivity, premature aging, and early cancer development will often have diffusely thin hair.

Differential diagnosis

Removing hairs and placing them on a microscope slide with mounting fluid will allow demonstration of the particular type of structural hair defect.[18] Many rare forms of diffuse congenital hair loss are associated with syndromes, and complete examination of the child is necessary for accurate diagnosis (Figure 15.21). The differential diagnosis of this type of hair loss is given in Box 15.5.

Acquired Diffuse Alopecia

Diffuse hair loss with onset in childhood after a period of normal hair growth is rare. It usually results from telogen effluvium or cancer chemotherapy. In other children with diffuse hair loss a careful search for endocrine, chemical, and nutritional abnormalities is warranted (Box 15.6). In these children, a rigorous and detailed history should be taken and appropriate laboratory studies ordered if the clinical data so indicate. Because most of the endocrine, chemical, and nutritional causes are correctable, the clinician should

Fig. 15.21 Cone-shaped teeth in a child with hypohidrotic ectodermal dysplasia.

Fig. 15.20 Broken hairs in Netherton's syndrome.

Box 15.5 Differential diagnosis of congenital diffuse hair loss

Hair shaft defects
Trichorrhexis nodosa (broomstick fractures)
   Familial form
   Argininosuccinic aciduria
Pili torti (twisted hair)
   Classic form
   Menkes' syndrome
Monilethrix (beaded hair)
Trichorrhexis invaginata (bamboo hair)
   Netherton's syndrome

Absent or sparse hair
Atrichia congenita
Ectodermal dysplasias
Photosensitivity disorders
Premature aging disorders
Premature cancer disorders

Box 15.6 Differential Diagnosis of Acquired Diffuse Hair Loss

Telogen effluvium

Endocrine
Hypothyroidism
Hypopituitarism
Hypoparathyroidism
Diabetes mellitus

Androgenetic alopecia
Male pattern in adolescents

Chemical
Thallium poisoning (rat poison)
Antithyroid drugs
Heparin
Coumarin
Antimetabolites (e.g. cyclophosphamide)

Nutritional
Hypervitaminosis A
Acrodermatitis enteropathica (zinc deficiency)
Marasmus

---

consider undertaking a thorough laboratory evaluation in such children.

Telogen Effluvium

Telogen effluvium is the name given to the acquired diffuse alopecia that results from rapid conversion of scalp hairs from the growing state to the resting state (Figs 15.22, 15.23).[19] In physiologic circumstances an infant or child has 85% of scalp hair in a growing, or anagen, state and only 15% of hair in a resting, or telogen, state. Each individual scalp hair grows for

Fig. 15.22 Acquired diffuse nonscarring alopecia in telogen effluvium.

Fig. 15.23 Telogen effluvium following hospitalization.

3–5 years, then regresses over 2 or 3 weeks, and rests for 3 months. This growth throughout the scalp is asynchronous in that the majority of hairs are growing at any time of observation. Acutely stressful events, such

as birth, auto accidents, illnesses with high fever, and acute psychiatric problems, may result in a rapid conversion of growing hairs to resting hairs. Following the event by 2–4 months, the hairs are shed and usually continue to shed over 3–4 months. Each hair shed is a resting hair and will be replaced by a normal growing hair. In the newborn, the hairs are shed in two phases from the frontal scalp to the occipital scalp and are not asynchronous in growth phase until about 12 months of age.

Diagnosis of telogen effluvium can be made by evaluation of the trichogram. This is performed by plucking at least 50 hairs from a child's scalp and examining the roots to determine whether they are growing or resting. This is best done by cutting away the remainder of the hairs and mounting the roots in a commercial slide-mounting medium. A growing, or anagen, hair will have a pigmented core and a bulbous root that is larger in diameter than the hair shaft. Often, the external root sheath is present. In a telogen, or resting, hair, the external root sheath is absent or fragmented, pigment is often absent, and the root of the hair is narrower than the caliber of the other hair and frequently curved. One can reassure the patient with telogen effluvium that complete regrowth is possible. Telogen effluvium has been reported after surgery, crash diets, and the use of anticoagulants and antithyroid drugs. Anagen effluvium, in which growing hairs are lost, is an expected result of cancer treatment in children in which the antimetabolites interfere with hair growth, or radiation to the head injures the growing hair.

Androgenetic Alopecia (Male pattern hair loss)

Androgenetic alopecia is an androgen-dependent hereditary disorder of hair loss. It may be seen in 14% of healthy boys 15–17 years of age. It is characterized by hair loss in the bitemporal, frontal, midscalp, vertex, or a combination of these regions of the scalp. Topical minoxidil 5% applied daily and oral finasteride 1 mg/day are FDA approved for the treatment of androgenetic alopecia in males greater than 18 years of age.[20]

EXCESSIVE HAIR

Excessive hair may be congenital or acquired.

Congenital Hypertrichosis

Clinical features

Excessive hair may be generalized (hypertrichosis lanuginosa) or circumscribed (nevoid hypertrichosis). Excessive body hair in the newborn may be a transient problem, especially in premature infants, and resolves by 6 months of age, or may represent the rare hypertrichosis lanuginosa in which long, fine lanugo hairs cover the entire glabrous skin (Fig. 15.24). Hypertrichosis lanuginosa is thought to be autosomal dominant (Fig.15.25), but most cases are sporadic.[21] Congenital hypothyroidism may also demonstrate excessive body hair. Circumscribed hypertrichosis may be seen as one to six patches of excessive, long hair over various body regions (Figs 15.26, 15.27). It is usually persistent, but spontaneous remission has been reported.[22] When in the midline, circumscribed hypertrichosis may be associated with nervous system abnormalities. Hypertrichosis over the lumbosacral spine (the 'human tail') may be a clue to spina bifida; over the occiput it may indicate a meningocele or encephalocele. Facial hypertrichosis may be seen in a number of syndromes listed in Box 15.7.

Differential diagnosis

Circumscribed areas of hypertrichosis must be differentiated from congenital smooth muscle and pilar nevus and congenital pigmented nevi (Box 15.8). Differentiating hypertrichosis lanuginosa from the transient lanugo overgrowth may be difficult in the first few months of life, although the body and facial hairs in hypertrichosis lanuginosa are longer, often reaching 2 inches in length.

Pathogenesis

In nevoid hypertrichosis, excessive numbers of hair follicles are found. In hypertrichosis lanuginosa, body

Fig. 15.24 Hypertrichosis lanuginosa.

Fig. 15.25 Hypertrichosis lanuginosa.

Fig. 15.26 Congenital circumscribed (nevoid) hypertrichosis.

Fig. 15.27 Localized congenital hypertrichosis.

Box 15.7 Syndromes with hypertrichosis
Cornelia de Lange's syndrome
Rubinstein-Taybi syndrome
Gingival hyperplasia with hypertrichosis
Winchester syndrome
Recessive dystrophic epidermolysis bullosa
Fetal hydantoin syndrome
Erythrohepatic porphyria

Box 15.8 Differential diagnosis of circumscribed congenital hypertrichosis
Congenital pigmented nevus
Pilar and smooth muscle hamartoma
Nevoid hypertrichosis
Midline nevoid hypertrichosis with spinal or central nervous system malformations

hairs appear as terminal hairs rather than vellus hairs. Endocrine evaluations are normal.

Treatment

The treatment options for either diffuse or circumscribed hypertrichosis include cutting or shaving, depilatories, electrolysis,[23] or laser.[24,25] The best option for any individual will depend on the degree of excess hair. Shaving, cutting, and depilatories are the simplest and cheapest, but have to be done repeatedly. Electrolysis is slow and somewhat painful, but permanent. Laser is faster and less painful than electrolysis, but is more expensive and may not be permanent.

Patient education

In circumscribed hypertrichosis, the clinician should explain that a malformation has taken place, with excessive follicular structures in that segment of skin. In hypertrichosis lanuginosa, genetic counseling may be useful.

Follow-up visits

Support and counseling are very useful for parents and children, and regularly scheduled visits are useful.

Acquired Excessive Hair (Hirsutism)

Clinical features

Hirsutism is the growth of terminal hair in part or all of the male sexual pattern. It is observed predominantly in adolescent females. In Mediterranean races, females may have some male pattern hair, and it may be impossible to distinguish clinically from true hirsutism.[26] Asian females, in contrast, have no racial pattern of hirsutism. Excessive facial hair in the beard or moustache area may be accompanied by excessively long body hairs. Other features of virilization may be seen, such as increased muscle mass, clitoral hypertrophy, and deepening of the voice. A history of abnormal menses is often obtained.

Differential diagnosis

Racial forms that mimic hirsutism lack other signs of virilization, have female family members with similar findings, and lack endocrine abnormalities (Box 15.9). Children and adolescents with congenital erythro-

Box 15.9 Conditions resulting in hirsutism

Racial hirsutism

Polycystic ovaries

Ovarian tumors

Congenital adrenal hyperplasia

Cushing's syndrome

Exogenous androgens

poietic porphyria or porphyria cutanea tarda may have facial hirsutism, but they usually have a history of photosensitivity and scars from previous skin lesions.

Pathogenesis

Hirsutism is androgen dependent, and a careful gynecologic and endocrine evaluation will detect underlying disease. Hyperandrogenism should be considered in any female with hirsutism (see Box 15.9).[27] Normal testosterone production by the female is 50% adrenal and 50% ovarian. Although the skin does not produce androgens from cholesterol, it is capable of metabolizing weaker androgens to more potent androgens such as dihydrotestosterone. Most patients with moderate to severe hirsutism, and 50% of those with mild hirsutism, will demonstrate elevated levels of either serum free testosterone or dihydroepiandrosterone.[27]

Treatment

Screening evaluation for hyperandrogenism should include measurements of serum free testosterone, and dehydroepiandrosterone.[27] Treatment depends on the underlying endocrine abnormality and whether it is of ovarian or adrenal origin. Treatment options include hormonal suppression to decrease androgen production, administration of antiandrogens, and physical methods of hair removal.

Patient education

The clinician should explain to the patient and family that hirsutism is just one feature of an endocrine disorder, and that correcting the underlying endocrine disease is required.

Follow-up visits

Follow-up 2 weeks after gynecologic or endocrine consultation is obtained is useful.

Fig. 15.28 Unmanageable hair.

UNMANAGEABLE HAIR

The uncombable hair syndrome, woolly hair, and woolly hair nevus result in hair that is difficult to comb. In the uncombable hair syndrome (pili triangulati et canaliculi), an autosomal dominant condition, the entire scalp hair is blond or silvery and does not lay flat when combed (Fig. 15.28).[28] The characteristic hair shaft abnormality may be seen by either light or scanning electron microscopy of hairs cut in cross-section.[28] Generalized woolly hair is tightly curled scalp hair differing considerably from that of other family members.[29] In woolly hair nevus there are one to three patches of scalp hair that are curly and coarse, different from the remaining hair.[30] Also, the cowlick of long, straight hairs over the scalp vertex is seen in 7% of children.[31]

SCALP WHORLS

A single whorl in the parietal scalp is found in 98% of children. In 45% it is in the midline, in 40% to the right of midline, and to the left in the remainder.[31] Abnormal locations of scalp whorls may be clues to central nervous system disease.[31,32] For example, Down syndrome, trisomy 13, Prader-Willi syndrome, and Rubinstein-Taybi syndrome show anterior scalp whorls, whereas malformations of cranial bones often display widely spaced biparietal whorls.[31]

REFERENCES

1. Tan E, Tay Y-K, Giam Y-C. A clinical study of alopecia areata in Singapore. Pediatr Dermatol 2003; 19:298–302.
2. Sharma VK, Kumar B, Dawn G. A clinical study of childhood alopecia areata in Chandigarh, India. Pediatr Dermatol 1996; 13:372–377.
3. Mandini S, Shapiro J. Alopecia areata update. J Am Acad Dermatol 2000; 42:549.
4. Norris D. Alopecia areata: current state of knowledge. J Am Acad Dermatol 2004; 51:S16–S17.
5. Gilhar A, Kalish RS. Alopecia areata: a tissue specific autoimmune disease of the hair follicle. Autoimmunity Rev 2006; 5:64–69.
6. Whiting DA. Histopathology of alopecia areata in horizontal sections of scalp biopsies. J Invest Dermatol 1995; 104:S26–S27.
7. Peereboom-Wynia JD, Beek CH, Mulder PG, et al. The trichogram as a prognostic tool in alopecia areata. Acta Derm Venereol 1993; 73:280–282.
8. Tay YK, Levy ML, Metry DW. Trichotillomania in childhood: case series and review. Pediatrics 2004; 113:e494–e498.
9. Messinger ML, Cheng TL. Trichotillomania. Pediatr Rev 1999; 20:249–250.
10. Bruce TO, Barwick LW, Wright HH. Diagnosis and management of trichotillomania in children and adolescents. Paediatr Drugs 2005; 7:365–376.
11. Hantash BM, Schwartz RA. Traction alopecia in children. Cutis 2003; 71:18–20.
12. Weiss G, Shermer A, Trau H. Yellowish, verrucous lesions on the scalp. Am Fam Physician 2005; 71:961–962.
13. Kruk-Jeromin J, Janik J, Rykala J. Aplasia cutis congenita of the scalp. Dermatol Surg 1998; 5:549–553.
14. Blunt K, Quan V, Carr D, et al. Aplasia cutis congenita: a clinical review and associated defects. Neonatal Netw 1992; 11:17–27.
15. Santibanez-Gallerani A, Marshall D, Duarte AM, et al. Should nevus sebaceus of Jadassohn in children be excised? A study of 757 cases, and literature review. J Craniofac Surg 2003; 14:658–660.
16. de Berker D. Congenital hypotrichosis. Int J Dermatol 1999; 38:S25–S33.
17. Sprecher E. Genetic hair and nail disorders. Clin Dermatol 2005; 23:47–55.
18. Smith VV, Anderson G, Malone M, et al. Light microscopic examination of scalp hair samples as an aid in the diagnosis of paediatric disorders: retrospective review of more than 300 cases from a single centre. J Clin Pathol 2005; 58:1294–1298.
19. Harrison S, Sinclair R. Telogen effluvium. Clin Exp Dermatol 2002; 27:389–395.
20. Olsen EA, Messenger AG, Shapiro J, et al. Evaluation and treatment of male and female pattern hair loss. J Am Acad Dermatol 2005; 52:301–311.
21. Lee JJ, Im SB, Kim DK. Hypertrichosis universalis congenita: a separate entity, or the same as gingival fibromatosis. Pediatr Dermatol 1993; 10:263–266.
22. Vergani R, Betti R, Martino P, et al. Giant nevoid hypertrichosis in an Iranian girl. Pediatr Dermatol 2002; 19:64–66.
23. Richards RN. Electrolysis for the treatment of hypertrichosis and hirsutism. Skin Ther Lett 1999; 4:3–4.
24. Littler CM. Laser hair removal in a patient with hypertrichosis lanuginosa congenita. Dermatol Surg 1997; 23:705–707.
25. Haedersdal H, Wulf HC. Evidence-based review of hair removal using lasers and light sources. J Eur Acad Dermatol Venereol 2006; 20:9–20.
26. Young R, Sinclair R. Hirsuties. I: Diagnosis. Australas J Dermatol 1998; 39:24–28.
27. Curran DR, Moore C. What is the best approach to the evaluation of hirsutism? J Fam Pract 2005; 54:465–467.
28. Wagner AM, Cunningham BB, Weinstein JM, et al. Uncombable hair syndrome: light microscopy diagnosis. Pediatr Dermatol 2005; 22:369–370.
29. Chen C, LeBoit PE, Price VH. Woolly hair in 4 members of a Chinese family. J Am Acad Dermatol 2006; 54:165–166,
30. Kumaran S, Dogra S, Handa S, et al. Woolly hair nevus. Pediatr Dermatol 2004; 21:609–610.
31. Samlaska CP, James WD, Sperling LC. Scalp whorls. J Am Acad Dermatol 1989; 21:553–556.
32. Furdon SA, Clark DA. Scalp hair characteristics in the newborn infant. Adv Neonatal Care 2003; 3:286–296.

Chapter 16 | Nail Disorders

Nail disorders are uncommon in children. However, nail changes may be useful in the clinical identification of systemic disorders. Normal variations are important to recognize and distinguish from nail disease. Concave nail shapes are normal from birth to 3 years of age.[1,2] Normal nails may have a few small pits in the nail plate. Scattered white spots are common in the nail plate and are caused by minor trauma.[1,2] Longitudinal ridging is also common in normal nails and worsens with age.

DISRUPTION OF THE NAIL SURFACE

Clinical Features

Changes in the surface of the nail that occur in childhood include pitting, scaling, longitudinal ridging, transverse ridges, or splitting (Fig. 16.1).[1,2] Pitting is predominantly seen in psoriasis and alopecia areata.[1-6] Pitting is the most common nail change seen in psoriasis (Fig. 16.2) and alopecia areata (Fig.16.3).[1-6] Pits are more numerous in alopecia areata, but it is often difficult to distinguish between the nail pitting of alopecia areata and psoriasis. Roughening and splitting of the nail surface (trachyonychia) is seen in idiopathic trachyonychia (20-nail dystrophy),[1,2,7] psoriasis,[1-4] alopecia areata,[1,2,5,6] lichen planus,[1,2,8] lichen striatus,[9] trauma[1,2] dermatitis of the digits,[1,2] and in some of the ectodermal dysplasias.[1,2] Transverse ridges (Beau's lines) are seen after a severe illness,[1,2] hand-foot-and-mouth disease,[10] a toxic event such as cancer chemotherapy,[11] or from a nervous habit of nail picking.[1,2,12,13] Multiple transverse ridges from repeated nail self-trauma (Fig. 16.4) may weaken the nail plate and lead to central splitting (Fig. 16.5).[1,2,12,13] This is particularly seen on the thumbnails of children (median nail dystrophy) and is associated with disruption of the cuticle.

Differential Diagnosis

When a disturbance of the nail surface is seen, onychomycosis is often considered in the differential diagnosis. Onychomycosis, although still uncommon in children is becoming more frequently seen and usually affects nails by producing thickening and surface roughening.[1,2,14] A potassium hydroxide (KOH) examination and fungal culture will help differentiate.

Pathogenesis

Injury to the germinative cells of the nail is the cause of disturbances of the nail surface, whether from inflammation, trauma, toxins, or chemotherapeutic agents.

Treatment

Treatment is difficult. If trauma is identified, behavior modification may help. Recovery is likely from all causes.

Patient Education

If self-trauma is the cause, open discussion with the patient regarding alternative habits is recommended. Reassurance that eventual recovery will occur should be given.

Follow-up Visits

A follow-up visit in 4–6 weeks may be useful in determining the course of disease.

THICK NAILS

Clinical Features

Nails thicken in proliferative epidermal disease. In psoriasis and lichen planus of children, all 20 nails

Fig. 16.1 Trachyonychia. Disruption of the nail surface with longitudinal ridging.

Fig. 16.2 Pitting of the nail in childhood psoriasis.

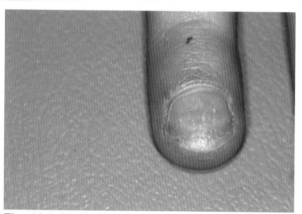

Fig. 16.3 Pitting of the nail in a child with alopecia areata.

Fig. 16.4 Median nail dystrophy. Multiple medial transverse grooves from repeated self-trauma.

Fig. 16.5 Central splitting of the nail from repeated self-trauma.

may be involved.[1–8] In psoriasis, thickening begins distally and is associated with distal nail separation (onycholysis), giving a yellow color to the nails (Fig. 16.6).[1–4] The entire nail plate may then be involved (Fig.16.7). Pitting of the nail surface also occurs (Fig. 16.8). In lichen planus there is thickening of the nails, with a pinched-up central ridge and synechia formation over the nail surface (Fig.16.9).[1,2,8]

In idiopathic trachyonychia[7] the child has thickened nails with exaggerated longitudinal ridges (Figs 16.10, 16.11). At least in some children, this disease may be a hereditary disorder. Trachyonychia of all 20 nails may be the presenting sign of alopecia areata, lichen planus, or psoriasis. Long-term follow-up is required to determine the development of associated features.[1–8]

Fig. 16.6 Psoriasis of the nail. Yellowing within nail represents separation of the nail plate from the nail bed.

Fig. 16.7 Involvement of entire nail in a child with psoriasis.

Fig. 16.8 Psoriasis of the nails. Note uninvolved nail.

Fig. 16.9 Lichen planus of the nail. Tricho-onychotic deformity with lichen planus lesion of the penis.

Fig. 16.10 Idiopathic trachyonychia. Exaggerated longitudinal ridging and rough surface of all 20 nails.

Psoriasis, lichen planus, and idiopathic trachyonychia account for most cases of thick nails (Fig.16.12).[1–8] Nails may be thickened, shiny, and contain horizontal ridges in dermatitis that involves the hands and cuti-cular skin (Fig. 16.13).[1,2] In pachyonychia congenita, an autosomal dominant disorder, thickened nails that are present at birth will become even thicker by age 2 or 3 years (Figs 16.14, 16.15).[15] Dermatophyte

Fig. 16.11 Idiopathic trahyonychia that progressed to thickening of the nails.

Fig. 16.12 Idiopathic trachyonychia with thickened, longitudinally ridged nails.

Fig. 16.13 Nail surface roughness and scale in a child with eczema.

Fig. 16.14 Pachyonychia congenita with distal thickening of fingernails.

Fig. 16.15 Pachyonychia congenita type II. Distal thickening of the toenails associated with painful circumscribed keratoses of the feet.

Fig. 16.16 Onychomycosis. Thickening and whitening of toenail.

infections of the nail (onychomycosis) will also thicken the nails. However, these infections will usually involve only one or two nails (Fig. 16.16).[1,2,14] Injury to the nail may heal with a thickened nail (Fig.16.17).

Differential Diagnosis

Conditions to be considered in the differential diagnosis of thick nails are listed in Box 16.1. Longitudinal nail biopsy may be useful in differentiating nail dis-

Fig. 16.17 Thickened fingernail after trumatic avulsion of the nail.

Box 16.1 Differential diagnosis of thick nails
Psoriasis
Lichen planus
Onychomycosis
Idiopathic trachyonychia
Dermatitis
Pachyonychia congenita
Ectodermal dysplasia
Palmoplantar keratodermas
Focal dermal hypoplasia
Dyskeratosis congenita
Norwegian scabies

orders.[16] Involvement of all 20 nails should suggest psoriasis, alopecia areata, lichen planus, or idiopathic trachyonychia but not fungal infection. KOH examination and fungal culture of will differentiate. Finding characteristic papulosquamous skin lesions will help in the diagnosis of psoriasis and lichen planus.

Pathogenesis

The increased turnover time in the nail matrix results in a thickened, often dystrophic nail. This occurs primarily in psoriasis and lichen planus. Pachyonychia congenita is caused by mutations in keratins 6a, 6b, 16, and 17.[15]

Treatment

There is no satisfactory treatment for all hypertrophic disorders of the nail but tazatotene 0.1% gel is helpful in the treatment of psoriatic nail disease.[17] In dermatophyte infection, itraconazole pulsed therapy is effective in the majority of cases.[14] Itraconazole is given at a dose of 3–5 mg/kg/day for 1 week followed by 3 weeks without treatment. This regimen is repeated, and then a third and final week of treatment is given. Terbinafine, 3–5 mg/kg given daily for 6 weeks for fingernails and 12 weeks for toenails, may also be used.[14]

Patient Education

The clinician must be careful to explain to the patient and family that nail thickening merely reflects overgrowth of nail cells and that it does not represent a specific disease.

Follow-up Visits

Visits every 6 months may be useful in following the course of these conditions.

THIN OR ATROPHIC NAILS

Clinical Features

Poorly developed or absent nails are characteristic of a wide variety of congenital syndromes.[1,2,18] All babies' nails are normally thin until 3–4 years of life, at times making the diagnosis of thin or atrophic nail difficult early in life. These nail-plate abnormalities generally reflect nail matrix disorders. Most often this is the result of ectodermal dysplasia (Fig. 16.18), but intrauterine injury to the nail, such as that caused by epidermolysis bullosa, may be responsible. Usually, most or all of the nails are affected. The nails are often narrow, and the nail plate is thin and fragile.

Fig. 16.18 Thin, hypoplastic nail in ectodermal dysplasia.

Fig. 16.19 Thin, hypoplastic thumbnail and dislocated patella in nail-patella syndrome.

Congenital anonychia, or complete absence of some or all nails, has been described as an isolated dominant or sometimes recessive condition, or associated with other congenital ectodermal defects.[19] With anonychia, neither the nail plate nor the nail bed is present.

The nail-patella syndrome (NPS) deserves special comment. It is thought to be an autosomal dominant syndrome with both ectodermal and mesodermal manifestations.[18] The nail matrix of usually the thumb, index fingers, and great toes is hypoplastic (Fig. 16.19). Occasionally, it is absent. Other nails may be involved. The lunula is often characteristically triangular. In addition, there are multiple bone abnormalities: rudimentary or absent patellae, bony spurs on the posterior iliac crest, subluxation of the elbows, and thickening of the scapulae are seen. Other anomalies described include skin laxity, heterochromia irides, glaucoma, and proteinuria. NPS is caused by mutations in the LMX1B gene which encodes the LMX1B protein which is involved in the dorsoventral patterning of the limbs.[18,20]

Periodic shedding of one or more nails is inherited as an autosomal dominant trait. This is a rare problem, and during the period of regrowth the nails may be dystrophic.[21]

The more important causes of acquired thin or atrophic nails include trauma, infection, lichen planus, erythema multiforme, and bullous drug eruptions. Poor acral circulation, such as in Raynaud's disease or vascular malformations, may also contribute.

Differential Diagnosis

The clinician must first determine whether the nail disorder is congenital or acquired. Most often, the associated clinical features are very useful in distinguishing one cause of nail disease or atrophy from another. Box 16.2 lists the conditions to be considered in the differential diagnosis of thin or atrophic nails.

Treatment

There is no treatment.

Patient Education

The clinician should emphasize to the patient and family that the cells responsible for nail growth are poorly formed or injured.

Follow-up Visits

Follow-up visits are unnecessary.

Box 16.2 Differential diagnosis of thin, absent, or atrophic nails

Congenital
Ectodermal dysplasia (anhidrotic, hidrotic)*
Epidermolysis bullosa
Incontinentia pigmenti
Nail-patella syndrome*
Acrodermatitis enteropathica
Anonychia with or without ectrodactyly*
Coffin-Siris syndrome*
Hallermann-Streiff syndrome*
Progeria

Acquired
Trauma
Infection
Lichen planus
Erythema multiforme
Focal dermal hypoplasia
Ellis-van Creveld syndrome (chondroectodermal dysplasia)
Turner's syndrome
Dyskeratosis congenita
Trisomy 13
Periodic shedding
Severe Raynaud's phenomenon
Vascular disease
Bullous drug eruptions

May be absent from birth.

Fig. 16.20 *Candida*-related paronychia. Swelling and redness of the proximal nail fold in child who is a thumb sucker.

PARONYCHIA

Clinical Features

Acute paronychia is most often caused by *Staphylococcus aureus*.[1,2,22] Occasionally, Gram-negative organisms such as *Pseudomonas* and *Proteus* are implicated. This is a common, painful infection of the nail fold in which the red, inflamed, swollen periungual tissue has a purulent exudate. Herpes simplex infection may also occur in the paronychial area (herpetic whitlow) and is distinguished by grouped vesicles on an erythematous base.[1,2,22]

Chronic paronychia is a difficult but common problem, primarily in children who are thumb suckers, nail biters, nail pickers and patients with type I diabetes mellitus.[1,2,15,22,23] It appears as dull-red swelling of the cuticle area that is usually not tender. Hobbies and habits that recurrently traumatize the nail fold are important causes. Chronic or recurrent dermatitis

Fig. 16.21 Nail changes that accompany *Candida* paronychia.

often occurs around the nail folds and may be the underlying cause. The nail fold is red, indurated, and raised, and the cuticle margin is lost (Fig. 16.20). Often, there is proximal separation of the nail plate from the nail bed and nail surface changes (Fig. 16.21). *C. albicans* can be cultured from 95% of patients with chronic paronychia.[2,22]

Differential Diagnosis

Paronychia is so characteristic that it is not easily confused with other conditions.

Pathogenesis

Alterations in the integrity of the cuticle area, such as maceration and trauma, alter the epidermal barrier and allow microbial invasion.

Treatment

Treatment is complicated by the fact that avoiding the underlying cause may be extremely difficult. Incision and drainage and systemic antibiotics are the usual treatments for acute bacterial paronychia. However, there are no studies comparing the efficacy of either treatment alone versus each other or versus combination therapy.[24] Topical antifungal agents with activity against *Candida* and topical steroids have both been shown to be effective.[22,25,26] Aspiration of occluding material by children who are thumb suckers must be avoided by covering the thumb with a cotton sock and taping it around the wrist.

Patient Education

Elimination or reduction of the causes of maceration and trauma should be emphasized.

Follow-up Visits

A visit in 1 month will be useful to determine the response to therapy.

INGROWN TOENAILS

Clinical Features

The large toes have a particular predilection for penetration of their nails into the lateral nail fold, producing a tender and sometimes erythematous swelling (Fig. 16.22). In infants this may appear at 1–2 months

Fig. 16.22 Ingrown toenails with lateral nail-fold hypertrophy

of age, with hypertrophy of the lateral nail folds.[27] Limping and discomfort on walking are frequent complaints. Purulence is occasionally seen secondary to bacterial invasion, usually due to *S. aureus*.

Differential Diagnosis

An ingrown toenail is usually so characteristic that it is not confused with other processes.

Pathogenesis

Ingrown toenails are caused by the penetration of ragged edges of the nail plate into the lateral nail fold, giving rise to a foreign body inflammatory response with eventual formation of granulation tissue.[27,28] Tight-fitting shoes and improper nail cutting promote crowding of the nail plate.[28] In infants, asynchronous growth of the nail plate and the lateral nail folds may produce the penetration of the edge of the nail plate within the nail fold.[27]

Treatment

The majority of cases resolve with simple local measures.[28] In infants these include minimization of

---

Box 16.3 Causes of specific color changes in nails	
Black	**Yellow**
Peutz-Jeghers syndrome	Yellow nail syndrome
Vitamin B deficiency	Onycholysis
Pinta	**Red lunulae**
Ammoniated mercuric sulfide	Collagen vascular diseases
Hair dyes	Systemic lupus erythematosus
Film developer	Rheumatoid arthritis
Irradiation	Carbon monoxide poisoning
Junctional nevus	Cardiac failure
Malignant melanoma	Cirrhosis
Fungus	Psoriasis
	Idiopathic trachyonychia
Blue lunulae	**Gray**
Antimalarials	Silver salts
Wilson's disease	Phenolphthalein
Purpura	Malignant melanoma
Cyanosis	**White**
Argyria	Arsenic (Mees' lines)
	Partial onycholysis
Green	Leukonychia (hereditary, traumatic, idiopathic)
Pseudomonas	Hypoalbuminemia
Aspergillus	**Brown**
	Resorcinol (nail lacquer)
Red	Film developer
Resorcinol (nail lacquer)	Fungus infection
Hemorrhage	Tobacco staining
Half-and-half nail of renal disease	

pressure by wearing loose-fitting shoes, proper trimming of the nails, soaking of the foot, and using cotton to prevent the nail edge from penetrating the skin.[27] Chronic recurrences unresponsive to conservative therapy require surgery. The best results are obtained by removal of the involved portion of the nail in conjunction with phenolization of the nail matrix to prevent regrowth of the removed nail.[28]

Patient Education

Instructions in cutting the toenails are invaluable. The lateral margins must remain smooth. One should not cut the toenail until it grows beyond the distal end of the lateral nail fold. Trimming the nail straight across rather than in an arc is required. Patients and family should be instructed to avoid tight-fitting shoes. For infants, the clinician should explain to the family that a slow-growing nail plate penetrates a rapidly growing lateral nail fold.

Follow-up Visits

A visit in 1 month is useful in evaluating therapy and reemphasizing toenail care.

COLOR CHANGES IN THE NAIL

It is beyond the scope of this chapter to discuss nail color changes in detail, but Box 16.3 lists the disorders to be considered when specific color changes in the nail are encountered. Particular consideration should be given to hemorrhage into the nail (Fig. 16.23) which may be the result of trauma, including biting.

Fig. 16.23 Hemorrhage into fingernails as result of biting the child's nails as 'punishment.'

REFERENCES

1. Noronha PA, Zubkiv B. Nails and nail disorders in children and adults. Am Fam Physician 1997; 55:2129–140.
2. Pappert AS, Scher RK, Cohen JL. Nail disorders in children. Pediatr Clin North Am 1991; 38:921–940.
3. Kumar B, Jain R, Sandhu K, et al. Epidemiology of childhood psoriasis: a study of 419 patients from northern India. Int J Dermatol 2004; 43:654–658.
4. Salomon J, Szepietowski JC, Proniewicz A. Psoriatic nails: a prospective clinical study. J Cutan Med Surg 2003; 7:317–321.
5. Tan E, Tay YK, Goh CL, et al. The pattern and profile of alopecia areata in Singapore – a study of 219 Asians. Int J Dermatol 2002; 41:748–753.
6. Tosti A, Morelli R, Bardazzu F, et al. Prevalence of nail abnormalities in children with alopecia areata. Pediatr Dermatol 1994; 11:112–115.
7. Scheinfeld NS. Trachyonychia: a case report and review of manifestations, associations, and treatments. Cutis 2003; 71:299–302.
8. Peluso AM, Tosti A, Piraccini BM, et al. Lichen planus limited to the nails in childhood: case report and literature review. Pediatr Dermatol 1993; 10:36–39.
9. Kavak A, Kutluay L. Nail involvement in lichen striatus. Pediatr Dermatol 2002; 19:136–138.
10. Clementz GC, Mancini AJ. Nail matrix arrest following hand-foot-mouth disease: a report of five children. Pediatr Dermatol 2000; 17:7–11.
11. Guillot B, Bessis D, Dereure O. Mucocutaneous side effects of antineoplastic chemotherapy. Expert Opin Drug Saf 2004; 3:579–587.
12. Griego RD, Orengo IF, Scher RK. Median nail dystrophy and habit tic deformity: are they different forms of the same disorder? Int J Dermatol 1995; 34:799–800.
13. Lubitz L. Nail biting, thumb sucking and other irritating behaviours in childhood. Aust Fam Physician 1992; 21:1090–1094.
14. Gupta AK, Skinner AR. Onychomycosis in children: a brief overview with treatment strategies. Pediatr Dermatol 2004; 21:74–79.
15. Smith FJ, Liao H, Cassidy AJ, et al. The genetic basis of pachyonychia congenita. J Investig Dermato Symp Proc 2005; 10:21–30.
16. Grover C, Khandpur S, Reddy BS, et al. Longitudinal nail biopsy: utility in 20-nail dystrophy. Dermatol Surg 2003; 29:1125–1129,
17. Scher RK, Stiller M, Zhu YI. Tazarotene 0.1% gel in the treatment of fingernail psoriasis: a double-blind, randaomized, vehicle-controlled study. Cutis 2001; 68:355–358.
18. Fistarol SK, Itin PH. Nail changes in genodermatosis. Eur J Dermatol 2002; 12:119–128.
19. al Hawsawi K, al Aboud K, Alfadley A, et al. Anonychia congenita totalis: a case report and review of the literature. Int J Dermatol 2002; 41:397–398.
20. McIntosh I, Dunston JA, Liu L, et al. Nail-patella syndrome revisited: 50 years after linkage. Ann Hum Genet 2005; 69:349–363.
21. Martin S, Rudolph AH. Familial dystrophic periodic shedding of the nails. Cutis 1980; 25:622–623.
22. Rockwell PG. Acute and chronic paronychia. Am Fam Physician 2001; 63:1113–1116.
23. Kapellen TM, Galler A, Kiess W. Higher frequency of paronychia (nail bed infections) in pediatric and adolescent

patients with type I diabetes mellitus than in non-diabetic peers. J Pediatr Endocrinol Metab 200316:751–758.

24. Shaw J, Body R. Best evidence topic report. Incision and drainage preferable to oral antibiotics in acute paronychial nail infection. Emerg Med J 2005; 22:813–814.

25. Tosti A, Piraccini BM, Ghetti E, et al. Topical steroids versus systemic antifungals in the treatment of chronic paronychia: an open, randomized double-blind and double dummy study. J Am Acad Dermatol 2002; 47:73–76.

26. Daniel CR 3rd, Daniel MP, Danies J, et al. Managing simple chronic paronychia and onycholysis with ciclopirox 0.77% and an irritant-avoidance regimen. Cutis 2004; 73:81–85.

27. Baran R, Bureau H. Congenital malalignment of the big toenail as a cause of ingrowing toenail in infancy. Pathology and treatment (a study of thirty cases). Clin Exp Dermatol 1983; 8:619–623.

28. Rounding C, Bloomfield S. Surgical treatments for ingrowing toenails. The Cochrane Database of Systemic Reviews. Issue 1 Art NO:CD001541. DOI:10.1002/14651858.CD001541.pub 2, 2003.

Chapter 17

Disorders of Pigmentation: the White Lesions and the Brown Lesions

An infant's skin color is always light at birth and becomes darker with age. Hyperpigmentation of the scrotum and of the linea alba is common in dark-skinned infants. Focal pigmentary changes are very common in infants and children. Loss of skin color or increase in skin color in an infant or child may cause concern in parents. Mongolian spots are expected in dark-skinned newborns and café-au-lait spots are very common. Hypopigmented lesions, in contrast, are uncommon in infants, with piebaldism or ash-leaf macules occurring in less than 1% of babies. Alterations in skin color in an infant or child are often the earliest clues to genetic diseases, such as the hypopigmented macules in tuberous sclerosis and café-au-lait spots in neurofibromatosis. Acquired pigmentary changes are also common. This chapter is divided into discussions of white lesions and brown lesions.

WHITE LESIONS

Congenital Circumscribed Flat Hypopigmentation or Depigmentation

Localized areas of hypopigmented or depigmented skin are uncommon in infants and newborns. A hypopigmented area of the skin is found in approximately 8 per 1000 live births, and a hypopigmented tuft of hair is found in 3 per 1000 live births (Figs 17.1, 17.2).[1]

Piebaldism and Waardenburg's syndrome

Clinical features: *Piebaldism* is the name designated to circumscribed areas of absence of pigment in the newborn.[2] This disorder is transmitted in an autosomal dominant pattern. Although completely devoid of melanocytes, the white patches of skin may be difficult to detect at birth because of the light color of most newborn skin. The use of a Wood's lamp to examine the infant's skin may accentuate differences in color. A depigmented tuft of hair, usually in the frontal region, may also be seen.

Waardenburg's syndrome patients exhibit a white forelock, dystopia canthorum, white patches on the skin, heterochromia of the irises, sensorineural deafness in one or both ears, and other defects.[2] There are four types of Waardenburg's syndrome. Type II does not exhibit dystopia canthorum but is more likely to have sensorineural hearing loss and heterochromia iridis than type I. In addition to the typical features of Waardenburg's type I, type III exhibits musculoskeletal abnormalities, and type IV is associated with Hirschsprung's disease.[2] Types I, II, and III are autosomal dominant and type IV is autosomal recessive.[2]

Differential diagnosis: The differential diagnosis of congenital circumscribed depigmentation includes the depigmented macules of piebaldism and Waardenburg's syndrome, ash-leaf or hypopigmented macules, nevus depigmentosus, and nevus anemicus. It is at times difficult in the newborn to distinguish hypopigmented macules from totally depigmented macules. Depigmented macules appear totally white when examined with a Wood's lamp, while hypopigmented macules are noted to have some color. Biopsy of a depigmented lesion will reveal a total lack of melanocytes, whereas melanocytes will be present in a hypopigmented macule. A family history of piebaldism, Waardenburg's syndrome, or tuberous sclerosis is very helpful. Nevus depigmentosus is a congenital localized area of hypopigmentation secondary to hypofunctional melanocytes, whereas nevus anemicus is a hypopigmented macule caused by alterations in vascular tone. Nevus anemicus can be differentiated by loss of the borders by pressing with a glass microscope slide.

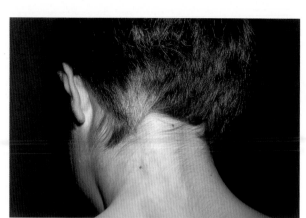

Fig. 17.1 Piebaldism. Segmental white patch on the neck with a tuft of white hair present from birth.

Fig. 17.2 Piebaldism. Symmetrical, depigmented patches on both sides of the trunk.

Pathogenesis: The majority of patients with piebaldism have mutations in the *c-kit* proto-oncogene, which encodes for a transmembrane tyrosine kinase cell

surface receptor for stem cell factor.[2] In patients who have normal *c-kit*, heterozygous mutations in SLUG have been identified. SLUG is a downstream molecular target of the *c*-kit signaling pathway. Some patients with piebaldism lack mutations in both *c-kit* and SLUG and their genetic abnormality remains to be identified. Waardenburg's syndrome types I and III are caused by mutations in the *pax*-3 gene.[2] Type II is caused by mutations in the MITF gene, homozygous deletions in SLUG, as well as other unidentified abnormalities.[3] Type IV is caused by mutations in either the EDN3, EDNRB, or SOX10 genes.[2] These genes are all involved in embryonic migration and survival of cells in the organs affected in these syndromes.

Treatment: There is no treatment for the depigmentation of skin or hair in piebaldism or Waardenburg's syndrome. Patients with Waardenburg's syndrome should be referred to the appropriate specialists, depending on their associated problems.

Patient education: The genetic nature of these diseases should be explained to the patient and family. Those with Waardenburg's syndrome should be told of the associated difficulties.

Follow-up visits: No follow-up visits are necessary for the skin changes. Follow-up of a patient with Waardenburg's syndrome depends on the associated features.

White patches of tuberous sclerosis (ash-leaf macules)

Clinical features: The white spots of tuberous sclerosis appear as hypopigmented macules, which may be lance-ovate (ash-leaf macules), polygonal (thumb-print), or confetti-shaped (Figs 17.3, 17.4).[4,5] The macules range in size from 0.1 to 12 cm at their greatest diameter.[4,5] In the newborn period they may be the only sign of tuberous sclerosis, and in families in which this condition occurs, involvement of the newborn infant may be first suspected by the presence of these lesions. A Wood's lamp examination is often necessary to detect the lesions in the newborn. They may be found anywhere on the skin but are most predominant on the posterior trunk and the extremities. Hypopigmented macules by themselves are not diagnostic of tuberous sclerosis because 2–3 per 1000 otherwise normal newborns and 5% of Caucasians under age 45 years will also demonstrate these

Fig. 17.3 Ash-leaf hypopigmented macule of tuberous sclerosis.

Fig. 17.4 Two ash-leaf macules of tuberous sclerosis. Note different shapes.

Fig. 17.5 Facial angiofibromas of tuberous sclerosis that mimic acne.

Fig. 17.6 Shagreen patch on sacral skin (tuberous sclerosis).

patches.[1,6] However, less than 1% of people will have two hypopigmented macules, and greater than three is exceedingly rare.[6]

The other signs and symptoms of tuberous sclerosis do not appear until later in life.[4,5] The angiofibromas found on the nose and face, which may mimic acne, usually begin to appear between the ages of 2 and 10 years (Fig. 17.5). Seizure disorders usually appear within the first year of life, but renal tumors and periungual fibromas usually appear after adolescence. A large connective tissue nevus, designated as a shagreen patch (Figs 17.6, 17.7), is seen in almost half of patients.[4,5] It may be present at birth, or it may become more apparent as the child becomes older. It is skin-colored to ivory-colored and feels thickened (Fig. 17.8). The fibrous forehead plaque present in 20% of patients (Fig. 17.9) is also one of the major features of tuberous sclerosis (Figs 17.10, 17.11; Box 17.1).[4]

Fig. 17.7 Shagreen patch on back of child with tuberous sclerosis.

Differential diagnosis: The differential diagnosis of hypopigmented macules in the newborn includes nevus depigmentosus, nevus anemicus, piebaldism,

Fig. 17.8 Red forehead plaque of tuberous sclerosis.

Fig. 17.9 Flesh-colored forehead plaque of tuberous sclerosis.

Fig. 17.10 Periungual fibrous nodules (Koenen's tumors) on the toes of an adolescent with tuberous sclerosis.

and hypomelanosis of Ito. Nevus depigmentosus is generally a larger segmental area of hypopigmentation. The involved skin in piebaldism and Waardenburg's syndrome is totally depigmented. The areas of hypopigmentation in hypomelanosis of Ito are swirled and may cover a large portion of the body. In an infant without a family history of tuberous sclerosis, other criteria must be present to establish the diagnosis (see Box 17.1).[4–6]

Pathogenesis: Tuberous sclerosis is an autosomal dominant condition with nearly 100% penetrance.[4,7] Often, a characteristic family history is difficult to obtain. The spontaneous mutation rate is as high as 65–75%.[4,7] Tuberous sclerosis is caused by mutations in the genes coding for the proteins hamartin (TS1) or tuberin (TS2). Similar phenotypes are seen with mutations in either gene.[4]

Fig. 17.11 Gingival fibrous tumors in tuberous sclerosis.

Treatment: There is no effective treatment for the hypopigmented macules. Although these lesions do contain melanocytes, they are hypofunctional; there-

Box 17.1 Diagnostic criteria for tuberous sclerosis

Major features

Facial angiofibromas or forehead plaque

Nontraumatic ungual or periungual fibroma

Hypomelanotic macules (three or more)

Shagreen patch

Multiple retinal nodular hamartomas

Cortical tuber

Subependymal giant-cell astrocytoma

Cardiac rhabdomyoma (single or multiple)

Lymphangiomatosis

Renal angiolipoma

Minor features

Multiple, randomly distributed enamel pits in dental enamel

Hamartomatous rectal polyps

Bone cysts

Cerebral white matter radial migration lines

Gingival fibromas

Nonrenal hamartoma

Retinal achromic patch

Confetti skin lesions

Multiple renal cysts

Definite tuberous sclerosis complex

Either two major features or one major feature plus two minor features

Probable tuberous sclerosis complex

One major plus one minor feature

Possible tuberous sclerosis complex

Either one major or two or more minor features

fore, they are more susceptible to ultraviolet radiation (UVR) and should be protected from excess sunlight. Children in whom the diagnosis of tuberous sclerosis has been documented are best managed in an appropriate multispecialty clinic.

Patient education: For those children with a family history of tuberous sclerosis and hypopigmented macules, the family should be told that it is highly likely that the child has tuberous sclerosis. In families without a history of tuberous sclerosis, discussion should be based on the number of hypopigmented macules present. A child with three or more hypopigmented macules is likely to have tuberous sclerosis and should be referred to the appropriate multispecialty clinic for evaluation for other stigmata of the disease. A child with one hypopigmented macule is less likely to have tuberous sclerosis. The parents

should be told about the other findings associated with tuberous sclerosis.

Follow-up visits: Infants likely to have tuberous sclerosis should be followed in a multispecialty clinic. Infants with one or two hypopigmented macules should be evaluated on a yearly basis.

Nevus depigmentosus

Clinical features: Nevus depigmentosus generally presents at birth, or within several months after birth as a unilateral, localized, quasidermatomal patch of hypopigmentation (Fig. 17.12).[8,9] The borders may be regular or irregular and at times the lesions may be whorled. A negative family history for hypopigmented birthmarks is usually obtained.

Fig. 17.12 Nevus depigmentosus. Quasidermatomal hypopigmentation.

Differential diagnosis: The differential diagnosis of nevus depigmentosus is the same as that for hypopigmented macules (Box 17.2).

Pathogenesis: Nevus depigmentosus should be considered a birthmark consisting of hypofunctional melanocytes.[8] In general, hypofunctioning melanocytes produce and transfer less melanin to the surrounding keratinocytes. Therefore, the skin supplied by these melanocytes appears lighter than normal skin.

Treatment: As with the other forms of congenital hypopigmentation, there is no effective treatment. Because of the hypopigmentation in these areas, they should be chronically protected from excess UVR.

Box 17.2 Differential diagnosis of patchy pigment loss in children

Postinflammatory hypopigmentation

Pityriasis alba

Tinea versicolor

Vitiligo

White spots (ash-leaf macules), with or without tuberous sclerosis

Halo nevus

Piebaldism

Morphea

Lichen sclerosus

Hypomelanosis of Ito

Waardenburg's syndrome

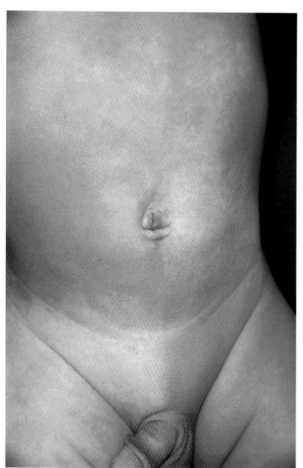

Fig. 17.13 Hypomelanosis of Ito. Whorls of hypopigmentation of the trunk with demarcation at midline.

Fig. 17.14 Hypomelanosis of Ito. Whorls of hypopigmentation extending down an extremity.

Patient education: Parents should be informed of the chronicity and benign nature of this birthmark. They should be told that the involved area of skin will be more sensitive to UVR than the child's normal skin, and that the area should be protected from excess sunlight.

Follow-up visits: Follow-up visits are not necessary.

Hypomelanosis of Ito

Clinical features: Newborns with hypomelanosis of Ito have bizarre hypopigmented swirls on their skin that follow Blaschko's lines (Figs 17.13, 17.14). The hypopigmentation may be quite extensive, involving an entire half of the body, or in some circumstances it may even be found bilaterally. Patients with hypomelanosis of Ito may have associated neurologic, skeletal, and/or ocular abnormalities. Because it is not a single entity, but a cutaneous sign of mosaicism, the exact incidence is unknown.[10]

Differential diagnosis: The differential diagnosis of hypomelanosis of Ito is the same as that for hypopigmented macules, but it is distinguished by the whorled pattern following Blaschko's lines and by involvement of an extensive portion of the body. Hypomelanosis of Ito is often confused with incontinentia pigmenti, linear and whorled hypermelanosis, or the linear hypermelanosis associated with the Proteus syndrome, all of which follow Blaschko's lines and have sharp midline demarcation of pigmentation. Hypomelanosis is lighter than normal skin color, rather than darker. Rarely, patients with incontinentia pigmenti will also have whorled hypopigmentation, making differentiation from hypomelanosis of Ito difficult.

Pathogenesis: The hypopigmentation is secondary to hypofunctioning of melanocytes. It is thought that a mishap early in embryogenesis is responsible for mosaicism, with two distinct genetically different melanocyte populations produced. Hypomelanosis of Ito is a non-specific, descriptive term applied to individuals with extensive areas of whorled pigmentation but without a consistent genetic defect.[10]

Treatment. As with the other hypopigmented and depigmented problems, no treatment is available for the pigmentary changes. Associated neurologic, skeletal, or ophthalmologic problems should be referred to the appropriate specialist.

Fig. 17.15 Nevus anemicus. Hypopigmented macule that disappears with pressure on the surrounding skin.

Patient education: The clinician should inform the parents that the number of infants who will have associated problems is unknown. They should also be told that no specific genetic defect has been identified.

Follow-up visits: Follow-up will depend on the associated abnormalities.

Nevus anemicus

Clinical features: Nevus anemicus presents as a solitary, localized, hypopigmented macule (Fig. 17.15).[11]

Differential diagnosis: Nevus anemicus is separated from the other forms of congenital hypopigmentation by diascopy. This will cause blanching of the surrounding normal skin and obscure the original borders of the lesion.

Pathogenesis: Unlike the other congenital hypopigmented macules, nevus anemicus is a problem of vascular control and not of melanocytes. The defect is thought to be a localized vascular hypersensitivity to catecholamines via α-adrenergic receptors.[11] Injection of α-blocking agents will temporarily return the skin to normal color.

Treatment: No treatment is necessary.

Patient education: The benign nature of the disorder should be discussed.

Follow-up visits: No follow-up visits are necessary.

Fig. 17.16 Generalized vitiligo. Involvement of perineal and inguinal skin. Note the distinct borders.

Fig. 17.17 Vitiligo involving the lips.

Fig. 17.18 Symmetric acral vitiligo.

Fig. 17.19 Vitiligo of eyelashes and eyebrow in Vogt-Koyanagi-Harada syndrome.

Acquired Circumscribed Flat Hypopigmentation or Depigmentation

Vitiligo

Clinical features: Vitiligo is a patchy loss of skin pigment. The patches are flat, completely depigmented, and have distinct borders (Figs 17.16, 17.17). Five percent of patients will have inflammatory vitiligo with raised erythematous borders. In dark-skinned patients, hypopigmented skin can be seen between the depigmented and normal skin (trichrome vitiligo). Hair within the patch of vitiligo is often depigmented as well. Fifty percent of cases of vitiligo start before the age of 18 years.[12] Vitiligo may be divided into generalized or segmental types. Generalized vitiligo usually begins acrally and symmetrically (Fig. 17.18). The extensor surface of the extremities and the face and neck are the areas most commonly involved. Generalized vitiligo continues to spread and develop new lesions for years, although most patients will have less than 20% of the body surface involved.[13] Generalized vitiligo is associated with other autoimmune diseases, but they are rarely seen in childhood, and random screening should not be performed. Generalized vitiligo is the most common form seen in children, although segmental vitiligo is more common in children than in adults.[12] Segmental vitiligo affects only one part of the body. It spreads rapidly in that area and then stabilizes, usually within 1 year. It is not associated with autoimmune diseases. Vitiligo of the face, eyelashes, and scalp hair in association with uveitis, dysacousis, and alopecia areata occurs in the rare Vogt-Koyanagi-Harada syndrome (Fig. 17.19).[12] Complete spontaneous repigmentation is unusual in vitiligo. Pigmentation returns first around hair follicles. In black and other dark-skinned children, vitiligo produces great distress (Figs 17.20, 17.21).

Differential diagnosis: The conditions to be considered in the differential diagnosis of vitiligo are listed in Box 17.2. In contrast to vitiligo, the

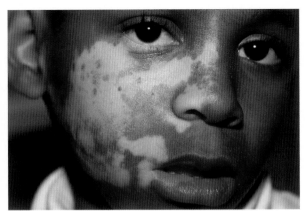

Fig. 17.20 Rapidly progressing segmental vitiligo.

abnormally pigmented areas of pityriasis alba and tinea versicolor are hypopigmented rather than depigmented and often have scaling and indistinct borders. In postinflammatory hypopigmentation, irregular mottling of both hyperpigmented and hypopigmented areas is often seen. In piebaldism, lesions are present from birth. Patients with morphea and lichen sclerosus have immobilized skin and hypopigmentation.

Pathogenesis: An infiltrate of T lymphocytes is seen in early vitiligo lesions.[14] Long-standing inactive lesions of vitiligo always lack melanocytes.[14] Several theories have been postulated to explain the cause of vitiligo.[12] These include the autoimmune, autocytotoxic, neural, and genetic theories. It is likely that vitiligo is a heterogeneous disorder with portions of all theories being correct in a given subset of patients.

Treatment: There is no entirely satisfactory treatment, and not all children will want treatment. Desire for treatment will depend on the age of the patient, location and extent of the disease, and cultural beliefs. Patients not wishing therapy should be advised about the lack of natural protection from the sun and the need for photoprotection. Cover-up cosmetics that match the child's skin color may be very beneficial for cosmetically sensitive areas.

For those children who desire therapy, initial therapy is based on the extent of the body surface involved. If less than 25% of the body surface area is involved, topical therapy should be attempted. Topical glucocorticosteroids have been used for decades. Potent topical steroid are equally effective as superpotent topical steroid and have less risk for the development of side effects.[15] The topical immunomodulators (pimecrolimus and tacrolimus) have been successfully employed in the treatment of

Fig. 17.21 (A) Symmetric acral vitiligo before PUVA treatment. **(B)** Same patient shows perifollicular pattern of repigmentation during PUVA therapy.

vitiligo.[14] Because of the risk of telangiectasia and atrophy with the use of topical steroids, topical immunomodulators are preferred by many authorities.[14] Topical calcipotriol has also been used, but it is not very effective as a single agent.[14]

For children with >25% of the body surface area involved or in those children that have failed topical therapy and wish further treatment, phototherapy should be employed. Narrow-band UVB (UVB 311 nm) is as effective as psoralens plus UVA (PUVA) and has minimal side effects. Therefore, it is the recommended type of phototherapy for childhood vitiligo.[14]

In chronic, stable vitiligo unresponsive to other therapies, surgical transplantation of melanocytes may be performed.[14] Repigmentation in vitiligo is a very slow process. It may take 2–6 months to see an initial response. Treatments may need to be continued or intermittently restarted for years. One hundred percent repigmentation is very unlikely.

Fig. 17.22 Pityriasis alba. White, slightly scaly patches with indistinct borders on child's cheek.

Patient education: The clinician should discuss the natural history of vitiligo with the child and family and should also emphasize the need to follow a strict regimen in those motivated to undergo therapy.
Follow-up visits: During therapy, visits every 2 months are advisable to assess repigmentation and side effects of therapy.

Pityriasis alba

Clinical features: Pityriasis alba is characterized by multiple oval, scaly, flat, hypopigmented patches on the face, extensor surface of arms, and upper trunk (Fig. 17.22).[16] The lesions range 5–50 mm in diameter, and multiple patches may be seen. The borders are indistinct. Pityriasis alba occurs predominantly between the ages of 3 and 16 years, and up to 40% of all children may be affected. The lesions do not itch, and medical help is sought because of the child's appearance. It is particularly distressing in dark-skinned children. It is a chronic dermatitis and may be recurrent over several years. Most authors regard this as a form of atopic dermatitis.

Differential diagnosis: Pityriasis alba most closely mimics tinea versicolor, which can be excluded by findings in a negative potassium hydroxide (KOH) examination. (See Box 17.2 for the list of conditions to be considered in the differential diagnosis.)

Pathogenesis: On pathologic examination, the lesion resembles that seen in chronic dermatitis. Hyperkeratosis, parakeratosis, spongiotic edema, and a lymphocytic infiltrate are seen. The cause of the hypopigmentation is not known, but it is likely related to

inflammatory mediators that inhibit melanocyte function.

Treatment: There is no satisfactory treatment for pityriasis alba. Bland lubricants and topical glucocorticosteroids have some influence on the disorder.

Patient education: The natural history of this disorder should be emphasized.
Follow-up visits: Follow-up visits should be scheduled at monthly intervals if a treatment program is considered.

Postinflammatory hypopigmentation

Clinical features: After any inflammatory skin disease or injury to the skin, irregular hypopigmented areas may appear. The hypopigmentation is most obvious in dark-skinned people. The hypopigmented blotches

Fig. 17.23 Postinflammatory hypopigmentation with numerous hypopigmented patches on child's back.

Fig. 17.24 Blotchy hypopigmentation after treatment for atopic dermatitis.

are usually in a mottled pattern and may be associated with hyperpigmented areas (Figs 17.23, 17.24). They resolve several months after the inflammatory disorder.

Differential diagnosis: Blotchy hypopigmentation associated with hyperpigmentation, and a history of a preceding inflammatory dermatosis differentiate this form of hypopigmentation (see Box 17.2).

Box 17.3 Classification of oculocutaneous albinism

OCA1 (Tyrosinase related)
No tyrosinase activity OCA1A

Residual tyrosinase activity

    Yellow OCA1B

    Minimal pigment OCA1MP

    Temperature-sensitive OCA1TP

OCA2
P gene

OCA3
TRP-1

OCA4
MATP

Defects in melanosomes and other lysosomal-like structures

Hermansky-Pudlak syndrome

HPS2
β-3A subunit of Ap3

HPS-7
DTNPB1 gene

Chediak-Higashi syndrome
CHS-1 gene

Fig. 17.25 OCA1. Newborn with hair and skin totally devoid of pigmentation.

Pathogenesis: Inflammatory injury to melanocytes and epidermal cells results in decreased pigment production and transfer.

Treatment: Treatment is not necessary.

Patient education: The patient should be informed of the nature of the pigment loss and told that recovery is expected.

Follow-up visits: Follow-up visits are unnecessary.

Diffuse hypopigmentation or depigmentation: albinism

Clinical features: Albinism can be separated into those individuals with eye, skin, and hair abnormalities (oculocutaneous albinism [OCA]) and those with only eye involvement (ocular albinism [OA]). There are four classes of OCA (Box 17.3).[17] All variants of OCA have defects in melanin synthesis, resulting in reduction or total absence of pigmentation (Fig. 17.25).[17] All newborns with OCA1 have fine white hair, pink skin, blue irides, severe nystagmus, and photophobia. The skin and hair in patients with OCA1A will remain white their entire life. Patients with variants of OCA1 may develop darker hair, skin, and eyes; freckles; lentigines; and nevi. In the other classes of OCA, hair and skin pigment may be present at birth and increase with age. Pigmented nevi and freckles commonly develop in these patients. The phenotypic expression of these forms of OCA is quite variable. Hermansky-Pudlak syndrome (HPS) is albinism associated with bleeding caused by abnormal platelet aggregation, whereas Chediak-Higashi is albinism associated with susceptibility to infection as a result of dysfunctional leukocyte degranulation.

Differential diagnosis: The diagnosis of OCA1 in a child with white skin and hair and blue eyes is usually obvious. The other classes may be difficult to diagnose in light-skinned whites. The major differential is between the classes of OCA.

Pathogenesis: OCA1 is caused by mutations in the genes encoding for the protein tyrosinase.[17] OCA1A is due to complete lack of functional tyrosinase. In the variants of OCA1, partial tyrosinase function remains. Tyrosinase is a major enzyme necessary for the formation of the pigment melanin. OCA2 is caused by defects in the P gene.[24] The function of this gene product has not yet been determined, but may be involved in the regulation of melanosomal pH or melanosome trafficking.[17] OCA3 is caused by mutations in the gene coding for the protein TRP-1. TRP-1 is another enzyme involved in the formation of melanin. OCA4 is caused by mutations in the gene encoding for a membrane-asscoiated protein transporter (MATP). Its exact function is still unknown. There are 15 known varieties of Hermansky-Pudlak syndrome identified in mice and 8 types in humans. There are only 2 types of the Hermansky-Pudlak syndrome in which the genes have been identified. In HPS-2 the abnormal gene is AP3B1 which encodes the β-3A sub unit of AP3. It functions in cargo selection and vesicle trafficking to lysosomal structures. In HPS-7, the abnormal gene is DTNBP1 which encodes a protein which binds to α and β dystrobrevin. Chediak-Higashi syndrome is caused by mutations in the CHS1 gene. Its protein product is also thought to play a role in vesicle transport. Patients with Hermansky-Pudlak syndrome or the Chediak-Higashi syndrome have defects in melanosomes and other lysosomal-like structures.

Treatment: No treatment is available for the pigmentary changes. Because of the lack of pigmentation, sun protection is required for all children with albinism.

Patient education: The family should be referred to an ophthalmologist and to the appropriate specialists for genetic counseling and identification of the class of OCA expressed. The need for photoprotection should be stressed.

Follow-up visits: Follow-up visits are determined by the type of OCA and the degree of ocular involvement.

BROWN LESIONS

In considering a hyperpigmented state, one should first determine whether the hyperpigmentation is circumscribed or diffuse.

Circumscribed Flat Hyperpigmentation

Clinical features

Freckles: Freckles are small, 1–5 mm, light-brown, pigmented macules that are UVR responsive and occur in sun-exposed skin (Fig. 17.26). They are autosomal dominant and first appear at age 3–5 years,

Fig. 17.26 Freckles. Note the sunburn between freckled areas.

Fig. 17.27 Lip lentigines not associated with the Peutz-Jeghers syndrome.

Fig. 17.28 Lip lentigines in an adolescent with the Peutz-Jeghers syndrome.

predominantly on the face and extensor surface of the extremities. They are most frequent in fair-skinned, light or red-haired, blue-eyed children.[18] They become less common with age.

Lentigines: Lentigines are brown or brown-black, 1–2 mm macules found sparsely scattered over the body, including the mucous membranes (Fig. 17.27).[19,20] They do not change with sun exposure. They usually first appear during school age. Lentigines on the lips (Fig. 17.28) are also seen in the autosomal dominant Peutz-Jeghers syndrome associated with multiple bowel polyps and an increased risk of gastrointestinal and genitourinary carcinomas.[21] Multiple lentigines are associated with cardiac abnormalities in the so-called LEOPARD syndrome (*l*entigines, *e*lectrocardiograph abnormalities, *o*cular hypertelorism, *p*ulmonary stenosis, *a*bnormalities of the genitalia, growth *r*etardation, *d*eafness) (Fig. 17.29).[22] Central facial lentigines have been described in association with cardiac defects and malignancies in the NAME (Carney complex) syndrome (*n*evi, *a*trial myxomas, *m*yxoid neurofibroma, *e*phelides).[23] Generalized lentigines

Box 17.4 Diagnostic criteria for neurofibromatosis type 1
Two or more of the following must be found:
Six or more café-au-lait spots greater than 5 mm in diameter in prepubertal children; greater than 1.5 mm in postpubertal children
Two or more neurofibromas of any type
One plexiform neurofibroma
Axillary freckling
Inguinal freckling
Two or more Lisch nodules (iris hamartomas)
Distinctive osseous lesion, such as sphenoid dysplasia or thinning of a long bone, with or without pseudoarthrosis
A first-degree relative with NF-1

may also be seen in children without any associated systemic defects.[24]

Café-au-lait spots: Café-au-lait spots are tan, flat, oval macules with distinct borders (Fig. 17.30). They frequently have a diameter greater than 0.5 cm. Multiple café-au-lait spots occur in type 1 neurofibromatosis (NF-1) (Box 17.4). In children age 6 or older, café-au-lait macules over 0.5 cm are a major criterion for NF-1 (see Box 17.4) (Figs 17.31, 17.32).[4] Rarely, families have autosomal-dominant, multiple, café-au-lait macules without other stigmata of neurofibromatosis.[25] Café-au-lait spots are rarely present at birth, but increase in number with age through the teen years. They are seen in 25–35% of children between the ages of 4 and 18 years.[25,26] Large, solitary café-au-lait macules are usually an isolated finding,[27]

Fig. 17.29 Child with multiple lentigines and the LEOPARD syndrome. Note scars from repair of pulmonary stenosis.

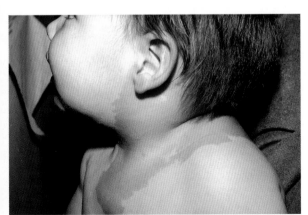

Fig. 17.30 Café-au-lait spot. Large lesion on a child's neck.

Fig. 17.31 Numerous café-au-lait spots on the abdomen and chest of a child with neurofibromatosis type 1.

Fig. 17.32 Numerous café-au-lait spots in a child's axilla in neurofibromatosis type 1.

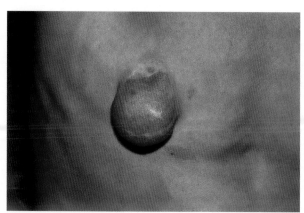

Fig. 17.33 Soft cutaneous neurofibroma surrounded by café-au-lait spots in an adolescent with neurofibromatosis type 1.

Fig. 17.34 Soft neurofibroma on buttock of infant with NF-1

Fig. 17.35 Proteus syndrome. Port-wine stain on child with multiple CALMs.

Fig. 17.36 Proteus syndrome. Overgrowth of second and third toes on one foot.

Fig. 17.37 Mongolian spots. Extensive lesions over the back and buttocks.

but may also be seen in the McCune-Albright and Proteus syndromes.[28,29] McCune-Albright syndrome is characterized by the association of a giant café-au-lait macule with precocious puberty and polyostotic fibrous dysplasia.[28] The Proteus syndrome can be mistaken for NF-1 because of the skeletal overgrowth and large hamartomas that are confused with plexiform neurofibromas.[29] In NF-1, more café-au-lait spots appear with age and may be accompanied by soft cutaneous neurofibromas (Figs 17.33–17.36).

Mongolian spots: The mongolian spot is a blue-black macule found over the lumbosacral area in up to 90% of Asian, black, and American Indian babies. They are occasionally noted over the shoulders and back and may extend over the buttocks and extremities (Fig. 17.37).[30] As the normal skin pigment darkens, the mongolian spot becomes less obvious, but lesions are persistent throughout life.

Nevus of Ota, nevus of Ito: Flat, blue-black, speckled pigmentary discoloration may be noted in the skin surrounding the eye (nevus of Ota) (Fig. 17.38) or around the chest and shoulder (nevus of Ito). Most cases are present at birth, but some are acquired.[31] The sclera may be involved in nevus of Ota.

Linear and whorled nevoid hypermelanosis: Hypermelanotic macules arranged in streaks corresponding to Blaschko's lines, with sharp demarcation at the midline, characterize linear and whorled nevoid hypermelanosis (Figs 17.39, 17.40).[32]

Postinflammatory hyperpigmentation: In children with dark skin, any inflammatory skin disorder may heal

Fig. 17.39 Linear and whorled hypermelanosis. Brown whorls over the trunk of a child.

Fig. 17.40 Linear and whorled hypermelanosis. Brown whorls over the trunk of a child.

with hyperpigmentation. Often the pigmentation persists for months.

Differential diagnosis

Freckles are small, acquired, sun-responsive macules, whereas lentigines and café-au-lait macules are not related to sun exposure. Café-au-lait macules are larger and lighter brown than lentigines. Skin biopsy may differentiate the acquired flat pigmented lesions from one another, but should only be done if it will help delineate one of the associated genetic syndromes. Mongolian spots, nevus of Ota, and nevus of Ito are blue-black, with location being used to differentiate. Linear and whorled nevoid hypermelanosis is obvious by the extent of the condition and the pigmentation occurring along the lines of Blaschko. Unlike incontinentia pigmenti, linear and whorled nevoid hypermelanosis is not preceded by a vesicular or

Fig. 17.38 Nevus of Ota. Speckled blue macules in the periorbital skin and sclera.

Box 17.5 Differential diagnosis of circumscribed, flat, pigmented lesions

Acquired
Freckles
Lentigo
Café-au-lait spot
Junctional melanocytic nevi
Postinflammatory hyperpigmentation

Congenital
Mongolian spot
Nevus of Ota, nevus of Ito
Linear and whorled nevoid hypermelanosis

verrucous stage. The conditions to be included in the differential diagnosis are listed in Box 17.5.

Pathogenesis

Freckles: Freckles are areas with increased pigment secondary to sun exposure. Sixty percent of patients with freckles have specific polymorphisms of the melanocortin-1 receptor.[33]

Lentigines: In lentigines, increased numbers of melanocytes are dispersed along the basal layer of the epidermis, and the epidermal rete ridges are elongated. The majority of cases of Peutz-Jeghers syndrome are caused by mutations in the LKB1/STK11 gene, which encodes a multifunctional serine-threonine kinase.[21] The Carney complex is caused by mutations in the PRKAR1A gene, which encodes for the R1 alpha regulatory subunit of the cyclic-AMP-dependent protein kinase A.[23] The genetic defect in the LEOPARD is in the PTPN11 gene which encodes the protein tyrosine phosphatase SHP-2.[22]

Café-au-lait spots: In café-au-lait spots, melanocyte activity is increased, as is the melanin in melanocytes and in epidermal cells. The number of melanocytes is not increased. Despite this in vivo increase in function, no differences have been demonstrated in vitro in melanocytes grown from café-au-lait macules compared with melanocytes from normal skin. Neurofibromatosis is an autosomal dominant disease caused by mutations in the gene that encodes a protein, neurofibromin, which acts as a tumor suppressor.[4] The McCune-Albright syndrome is due to a dominant somatic mutation in the Gs alpha gene which leads to a constitutively activated adenyl cyclase.[28]

Mongolian spots: The pathology of mongolian spots consists of spindle-shaped cells that contain pigment and are located between collagen fibers deep within the dermis.

Nevus of Ota, nevus of Ito: Similar to mongolian spots, nevus of Ota and nevus of Ito have spindle-shaped melanocytes found within the dermis.

Linear and whorled nevoid hypermelanosis: With linear and whorled nevoid hypermelanosis, epidermal melanocytes are increased in number and keratinocytes have increased melanin in the affected area. It is thought that two genetically distinct populations of melanocytes are produced. Chromosomal mosaicism with trisomy 20 has been identified in one patient with linear and whorled nevoid hypermelanosis.[34]

Postinflammatory hyperpigmentation: With postinflammatory hyperpigmentation, the excess pigment is related to loss of pigment from damaged epidermal keratinocytes and melanocytes into the dermis, where the large polymer melanin sits free in the dermis or is engulfed by macrophages to form melanophages. Breakdown of the dermal pigment is slow.

Treatment

No treatment is necessary, but cosmetically bothersome lesions may be treated with any of the q-switched lasers.[35]

Patient education

The common and benign nature of these pigmented areas should be emphasized. Parents of children with macular pigmentary disorders should be told of the possibility of any associated systemic syndromes.

Follow-up visits

Children likely to have associated syndromes should be referred for genetic evaluation; otherwise, follow-up visits are unnecessary.

Melanocytic Nevi

There are two distinct forms of melanocytic nevi with entirely different natural histories. These are congenital melanocytic nevi (CMN) and acquired nevi. They will be considered separately.

Congenital melanocytic nevi

Clinical features: Skin-colored to tan, or brown-black, solitary papules with smooth surfaces represent CMN. Multiple classifications of CMN have been used. The most common classification of CMN is based on the size of the lesion.[36] Lesions <1.5 cm in greatest diameter are considered small. Lesions 1.5–20 cm in greatest diameter are considered medium, with those over 20 cm in greatest diameter considered large. We prefer an alternative classification which defines large as covering greater than 5% of the body surface area.[37] Also, there are no data to support any difference in natural history between small CMN and medium CMN. Most CMN are small at birth, measuring less than 1.5 cm in greatest diameter (Fig. 17.41).[36] Large melanocytic nevi are very uncommon, occurring in 1 in 20 000 live births.[36]

Large melanocytic nevi are often not uniform in color and may contain flat tan areas, brown areas, blue-black plaques, and pigmented, long, thick hair (Figs 17.42, 17.43). Numerous smaller nevi located at skin sites distant from the large nevi are found. These 'satellite lesions' are more often uniform in color and may arise throughout childhood. Neurocutaneous melanosis is the association of a giant CMN overlying the scalp or spine, with central nervous system (CNS) involvement. The results of magnetic resonance imaging of the brain are abnormal in approximately 25% of these children, but only 1–2% will be symptomatic.[38] Erosions and ulcerations may be seen in neonates with large CMN, but these are not changes that signal malignancy.[38] A variant of CMN is the nevus spilus.[39] Nevus spilus is a café-au-lait macule studded with small, dark, raised nevi (Fig. 17.44).

Fig. 17.41 Small congenital nevus.

Fig. 17.42 Large congenital nevus with long, pigmented hair and a mixture of tan, brown, and blue within the lesion.

Fig. 17.43 Large congenital nevus in the so called 'bathing suit' distribution.

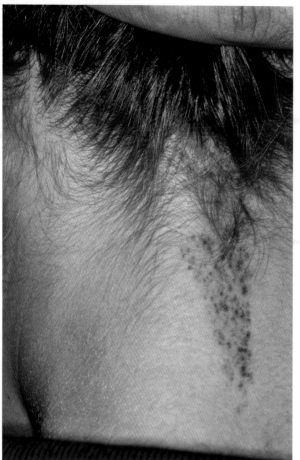

Fig. 17.44 Nevus spilus. Flat, tan lesion containing numerous small, dark brown areas.

Differential diagnosis: Occasionally, a congenital melanocytic nevus will be flat at birth and will appear as a café-au-lait macule, but with time it becomes raised. Congenital smooth muscle and pilar hamartomas may also present as light-brown plaques with fine hair and may be difficult to distinguish from CMN. Histological examination will differentiate.

Pathogenesis: Nests of pigment cells are found within the epidermis and dermis. Sometimes the pigment cells are large and unusually shaped, making it difficult to distinguish benign from malignant changes.[36] In giant CMN, pigment cells may populate the entire dermis and extend around hair and eccrine sweat structures. Most authorities consider congenital nevocellular nevi to be developmental errors in pigment-cell proliferation and migration. The pathogenesis of CMN is unknown.

Treatment: The management of large CMN is controversial. Patients with large CMN are at risk for the development of melanoma; however, many of these melanomas do not always occur in the skin.[36] In these instances, removal of the CMN from the skin would not be beneficial. Currently it is advisable to take into consideration the potential for cosmetic improvement and surgical risk before recommending removal of such lesions. There is no compelling reason to remove these in the child's first year. Small lesions can be removed during adolescence. There is no urgency to remove small congenital nevi before puberty. Lifelong observation of small and medium CMN is an acceptable option.[36] There is a very small risk of melanoma arising in a small congenital nevus in late adolescence or in young adults.[36]

Patient education: There is no uniform agreement among authorities as to the best management for congenital nevi, and the clinician should explain to the parents both the positive and negative reasons for treatment. CMN will grow proportionately with the child, and this should not be a concern. Satellite lesions may continue to develop throughout childhood. Any change in one portion of the CMN should be evaluated to determine the need for biopsy. In patients with large CMN overlying the scalp and spine, the small risk of neurocutaneous melanosis should be discussed.

Follow-up visits: Yearly visits are recommended for large CMN, and additional visits are recommended any time there is a nonproportional change in the birthmark. Children with large CMN overlying the scalp or spine should be evaluated by a neurologist if there are any signs of CNS or developmental abnormalities.

Acquired melanocytic nevi (common moles)

Clinical features: The development of acquired melanocytic nevi in white children is related to genetic susceptibility and sun exposure.[41-43] This is not true for nonwhite children, who develop fewer nevi.[44] There are families in which members develop numerous, atypical nevi beginning in childhood. Members of these families are at markedly increased risk for the development of melanoma.[45] In white skin the development of moles is related to skin type, hair and eye color, freckles, and sun exposure.[41-45] Those children with light skin, light hair and eye color, many freckles,

Fig. 17.45 Congenital nevus involving toe and toenail plate in child.

and a history of numerous sunburns develop the highest number of nevi.[41–45] Children with similar genetic backgrounds who are exposed to more UVR will develop more nevi.[41]

To differentiate benign moles from melanoma, it is important to understand the changes that occur during the development of common acquired nevi.[46] Acquired melanocytic nevi begin as flat, well-demarcated, brown to brown-black lesions (Fig. 17.45). These are called *junctional melanocytic nevi*. They characteristically have regular borders and may have a light-brown rim (rim mole) and/or a dark-brown center. Rim moles are commonly seen in the scalp. They usually measure 2–5 mm but may occasionally be larger. Most nevi found in infants and children are junctional nevi. Enlargement and darkening of nevi with growth spurts and puberty is also a common event.

Approximately 20% of junctional melanocytic nevi will progress to compound melanocytic nevi, which

Fig. 17.46 Back of an adolescent with multiple benign junctional and compound nevi.

Fig. 17.47 Compound nevus, darker in the center.

Fig. 17.48 Compound nevus with different brown zones.

Fig. 17.49 Nonpigmented intradermal nevus of the scalp.

appear as small, raised, dome-shaped, brown to brown-black papules (see Fig. 17.33). There are several frequent clinical variants of compound nevi. In some of these, the center will be raised and darker than the periphery (fried egg mole) (Fig. 17.46). Compound nevi may also appear skin colored, with little melanin production (Figs 17.47–17.49). Neither of these changes is worrisome.

Dermal nevi are usually few in number before the preadolescent growth period, averaging one or two. A less common type of dermal nevi is the so called *Becker's nevus*. This is a large, pigmented, hairy nevus that occurs most commonly over the shoulder and is often first noticed in adolescence (Figs 17.50, 17.51).[47] It may be seen in other locations.

A halo may appear around a nevus that is regressing in childhood (Fig. 17.52), producing the 'halo nevus.'[48] This change may occur during any stage of nevus development. Multiple halo nevi may be seen in an individual, and this is at times associated with vitiligo.

There are two other uncommon types of benign nevi that are sometimes confused with melanoma. The Spitz nevus begins as a solitary red or red-brown nodule, usually on the extremities or face (Figs 17.53–17.55).[49] Blue nevi are blue to blue-black, 4–10 mm solitary papules (Figs 17.56, 17.57).

ATYPICAL NEVI. No single change takes place when a common nevus becomes malignant, but rather a spectrum of changes are encompassed by the so called *atypical* or *dysplastic nevus*. Clinically, these lesions are usually over 5 mm in diameter, with a variegated tan to brown color on a pink background and an impalpable, irregular, ill-defined border (Fig. 17.58). They occur in the familial melanoma syndrome and in patients with melanoma who do not have a family history of melanoma or the clinical phenotype of the

Fig. 17.50 Becker's nevus on the back and arm of an adolescent male.

Fig. 17.51 Becker's nevus of one side of chest in adolescent male.

Fig. 17.52 Halo nevus. Loss of pigment around regressing central intradermal nevus.

Fig. 17.53 Spitz nevus. Red papule on the face of a child.

Fig. 17.54 Spitz nevus. Red papule on the face of a child.

Fig. 17.55 Spitz nevus with fine scale on surface.

Fig. 17.56 Blue nevus. Blue-black papule on a child's shoulder.

Fig. 17.57 Blue nevus in umbilicus.

Fig. 17.58 Atypical nevus with irregular borders and pink background.

familial melanoma syndrome. They may also be seen as isolated moles occurring in the general population.

Box 17.6 ABCDs of melanoma detection

Asymmetry: the lesion is not round, but has an irregular shape

Border: the border is not even, but notched and irregular

Color: areas of red, white, and/or blue within a brown area

Diameter: greater than 10 mm

Evolution: a rapid change in any of these parameters over a few weeks is a matter for concern.

MALIGNANT MELANOMA. Malignant melanomas are rare in childhood, and although still uncommon they are being seen with increased frequency in adolescents, but not in prepubertal children.[50] One must be familiar with the ABCDEs of melanoma (Box 17.6), but at times these characteristics can be difficult to apply to prepubertal children (Fig. 17.59). Some pigmented nevi in children will be asymmetrical with irregular borders. Changes in color must also be

Fig. 17.59 Severely atypical nevus with marked abnormalities in symmetry and borders.

Fig. 17.60 Malignant melanoma on the chest of an adolescent male.

evaluated carefully. The pigmented lesion that changes from light-brown to dark-brown is not a cause for worry. Within a single brown lesion the appearance of red, white, and blue colors (Fig. 17.60) is a worrisome change. The most important clinical feature is rapid, progressive growth of a pigmented lesion disproportionate to the other nevi. Ulceration and bleeding are far-advanced signs. In familial malignant melanoma, multiple primary melanomas may be found, usually first appearing in late adolescence or early adult life.[51] There is a correlation with skin type, large numbers of nevi, and a history of excess sun exposure in childhood and melanoma later in life.[41–45]

Differential diagnosis: The conditions to be considered in the differential diagnosis of circumscribed, acquired pigmented lesions are listed in Box 17.7. Histology will differentiate these pigmented lesions from one another.

Box 17.7 Differential diagnosis of circumscribed, acquired pigmented lesions
Junctional melanocytic nevus
Dermal melanocytic nevus
Compound melanocytic nevus
Atypical melanocytic nevus
Spitz nevus
Blue nevus
Malignant melanoma
Pyogenic granuloma
Mastocytoma
Dermatofibroma
Juvenile xanthogranuloma

Pathogenesis – junctional, compound, and dermal melanocytic nevi: Clumps of increased numbers of melanocytes are located at the dermal–epidermal junction in junctional nevi. Dermal melanocytic nevi represent accumulations of groups of melanocytes within the mid to upper dermis. When associated with clumps of melanocytes at the dermal–epidermal junction, such a nevus is called a *compound nevus*. Development of these types of nevi is related to genetic background and amount of sun exposure. Spitz nevi are composed of collections of melanocytes with irregular cytoplasmic and nuclear shapes and are located throughout the dermis. These nevi are associated with a proliferation of blood vessels. The bizarre nuclear shapes often result in confusion with melanoma. These histologic changes are categorized as *spindle* and *epithelioid*. Not all histologically spindle and epithelioid nevi are red-brown papules. Therefore, when a pathology report indicates a spindle and epithelioid nevus, clinical correlation is extremely important.

Atypical nevi display architectural atypia and cytologic dysplasia. These changes encompass a wide spectrum between common nevi and melanoma.

In malignant melanomas, the tumor originates at the dermal–epidermal junction and has a radial growth phase before it demonstrates a vertical growth phase. The tumor cells within a melanoma show great variation in size and shape, and invade epidermal structures. The depth of invasion is an important prognostic factor and is the basis for histologic classifications of melanomas. Familial melanoma has been linked to the cell cycle regulator CDKN2A gene, which encodes for the p16 tumor suppressor (p16INK4A) and the alternate reading frame (p14ARF).[52,53] Mutations in the cyclin-dependent kinase-4 (CDK4) also cause familial melanoma.[52,53] There are compelling data to support a role of sunlight in melanomas. An experienced dermatopathologist should review the histology of all pigmented lesions in which the diagnosis of melanoma is considered.

A blue nevus represents clumps of mature melanocytes located in the deep dermis.

Becker's nevus is considered a hamartoma of hair follicles and associated arrector pilae muscles. In Becker's nevus the number of melanocytes is slightly increased, and melanin is seen throughout the epidermis.

Treatment: In any raised pigmented lesion in which melanoma is suspected, surgical excision is the treatment of choice. Although malignant melanoma is rare in childhood it is becoming more common in adolescents.[50] Therefore, a high index of suspicion of malignant melanoma should be maintained for any rapidly growing pigmented skin lesion in postpubertal children. Any excised skin lesion, particularly pigmented skin lesions, should be sent to a pathologist. In childhood or adolescence it is unnecessary to remove common melanocytic nevi that are uniform in shape and color.

Patient education: Families with familial melanoma traits and with sporadic melanomas must be counseled regarding the high risk for the development of melanoma, the importance of routine follow-up, and the need for excision of any changing lesion. Parents of children with light skin, light hair, blue eyes, and freckles need to be told of the correlation between sun exposure in childhood and the increased risk of developing melanoma later in life. Proper sun protection programs should be discussed. The risk of melanoma in a child who has a solitary atypical nevus without a family history of melanoma is unknown. If a lesion is removed, the nature of the lesion can be explained to the patient after confirmation by the pathologist.

Follow-up visits: Adolescents with the familial melanoma syndrome or with a family history of sporadic melanoma should be followed yearly. If a lesion has been excised, a visit 1–2 weeks after surgical removal is necessary to inform the patient of the diagnosis and suggested further treatment, if any.

Acanthosis Nigricans

Clinical features

Acanthosis nigricans is characterized by hyperpigmentation and a velvety thickening of irregular, linear folds of skin of the posterior neck and the axilla (Figs 17.61, 17.62). It is common in Native American, African-American, and Hispanic adolescents.[54–56] Often, parents complain that their child's skin is dirty and cannot be cleaned. Small papillomatous growths (skin tags) may be found within the irregular folds. Acanthosis nigricans also can be found in other skin areas, such as elbows, inguinal creases, areolae, and knuckles. It is associated with obesity and correlates well with hyperinsulinemia and insulin resistance.[54–58] With obesity, the age of onset correlates with the onset of obesity. Less commonly it is associated with other endocrinologic abnormalities and with various craniofacial syndromes.[59]

Fig. 17.61 Acanthosis nigricans of a child's axilla. Velvety, brown rows of hyperpigmentation.

Fig. 17.62 Acanthosis nigricans of a child's neck.

Differential diagnosis

Acanthosis nigricans is so distinctive that it is seldom misdiagnosed. A lichenified chronic dermatitis may mimic it.

Pathogenesis

The epidermis is papillomatous with no abnormality of pigmentation. The majority of children with acanthosis nigricans will have obesity and insulin resistance.[54-58]

Treatment

In obese adolescents, weight loss has resulted in reversal of the acanthosis nigricans and may decrease the risk for future problems associated with type II diabetes mellitus.[58]

Patient education

Parents should be told that acanthosis nigricans is not dirt and is unrelated to hygiene. If the child is obese, the relationship of the skin condition to obesity should be emphasized, and the institution of a weight-control program should be considered. Nonobese children with signs of associated hyperandrogenism should be referred for endocrine evaluation.

Follow-up visits

Follow-up visits should be determined by therapy.

Box 17.8 Differential diagnosis of diffuse hyperpigmentation

Addison's disease

Acromegaly

Cushing's syndrome of pituitary origin

Thyrotoxicosis

ACTH administration

Subacute bacterial endocarditis

Lymphomas and leukemia

Scleroderma, dermatomyositis

Renal failure

Hemochromatosis

Familial progressive hyperpigmentation

Chronic arsenism

Argyria

Diffuse Hyperpigmentation

Diffuse hyperpigmentation is rare in infancy and childhood. Pigmentation of the scrotum, linea alba, and palmar creases may occur. Diffuse hyperpigmentation may occur as a result of endocrine disturbances, such as adrenal insufficiency, with overproduction of adrenocorticotropic hormone (ACTH) and its melanocyte-stimulating fragments, or hyperfunction of the pituitary. Box 17.8 lists the conditions to be included in the differential diagnosis of diffuse hyperpigmentation.

REFERENCES

1. Alper JC, Holmes LB. The incidence and significance of birthmarks in a cohort of 4641 newborns. Pediatr Dermatol 1983; 1:58–68.
2. Thomas I, Kihiczak GG, Fox MD, et al. Piebaldism: an update. Int J Dermatol 2004; 43:716–719.
3. Sanchez-Martin M, Perez-Losada J, Rodriquez-Garcia A, et al. Deletion of the SLUG (SNA12) gene results in human piebaldism. Am J Med Genet 2003; 122A:125–132.
4. Arbuckle HA, Morelli JG. Pigmentary disorders: update on neurofibromatosis-1 and tuberous sclerosis, Curr Opin Pediatr 2000; 12:354–358.
5. Jozwiak S, Schwartz RA, Janniger CK, et al. Skin lesions in children with tuberous sclerosis complex: the prevalence, natural course and diagnostic significance. Int J Dermatol 1998; 37:911–917.
6. Vanderhooft SL, Francis JS, Pagon RA, et al. Prevalence of hypopigmented macules in a healthy population. J Pediatr 1996; 129:355–361.
7. Sparagna SP, Roach ES. Tuberous sclerosis complex. Curr Opin Neurol 2000; 13:115–119.
8. Lee HS, Chun YS, Hann SK. Nevus depigmentosus: clinical features and histopathologic characteristics in 67 patients. J Am Acad Dermatol 1999; 40:21–26.
9. DiLernia V. Segmental nevus depigmentosus: analysis of 20 patients. Pediatr Dermatol 1999; 16:349–353.
10. Rutland BM, Edgar MA, Horenstien MG. Hypomelanosis of Ito associated with precocious puberty. Pediatr Neurol 2006; 34:51–54.
11. Ahkami RN, Schwartz RA. Nevus anemicus. Dermatology 1999; 198:327–329.
12. Herane MI. Vitiligo and leukoderma in children. Clin Dermatol 2003; 21:283–295.
13. Handa S, Kaur I. Vitiligo: clinical findings in 1436 patients. Int J Dermatol 1999; 26:653–657.
14. Grimes PE. New insights and new therapies in vitiligo. JAMA 2005; 293:730–735.
15. Njoo MD, et al. Nonsurgical repigmentation therapies in vitiligo: meta-analysis of the literature. Arch Dermatol 1998; 134:1532–1540.
16. Lin RL, Janniger CK. Pityriasis alba. Cutis 2005; 76:21–24.
17. Tomita Y, Suzuki T. Genetics of pigmentary disorders. Am J Med Genet 2004; 131C:75–81.
18. Bastiens M, Hoefnagel J, Westendorp R, et al. Solar lentigines are strongly related to sun exposure in contrast to ephelides. Pigment Cell Res 2004; 17:225–229.
19. Okulicz JK, Schwartz RA, Joswiak S. Lentigo. Cutis 2001; 67:367–370.

20. Cicek Y, Ertas U. The normal and pathological pigmentation of oral mucous membrane: a review. J Contemp Dent Pract 2003; 15:76–86.
21. Launonen V. Mutations in the human LKB1/STK11 gene. Hum Mutat 2005; 26:291–297.
22. Digilio MC, Sarkozy A, de Zorzi A, et al. LEOPARD syndrome: clinical diagnosis in the first year of life. Am J Med Genet 2006; 40:740–746.
23. Wilkes D, McDermott DA, Basson CT. Clinical phenotypes and molecular genetic mechanisms of Carney complex. Lancet Oncol 2005; 6:501–508.
24. Chong WS, Klanwarin W, Giam YC. Generalized lentiginosis in two children lacking systemic associations: case report and review of the literature. Pediatr Dermatol 2004; 21:39–45.
25. Landau M, Krafchick BR. The diagnostic value of café-au-lait macules. J Am Acad Dermatol 1999; 40:877–890.
26. Cohen JB, Janniger CK, Schwartz RA. Café-au-lait spots. Cutis 2000; 66:2224.
27. Nguyen JT, Yan AC, James WD. Large solitary café-au-lait spots: a report of 5 cases and review of the literature. Cutis 2004; 73:311–314.
28. Lumbruso S, Paris F, Sultan C. McCune-Albright syndrome: molecular genetics. J Pediatr Endocrinol Metab 2002; 15(Suppl 3):875–882.
29. Turner JT, Cohen MM Jr, Biesecker LG. Reassessment of the Proteus syndrome literature: application of diagnostic criteria. Am J Med Genet 2004; 130:111–122.
30. Cordova A. The mongolian spot: a study of ethnic differences and a literature review. Clin Pediatr 1981; 20:714–719.
31. Chan HH, Kono T. Nevus of Ota: clinical aspects and management. Skin Med 2003; 2:89–96.
32. Nehal KS, De Benito R, Orlow SJ. Analysis of 54 cases of hypopigmentation and hyperpigmentation along the lines of Blaschko. Arch Dermatol 1996; 132:1167–1170.
33. Bastiaens M, ter Huurne J, Gruis N, et al. The melanocortin-1-receptor gene is the major freckle gene. Hum Mol Genet 2001; 10:1701–1708.
34. Hartmann A, Hofmann UB, Hoehn H, et al. Postnatal confirmation of prenatally diagnosed trisomy 20 mosaicism in a patient with linear and whorled nevoid hypermelanosis. Pediatr Dermatol 2004; 21:636–641.
35. Chan HH, Kono T. The use of lasers and intense pulsed light sources for the treatment of pigmentary lesions. Skin Therapy Lett 2004; 9:5–7.
36. Tannous ZS, Mihm MC Jr, Sober AJ, Duncan LM. Congenital melanocytic nevi: clinical and histopathologic features, risk of melanoma, and clinical management. J Am Acad Dermatol. 2005; 52:197–203.
37. Swerdlow AJ, Green A. Melanocytic naevi and melanoma: an epidemiological perspective. Br J Dermatol. 1987; 117:137–46.
38. Plikaitis CM, David LR, Argenta LC. Neurocutaneous melanosis: clinical presentations. J Craniofac Surg. 2005; 16:921–5.
39. Giam YC, Williams ML, Leboit PE, et al. Neonatal erosions and ulcerations in giant congenital melanocytic nevi. Pediatr Dermatol. 1999; 16:354–8.
40. Schaffer JV, Orlow SJ, Lazova R, Bolognia JL. Speckled lentiginous nevus: within the spectrum of congenital melanocytic nevi. Arch Dermatol. 2001; 137:172–8.

41. English DR, Milne E, Simpson JA. Ultraviolet radiation at places of residence and the development of melanocytic nevi in children (Australia). Cancer Causes Control. 2006; 17:103–7.
42. Whiteman DC, Brown RM, Purdie DM, Hughes MC. Melanocytic nevi in very young children: the role of phenotype, sun exposure, and sun protection. J Am Acad Dermatol. 2005; 52:40–7.
43. Bauer J, Buttner P, Wiecker TS, et al. Risk factors of incident melanocytic nevi: a longitudinal study in a cohort of 1,232 young German children. Int J Cancer. 2005; 115:121–6.
44. Gallagher RP, Rivers JK, Yang CP, et al. Melanocytic nevus density in Asian, Indo-Pakistani, and white children: the Vancouver Mole Study. J Am Acad Dermatol. 1991; 25:507–12.
45. Bauer J, Garbe C. Acquired melanocytic nevi as risk factor for melanoma development. A comprehensive review of epidemiological data. Pigment Cell Res. 2003; 16:297–306.
46. Morelli JG, Weston WL. Sun, kids, moles, and melanoma. Contemp Pediatr 1999; 16:65–73.
47. Danarti R, Konig A, Salhi A,et al. Becker's nevus syndrome revisited. J Am Acad Dermatol. 2004; 51:965–9.
48. Lai C, Lockhart S, Mallory SB. Typical halo nevi in childhood: is a biopsy necessary? J Pediatr. 2001; 138:283–4.
49. Cesinaro AM, Foroni M, Sighinolfi P, et al. Spitz nevus is relatively frequent in adults: a clinico-pathologic study of 247 cases related to patient's age. Am J Dermatopathol. 2005; 27:469–75.
50. Huynh PM, Grant-Kels JM, Grin CM. Childhood melanoma: update and treatment. Int J Dermatol. 2005; 44:715–23.
51. Greene MH. The genetics of hereditary melanoma and nevi. Cancer. 1999; 86:2464–77.
52. Molven A, Grimstvedt MB, Steine SJ, et al. A large Norwegian family with inherited malignant melanoma, multiple atypical nevi, and CDK4 mutation. Genes Chromosomes Cancer. 2005; 44:10–18.
53. Pho L, Grossman D, Leachman SA. Melanoma genetics: a review of genetic factors and clinical phenotypes in familial melanoma. Curr Opin Oncol. 2006; 18:173–9.
54. Stuart CA, Driscoll MS, Lundquist KF, et al. Acanthosis nigricans. J Basic Clin Physiol Pharmacol. 1998; 9:407–18.
55. Grinstein G, Muzumdar R, Aponte L, Vuguin P, Saenger P, DiMartino-Nardi J. Presentation and 5-year follow-up of type 2 diabetes mellitus in African-American and Caribbean-Hispanic adolescents. Horm Res. 2003; 60:121–6.
56. Stoddart ML, Blevins KS, Lee ET, et al. Association of acanthosis nigricans with hyperinsulinemia compared with other selected risk factors for type 2 diabetes in Cherokee Indians: the Cherokee Diabetes Study. Diabetes Care. 2002; 25:1009–14.
57. Litonjua P, Pinero-Pilona A, Aviles-Santa L, Raskin P. Prevalence of acanthosis nigricans in newly-diagnosed type 2 diabetes. Endocr Pract. 2004; 10:101–6.
58. Bindler RM, Bruya MA. Evidence for identifying children at risk for being overweight, cardiovascular disease, and type 2 diabetes in primary care. J Pediatr Health Care. 2006; 20:82–7.
59. Torley D, Bellus GA, Munro CS. Genes, growth factors and acanthosis nigricans. Br J Dermatol. 2002; 147:1096–101.

Immobile and Hypermobile Skin

Certain skin changes are distinguished by palpation rather than by visual assessment of morphology. Skin mobility and elasticity are two qualities that are distinguished by this method.

Skin that is immobile is fixed to the underlying fascia and sometimes to muscle or bone. A growth or nodule that is fixed to the underlying fascia might indicate a malignant tumor in childhood. Far more common, however, are fibrous thickenings that attach the dermis to the fascia, as in the various types of morphea. Testing for this feature is performed by grasping the skin with the thumb and fore-finger and determining its movement. Hypermobile skin is often associated with hypermobile joints and brings to mind the various forms of the Ehlers-Danlos syndrome.

SKIN THICKENINGS

Skin may become thickened and immobile in certain areas. Nodules are not formed, but the thickened, slightly raised, or slightly depressed area can be appreciated on palpation.

MORPHEA

Clinical Features

Localized thickening of the skin should be called *morphea*. Rheumatologists use the term localized scleroderma,[1] but this can be confusing to patients and parents who search the internet and develop concern that their condition may be progressive systemic sclerosis. This causes the family undue worry. The classifications of morphea are listed in Box 18.1. Circumscribed areas of morphea may occur as solitary or multiple oval lesions, or as a linear lesion (Fig. 18.1).[1-3] The majority of children will have either linear or plaque-type morphea.[1-3] The mean age of development is approximately 7 years.[1] Females are more commonly affected.[1] Atrophy of an extremity, digital contracture, or facial hemiatrophy (Parry-Romberg syndrome) may occur (Fig. 18.2).[1-3] Linear lesions of the forehead often extend into the frontal scalp, producing a scarring hair loss (en coup de sabre) (Fig. 18.3).[1-3] En coup de sabre has been associated with ophthalmologic and neurologic abnormalities.[1,4] The immobile area will be exaggerated by having the child wrinkle the forehead. The surface of the immobile, bound-down skin of morphea is often shiny and hypopigmented (Fig. 18.4), and it may be surrounded by a violaceous hue (lilac) or a brown border (Fig. 18.5).[2,3] Guttate morphea may present with a depressed, dusky appearing, slightly thickened area that is not completely bound down (Fig. 18.6).[1-4] Large plaques and linear lesions may be seen (Figs 18.7–18.9). Some children have lesions of guttate morphea and linear morphea simultaneously. Concurrent lesions of morphea and lichen sclerosus (LS) have also been noted in childhood. About one-third of children with morphea have arthralgias.[2] ANA is positive in over 40% of patients, but these children do not develop SLE.[1] The eosinophil count may be elevated, especially in eosinophilic fasciitis.[1,3]

Deep morphea consists of subcutaneous morphea, eosinophilic fasciitis, and pansclerotic morphea. Subcutaneous morphea and eosinophilic fasciitis may represent the same entity. There is often diffuse thickening of the skin in an irregular surface pattern, leading to a 'lumpy-bumpy' skin appearance.[2,3] Children with eosinophilic fasciitis often progress to scleroderma-like fibrosis of the skin with sparing of distal areas.

Box 18.1 Classification of morphea

Plaque	Generalized
Guttate	Bullous
Linear	Deep
Nodular	Pan-Sclerotic

Fig. 18.1 Linear morphea (scleroderma). White, bound-down plaque extending down the left hand and fifth finger.

Fig. 18.2 Hyperpigmentation and facial atrophy.

Fig. 18.3 Linear scleroderma of the forehead in a child.

Fig. 18.4 Residual hypopigmentation following linear morphea on the leg.

Fig. 18.5 Lilac borders with white center of an 'active' lesion.

Differential Diagnosis

Lichen sclerosus has many features that overlap those of morphea, but its characteristic epidermal thinning and lichenoid papules help differentiate it from morphea. Atrophoderma may mimic morphea and is differentiated by the characteristic well-demarcated areas with cliff-drop borders, which are usually seen on the trunk. Progressive systemic sclerosis is rare in childhood and usually presents with severe acral and orofacial sclerosis.[3]

The dusky lesions of early morphea often appear slightly depressed, and only with the evolution of lesions such that some become 'bound down' will the diagnosis be certain. An excisional skin biopsy down to and including fascia may be diagnostic.

Fig. 18.7 Morphea on child's abdomen. Note lilac-colored border, brownish areas, and white areas within the same lesion.

Fig. 18.6 Slightly depressed, tan, slightly bound-down lesions of early morphea.

Fig. 18.8 Linear morphea on back of neck of adolescent boy.

Fig. 18.9 Linear morphea on submandibular skin.

Pathogenesis

The mechanism of the disease is unknown, but it is thought to be of autoimmune nature and the debate over the role of *Borrelia burgdorferi* infection continues.[5–8] An inflammatory stage precedes the sclerotic stage and is characterized by a predominantly lymphocytic infiltrate around dermal blood vessels and collagen bundles. In the sclerotic stage, thickened dermal collagen replaces the subcutaneous fat. Injury to the underlying muscle fibers, with separation and inflammation of muscle, occurs in linear forms. In eosinophilic fasciitis, thickening and inflammation of the fascia is diagnostic.[3] The inflammation often demonstrates an excess of eosinophils. Fibrous replacement of the subcutaneous fat may be minimal.

Treatment

There is no specific treatment. Topical calcipotriene ointment, with and without occlusion; topical imiquimod; UVA1, alone or in combination with calcipotriene ointment; low-dose broad-band UVA; PUVA;

methotrexate; and systemic steroids have all been demonstrated to be effective treatments.[3,9–15] Physical therapy may be of benefit in linear morphea. There are no comparative treatment studies.

Patient Education

The duration of lesion activity is 3–5 years, followed by softening of the skin. Residual pigmentary changes may last several years longer.[1–3] Atrophy of the limbs or facial hemiatrophy will persist.

Follow-up Visits

Examination at 3-month intervals is useful to determine whether systemic symptoms or signs have appeared.

Fig. 18.10 Lichen sclerosus (LS) of a child's vulva.

LICHEN SCLEROSUS

Clinical Features

The white papules and immobile plaques of LS occur primarily in the anogenital area in grade-school age or

Fig. 18.11 Hemorrhagic areas within vulvar LS. Mistaken for child abuse.

Fig. 18.12 Extragenital LS of the neck. Telangiectasia and fine wrinkling within the white area.

Fig. 18.13 White patch of LS on neck of adolescent girl.

adolescent girls.[16,17] LS is 5–10 times more common in girls (Fig. 18.10).[16,17] Purpura, vesicles, and telangiectasia may be seen within the plaques in the genital area (Fig.18.11). As the lesions age, the skin surface becomes thinned and finely wrinkled. Bleeding may occur.[16,18] Ulcerations and excoriations may be superimposed on these primary lesions. The anogenital lesions in girls tend to surround both the vulva and the anus in a figure-eight pattern.[16,17] Itching and burning of the skin are frequent complaints. Painful defecation, constipation, bloody stools, and encopresis may be reported.[16,17]

Extragenital lesions appear as asymptomatic white papules on the upper back or upper chest (Figs 18.12, 18.13) and occasionally on the face or extremities.[16] About one-fourth of patients with anogenital lesions will also have distal extragenital lesions. The isomorphic phenomenon occurs in LS, and lesions may develop in surgical scars or other sites of skin trauma. Coexistence of LS with morphea is observed in children.[2] Familial cases have been documented, and it may be useful to examine siblings or parents.[16]

Differential Diagnosis

Skin immobility suggests localized scleroderma, but the atrophic wrinkled epidermis, the white color, and papular lesions help distinguish it from scleroderma. Anogenital lesions may be confused with sexual abuse, and abuse investigations may be incorrectly initiated.[16] In LS, the hymen is never involved, whereas it may reveal injury in sexual abuse. Also, candidiasis, intertrigo, or irritant dermatitis may be confused with LS. Atrophic areas of lichen planus may mimic LS, but the purple papular border of lichen planus is a useful differentiating feature.

Pathogenesis

In LS, the dermis is sclerotic and thickened and the epidermis is thinned and atrophic.[16] A bandlike accumulation of lymphocytes is present in the mid-dermis, and features of epidermal injury are also seen. Atrophy of the epidermis and hydropic degeneration of the basal epidermal cells are present.[16] Hyperkeratosis occurs, so that the stratum corneum layer is much thicker than the remainder of the epidermis.[16] Edema and homogenization of collagen in the upper dermis are also seen. As the lesions progress, the collagen of the lower dermis thickens, mimicking

circumscribed morphea. The mechanism of this inflammatory disease is unknown.

Treatment

Without treatment the majority of patients will improve symptomatically by puberty but symptoms may recur intermittently throughout life.[16,17,19] There is no specific treatment, but superpotent topical glucocorticosteroid ointments applied two times daily for 2 weeks will improve symptoms and clinical appearance.[16,17,19] Repeat 2-week courses of superpotent topical steroids may be used if symptoms return. Topical tacrolimus and pimecrolimus have also been used.[20,21] Topical lubricants may relieve the symptoms. Cleanliness of the anogenital area is useful in preventing superimposed infection. For bleeding telangiectatic vessels, the vascular-specific pulsed dye laser at 585 nm has been useful.[18]

Patient Education

It is helpful to explain to patients that the course of LS is irregularly progressive, although lesions may remain stable for long periods. The clinician should emphasize that by puberty most children will have spontaneous improvement.[16,17,19] Patients should be informed that areas of whitish thickening (leukoplakia) may appear on the mucosa or adjacent mucosal surfaces, and that these may progress to carcinoma. Carcinomas have been reported in childhood, but they are exceedingly rare.[22]

Follow-up Visits

Yearly examinations are useful to monitor the progress of the disease and examine lesions for possible malignant changes, which require biopsy.

EHLERS-DANLOS SYNDROME
Clinical Features

Ehlers-Danlos syndrome (EDS) is a phenotype in which there is excessive stretching of skin and joints.[15–18] Six different subtypes of Ehlers-Danlos syndrome have been described, with most forms having autosomal dominant inheritance (Table 18.1).[23–25] The increase in skin stretchability is often spectacular; however, the skin returns to its normal position (Figs 18.14, 18.15). Skin fragility is a major problem,

Table 18.1 Subtypes of Ehlers-Danlos syndrome and their clinical features

Subtype	Old name	Inheritance	Skin/joints	Other	Gene defect
Classical	Gravis type I Mitis type II	AD	Hyperextensible, lax skin and joints	Hernias, scars, varicosities	Col 5A1 or 5A2
Hypermobility	Hypermobile type III	AD	Hyperextensible, lax hands and feet		Col 1A2 or 3A1
Vascular	Arterial-ecchymotic type IV	AD	Pale, thin, prominent veins, ecchymoses	Bowel and/or aortic rupture	Col 3A1
Kyphoscoliosis	Ocular-sclerotic type VI	AR	Hyperextensible skin, lax joints	Ocular globe rupture	Lysyl hydroxylase
Arthrochalasia	Arthro-chalasia multiplex congenita type VIIA and type VIIB	AD	Lax joints, congenital hip dislocation	Bruising	Col 1A1 or 1A2
Dermatosparaxis	Dermato-spraxis type VIIC	AR	Skin fragility, sagging skin	Premature fetal membrane rupture	Procol I n-terminal peptidase

AD, Autosomal dominant; AR, autosomal recessive.

Fig. 18.14 Hyperextensible, lax joints of a child with Ehlers-Danlos syndrome I.

Fig. 18.15 Hyperextensible, lax joints of an adolescent with Ehlers-Danlos syndrome I.

and slow healing is very common.[23–25] Skin injury often results in large hematomas that heal with a fibrotic nodule covered by thin, wrinkled epidermis. These are usually prominent over the lower part of the legs (Figs 18.16, 18.17). These nodules may calcify. Wound dehiscence is observed in at least one-third of these lesions (Fig. 18.18). Easily visible veins and epistaxis are also noted. Hyperextensible joints may result in subluxation of the joints, particularly of the shoulders, elbows, hips, and knees (see Fig. 18.14). Flat feet, kyphosis, and scoliosis may occur. Back pain may become a problem with age, and weakness, muscle cramps, and arthritis may eventuate.[26] Jaw pain or jaw clicking is common.[26]

Fig. 18.16 Large 'fish mouth' scars on the knees of a child with Ehlers-Danlos type I.

Fig. 18.18 Poorly healing wound on leg of child with Ehlers-Danlos.

Fig. 18.17 Purple-brown skin on leg of child with Ehlers-Danlos type I.

Other symptoms vary depending on type. The vascular type is the most symptomatic. Hematemesis and bleeding in the lower intestine may occur. Menorrhagia may be seen. Aortic aneurysms and rupture, arteriovenous fistula, retinal detachment, lens abnormalities, and myopia have been described.[23–25] Premature births and miscarriages are common.

Differential Diagnosis

The hyperextensible skin is characteristic and usually is not confused with other disorders.

Pathogenesis

The common problem in all six subtypes is faulty formation of collagen.[23–25] Because collagen limits the stretchability of skin, joints, and blood vessels, defect-ive collagen results in hyperextensible skin and joints and fragile blood vessels. The genetic defects have now been identified for all six types of Ehlers-Danlos (see Table 18.1). Autosomal recessive tenascin x abnormalities have been demonstrated to cause an EDS phenotype although abnormal scarring is not present.[27]

Treatment

Protective measures to prevent skin trauma, particularly during the toddler stage, are most useful. Pediatric orthopedic and ophthalmologic care is recommended. Otherwise, no satisfactory treatment is available.

Patient Education

Informed genetic counseling should be given if a parent is affected. The expectation of premature birth should be emphasized. The skeletal and eye difficulties that may occur as the child grows should also be stressed.

Follow-up Visits

Yearly ophthalmologic and orthopedic examinations are recommended.

REFERENCES

1. Zulian F, Athreya BH, Laxer R, et al. Juvenile localized scleroderma: clinical and epidemiological features in 750 children. An international study. Rheumatology 2005; 45(1):614–620.
2. Krafchik BR. Localized morphea in children. Adv Exp Med Biol 1999; 455:49.
3. Nelson AM. Localized scleroderma including morphea, linear scleroderma and eosinophilic fasciitis. Curr Probl Pediatr 1996; 26:318.
4. Drolet B. Linear scleroderma en coup de sabre with associated neurologic abnormalities. Pediatrics 2005; 2006; 117(1):e132–e136.
5. Salpietro DC, Merlino MV, Bruglia S, et al. Linear scleroderma 'en coup de sabre' associated with facial atropy in a patient seropositive of *Borrelia burgdorferi*: a true case or molecular mimicry. Pediatr Allergy Immunol 2004; 15:570.
6. Weide B, Schittek B, Klyscz T, et al. Morphea is neither associated with features of *Borrelia burgdorferi* infection, nor is this agent detectable in skin lesions by polymerase chain reaction, Br J Dermatol 2000; 143:780.
7. Ozkan S, Atabey N, Fetil E, et al. Evidence for *Borrelia burgdorferi* in morphea and lichen sclerosus. Int J Dermatol 2000; 39:278.
8. Weide B, Walz T, Garbe C. Is morphea caused by *Borrelia burgdorferi*? A review. Br J Dermatol 2000; 142:636.
9. Dytoc M, Ting PT, Man J, et al. First case series on the use of imiquimod for morphea. Br J Dermatol 2005; 153:815.
10. Kreuter A, Gambichler T, Avermaete A, et al. Combined treatment with calcipotriol ointment and low-dose ultraviolet A1 phototherapy in childhood morphea. Pediatr Dermatol 2001; 18:241.
11. Cunninghan BB, Landells ID, Langman C, et al. Topical calcipotriene for morphea/linear scleroderma. J Am Acad Dermatol 1998; 39:211.
12. Gruss CJ, Von Kobletzki G, Behrens-Williams SC, et al. Effects of low-dose ultraviolet A-1 phototherapy on morphea. Photodermatol Photoimmumol Photomed 2001; 4:149–155.
13. Stege H, Berneburg M, Humke S, et al. High-dose UVA1 radiation therapy for localized scleroderma. J Am Acad Dermatol 1997; 36:938.
14. El-Mofty M, Zaher H, Bosselia M, et al. Low-dose broad-band UVA in morphea using a new method for evaluation. Photodermatol Photoimmunol Photomed 2000; 16:43.
15. Kershcer M, Meurer M, Sander C, et al. PUVA bath photochemotherapy for localized scleroderma. Evaluation of 17 consecutive patients. Arch Dermatol 1996; 132:1280–1282.
16. Powell JJ, Wojnarowska F. Childhood vulvar lichen sclerosus: an increasingly common problem. J Am Acad Dermatol 2001; 44:803.
17. Powell JJ, Wojnarowska F. Lichen sclerosus. Lancet 1999; 353:1777.
18. Rabinowitz LG. Lichen sclerosus et atrophicus treatment with the 585-nm flashlamp-pumped pulsed dye laser. Arch Dermatol 1993; 129:381.
19. Powell J, Wojnarowska F. Childhood vulvar lichen sclerosus. The course after puberty. J Reprod Med 2002; 47:706.
20. Bohm M, Frieling U, Luger TA, et al. Successful treatment of anogenital lichen sclerosus with topical tacrolimus. Arch Dermatol 2004; 140:1169.
21. Boms S, Gambichler T, Freitag M, et al. Pimecrolimus 1% cream for anogenital lichen sclerosus in childhood. BMC Dermatol 2004; 14:14.
22. Carlson JA, et al. Vulvar lichen sclerosus and squamous cell carcinoma: a cohort, case control, and investigational study with historical perspective; implications for chronic inflammation and sclerosis in the development of neoplasia. Human Pathol 1998; 29:932.
23. Hamel BCJ. Ehlers-Danlos syndrome. Netherland J Med 2004; 62:140.
24. Reichel JL, et al. What syndrome is this? Pediatr Dermatol 2001; 18:156.
25. Mao J-R, Bristow J. The Ehlers-Danlos syndrome: on beyond collagens. J Clin Invest 2001; 107:1063.
26. Stanitski DF, et al. Orthopaedic manifestations of EhlersDanlos syndrome. Clin Ortho Related Res 2000; 376:213.
27. Bristow J, Carey W, Egging D, et al. Tenascin-X, collagen, elastin and the Ehlers-Danlos syndrome. Am J Gent C Semin Med Genet 2005; 15:139.

Genodermatoses

There are hundreds of hereditary skin diseases, and the discussion of all of them is beyond the scope of this textbook. Several of the common genodermatoses are considered in other chapters: the neurocutaneous disorders in Chapter 17, genetic nail disorders in Chapter 16, genetic hair disorders in Chapter 15, photodermatoses in Chapter 10, and vascular lesions in Chapter 14. There are uncommon types of hereditary skin diseases that may be encountered in practice. Comprehensive textbooks and atlases may assist diagnosis of less common skin disorders.[1,2] In addition, access is available to large databases of genetic mutations[3] and laboratories, which can confirm the specific mutation.[4,5]

More common conditions are considered here because they are important in the differential diagnosis and they are life-long problems for the affected individuals. Included in this chapter are the disorders of keratinization, including the ichthyoses and Darier's disease, the mechanobullous diseases, and ectodermal dysplasias. Acrodermatitis enteropathica is also included in this chapter, although it is separate from the three major categories.

ICHTHYOSIS

Ichthyosis is a term used to describe excessive scaling of the skin, which may be 'fish scale like.'[6] Although normal infants born after 40–42 weeks of gestation will display some thin scales and mild peeling of skin, as will the postmature infant, the scaling in the forms of ichthyosis is usually generalized and the scales are thick. At least 15 different genes have been associated with ichthyosis[6–8] and more may be found in the future. The genes affecting ichthyosis control structural proteins, lipid metabolism, protein catabolism, peroxisomal transport and processing, and DNA repair.[6] Four major hereditary types of ichthyosis will be described below. Lamellar and bullous types of ichthyosis usually present at birth with severe scaling. Ichthyosis vulgaris and X-linked ichthyosis may be present in the neonate or may present later in childhood. Harlequin ichthyosis is a severe but extremely rare form of ichthyosis where infants are born with severe ichthyosis associated with 'armor-like' thick yellow plates of scale separated by deep red fissures.[9–11] Ichthyosis may also present at birth with an infant who is born with a shiny, translucent membrane called a collodion membrane (see Ch. 21).[6]

Clinical Features

Ichthyosis vulgaris

Ichthyosis vulgaris is inherited as a semidominant disease that may be as frequent as 1 in 250 individuals.[7] In a semidominant disease an individual with a mutation on one allele may have a less severe disease than an individual with mutations on both alleles. Fine scales usually become prominent by 6 months to 1 year of age.[12] The scales are most prominent over the lower legs (Figs 19.1, 19.2), trunk (Fig. 19.3), and buttocks. Dry, follicular, horny plugs (keratosis pilaris) are present on the extensor extremities and may be widespread. Palms and soles show an increased number of skin creases. The entire skin surface is dry. Water retention by the stratum corneum is minimal.[13] Some children may have associated atopic dermatitis.[14] The skin in ichthyosis vulgaris usually remains normal throughout the newborn period.

X-Linked ichthyosis

X-linked ichthyosis may appear at birth but usually presents in infancy with scales over the posterior

Fig. 19.2 Ichthyosis vulgaris. Prominent scales over the lower legs in a 12-year-old.

Fig. 19.1 Ichthyosis vulgaris. Scales over the lower legs in a toddler.

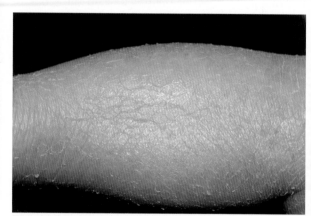

Fig. 19.3 Ichthyosis vulgaris. Fine scales on infant's arm.

Fig. 19.4 X-Linked ichthyosis. Darkened scales with sparing of antecubital fossa.

Fig. 19.5 X-linked ichthyosis. Large, dark, platelike scales on arm.

neck, upper trunk, and extensor surfaces of the extremities.[12] As the child ages, the scales often become thicker and a dirty-yellow or brown color (Figs 19.4, 19.5). The antecubital and popliteal fossae may be spared (see Fig. 19.4). Scaling is usually mild during the first 30 days of life, and the skin is a normal color.

Palms and soles are spared, in contrast to the other forms of ichthyosis. The incidence is thought to be in the range of 1 in 2000–9500 males.[6] The cause for this disorder is a mutation in the enzyme steroid sulfatase, which is localized to the distal short arm of the X chromosome.[6] The mother of an infant with X-linked ichthyosis may fail to initiate or progress in her labor because the steroid sulfatase deficiency in the fetal placenta will cause low levels of estrogen.[15]

Lamellar ichthyosis and congenital nonbullous ichthyosiform erythroderma

Both lamellar ichthyosis and congenital nonbullous ichthyosiform erythroderma are most commonly autosomal recessive traits. Two separate clinical disease entities exist which are caused by at least five different genes.[6,12] Individuals with nonbullous congenital ichthyosiform erythroderma have generalized fine scales on erythematous skin. Those with lamellar ichthyosis have larger, darker, platelike scales, with or without erythematous skin (Figs 19.6, 19.7). Patients with lamellar ichthyosis have been associated with a gene defect in transglutaminase-1 gene (TGM-1) or a ATP-binding casette transporter gene, ABCA12.[6] Congenital nonbullous ichthyosiform erythroderma can also be associated with the TGM-1 gene as well as genes associated with lipoxygenase genes ALOX12 and ALOXE3 or additional genes.[6] With either condition, the affected baby can be born with a collodion membrane, and the two conditions may not be able to be distinguished in neonates.[12] Severe water and electrolyte imbalance may develop.[16] The erythroderma may fade during childhood in some infants (Fig. 19.8). Ectropion and eclabium may be present at birth or appear shortly after in patients with lamellar

Fig. 19.6 Lamellar ichthyosis. Thickened, shiny skin without erythema in child.

Fig. 19.8 Lamellar ichthyosis versus epidermolytic hyperkeratosis.

Fig. 19.7 Lamellar ichthyosis. Thickened scales in scalp and shiny, thickened skin of ear and face in toddler.

ichthyosis.[12] The palms and soles in these patients may be greatly thickened. Skin biopsy after the collodion membrane is shed will demonstrate hyperkeratosis but is otherwise not diagnostic.[12]

Fig. 19.9 Epidermolytic hyperkeratosis. Hyperkeratosis of palms and deep fissures of creases.

Fig. 19.10 Epidermolytic hyperkeratosis. Thickened, malodorous skin on legs and ankles.

Bullous ichthyosis (congenital bullous ichthyosiform erythroderma, epidermolytic hyperkeratosis)

Epidermolytic hyperkeratosis, an autosomal dominant disorder, is characterized by extensive scaling at birth, erythroderma, and recurrent episodes of bullae formation (Figs 19.9–19.11). Epidermolytic hyperkeratosis is caused by a defect in the suprabasal epidermis causing aggregation of keratins K1 and K10.[6,8,17] The blisters represent lysis of the epidermal granular layer, and secondary infection with *Staphylococcus aureus* becomes a major difficulty in the neonatal period and during infancy. As the child ages, the involvement becomes more limited in extent. By school age, thick, warty, dirty-yellow scales with malodorous excessive bacterial colonization of the skin will have developed on the palms, soles, elbows, and knees. Skin biopsy will reveal enlargement of the granular cell layer with bizarre vacuolization of the epidermal granular cells.[12] A related autosomal dominant condition called *bullous ichthyosis of Siemens* demonstrates similar but milder findings, with more superficial bullae and is associated with defects in keratin K2e.[8,17] Widespread epidermal nevi that show pathologic changes of epidermolytic hyperkeratosis (EHK), such as ichthyosis hystrix and systematized epidermal nevi, may show histologic changes similar to EHK.[18] These nevi may represent mosaicism for epidermolytic hyperkeratosis, with the affected skin showing the gene mutation for keratins K1 or K10 and the unaffected intervening skin displaying normal keratins.[18]

Differential Diagnosis

At birth, lamellar and bullous types of ichthyosis may be difficult to distinguish from one another. The hereditary pattern and skin biopsy may help. If an indi-

Fig. 19.11 Epidermolytic hyperkeratosis.

vidual with ichthyosis has corneal opacities and sparing of the palms and soles, the diagnosis is likely to be X-linked ichthyosis. If an ectropion and eclabium are present, it is likely to be lamellar ichthyosis; and recurrent bullous episodes will distinguish epidermolytic hyperkeratosis. Measurement of steroid sulfatase activity may be useful in the diagnosis of X-linked ichthyosis.

Ichthyosis vulgaris in its mild form may be difficult to distinguish from dry skin, but the extensive distribution of scales, particularly scaling over the buttocks and lower legs, increased palmar creases, and skin biopsy will differentiate ichthyosis vulgaris from dry skin. Scaling disorders with the appearance of ichthyosis can be associated with many disorders.[6]

Pathogenesis

The clinical presentation and skin biopsy may be able to group the patient into a specific diagnostic category of ichthyosis. In ichthyosis vulgaris there is a thin or absent granular cell layer in addition to the hyperkeratosis. X-linked ichthyosis demonstrates hyperkeratosis with an otherwise normal-appearing epidermis. Vacuolization and separation of the granular cell layer with blister cavity formation are associated with the hyperkeratosis in bullous ichthyosis. Similar findings in the more superficial epidermis are found in bullous ichthyosis of Siemens. Lamellar ichthyosis may demonstrate hyperkeratosis, acanthosis, and a mild chronic inflammatory infiltrate.

Molecular diagnosis may accurately confirm the diagnosis, if available.[3-5] Classification of the specific disease, the expected severity of the disease and the genetic transmission of the disease may be important if the parents are considering additional children. Although we have recently gained increased knowledge about the molecular defects in many of the ichthyoses, we are currently unable to direct therapy based upon the protein or enzyme defect.

Treatment

There is no satisfactory treatment for the ichthyosis. In ichthyosis vulgaris and X-linked ichthyosis, hydration of the skin twice daily and the generous use of lubricants will control the dryness and scaling. The use of alpha-hydroxy acids such as lactic acid 5% ointment or 12% ammonium lactate lotion applied once or more daily may be helpful in the more severe ichthyoses, although many patients do as well with bland lubricants alone. In bullous ichthyoses, systemic antistaphylococcal antibiotics are required to treat the infectious episodes.

In ichthyosis, great caution must be used in applying therapy to the skin of an affected infant or child. Because of the larger surface area per body weight, systemic toxicity and side effects can be seen and acidosis can occur secondary to topical therapy. The clinician should recognize that both the active medication and the vehicle for the medication could cause significant toxicity in the infant with ichthyosis.

The synthetic retinoids given orally have shown promise in management of ichthyosis, but their use is restricted by long-term effects on growing bones.[19,20]

Patient Education

The genetic nature of the ichthyoses and the methods of controlling these disorders should be emphasized to the family by the clinician. Good supportive relationships should be established with these patients. Genetic documentation of the specific defects may currently help in future family planning and in the future for specific gene-based therapies.

Follow-up Visits

A visit 1 week after discharge from the newborn nursery is useful in evaluating therapy. Thereafter, routine visits for pediatric care and additional visits may be necessary depending on the severity of the ichthyosis.

NETHERTON'S SYNDROME

Netherton's syndrome is a severe, autosomal recessive disorder characterized by congenital ichthyosis with defective cornification. These children have a specific hair shaft defect (trichorrhexis invaginata, or 'bamboo hair') (see Ch. 15, Figs 15.15, 15.16) and severe atopic manifestations including atopic derma-

Fig. 19.12 Netherton's syndrome. Red, scaly skin of child's arm.

Fig. 19.13 Netherton's syndrome. Short broken hairs and red scaly skin.

titis and hay fever, with high serum IgE levels and hypereosinophilia (Figs. 19.12, 19.13). In addition, infants with Netherton's syndrome may have severe failure to thrive, infections, and hypernatremic dehydration, which result in high postnatal mortality. The genetic cause of this disease is a mutation in SPINK5, which encodes the serine protease inhibitor LEKTI.[21] SPINK5 appears to play a critical role in epidermal barrier function and the extent of serine proteinase activation correlates with the degree of barrier dysfunction.[22]

Fig.19.14 Epidermolysis bullosa simplex, Weber-Cockayne type. Minor trauma on playground equipment induced blisters of the palms.

EPIDERMOLYSIS BULLOSA

Epidermolysis bullosa is a term used to describe a group of inherited skin conditions associated with blister formation after mild trauma. This condition can be associated with defects of many different proteins present at the junction of the dermis and epidermis or within the epidermis or dermis. The severity of the disease may be associated with not only the specific proteins involved, but also the specific mutation associated with the gene encoding that protein. Epidermolysis bullosa can be divided into nonscarring and scarring types. The nonscarring types include those with intraepidermal separation and junctional separation, whereas the scarring (dystrophic) form includes the subepidermal types. The disease is uncommon but potentially life-threatening to newborns and infants. Correct diagnosis in the newborn period can be difficult and depends on a combination of clinical, histologic, and molecular biology techniques.[23-25] In all forms of epidermolysis bullosa, evolution of clinical lesions during the first 30 days of life may make the diagnosis difficult. A family history of childhood blistering diseases is often absent, and the clinician must depend on the findings in the affected baby.[23,25] Extreme care must be taken to obtain a biopsy of an induced blister and not an old or established blister. Induction of a blister with a pencil eraser or a suction device is the most reliable method.[23] Optimally, the biopsy specimen should be examined by immunofluorescent mapping, and electron microscopy can be used to confirm the diagnosis.[23]

Clinical Features

Nonscarring types of epidermolysis bullosa

Epidermolysis bullosa simplex: Epidermolysis bullosa simplex is dominantly inherited and may be generalized or localized.[23,25] The most common form is localized to the hands and feet (Figs 19.14, 19.15) and often is not present at birth. This form, which causes recurrent blisters on the hands and feet, is called Weber-Cockayne disease. Blisters of the hands and feet first occur in late childhood or adolescence,

Fig. 19.15 Epidermolysis bullosa simplex, Weber-Cockayne type.

Fig. 19.16 Epidermolysis bullosa simplex, Weber-Cockayne type. Painful blisters on the foot of a child after a run.

Fig. 19.17 Epidermolysis bullosa simplex, Koebner type. Discrete blisters on a toddler's foot.

Fig. 19.18 Epidermolysis bullosa simplex, Dowling-Meara type. Grouped blisters on the leg of a child.

Fig. 19.19 Epidermolysis bullosa simplex, Dowling-Meara type. Grouped blisters on the arm of a child.

when the child experiences minor frictional trauma (Fig. 19.16). It often has its onset in warm weather.

Epidermolysis bullosa simplex may also be generalized, with lesions present at birth or, more likely, the appearance of blisters at 6–12 months of age.[23,25] These lesions are more numerous on the distal extremities but may also be seen on elbows and knees.

The condition is autosomal dominant and worsens in warm weather. In the Koebner type of generalized epidermolysis bullosa simplex, the lesions are discrete

Fig. 19.20 Junctional epidermolysis bullosa. Newborn with a few scattered blisters.

Fig. 19.22 Junctional epidermolysis bullosa. Nonhealing granulation tissue at blister site on child's ear.

Fig. 19.21 Junctional epidermolysis bullosa. Severe oral erosions in an infant.

Fig. 19.23 Scarring (dystrophic) epidermolysis bullosa. Hemorrhagic bulla.

epidermolysis bullosa are recognized.[23,25] Both will present at birth with very few lesions (Fig. 19.20). Mucous membrane lesions appear within the first month of life in the lethal form and are absent or minimal in the milder form. Oral mucosa becomes severely affected in the lethal form (Fig. 19.21), interfering with eating and often resulting in failure to thrive.[23,25] Nonhealing granulation tissue may develop over bony prominences such as the spine, ear, or midface (Fig. 19.22) [23,25] Secondary bacterial infection can be severe. The majority of lesions heal without scarring, but lateral extension of large bullae can result in hemorrhage and healing with scarring.

Scarring (dystrophic) forms of epidermolysis bullosa

In epidermolysis bullosa of the recessive dystrophic type, hemorrhagic bullae appear on the skin at birth

(Fig. 19.17), and in the Dowling-Meara type they are grouped (Figs 19.18, 19.19).[23,25]

Junctional epidermolysis bullosa: A generalized, often fatal form (Herlitz) and a milder form of junctional

Fig. 19.24 Scarring (dystrophic) epidermolysis bullosa. Hemorrhagic bulla.

Fig. 19.25 Dystrophic epidermolysis bullosa, recessive. Hemorrhagic blister on newborn.

Fig. 19.26 Recessive dystrophic epidermolysis bullosa. Multiple white milia at border of scar.

Fig. 19.27 Recessive dystrophic epidermolysis bullosa. Missing toenails and scarring.

or shortly after (Fig. 19.23).[25] Removal of the blister roof leaves a raw, bleeding base that heals with scar formation (Figs 19.24, 19.25). Healing scars often entrap islands of epithelium, producing milia that appear as tiny white cysts within scars (Figs 19.26, 19.27).[23,25] Scarring is sufficiently severe to result in replacement of nails and pseudowebbing of all digits, leading eventually to a clublike appearance of hands and feet (Fig. 19.28).[25] Scarring alopecia of the scalp will develop. Severe scarring of the eyelid may occur.[25] Blisters and erosions of the oral mucosa result in limitation of eating, immobilization of the tongue, and esophageal stricture with resultant dysphagia in 76% of cases.[25] Laryngeal bullae will produce respiratory stridor.[25] The teeth may be malformed and carious (Fig. 19.29). Anemia caused by chronic blood loss and malnutrition occurs, and failure to thrive will commonly develop.[25] Secondary bacterial or candidal infection of the skin is frequent. In adolescent years,

squamous cell carcinoma may arise in atrophic scars of the skin (Fig. 19.30) or in leukoplakic areas of the mucous membranes.[23,25]

In epidermolysis bullosa of the dominant dystrophic type, hemorrhagic bullae are seen at birth, and erosions caused by intrauterine blister formation may be observed at delivery.[23,25] Intrauterine erosions are frequently found over the dorsa of the feet and the anterior lower legs. As the child ages, atrophic scars and milia appear (Fig. 19.31). Mucous membrane involvement is less common than in the recessive dystrophic type and when present is quite mild.[25] Ichthyosis, keratosis pilaris, thickened nails, and hyperhidrosis may develop. Nails may be shed and replaced by scars (Fig. 19.32), but pseudowebbing does not occur.[25] Scarring alopecia is absent, and anemia and failure to thrive are rarely seen.[25]

A variant, also dominantly inherited, characterized by white atrophic lesions without clinical blister for-

Fig. 19.28 Recessive dystrophic epidermolysis bullosa. Loss of toenails, pseudowebbing of digits, and new blisters.

Fig. 19.29 Recessive dystrophic epidermolysis bullosa. Loss of teeth and restriction of mouth opening in child.

Fig. 19.30 Recessive dystrophic epidermolysis bullosa. Huge verrucous growth on hand of adolescent represents squamous cell carcinoma.

Fig. 19.31 Dominant dystrophic epidermolysis bullosa. Blister, scar formation, milia, and loss of a fingernail in infant.

Fig. 19.32 Dominant dystrophic epidermolysis bullosa. Loss of toenails, active blisters, but no pseudowebbing in adolescent.

Fig. 19.33 Gene mutations in epidermolysis bullosa. (From Marinkovich MP. Protein–protein interactions at the dermal–epidermal BMZ. In: Barker J, McGrath J, eds. Cell adhesion and migration in skin disease. Amsterdam: Harwood Academic Publishers; 2001.)

mation, is called albopapuloid form.[25] Numerous milia and hypopigmented scars are seen, predominantly on the trunk rather than the extremities.

Differential Diagnosis

The ease of blistering skin by suction or friction will differentiate epidermolysis bullosa from friction blisters or spontaneous blistering disease.[23,25] At birth, obstetric injuries are frequently confused because of the hemorrhagic blisters and eroded, raw areas. Urinary uroporphyrins will distinguish porphyria cutanea tarda from epidermolysis bullosa. The forms of epidermolysis bullosa may be differentiated from one another by the inheritance pattern, with a skin biopsy specimen examined by electron microscopy, or by molecular genetic analysis.[23,25]

Pathogenesis

The mechanism of epidermolysis bullosa is known to be due to gene mutations encoding structural proteins: keratin 5, keratin 14, or plectin in epidermolysis bullosa simplex; laminin 5, BP180, or α6β4 integrin in junctional epidermolysis bullosa and collagen VII in dystrophic forms of epidermolysis bullosa (Fig. 19.33).[23,25] They are distinguished by ultrastructural examination of the skin biopsy specimen. Recurrent bullous eruption of the hands and feet demonstrates a separation of epidermal cells just above the basal layer. Epidermolysis bullosa simplex separates the basal cells within the basal layer. In junctional epidermolysis bullosa, the separation occurs just below the plasma membrane of the basal cells and above the basal lamina of the dermis.[23–25] The scarring forms show a separation below the basal lamina in the dermis. In epidermolysis bullosa dystrophica, recessive type, the anchoring fibrils, which support the basal lamina, are missing.[23–25]

The severity and clinical presentation of the different types of epidermolysis bullosa not only depend on the specific gene involved but also specific mutations on that gene. Mutations in the evolutionarily conserved regions of the gene may produce more severe clinical disease than mutations that do not involve the conserved region. This is specifically seen in epidermolysis bullosa-Dowling-Meara, in which the mutations are in the highly conserved region of the keratin genes.[23-25] Patients who have premature termination type of mutations usually have more severe disease than those patients that have structural mutations of the same gene.[23,24]

Treatment

Treatment is symptomatic and supportive.[23,25] Several epidermolysis bullosa pediatric dermatology centers have developed across the United States. Each center has teams of physicians and support personnel who are knowledgeable about caring for children with the multiple complications of epidermolysis bullosa. One of the centers for epidermolysis bullosa may be consulted for a comprehensive care program. For the scarring and junctional forms, skilled nursing and general healthcare are required. For the newborn infant, small, frequent feedings with a soft nipple are indicated. Gentle handling; aggressive lubrication to prevent friction; soft, loose-fitting clothing; gentle sponge baths; cotton diapers; and a sheepskin pad for the crib should be instituted. Large blisters can be opened with sterile scissors and the roof allowed to collapse by gently compressing out the fluid. Blisters and erosions should have a topical lubricant applied gently to the surface to accelerate healing and prevent additional friction to the area.

For infants and children, a passive physical therapy program should be instituted. Water beds, egg-crate padding, or sheepskin is useful for sleep. Keeping the room cool will reduce blistering and the accompanying pruritus. Wound dressings may be useful for large nonhealing erosions. Keratinocyte-cultured autografts have been successful in severe nonhealing areas.[26] If anemia is present, vitamin supplements, iron, or transfusions may be required. Protein and caloric requirements may be twice that recommended for size because of ongoing skin or mucosal losses. Fluids should be lukewarm, and acidic juices should be avoided. Nutritional supplements or possibly a gastrostomy tube may be considered. Wholegrain breads and cereals may reduce constipation, which can be a major problem. A multidisciplinary approach is required in the scarring forms to deal with problems such as esophageal strictures, dental disease, pseudodactyly, laryngeal disorders, urethral meatal stenosis, conjunctival scarring, and psychosocial problems.

Patient Education

Much support is required for parents and patients with these disorders, which are chronic, frustrating and, in the dystrophic form, severely debilitating. Patients and family members should be provided with a checklist of steps to reduce friction, and they should be instructed by persons skilled in nursing techniques. Lay support groups, DEBRA (Dystrophic Epidermolysis Bullosa Research Association) of America, Inc. (http://www.debra.org/), and the Epidermolysis Bullosa Medical Research Foundation (http://www.ebkids.org) have excellent information available for parents and a North American network of local support groups to help families with children who have epidermolysis bullosa. Future therapy using gene transfer technology may be helpful and give hope for the patients who are most severely involved.[27-31]

Follow-up Visits

A regular schedule of visits is required to monitor anemia and secondary infections. After birth, visits should be weekly or biweekly. Routine immunizations and well baby care are needed. Arrangements for annual evaluations at one of the pediatric centers of epidermolysis bullosa care may be beneficial for the patient and their families.

ECTODERMAL DYSPLASIAS

There are considered to be over 200 different ectodermal dysplasias of which about 30 have been studied at the molecular level.[32] The ones most frequently seen include incontinentia pigmenti, hypohidrotic and hidrotic forms of ectodermal dysplasia, Goltz syndrome, the palmoplantar keratodermas, and Darier's disease. Ectodermal dysplasias are genetic disorders of the embryonic ectoderm that have defects involving at least two of the structures associated with skin, hair, teeth, nails, and/or sweating. Skin defects include ichthyosis, pigmentary abnormalities, and hypoplasias or aplasias. Sparse or absent scalp or other hair may be found. Ichthyosis with sparse hair is a frequent combination in Netherton's syndrome, the keratitis-ichthyosis deafness syndrome, and other forms of ichthyosis.[6] Teeth may be cone-shaped, sparse, or absent. Nails may be thickened, thinned, or hypoplastic. Sweating is usually diminished, but hypohidrosis may be patchy and difficult to detect.

Fig. 19.34 Incontinentia pigmenti. Linear vesicles and crust in affected newborn girl.

Fig. 19.35 Incontinentia pigmenti. Warty, linear growths at site of previous blisters.

Fig. 19.36 Incontinentia pigmenti. Whorled pigmentation of extremity in sites of previous blisters.

Fig. 19.37 Incontinentia pigment. Whorled, brown-pigmented streaks on abdominal skin where no prior blisters were noted.

Fig. 19.38 Incontinentia pigmenti. Missing teeth in affected child.

Incontinentia pigmenti

Clinical features

Four distinct stages of skin changes occur in incontinentia pigmenti. First, linear rows of blisters on the extremities are seen (Fig. 19.34).[33] These blistering episodes may be observed in the neonatal period and recur over the first 4 months of life and are replaced by warty linear areas that may last until 1 year of age (Fig. 19.35).[33] Rows of brown pigmentation are then left (Fig. 19.36). In addition, swirls of brown pigmentation are found on the trunk and in areas where the blisters and warty lesions did not occur (Figs 19.37, 19.38).[33] The lesions may follow along the lines of Blaschko (see Chs 2, 21). The pigmentation fades as the child ages and is usually not seen after adolescence. Hypopigmented, scarred areas may develop afterwards.

Incontinentia pigmenti is a X-linked trait that is usually lethal to the male, which explains the female predominance in this disorder.[33,34] The gene responsible for incontinentia pigmenti encodes the 48 kDa NF-κB essential modulator (NEMO) protein, also referred to as IKKg, which is the essential modulator of nuclear factor κB (NF-κB).[34,35] Mental retardation, seizures, microcephaly, and other central nervous system disorders occur in up to 30% of the reported patients,[33] although it is our experience that the association is much lower. Ocular and skeletal anomalies may also be noted.

Differential diagnosis

In the blistering stage, herpes simplex or bullous impetigo may be confused with incontinentia pigmenti, but the linear arrangement of its blisters and appropriate cultures will distinguish it from these two disorders. The warty phase may mimic linear epidermal birthmarks or warts. The hyperpigmentation is uniquely arranged in whorls and is unlikely to be confused with other causes of hyperpigmentation.

Pathogenesis

Skin biopsy demonstrates an inflammatory dermatitis with subcorneal vesicles filled with numerous eosinophils.[33] The warty stage merely demonstrates hyperkeratosis and chronic inflammation in the dermis. In the pigmentary stage, melanin is found free in the dermis or engulfed by dermal macrophages, which accounts for the term incontinentia pigmenti..[33] Understanding the genetics of this condition should allow improved understanding of the acute der-matitis and peculiar linear arrangement of the lesions.[34,35]

Treatment

There is no satisfactory treatment.

Patient education

The clinician should emphasize that the disorder is inherited and describe the expected future cutaneous stages.

Follow-up visits

Routine infant care visits should be scheduled. Additional visits may be necessary, based on complications that arise.

Hypohidrotic and Hidrotic Ectodermal Dysplasias

Clinical features

Two common forms of ectodermal dysplasia have been recognized, the hypohidrotic form and the hidrotic form.[36] One of the forms was called the anhidrotic form but it should be called *hypohidrotic* because

Fig. 19.39 Hypohidrotic ectodermal dysplasia. Absence of eyebrows and lashes and darkened eyelids in newborn.

sweating may be markedly decreased but not absent. In each there is sparse scalp hair. In addition, a number of other uncommon and rare forms of ectodermal dysplasias have thin or absent hair.[32,36] Absence of the eyebrows and eyelashes in the newborn may be an important clue to the diagnosis (Fig. 19.39).[37] Other clinical findings may be less obvious.

In hypohidrotic ectodermal dysplasia, sweating is reduced or completely absent.[37] Such infants may present with fever of unknown origin or recurrent high fevers, due to inability to control body temperature through sweating, but are due to diminished nasal mucous glands. The facies of such children are very distinctive, with everted lips, prominent frontal ridges, a saddle nose, and absence of eyebrows and eyelashes. Temporary and permanent teeth are reduced in number or may be entirely absent. If teeth erupt, they are often cone shaped, and this may be observed by dental radiographs even in the pre-eruptive stage. Atrophic rhinitis and frequent upper respiratory symptoms may lead to the mistaken diagnosis of respiratory allergy.[37] Scalp hair is seldom totally absent, but it is very sparse and is often the first concern of the parents. Fingernails and toenails are normal in at least half of cases but may be thin or brittle. A careful genetic history should be obtained.

The hidrotic form is characterized by nail dystrophy as the most prominent clinical finding. The nails are thickened, slow growing, and brittle. Thick nails may be apparent early in infancy. In one-third of families, the only feature present is nail disease. As in the hypohidrotic form, the scalp hair is thin and sparse and eyebrows are thin, but sweating is normal. Teeth are often normal. The palms and soles may be diffusely thickened, and thickened skin over the knuckles, knees, and elbows may be prominently observed.

Differential diagnosis

The major conditions to be considered in the differential diagnosis are listed in Box 15.5. The findings of disorders of nails, skin, and teeth in the same patient in addition to the hair loss will suggest ectodermal dysplasia. Within a single family with ectodermal dysplasia, the features may be quite variable. To diagnose abnormalities of sweating, a combination of tests may be required.[38] Sweat pore counting using silicone rubber plastic imprints and silver nitrate staining is reliable but does not take into account functional sweating, which can be quantified by 0-phthaldialdehyde stains of induced sweating.[38]

Pathogenesis

Hypohidrotic and hidrotic ectodermal dysplasia are associated with genetic defects associated with cell–cell communication and signaling.[32,36] Hypohidrotic ectodermal dysplasia is most commonly inherited in an X-linked recessive pattern by a defect in the protein ectodysplasin, a tumor necrosis factor ligand, but other genetic variations are also possible.[32,36] The hidrotic form is usually inherited as an autosomal dominant condition and has been observed in a large French-Canadian family surnamed Clouston. The gene for the hidrotic form is associated with the connexin gene GJB6.[32,36] In the hypohidrotic form, sweat glands are absent or rudimentary, as are scalp hair follicles, sebaceous glands, and the mucous glands of the respiratory passages. Lack of sweating results in poor thermal control and high fevers. Lack of hair follicles is expressed as sparse hair, and lack of respiratory mucus produces frequent infections and watery rhinorrhea. Disordered keratinization is thought to be important in the hidrotic form to explain the nail disease and hyperkeratosis of the palms and soles.

Treatment

Fever control through the use of cool compresses is vital in the newborn or infant with recurrent fevers. There is no specific therapy otherwise available.[37] The use of wigs and dental corrective devices may be necessary.

Patient education

Genetic counseling is very useful to the patient and family, as is the explanation of the cause of the febrile responses and respiratory symptoms in the infant. Genetic testing may be important to confirm the specific genetic defect and for family counseling.

Follow-up visits

At least one follow-up visit within 4 weeks of the initial visit is most useful to re-explain the genetic factors and the symptoms of disease.

Focal Dermal Hypoplasia (Goltz Syndrome)
Clinical features

The hallmark of Goltz syndrome are linear, red, swirly streaks in the skin that represent the areas of focal

Fig. 19.40 Focal dermal hypoplasia. Linear and whorled red streaks on female infant.

Fig. 19.41 Focal dermal hypoplasia. Atrophic and scarred skin with hypopigmented patch in child.

Fig. 19.42 Focal dermal hypoplasia. Syndactyly of toes in child.

dermal hypoplasia (Fig. 19.40).[39,40] Atrophy, scarring areas, hypopigmentation (Fig. 19.41), and telangiectasias that follow the lines of Blaschko are seen. There may be yellow nodules in a linear pattern.[39,40] Small papillomatous growths on periorificial or intertriginous areas are found. In the oral mucosa or perineal area they may be mistaken for warts. Nails may be hypoplastic, short, or brittle. Hair is sparse. Teeth are sparse, and enamel defects are frequently found.[39,40]

Syndactyly, polydactyly, and a variety of other bony malformations are seen (Fig. 19.42). Lip pits, hemihypoplasia of the tongue, cleft lip, strabismus, colobomas, cataracts, neurosensory hearing loss, and mental retardation are common.[39,40]

Differential diagnosis

Many other ectodermal dysplasias will demonstrate some features in common with Goltz syndrome, but will not show the characteristics of focal dermal hypoplasia.[39] Sometimes, aplasia cutis congenita or intrauterine erosions of epidermolysis bullosa are mistaken for dermal hypoplasia, but a skin biopsy will distinguish. In focal dermal hypoplasia, a normal epidermis overlies subcutaneous fat with a rudimentary dermis present. In aplasia cutis, the epidermis is absent or effaced, and subcutaneous fat is diminished; in dystrophic epidermolysis bullosa, the sweat glands and hair follicles are present in a normal dermis with a loss of epidermis.

Pathogenesis

An X-linked dominant inheritance pattern is described with many sporadic cases. In a variant with microphthalmia, a deletion of Xp22 is described.[39]

Treatment

There is no available treatment. Consultation with, or referral to, a multidisciplinary genetics clinic may be of great assistance in assessment.

Patient education

The genetics of the disease should be discussed with the patient and family, including the likelihood of a great variety of bony, eye, and central nervous system disturbances.

Follow-up visits

The frequency of review should be determined by the associated defects.

Fig. 19.43 Diffuse palmoplantar keratoderma. All of child's palmar skin is thickened.

Fig. 19.44 Diffuse palmoplantar keratoderma. Involvement of sole of foot.

There are many genetic types and phenotypic patterns of hereditary palmoplantar keratodermas.[41-43] Thickening can be diffuse, involving the entire surface (Fig. 19.43); round and linear (Fig.s 19.44, 19.45); or striate (Fig. 19.46) or multiple discrete 1–2 mm papules (Fig. 19.47). Mutations can involve Keratins 1, 6b, 9, 14, 16, and 17 as well as desmoglein 1, loricrin and other genes.[41-43] Similar phenotypes can be seen with different mutations.[41,43] Palmoplantar keratodermas can be associated with deafness, and the clinician should consider hearing screening if hearing loss is suspected in affected children.[44]

Keratosis Follicularis (Darier-White Disease)

Clinical features

Keratosis follicularis is characterized by skin-colored to red-brown, keratotic 2–5 mm papules on the face, neck, scalp, chest, back (Figs 19.48–19.51), and prox-

Fig. 19.45 Oval and linear palmoplantar keratoderma. Child's palm has linear and oval plaques of thickening.

Fig. 19.46 Striate palmoplantar keratoderma. Linear streaks of epidermal thickening on fingers.

The Hereditary Palmoplantar Keratodermas

Some children are born with thickening of the palms and soles or develop thickening later in childhood.

Fig. 19.47 Punctate palmoplantar keratoderma. Adolescent has discrete thickened areas on palms.

Fig. 19.48 Keratosis follicularis. Numerous red, keratotic papules on adolescent's upper back.

Fig. 19.49 Keratosis follicularis. Confluent keratotic papules are tightly grouped in an area of more severe involvement.

Fig. 19.51 Keratosis follicularis (Darier's disease). Keratotic papules on trunk.

Fig. 19.50 Keratosis follicularis. Discrete brown, 'greasy-feeling' keratotic papules.

imal extremities.[45,46] The skin changes usually begin between the ages of 5 to 10 years, but the age of onset is variable. Over the tops of the hands, the skin changes

involve skin-colored, flat-topped papules; 0.1 mm punctate papules may be seen on the palms. There are longitudinal streaks of the nails, which terminate in a wedge-shaped split in the free end of the nail. Heat sensitivity is severe, with exacerbations in hot weather or after sun exposure. Severe bacterial or herpes simplex skin infections may occur in affected skin areas. Hypopigmented macules on the trunk and extremities are seen. The course often worsens during adolescence.[46]

Differential diagnosis

Inflamed lesions of keratosis pilaris can mimic keratosis follicularis, except that they are usually localized to the extensor proximal arms and legs. The lesions of keratosis pilaris are often much smaller, white, and likely to be dome shaped. A biopsy may be required to distinguish. Keratosis follicularis has focal areas of acantholytic dyskeratosis, whereas keratosis pilaris reveals a follicular keratotic plug in the body hair channel.

Pathogenesis

Keratosis follicularis is associated with mutations in ATP2A2, a gene that encodes the sarco/endoplasmic reticulum Ca^{2+}-ATPase isoform 2. Abnormalities in the function of this calcium pump are hypothesized to interfere with cell growth and differentiation calcium-dependent signaling processes.[47]

Treatment

Keeping the skin surface cool, sometimes with wet dressings, is helpful. Oral retinoids, such as isotretinoin at 0.5–1.0 mg/kg/day, during hot months may be useful. Oral antibiotics for bacterial superinfections should be used.

Fig. 19.52 Acrodermatitis enteropathica. Perioral erosions, scalp crusting, and hand erosions in infant.

Fig. 19.53 Acrodermatitis enteropathica. Erosive dermatitis on cheeks of infant.

Fig. 19.54 Chronic acrodermatitis enteropathica. Red plaques in genital area.

Fig. 19.55 Chronic acrodermatitis enteropathica. Scaly red areas on each ankle.

ACRODERMATITIS ENTEROPATHICA

Clinical Features

Acrodermatitis enteropathica is an autosomal recessive disorder of zinc transport.[48] It is not apparent at birth, but begins at 1–2 months of age in a formula-fed infant or after weaning in a breastfed infant.[48] The cutaneous findings demonstrate acral skin erosions, intermittent diarrhea, and failure to thrive.[48]

The erosions appear as red, moist areas over the distal extremities, including the hands and feet, and in the perioral and perineal areas (Figs 19.52, 19.53). Often, the cutaneous features precede the diarrhea by several weeks to several months. As the disorder continues, weight loss occurs, along with photophobia, apathy, irritability, anorexia, anemia, alopecia, thrush, and paronychia caused by *Candida albicans*. If the child survives the complications of malnutrition, the skin lesions become erythematous plaques with silvery scales that mimic psoriasis (Figs 19.54, 19.55).

Zinc deficiency can also be seen in premature and term infants who are fed a diet deficient in zinc. Occasionally, human breast milk can be low in zinc, allowing zinc deficiency in the totally breastfed infant.[49] This occurs more frequently in a premature infant.[49] Acquired zinc deficiency can be seen in organic acidurias, during hyperalimentation, and a variety of severe gastrointestinal disturbances.[50]

Measuring serum or plasma zinc levels affirms the diagnosis.[48,49] There are many sources of zinc contamination in rubber stoppers and glass tubes and other blood-collecting devices that produce falsely high zinc levels. Thus, the diagnosis may be obscured. Therefore, blood samples should be collected in acid-washed sterile plastic tubes, using acid-washed plastic syringes.

Differential Diagnosis

The lesions of acrodermatitis enteropathica are often mistaken for mucocutaneous candidiasis associated with an immune deficiency such as human immunodeficiency virus (HIV) infection. Measuring plasma or serum zinc levels will distinguish between the two. Often, protein–calorie malnutrition states are considered, but lesions usually develop in such patients after 6 months of age, and the nutritional history may distinguish between the two. Cystic fibrosis can present with loose stools and acral erythematous eruption.[51] Histiocytosis X will present with intertriginous erosions in infancy. Acquired zinc deficiency states, such as seen with prolonged parenteral hyperalimentation, will mimic acrodermatitis enteropathica. Necrolytic migratory erythema, seen with a glucagonoma, will also mimic the lesions of acrodermatitis enteropathica.[50]

Pathogenesis

Depletion of body zinc stores caused by faulty transport of zinc is responsible for the symptoms and signs of acrodermatitis enteropathica.[48,49,52] The mutated gene in acrodermatitis enteropathica is SLC39A4. This gene encodes a zinc transporter protein belonging to the zinc/iron-regulated-transporter-like-protein (ZIP) family.[53,54] The zinc deficiency is the result of depletion of total body stores. Zinc is a nutritionally essential trace element which functions as a cofactor for numerous enzymes, including those involved in DNA and RNA replication and protein synthesis.[55]

Treatment

Oral zinc sulfate, 1 mg/kg/day or more given twice a day, produces rapid clinical improvement.[56] Apathy disappears within 24 hours, and the skin lesions and diarrhea resolve within 7–14 days. Photophobia, alopecia, and growth failure are reversed over the ensuing months.

Patient Education

The hereditary inability to absorb zinc should be explained to the patient and family. It is not known whether lifetime maintenance with supplemental zinc is required.

Follow-up Visits

A visit 2 weeks after diagnosis is useful to repeat measurement of zinc levels and to evaluate the response to treatment. The measurement of plasma or serum zinc levels at monthly intervals is useful to monitor supplemental zinc requirements.

REFERENCES

1. Sybert V. Genetic skin disorders. New York: Oxford University Press; 1997.
2. Spitz J. Genodermatoses: a clinical guide to genetic skin disorders. 2nd edn. Philadelphia: Lippincott Williams & Wilkins; 2005.
3. Information NCfB. OMIM – Online Mendelian Inheritance in Man. Cited; Available from: http://www.ncbi.nlm.nih.gov/entrez/query.fcgi?db=OMIM
4. GeneDx. Cited; Available from: http://www.genedx.com
5. Genetests. Cited; Available from: http://www.genetests.org/servlet/access
6. Richard G. Molecular genetics of the ichthyoses. Am J Med Genet C Semin Med Genet 2004; 131C(1):32–44.
7. Smith FJ, Irvine AD, Terron-Kwiatkowski A, et al. Loss-of-function mutations in the gene encoding filaggrin cause ichthyosis vulgaris. Nat Genet 2006; 38(3):337–342.
8. Rugg EL, Leigh IM. The keratins and their disorders. Am J Med Genet C Semin Med Genet 2004; 131C(1):4–11.

9. Hovnanian A. Harlequin ichthyosis unmasked: a defect of lipid transport. J Clin Invest 2005; 115(7):1708–1710.

10. Akiyama M, Sugiyama-Nakagiri Y, Sakai K, et al. Mutations in lipid transporter ABCA12 in harlequin ichthyosis and functional recovery by corrective gene transfer. J Clin Invest 2005; 115(7):1777–1784.

11. Akiyama M, Sakai K, Sugiyama-Nakagiri Y, et al. Compound heterozygous mutations including a de novo missense mutation in ABCA12 led to a case of harlequin ichthyosis with moderate clinical severity. J Invest Dermatol 2006; 126(7):1518–1523.

12. Ammirati CT, Mallory SB. The major inherited disorders of cornification. New advances in pathogenesis. Dermatol Clin 1998;1 6(3):497–508.

13. Mukherjee S, Gupta AB. A statistical study on in vivo sorption and desorption of water in ichthyosis vulgaris. J Dermatol 1994; 21(2):78–83.

14. Palmer CN, Irvine AD, Terron-Kwiatkowski A, et al. Common loss-of-function variants of the epidermal barrier protein filaggrin are a major predisposing factor for atopic dermatitis. Nat Genet 2006;38(4):441–446.

15. Bradshaw KD, Carr BR. Placental sulfatase deficiency: maternal and fetal expression of steroid sulfatase deficiency and X-linked ichthyosis. Obstet Gynecol Surv 1986; 41(7):401–413.

16. Buyse L, Graves C, Marks R, et al. Collodion baby dehydration: the danger of high transepidermal water loss. Br J Dermatol 1993; 129(1):86–88.

17. Lane EB, McLean WH. Keratins and skin disorders. J Pathol 2004; 204(4):355–366.

18. Paller AS, Syder AJ, Chan YM, et al. Genetic and clinical mosaicism in a type of epidermal nevus. N Engl J Med 1994; 331(21):1408–1415.

19. Shwayder T. Disorders of keratinization: diagnosis and management. Am J Clin Dermatol 2004; 5(1):17–29.

20. DiGiovanna JJ, Robinson-Bostom L. Ichthyosis: etiology, diagnosis, and management. Am J Clin Dermatol 2003; 4(2):81–95.

21. Chavanas S, Bodemer C, Rochat A, et al. Mutations in SPINK5, encoding a serine protease inhibitor, cause Netherton syndrome. Nat Genet 2000; 25(2):141–142.

22. Hachem JP, Wagberg F, Schmuth M, et al. Serine protease activity and residual LEKTI Expression determine phenotype in Netherton syndrome. J Invest Dermatol 2006; 126(7):1609–1621.

23. Marinkovich MP, Herron GS, Khavari PA, et al. Inherited epidermolysis bullosa. 6th edn. New York: McGraw-Hill; 2003.

24. Uitto J, Richard G. Progress in epidermolysis bullosa: from eponyms to molecular genetic classification. Clin Dermatol 2005; 23(1):33–40.

25. Fine J-D, Bauer EA, McGuire J, et al. Epidermolysis bullosa. Baltimore: Johns Hopkins University Press; 1999.

26. Fivenson DP, Scherschun L, Choucair M, et al. Graftskin therapy in epidermolysis bullosa. J Am Acad Dermatol 2003; 48(6):886–892.

27. Ferrari S, Pellegrini G, Mavilio F, et al. Gene therapy approaches for epidermolysis bullosa. Clin Dermatol 2005; 23(4):430–436.

28. Ortiz-Urda S, Thyagarajan B, Keene DR, et al. PhiC31 integrase-mediated nonviral genetic correction of junctional epidermolysis bullosa. Hum Gene Ther 2003; 14(9):923–928.

29. Ortiz-Urda S, Lin Q, Green CL, et al. Injection of genetically engineered fibroblasts corrects regenerated human epidermolysis bullosa skin tissue. J Clin Invest 2003; 111(2):251–255.

30. Ortiz-Urda S, Thyagarajan B, Keene DR, et al. Stable nonviral genetic correction of inherited human skin disease. Nat Med 2002; 8(10):1166–170.

31. Robbins PB, Lin Q, Goodnough JB, et al. In vivo restoration of laminin 5 beta 3 expression and function in junctional epidermolysis bullosa. Proc Natl Acad Sci USA 2001; 98(9):5193–5198.

32. Itin PH, Fistarol SK. Ectodermal dysplasias. Am J Med Genet C Semin Med Genet 2004; 131C(1):45–51.

33. Bruckner AL. Incontinentia pigmenti: a window to the role of NF-kappaB function. Semin Cutan Med Surg 2004; 23(2):116–124.

34. Fusco F, Bardaro T, Fimiani G, et al. Molecular analysis of the genetic defect in a large cohort of IP patients and identification of novel NEMO mutations interfering with NF-kappaB activation. Hum Mol Genet 2004; 13(16):1763–1773.

35. Courtois G. The NF-kappaB signaling pathway in human genetic diseases. Cell Mol Life Sci 2005; 62(15):1682–1691.

36. Lamartine J. Towards a new classification of ectodermal dysplasias. Clin Exp Dermatol 2003; 28(4):351–355.

37. Masse JF, Perusse R. Ectodermal dysplasia. Arch Dis Child 1994; 71(1):1–2.

38. Berg D, Weingold DH, Abson KG, et al. Sweating in ectodermal dysplasia syndromes. A review. Arch Dermatol 1990; 126(8):1075–1079.

39. Kilmer SL, Grix AW Jr, Isseroff RR. Focal dermal hypoplasia: four cases with widely varying presentations. J Am Acad Dermatol 1993; 28(5 Pt 2):839–843.

40. Sacoor MF, Motswaledi MH. Three cases of focal dermal hypoplasia (Goltz syndrome). Clin Exp Dermatol 2005; 30(1):35–37.

41. Kimyai-Asadi A, Kotcher LB, Jih MH. The molecular basis of hereditary palmoplantar keratodermas. J Am Acad Dermatol 2002; 47(3):327–343; quiz 344–346.

42. Gedicke MM, Traupe H, Fischer B, et al. Towards characterization of palmoplantar keratoderma caused by gain-of-function mutation in loricrin: analysis of a family and review of the literature. Br J Dermatol 2006; 154(1):167–171.

43. Milingou M, Wood P, Masouye I, et al. Focal palmoplantar keratoderma caused by an autosomal dominant inherited mutation in the desmoglein 1 gene. Dermatology 2006; 212(2):117–122.

44. Montgomery JR, White TW, Martin BL, et al. A novel connexin 26 gene mutation associated with features of the keratitis-ichthyosis-deafness syndrome and the follicular occlusion triad. J Am Acad Dermatol 2004; 51(3):377–382.

45. Sehgal VN, Srivastava G. Darier's (Darier-White) disease/keratosis follicularis. Int J Dermatol 2005; 44(3):184–192.

46. Zeglaoui F, Zaraa I, Fazaa B, et al. Dyskeratosis follicularis disease: case reports and review of the literature. J Eur Acad Dermatol Venereol 2005; 19(1):114–117.

47. Byrne CR. The focal nature of Darier's disease lesions: calcium pumps, stress, and mutation? J Invest Dermatol 2006; 126(4):702–703.

48. Perafan-Riveros C, Franca LF, Alves AC, et al. Acrodermatitis enteropathica: case report and review of the literature. Pediatr Dermatol 2002; 19(5):426–431.

49. Young HS, Khan AS, Power S, et al. Case 4. Transient symptomatic zinc deficiency in a breast-fed premature infant: an acrodermatitis enteropathica-like eruption. Clin Exp Dermatol 2003; 28(1):109–110.

50. Sinclair SA, Reynolds NJ. Necrolytic migratory erythema and zinc deficiency. Br J Dermatol 1997; 136(5):783–785.
51. Darmstadt GL, Schmidt CP, Wechsler DS, et al. Dermatitis as a presenting sign of cystic fibrosis. Arch Dermatol 1992; 128(10):1358–1364.
52. Sandstrom B, Cederblad A, Lindblad BS, et al. Acrodermatitis enteropathica, zinc metabolism, copper status, and immune function. Arch Pediatr Adolesc Med 1994; 148(9):980–985.
53. Kury S, Dreno B, Bezieau S, et al. Identification of SLC39A4, a gene involved in acrodermatitis enteropathica. Nat Genet 2002; 31(3):239–240.
54. Kury S, Kharfi M, Kamoun R, et al. Mutation spectrum of human SLC39A4 in a panel of patients with acrodermatitis enteropathica. Hum Mutat 2003; 22(4):337–338.
55. McClung JP, Scrimgeour AG. Zinc: an essential trace element with potential benefits to soldiers. Mil Med 2005; 170(12):1048–1052.
56. Stevens J, Lubitz L. Symptomatic zinc deficiency in breast-fed term and premature infants. J Paediatr Child Health 1998; 34(1):97–100.

Drug Eruptions

There is an enormous variety of cutaneous reactions to drugs, with many different clinical patterns.[1–13] Common patterns include morbilliform eruptions, urticarial eruptions, and fixed drug eruptions. Vasculitic, lichenoid, purpuric, scarlatiniform, phototoxic, photoallergic, Sweet's syndrome, and acute generalized erythematous pustular (AGEP) eruptions have all been described in children.[1–13] Acneiform reactions and pigmentary disturbances are discussed in Chapters 3 and 16. The uncommon, but life-threatening drug eruptions include Stevens-Johnson syndrome (SJS), toxic epidermal necrolysis (TEN), the drug rash, eosinophilia, systemic symptoms (DRESS) syndrome,[3,7,13] widespread bullous reactions, and angioedema/anaphylaxis (see Ch. 14).[2,3,5,7] The same drug can cause very different skin eruption patterns in different patients. For example, ibuprofen can induce morbilliform eruptions, urticarial eruptions, SJS, lichenoid drug eruptions, photosensitivity, and fixed drug reactions.[1,2]

The diagnosis of a drug eruption is usually based on clinical suspicion and not confirmed by rechallenge studies. Evaluation of a drug eruption primarily depends on the drug reaction history profile (Box 20.1).[3,10] The specific morphology of the patient's skin lesions, and the relative frequency of similar reactions in the general population, are of assistance. Inadvertent and deliberate rechallenge reports implicate the drug with the specific skin reaction.[3,10] The timing of the eruption in relationship to the commencement of drug therapy may assist in establishing the association of the drug with the eruption. The onset of disease after ingestion of the drug varies from a few hours in urticarial reactions to as long as 3 months in DRESS syndrome and lichenoid reactions (Table 20.1). Specific medications have a higher frequency of drug eruptions and specific types of a drug eruption than other medications. The clinician should look for alternate explanations for the eruption, including infection or another primary illness. This is especially true in erythema nodosum[1] and exfoliative dermatitis in infants and children,[1] in which drugs rarely are the cause. Withdrawal of the suspected drug may help in the diagnosis.[3] However, removal of the suspected drug

---

Box 20.1 Drug reaction history profile

1. In clinical trials, the drug was 2× or greater more likely to cause a particular skin reaction than placebo.[3]
2. After the drug was approved, there were numerous reports of the particular skin reaction as an adverse event.[3]
3. Inadvertent rechallenge with the drug resulted in reappearance of the particular skin reaction.
4. Deliberate rechallenge resulted in reappearance of the cutaneous reaction.[10]

Table 20.1 Onset of drug eruption after ingestion of medication

Reaction	Time
Acute generalized erythematous pustulosis	Hours to 2 days
Urticaria	Hours to 7 days
Phototoxic eruptions	Hours to 7 days
Fixed drug eruption	1–7 days
Generalized pustular eruptions	1–21 days
Morbilliform eruptions	7–21 days
Scarlatiniform eruptions	7–21 days
Bullous drug reactions	7–21 days
Erythema nodosum eruptions	14–56 days
Stevens-Johnson syndrome	14–56 days
Toxic epidermal necrolysis	14–56 days
DRESS syndrome	30–100 days
Lichenoid eruptions	30–100 days

from the patient may not always result in rapid resolution of the drug eruption. Clearing is slow in the DRESS syndrome. Fortunately, the incidence of adverse drug reactions in infants and children appears to be less than in adults.[3,7] For a few drugs, the relative risk of a particular type of skin reaction is known (Table 20.2), but for many drug reactions, it is undetermined. The serious drug eruptions will be considered first.

STEVENS-JOHNSON SYNDROME AND TOXIC EPIDERMAL NECROLYSIS

Clinical Features

Because mucocutaneous features and etiologies of SJS and TEN may be indistinguishable, they will be

Table 20.2 Relative risk of life-threatening drug reactions* among anticonvulsants

Drug	Relative risk
Carbamazepine	120
Phenytoin	91
Phenobarbital	57
Lamotrigine	25
Valproic acid	24

Stevens-Johnson syndrome and toxic epidermal necrolysis.

considered here together. Both are serious, potentially life-threatening conditions characterized by large areas of epithelial necrosis.[1,3,4,6,7] Both are very uncommon in children with SJS estimated at 1 in 30 000 and TEN at 1 in 100 000. In SJS the necrosis is primarily mucosal and in TEN primarily in the skin but they can each have both mucosal and skin involvement. SJS, in

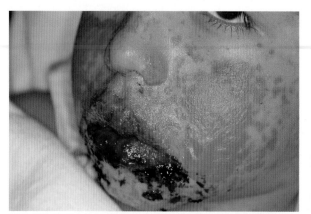

Fig. 20.1 Severe oral and skin involvement in SJS.

Fig. 20.2 Early oral involvement in Stevens-Johnson syndrome.

Fig. 20.3 Hemorrhagic crusts on the lips of a child with Stevens-Johnson syndrome.

contrast to erythema multiforme (EM), has a distinct prodrome lasting 1–14 days and is characterized by fever, headache, sore throat, malaise, and, sometimes, cough, vomiting, and diarrhea. Mucosal involvement is severe, with extensive mucosal necrosis, and it always involves at least two mucosal surfaces (Figs 20.1, 20.2). The oral mucosa (Fig. 20.3) and eyes (Fig. 20.4) are the most frequently involved, but vaginal and urethral necrosis and widespread gastrointestinal or lower respiratory tract necrosis may develop. An uncommon variant, sometimes called *recurrent oral erythema multiforme*, is limited to the oral mucosa. The initial cutaneous lesions mimic those found in EM (Fig. 20.5) but progress rapidly within hours from central blisters (Fig. 20.6) to severe epidermal necrosis (Fig. 20.7) with loss of the epidermis, leaving denuded skin. Large sheets of epidermis or mucosa may be lost (Fig. 20.8). The mouth is affected in every case of

SJS.[1,3,4,6,7] Hemorrhagic crusts often appear on the lips. Mucous membrane involvement often precipitates hospitalization in children because of severe limitation of the ability to eat. Redness, swelling, bullae, or denuded erosions may be seen on the conjunctivae, accom-

Fig. 20.5 Tender macules on the hands in SJS.

Fig. 20.4 Early eye involvement in Stevens-Johnson syndrome.

Fig. 20.6 Bullous macules with islands of uninvolved skin in Stevens-Johnson syndrome/toxic epidermal necrolysis overlap.

Fig. 20.7 Purple necrotic lesions in TEN.

Fig. 20.8 Extensive skin necrosis in TEN.

panied by pain and photophobia. Conjunctival scarring may be severe, and ocular complications are the most frequent long-term complications.[4,7]

TEN has similar cutaneous findings that may occur in the absence of mucosal involvement. Although lesions first begin on the extremities in a pattern similar to that noted in EM, extensive truncal and facial involvement soon follows. A large percentage of the skin may be lost, leading to complications similar to a thermal burn.[1] Healing with scarring and contractures may occur, and loss of hair and nails may ensue.[4,7] Permanent areas of depigmentation may develop.[4,7]

There may be considerable overlap in the clinical conditions of SJS and TEN.[9,11,13] SJS may be mucosal only, but more likely will have mucosal and necrotic skin lesions together. TEN may only involve skin but also may exhibit severe necrosis of oral mucosa. Attempts at classification of these two entities have been of help in clarifying the conditions, but the clinician should appreciate that there are overlapping clinical features and that early on it may be difficult to predict areas of involvement.[3,4,7–9,11,13] Most authorities now accept four major types of SJS/TEN. The typical SJS usually has only a few red macules with blisters, which accompany the mucous membrane involvement, and less than 10% of the body surface is involved. The 'overlap' SJS/TEN has 10–30% of body surface involved. Two types of TEN are recognized: one with 'spots' in which many red macules with blisters are seen involving more than 10% of the body surface, and one in which large confluent areas of skin are involved on the face and trunk and more than 30% of the body surface is involved. The course of SJS and TEN diseases is prolonged and accompanied by systemic symptoms of fever, dehydration, cough,

and lymphadenopathy. The child is often sick 3 or 4 weeks.[3,7–9] SJS and TEN are more likely to occur in children ages 2–10 years, which is younger than those with EM. Complications tend to be severe, with pseudomembrane formation of mucosa leading to mucosal scaring and loss of function in SJS.[3,7–9] As in a severe burn, fluid and electrolyte imbalance, renal and respiratory complications, and secondary bacterial infections complicate TEN.[3,7–9] Use of a severity scoring system such as SCORTEN may help with monitoring and response to therapy.[8]

Differential Diagnosis

All children who are suspected of having TEN, SJS or DRESS syndrome, should be biopsied. Paraneoplastic pemphigus may exactly mimic SJS.[13] Immunofluorescent examination of mucosal or skin biopsy will distinguish. SJS and TEN must be distinguished from staphylococcal scalded skin syndrome (SSSS), DRESS syndrome, and acute graft-versus-host disease by skin biopsy. SJS and TEN show full-thickness epidermal necrosis and subepidermal rather than intraepidermal blister formation (see Fig. 11.10).[13] In DRESS syndrome there is no epidermal necrosis but rather intense inflammation of the epidermis and dermis.[13] In graft-versus-host disease there is satellite cell necrosis in the epidermis and severe injury to cutaneous vessels not seen in SJS. Early in the course of disease, SJS may be confused with Kawasaki disease. In SJS there is necrosis of mucous membranes, whereas in Kawasaki disease there is redness and edema, but necrotic crusts and severe erosions are not seen. SJS may also be confused with the mucositis produced by chemotherapeutic agents in the child with cancer or with severe herpes stomatitis. Medication history and culture or rapid diagnostic test for herpes will distinguish.

Pathogenesis

In SJS and TEN there is increasing evidence that the toxic injury to keratinocytes and mucosal epithelial cells may be the result of genetic susceptibility to injury.[5,14] Almost all cases of SJS and TEN are related to drug ingestion, with nonsteroidal antiinflammatory agents, sulfonamides, and anticonvulsants the most often incriminated.[1–10] Because the skin is a large organ involved in drug detoxification, toxicity is thought to be related to the accumulation of arene oxides in keratinocytes as the result of cytochrome P-450 action on the parent drug.[5] The detoxification of arene oxides, which bind to keratinocyte ribonucleic acids (RNAs), depends on epoxide hydrolases, which may be genetically decreased in children susceptible to SJS or TEN. In a few children, infections with *Mycoplasma pneumoniae* or HSV have been associated with SJS.[4,7] The mechanism of epithelial damage with those infectious agents is not known.

Treatment

Patients with SJS or TEN require treatment as burn patients, preferably in a burn unit or a pediatric intensive care unit.[4,7,8] The offending drug must be discontinued.[4,7,8] Careful attention to fluid and electrolyte balance, respiratory toilet, fever control, and prevention of secondary bacterial infection of the denuded skin is required. Most affected children cannot eat or drink, and parenteral nutrition must be supplied.[4,7,8] The mortality rate is 1% in SJS but 30% in TEN. It is controversial whether systemic steroids 2 mg/kg/day or intravenous immunoglobulin therapy at 1.5–2.0 g/kg/day for 4 days is better than supportive care alone.[13–18] Ophthalmologic consultation should be obtained, and efforts to prevent conjunctival scarring should be initiated.[19]

Patient Education

With SJS and TEN, the drugs thought to be associated should be avoided and patients should be informed that they may be genetically susceptible to develop the condition. Each complication should be discussed with the patient and parents, making them aware of potential sequelae.

Follow-up Visits

For hospitalized patients, follow-up should be directed by their complications. Long-term follow-up will be required for those children who develop sequelae of mucosal or skin scarring.

DRESS SYNDROME

Clinical Features

DRESS syndrome, formerly known as the exfoliative dermatitis/fever/hepatitis/lymphadenopathy syndrome, is characterized by progressively widespread erythema (Fig. 20.9) with subsequent extensive scaling (Fig. 20.10) accompanied by fever, pronounced

Fig. 20.9 Red skin with islands of sparing in early DRESS syndrome.

Fig. 20.10 Extensive desquamation eventually develops in DRESS syndrome.

eosinophilia, atypical lymphocytes in the peripheral blood and skin, elevated liver enzymes, and finally generalized lymphadenopathy.[11,12] Hepatomegaly and occasionally splenomegaly will develop. Hepatic or renal

Box 20.2 Drugs associated With DRESS syndrome
Hydantoins
Carbamazepine
Allopurinol
Barbiturates
Penicillins
Sulfonamides
NSAIDs, including sulindac

impairment may eventually develop. Profound hypothyroidism has been seen in some affected children.[11,12] Progressive weight loss and protein loss may ensue. The most frequently implicated drugs are the hydantoin anticonvulsants (Box 20.2). Often, the drug is not suspected because the child has been receiving it for 1 or 2 months before skin involvement.[11,12]

Differential Diagnosis

DRESS syndrome may mimic lymphoma or chronic infections.[11,12] In some instances it may be difficult to distinguish from TEN, but epidermal necrosis is not prominent in skin biopsies of DRESS syndrome, whereas it is frequent in TEN.[13,14]

Pathogenesis

The hydantoin anticonvulsants are the most frequently implicated in DRESS syndrome, and phenobarbital and carbamazepine have also been associated (see Box 20.5 below).[6,11,12] Sulfonamides and minocycline antibiotics are less frequent causes. The mechanism of injury is not known, but drugs that are metabolized to arene oxide intermediates are believed to be directly toxic to cells.

Treatment

The suspected offending drug must be stopped, mindful that discontinuation of the drug very slowly results in reversal of symptoms over 3–6 weeks.[11,12,17] Many authorities recommend intravenous prednisolone or IVIG but there is no evidence demonstrating efficacy.[17] Early diagnosis may allow management as an outpatient, but later in the course hospitalization is necessary for hydration and nutritional support and wound care.

Patient Education

Parents and patients should be advised that the drug is causing all the symptoms including fever, enlarged lymph nodes, and organs and that withdrawing the drug is necessary but may require weeks for clearing. If caused by anticonvulsants, the child should avoid all aromatic anticonvulsants.[11,12]

Follow-up Visits

Frequent visits may be required if there are abnormalities in liver, renal, or thyroid function.

CLINICAL FEATURES

Commonly Seen Types of Drug Eruptions

Morbilliform drug eruptions

Cutaneous drug reactions often have specific patterns. The morbilliform (so-called *maculopapular eruption*) or exanthematous eruption is probably the most common of all drug-induced eruptions in children.[1,20–28] The term *morbilliform* means measles-like because of the development of a maculopapular erythematous

Fig. 20.11 Morbilliform drug eruption. Trimethoprim-sulfamethoxazole-induced eruption with confluence of lesions on the upper arms and buttocks.

Fig. 20.12 Morbilliform drug eruption. Trimethoprim-sulfamethoxazole-induced eruption with discrete macules and papules on the trunk and confluent erythema on the face.

Box 20.3 Drugs associated with morbilliform reactions

Antibiotics
Amoxicillin
Ampicillin
Cephalosporins
Chloramphenicol
Erythromycin
Gentamicin sulfate
Isoniazid
Penicillins
Sulfonamides
Trimethoprim
Trimethoprim-sulfamethoxazole combinations

NONSTEROIDAL ANTIINFLAMMATORY DRUGS (NSAIDs)
Ibuprofen
Meclofenamate sodium
Piroxicam
Sulindac
Zomepirac sodium

Anticonvulsants
Barbiturates
Carbamazepine
Phenytoin

Antifungals
Fluconazole
Ketoconazole

Others
Allopurinol
Alprazolam
Tacrolimus

rash that becomes confluent (Figs 20.11, 20.12). This rash often starts on the trunk and extends onto the extremities. It is frequently symmetric and often has areas of totally normal skin that are surrounded by the eruption. The initial macules may become papular, and then large plaques may form from the confluence of the individual lesions. The eruption typically lasts 7–14 days and may be associated with pruritus during that time. The patient may have associated fever, malaise, and arthralgias. Box 20.3 lists drugs associated with morbilliform drug eruptions; Table 20.3 lists the frequency of morbilliform rash to specific drugs.

Urticarial drug eruptions

Drug eruptions associated with hives are called *urticarial drug eruptions*. These present as edematous,

Table 20.3 Frequencies of drug morbilliform rash with antibiotic treatment

Drug	Frequency (%)
Cefaclor	12.3
Sulfonamides	8.5
Penicillins	7.4
Other cephalosporins	2.6

flat, erythematous papules that usually last less than 24 hours (Figs 20.13, 20.14). New lesions appear almost continuously.[20–28] The lesions may begin as small discrete papules that become confluent, large, figurate plaques (Figs 20.15, 20.16). Occasionally, the edema can be so intense in the center of the erythematous

Fig. 20.13 Urticarial drug eruption. Large urticarial plaques in a child treated with cefaclor.

Fig. 20.14 Mixed urticarial and morbilliform drug eruption. Trimethoprim-sulfamethoxazole-induced urticarial plaques on the left buttock with maculopapular lesions on the right buttock.

Fig. 20.15 Serum-sickness-like reaction to cefaclor. The urticarial lesions resolve with a dusky, bruised appearance. Note the swelling and edema involving the knee.

Fig. 20.16 Urticarial drug eruption. Confluent intense erythema with islands of normal skin in a patient treated with both phenobarbital and trimethoprim-sulfamethoxazole.

Box 20.4 Drugs commonly associated with urticarial drug eruptions
NSAIDs, especially ibuprofen
Cephalosporins, especially Ceclor
Acetylsalicylic acid
Antibiotics
Amoxicillin
Ampicillin
Penicillins
Sulfonamides
Trimethoprim-sulfamethoxazole
Asparaginase

papules and plaques that the center appears less erythematous than the periphery, giving a target appearance. Lesions may resolve, leaving a macular blue-brown appearance that looks like a bruise. The absence of epidermal injury and more typical urticarial papules and plaques on the rest of the body confirm that this is an urticarial drug eruption and not erythema multiforme. Box 20.4 lists the drugs associated with urticarial drug eruptions.

If the lesions show a deep extension with induration and swelling of the subcutaneous tissue, the reaction is called *angioedema*. If angioedema involves the mucous membranes, it can become life threatening secondary to airway obstruction.

One variant of urticaria is the serum-sickness-like reaction that clinically initially appears to resemble urticaria, often accompanied by angioedema. The child may develop fever, pruritus, arthritis, and/or arthralgias. As in urticaria, the large plaques may resolve with dusky to purple centers, giving the skin a bruised appearance. The affected child may appear severely ill and be very uncomfortable. Cephalosporins are most commonly reported to cause this type of drug eruption.[21–23]

Fixed drug eruptions

Fixed drug eruptions may present as solitary or multiple, sharply demarcated, erythematous lesions that go on to give an intense macular hyperpigmentation (Fig. 20,17).[29,30] The lesions may initially appear edematous, like urticaria, or become bullous (Fig. 20.18).

Fig. 20.18 Fixed drug eruption. Bullous reaction to tetracycline. The lesions have a necrotic, hyperpigmented epidermis with sharp demarcation of normal and involved skin.

Fig. 20.17 Fixed drug eruption. Trimethoprim-sulfamethoxazole-induced oval, erythematous macules with diffuse hyperpigmentation within several lesions.

Box 20.5 Drugs associated with fixed drug eruptions*
Trimethoprim-sulfamethoxazole
Acetaminophen
Barbiturates
Sulfonamides
Carbamazepine
Phenolphthalein
Tetracycline
Trimethoprim
Ciprofloxacin
Oral contraceptives
* First four listed are most frequent.

Over several days the edema and erythema will frequently decrease within the lesion, leaving a macular hyperpigmentation with sharply demarcated outlines in a figurate pattern. Rechallenges with the same medication may cause lesions in precisely the same spot and lesions on new locations as well. Box 20.5 lists the drugs that commonly cause fixed drug eruptions. Trimethoprim-sulfa, sulfonamides, and acetaminophen are the drugs that account for most childhood fixed drug eruptions.[1,29,30]

Uncommon Drug Reaction Patterns

Vasculitis

Palpable purpuric lesions associated with cutaneous necrotizing vasculitis can be associated with drugs.[1,27,28] The vasculitis is usually on the lower extremities in dependent areas but can occur anywhere on the body (Fig. 20.19). The lesions may begin as soft, small, erythematous or urticarial papules that blanch when

Fig. 20.20 AGEP. Pinpoint pustules on diffusely red skin with areas of scale.

pressure is applied over the skin. Over several hours to days, the lesions become firm and dark red-blue or purple. Box 20.6 lists drugs associated with vasculitis.

Acute generalized erythematous pustulosis

A rapid onset of widespread truncal redness with thousands of pinpoint (0.1 mm) pustules, followed by waves of desquamation, characterizes the distinct, uncommon reaction pattern of acute generalized erythematous pustulosis (AGEP) (Fig. 20.20).[1,31-33] It may begin within hours of starting the drug and certainly within a few days.[31,32] The child appears toxic and may have fever. Rapid reversal occurs with discontinuation of the drug. AGEP is particularly associated with amoxicillin, macrolide antibiotics, and anticonvulsants (Box 20.7).

Fig. 20.19 Vasculitis. Amoxicillin-induced lesions on legs.

Lichenoid drug eruptions

Slowly developing purple-red plaques characterize lichenoid eruptions (Fig 20.21).[1,28] The onset is often 1–3 months after starting the drug. The skin lesions may mimic lupus erythematosus or dermatomyositis. Diuretics and beta blockers are most often responsible (Box 20.8).

Box 20.6 Drugs associated with vasculitis
Allopurinol
Barbiturates and hydantoins
NSAIDs
Azithromycin
Gold
Penicillins
Sulfonamides
Diuretics, including thiazides and furosemide
Cimetidine
Thioureas
Coumadin

Box 20.7 Drugs associated with acute generalized erythematous pustulosis (AGEP)
Antibiotics, particularly amoxicillin, azithromycin, and erythromycin, and rarely, the cephalosporins
Anticonvulsants, such as carbamazepine
NSAIDs
Sulfonamides

Fig. 20.21 Lichenoid eruption of the hand in a child treated with thiazide diuretics.

Fig. 20.23 Tense bullae in a child treated with vancomycin.

Box 20.8 Drugs associated with lichenoid eruptions

Diuretics, such as furosemide and thiazides
Beta blockers
Antimalarials
Phenothiazine

Box 20.10 Drugs associated with widespread bullous reactions

Vancomycin	NSAIDs

Bullous drug reactions

In bullous drug reactions, tense bullae develop, usually on the extremities but often widespread (Fig. 20.23). They often begin within 2 weeks of starting the drug. Vancomycin is the most common cause of these eruptions (Box 20.10) and is associated with linear IgA deposits at the dermal–epidermal junction.[1]

Erythema nodosum reactions

Tender, ill-defined, red to dusky-red nodules are seen on the legs in erythema nodosum (Fig 20.22). The onset is abrupt and begins 2–5 weeks after starting the drug.[34] Oral contraceptives are most frequently implicated, but infectious causes are far more likely than drug reactions (Box 20.9).

Fig. 20.22 Erythema nodosum on the leg of a child taking NSAIDs.

Box 20.9 Drugs associated with erythema nodosum reactions

Oral contraceptives	Sulfonamides
NSAIDs	Opiates

Photosensitive drug eruptions

Drug photosensitivity reactions can be either phototoxic or photoallergic.[1] In either situation, a combination of topical or systemic medication and exposure to light is necessary.

Photoallergic reactions are less common than phototoxic reactions. The photoallergic reaction involves an immunologic response to a chemical (drug) that is altered by ultraviolet light. The body recognizes the altered form as a foreign antigen and develops an immunologic delayed hypersensitivity response. This process requires sufficient drug and light to produce adequate antigen for immunization.

Phototoxic reactions involve direct cutaneous injury by a drug after the drug is changed by light energy. Increased light energy or an increased amount of drug increases the risk of a phototoxic reaction.

Photosensitive eruptions are characterized by more intense dermatitis in the areas of greatest sun exposure. Often, the face, upper trunk, and extensor surfaces of the arms are involved. The lesions are usually

Fig. 20.24 Phototoxic reaction to psoralen-containing plant that caused marked hyperpigmentation of the hand.

Fig. 20.25 Acute sunburn phototoxic reaction in an adolescent receiving tetracycline.

Box 20.11 Drugs associated with phototoxic reactions
Coal tar derivatives
Furocoumarins found in plants
Furosemide
Griseofulvin
Ibuprofen
Methotrexate
Naproxen
Nifedipine
Para-aminobenzoic (PABA) esters
Phenothiazines
Psoralen
Sulfonamides
Tetracycline
Thiazides
Tretinoin

Box 20.12 Drugs associated with photoallergic reaction	
Fragrances and perfumes	Phenothiazines
PABA esters	Sulfonamides

sensitive drug reactions. Drugs responsible for photo-allergic reactions are listed in Box 20.12.

Sweet's syndrome reactions

Acute febrile neutrophilic dermatosis (Sweet's syndrome) is characterized by the abrupt onset of tender red plaques on the skin (Fig. 20.26).[36] It is rare, but with the increasing use of recombinant granulocyte stimulating factors the drug-induced eruption is far more frequent than the spontaneous disease (Box 20.13).

erythematous and edematous, with associated papules, vesicles, or oozing, weeping lesions. Increased skin fragility and scarring may be seen. Lesions may resolve with marked hyperpigmentation that may remain for months.

Phototoxic reactions are often painful, similar to severe sunburn (Figs 20.24, 20.25). Drugs responsible for phototoxic reactions are listed in Box 20.11.[1] Photoallergic reactions may be painful or have severe pruritus in the areas of the most intense sun exposure. Phototoxic reactions are dependent on both the amount of drug and the amount of light exposure. In addition to sunlight, fluorescent lamps or sunlight that comes through window glass may produce photo-

Fig. 20.26 Sweet's syndrome. Tender red plaques in an adolescent treated with Neupogen.

Box 20.13 Drugs associated with Sweet's syndrome
Granulocyte colony stimulating factor
Granulocyte-macrophage colony stimulating factor

DIFFERENTIAL DIAGNOSIS
Commonly Seen Types of Drug Reactions
Morbilliform drug eruptions

The onset of the eruption may occur after the offending drug is stopped. Morbilliform eruptions may fade over time, even with continuation of the responsible medication. Morbilliform drug eruptions caused by antimicrobial agents are often a diagnostic dilemma because the eruption may be a viral illness misdiagnosed as bacterial infection and treated with antibiotics. The morbilliform rash may be a viral exanthem. Some morbilliform eruptions are reproducible upon rechallenge. [10]

Urticarial drug eruptions

Urticarial lesions are usually pruritic, and at times it is difficult to separate an urticarial eruption from a morbilliform eruption early in the course of the condition (see Fig. 20.4). Urticarial lesions may occur immediately after exposure to the drug, or within several days. The individual urticarial lesions usually resolve over 24 hours, with new lesions arising. In the morbilliform drug eruption, individual lesions expand over several days, giving more of a confluent, macular-type eruption, whereas urticarial plaques are raised and indurated. Urticarial lesions commonly occur in children and are most often not associated with drugs (see Ch. 13). The serum-sickness-like reaction to drugs is not usually associated with circulating immune complexes, proteinuria, and lymphadenopathy, which are seen in a true serum-sickness reaction. The eruption usually begins 7 or more days after the drug is first given.

Fixed drug eruptions

Erythema multiforme, traumatic skin bruising, and pigmented lesions may be confused with fixed drug eruptions. Biopsy of the fixed drug lesion will often help to confirm the diagnosis. [13] A history of a previous episode with the drug should be sought. Rechallenge with the suspected medication may cause recurrences of similar lesions in the identical spot. The area of residual macular hyperpigmentation may take several months to resolve.

Uncommon Drug Reaction Patterns
Vasculitis

Drug-induced vasculitis can occur quickly after drug exposure or prolonged drug use. Because drugs are one of many causes of cutaneous vasculitis, other conditions inducing these lesions must be considered. Sepsis with bacterial emboli, and many viruses, can cause palpable purpura with very similar cutaneous appearances. Biopsy of an individual lesion can confirm the small-vessel vasculitis, and immunofluorescence examination of the biopsy should be negative in drug-related conditions; however, IgA or other immunoreactants may be found in infectious vasculitis.

The DRESS syndrome

Atopic dermatitis, severe contact dermatitis, or psoriasis may mimic the initial lesions. As the disease progresses, lymphoma, Epstein-Barr virus, human immunodeficiency virus (HIV) infections, or other chronic infections are often considered. A skin biopsy will sometimes differentiate. [13] Improvement after withdrawal of the suspected drug is definitive.

Acute generalized erythematous pustulosis

Pustular psoriasis may demonstrate the same gross morphology as AGEP, but the presence in skin biopsy samples of interstitial and angiocentric neutrophils in the drug reaction will distinguish. [13]

Lichenoid drug eruptions

The skin lesions may mimic lichen planus, lupus erythematosus, or dermatomyositis. The findings of skin biopsy will mimic other lichenoid eruptions, but immunofluorescent examinations are negative in drug reactions. [13]

Erythema nodosum reactions

Erythema nodosum reactions caused by infections are far more likely than those related to drug reactions. The histology is the same.

Bullous drug reactions

Immunobullous disorders or porphyrias may mimic drug-induced disease. Diuretics and nonsteroidal anti-inflammatory drugs (NSAIDs) may produce a pseudoporphyria syndrome that mimics porphyria cutanea tarda. Examination of plasma or urinary porphyrins will distinguish the porphyrias.

Biopsy for immunofluorescent examination will be negative in most drug-induced reactions and positive in immunobullous disorders. The exception is vancomycin-induced bullae in which linear IgA deposits are found along the dermal–epidermal junction, as found in linear IgA dermatosis. Improvement after withdrawal of the drug is definitive.

Photosensitive drug eruptions

Childhood dermatomyositis, lupus erythematosus, idiopathic photodermatosis, and erythropoietic protoporphyria may mimic photosensitive drug reactions. A skin biopsy for immunofluorescence is negative in drug reactions and often positive in collagen vascular diseases.

Sweet's syndrome reactions

Acute febrile neutrophilic dermatosis caused by acute myelogenous leukemias are rare and may be distinguished on skin biopsy by the presence of atypical myelogenous cells in the dermal infiltrate.

PATHOGENESIS

Drug reactions can occur secondary to immunologic or nonimmunologic reactions. Immunologic reactions require host immunologic pathways and are called *drug allergies*. The ability of a drug to elicit an immune reaction depends on many characteristics. Most drugs are small organic molecules with molecular weights less than 1000 daltons.[14] Because of their size, they are unable to elicit immune responses unless they bind to a larger molecule, which is usually a protein macromolecule. In this situation the drug functions as a hapten. Most drugs have little ability to form covalent bonds with macromolecules and are unable to form this type of immunologic antigen.

The host reacts to drugs in different manners. The body may respond differently to a drug given intravenously than to one applied topically. Patients may have variation in their ability to absorb or metabolize a given drug. The patient with infectious mononucleosis may be more likely to develop a morbilliform eruption to ampicillin.

The body's immunologic response to drugs may be immunoglobulin E (IgE)-dependent, which can be associated with pruritus, urticaria, bronchial spasm, and laryngeal edema. Drug eruptions may be associated with serum-sickness-like responses. Cytotoxic drug reactions can occur where the drug combines with the tissue, and that combination then becomes the target for antibodies or cellular-mediated cytotoxicity.

Most morbilliform reactions are reproducible and are believed to be immunologic but not IgE-mediated.[10] Nonimmunologic drug reactions can result through various modalities. Aspirin, opiates, and radiocontrast medications may directly release mast cell mediators, resulting in urticaria. Overdosage of a medicine may cause adverse cutaneous side effects by direct injury to cutaneous cells. Genetic inability to detoxify certain chemical compounds results in toxic metabolites that can also damage cutaneous cells. Direct activation of granulocytic cells by colony stimulating factors is responsible for Sweet's syndrome.

Secondary side effects of chemotherapy can include alopecia or particular types of rashes secondary to thrombocytopenia, or they can target specific areas of skin, as in acral erythema seen with cytotoxic agents. Antibiotics can destroy the normal bacterial flora, allowing overgrowth of other organisms.

Drugs may interact to compete for binding sites or cause metabolic changes. In addition, certain drugs, such as lithium, can exacerbate acne and psoriasis by activating neutrophils. Treatment with NSAIDs of a child with urticaria can exacerbate the urticaria.

Drug-induced urticaria can also be caused by IgE mechanisms, anti-IgE receptor antibodies, or circulating immune complexes. The IgE-dependent urticaria reactions usually occur within 36 hours of drug exposure, but they can occur within minutes. It usually begins 4–12 days after exposure to the drug, at which time an equilibrium has been achieved between antibody and drug antigen, allowing for the formation of immune complexes. The serum-sickness-type reaction is often accompanied by fever, hematuria, and arthralgia. Liver and neurologic injury may occur.

The pathophysiology of drug-associated cutaneous vasculitis is not clear, but immune complexes may be responsible. The lesions usually begin to resolve several days or weeks after the offending drug is removed.

The histologic picture for photoallergic contact dermatitis and phototoxic reaction is similar, with associated epidermal spongiosis, dermal edema, and inflammatory response. True phototoxicity is pathologically more like sunburn than a dermatitis.

The photosensitivity may be confirmed by a photopatch test in which the drug is readministered and multiple intensities of ultraviolet light exposure are given. Photosensitive reactions are usually in the ultraviolet A range. Photosensitive reactions often resolve with marked hyperpigmentation that may take several months to resolve.

TREATMENT

Removal of the offending drug is the usual first therapy. Drug eruption is easily diagnosed when one can identify a specific pattern of drug eruption with a known timely exposure to only a single medication, and that medication has been frequently associated with that specific type of eruption. The infant or child exposed to multiple medications over a short period offers a more difficult diagnostic and therapeutic dilemma. Depending on the severity of the drug reaction, none of the drugs, the most likely drug, or all of the drugs may need to be removed.

Morbilliform eruptions may fade with time, without drug removal, especially when associated with amoxicillin or ampicillin. Urticarial eruptions may respond to antihistamine therapy.

Anaphylaxis associated with urticarial eruptions and angioedema is a medical emergency. Immediate therapy should be started with 1:1000 aqueous epinephrine, 0.2–0.5 mL given subcutaneously, and intravenous fluids. Antihistamines and systemic steroids may also be required to maintain an adequate airway while the symptoms subside.

PATIENT EDUCATION

The parents of the affected child should be informed of the possible association of the cutaneous eruption and the specific drugs involved. The risk for the child from subsequent exposure to the specific or similar medications needs to be explained. For a severe reaction, the child may be instructed to wear a bracelet or necklace to alert examining healthcare workers to the suspected allergy. The parents should be informed of alternative forms of therapy that would avoid the offending agent.

The cause of the photosensitivity should be fully described to the family and child. If the drug that caused a phototoxic reaction is required, it may be continued if the ultraviolet light intensity can be decreased to a level that is not adequate to cause significant dermatitis. Children who develop a photo-toxic reaction to psoralen-containing plants, such as celery or limes, should avoid the combination of plant exposure and sun exposure. If possible, the photosensitizing drug should be totally withdrawn. If hyperpigmentation occurs, it may require months to resolve.

FOLLOW-UP VISITS

Follow-up visits are necessary to confirm the resolution of the eruption and recognize the response of the original illness that required drug therapy. The frequency and timing of the visits will depend on the severity of the original illness and the drug eruption.

The patient's medical records should document the possible drug-associated eruption to attempt avoidance of future exposures to the drug or related compounds. For penicillin-associated reactions, skin testing may be indicated to attempt to predict the future possibility of hypersensitivity reactions to the penicillins.

In children with photosensitive drug eruptions, additional follow-up visits for photopatch testing to confirm the diagnosis may be considered.

REFERENCES

1. Litt JZ. Litt's drug eruption reference manual: including drug interactions, 10th edn. New York: Taylor and Francis; 2005.
2. Diaz Jara M, Perez-Montero A, Garcia-Bira MT, et al. Allergic reactions due to ibuprofen in children. Pediatr Dermatol 2001; 18:66–67.
3. Nigen S, Knowles SR, Shear NH. Drug eruptions: approaching the diagnosis of drug-induced skin diseases. J Drugs Dermatol 2003; 2:278–299.
4. Lam NS, Yang NS, Yang YH, et al. Clinical characteristics of childhood erythema multiforme, Stevens-Johnson syndrome and toxic epidermal necrolysis in Taiwanese children. J Microbiol Immunol Infect 2004; 37:366–370.
5. Sullivan JR, Shear NH. The drug hypersensitivity syndrome: what is the pathogenesis? Arch Dermatol 2001; 137:357–364.
6. Rzany B, Correia O, Kelly JP, et al. Risk of Stevens-Johnson syndrome and toxic epidermal necrolysis during the first weeks of antiepileptic therapy: a case control study. Lancet 1999; 353:2190–2194.
7. Korman R, Koren G, Shear NH. Erythema multiforme, Stevens-Johnson syndrome and toxic epidermal necrolysis in children: a review of ten years experience. Drug Saf 2002; 25:965–972.
8. Kim SJ, Lee DP, Suh HS, et al. Toxic epidermal necrolysis: clinical course and SCORTEN-based comparison of mortality rate and treatment modalities in Korean patients. Acta Derm Venereol 2005; 85:497–502.
9. Roujeau JC. Clinical heterogeneity of drug hypersensitivity. Toxicology 2005; 209:123–129.
10. Lammintausta K, Kortekangas-Savolainen O. Oral challenge in patients with suspected cutaneous adverse drug reactions: findings in 784 patients during a 25-year period. Acta Derm Venereol 2005; 85:491–496.

11. Wolf R, Matz H, Marcos B, et al. Drug rash with eosinophilia and systemic symptoms vs. toxic epidermal necrolysis: the dilemma of classification. Clin Dermatol 200523:311–314.

12. Baruzzi A, Contin M, Barbara G, et al. Drug rash with eosinophilia and systemic symptoms secondary to phenobarbitone. Clin Neuropharmacol 2003; 26:177–178.

13. Bachot N, Rouheau JC. Differential diagnosis of severe cutaneous drug eruptions. Am J Clin Dermatol 2003; 4:561–572.

14. Crowson AN, Magro CM. Recent advances in the pathology of cutaneous drug eruptions. Dermatol Clin 1999; 17:537–560.

15. Trent JT, Kerdel FA. Intravenous immunoglobulin for the treatment of toxic epidermal necrolysis. Arch Dermatol 2003; 139:1081.

16. Prins C, Vittorio C, Padilla RS, et al. Effect of high-dose intravenous immunoglobulin therapy in Stevens-Johnson syndrome: a retrospective, multi-center study. Dermatology 2003; 207:96–99.

17. Tas S, Simmonart T. Management of drug rash with eosinophilia and systemic symptoms (DRESS syndrome): an update. Dermatology 2003; 206:353–356.

18. Bachot N, Revuz J, Roujeau JC. Intravenous immunoglobulin for Stevens-Johnson syndrome and toxic epidermal necrolysis: a prospective noncomparative study showing no benefit on mortality or progression. Arch Dermatol 2003; 139:33–36.

19. Di Pasqale MA, Espana EM, Liu DT, et al. Correlation of corneal complications with eyelid cicatricial pathologies in patients with Stevens-Johnson syndrome and toxic epidermal necrolysis syndrome. Ophthalmology 2005; 112:904–912.

20. Bousetta K, Ponvert C, Karila C, et al. Hypersensitivity reactions to paracetamol in children: a study of 25 cases. Allergy 2005; 60:1174–1177.

21. Ibia EO, Schwartz RH, Wiedermann RL. Antibiotic rashes in children: a survey in a private practice setting. Arch Dermatol 2000; 136:849–854.

22. Romano A. Recognizing antibacterial hypersensitivity in children. Paediatric Drugs 2000; 2:101–112.

23. Romano A, Gueant-Rodriguez RM, Viola M, et al. Diagnosing immediate reactions to cephalosporins. Clin Exp Allergy 2005; 35:1234–1242.

24. Agrawal S, Agarwalla A. Dapsone hypersensitivity syndrome: a clinico-epidemiological review. J Dermatol 2003; 32:883–889.

25. Menniti-Ippolito F, Traversa G, Da Cas R, et al. Niflumic acid and mucocutaneous reactions. Pediatrics 2006; 117:253–254.

26. Sturkenbloom M, Nicolosi A, Cantarutti L, et al. Incidence of mucocutaneous reactions in children treated with niflumic acid, other nonsteroidal antiinflammatory drugs or nonopioid analgesics. Pediatrics 2005; 116:e26–e33.

27. Carder KR. Hypersensitivity reactions in neonates and infants. Dermatol Ther 2005; 18:160–175.

28. Sanchex-Borges M, Capriles-Hulett A, Caballero-Fonseca F. Risk of skin reactions using ibuprofen-based medicines. Expert Opin Drug Saf 2005; 4:837–848.

29. Morelli JG, Tay YK, Rogers M, et al. Fixed drug eruptions in children. J Pediatr 1999; 134:365–367.

30. Nissinovitch M, Prous D, Ben Amitai D, et al. Fixed drug eruption in the genital area of 15 boys. Pediatr Dermatol 2002; 19:216–219.

31. Roujeau JC, Bioulac-Sage P, Bourseau C, et al. Acute generalized exanthematous pustulosis. Analysis of 63 cases. Arch Dermatol 1991; 127:1333–1338.

32. Lee UH, Yang JH, Choi JC, et al. Acute generalized exanthematous pustulosis in a six year old boy. J Dermatol 2004; 31:497–499.

33. Smith K, Norwwod C, Skelton H. Do the physical and histologic features and time course in acute generalized exanthematous pustulosis reflect a pattern of cytokine dysregulation? J Cutan Med Surg 2003; 7:7–12.

34. Kakourou T, Drosatou P, Psychou F, et al. Erythema nodosum in children: a prospective study. J Am Acad Dermatol 2001; 44:17–21.

35. Pruszkowski A, Bodemer C, Freitag S, et al. Neonatal and infantile erythrodermas. Arch Dermatol 2000; 136:875–879.

36. Herron MD, Coffin CM, Vanderhooft SL. Sweet syndrome in two children. Pediatr Dermatol 2005; 22:525–529.

Skin Diseases in Newborns

Skin lesions appearing in the first month of life usually prompt parents to seek medical advice. A thorough knowledge of fetal skin biology (see Ch. 1) and of cutaneous lesions of newborns is expected of those providing neonatal care.

This chapter is divided into five sections: neonatal skin care, transient skin disease in the newborn, birthmarks, common congenital malformations, and miscellaneous skin conditions in the newborn period. Many of the transient disorders of the newborn will be considered by their clinical features, differential diagnosis, and pathogenesis only because no treatment is required of these self-limited problems. Acne neonatorum is also discussed in Chapter 3, miliaria in Chapter 11, and pigmentary changes in Chapter 17.

NEONATAL SKIN CARE

The full-term newborn's skin feels very soft and smooth. The smooth texture and softness is related to the hydration of the epidermis and condition of the collagen and dermal matrix substances. At birth the full-term infant's skin is functionally mature. The barrier portion of the epidermis, the stratum corneum, is intact and effectively protects the infant.

Even though the infant's barrier function may be normal at birth, he or she is at increased risk for systemic toxicity of topically applied compounds (Box 21.1). The infant's surface area is great when compared to body mass. The infant's metabolism, excretion, distribution, and protein binding of chemical agents may be different from those of an adult. The premature infant is at much greater risk. The premature infant has markedly decreased epidermal barrier function and an even greater body surface area to body volume ratio. In addition, the immature organs of the premature infant may greatly change the metabolism, excretion, distribution, and protein binding of chemical agents. Local or systemic toxicity can occur in the premature infant from soaps, lotions, or other cleansing solutions that may not cause problems for the term infant.[1]

The skin of the mature infant often appears dry and cracked soon after birth (Figs 21.1–21.3). The stratum corneum, which has been accumulated in utero, has not yet shed. Fissures and bleeding may occur on the ankles and wrists. During this time, topical care should include moisturizing lotions or creams. The goal of therapy is to retain the soft, flexible texture of the infant's skin by hydrating and lubricating the epidermis. For infants in a dry environment, the moisturizers may need to be used indefinitely. Infants from a more humid environment may need only intermittent use of moisturizers.

The skin care of the premature infant is much more difficult and complex (Box 21.2).[1–3] Not only is the barrier portion of the epidermis absent or defective, but the skin has markedly increased fragility. Because of epidermal and dermal injury, the infant may have significant cutaneous pain that is accentuated by routine handling. The infant is at risk for developing sepsis from skin-associated organisms.[4] Many studies have looked at developing the best methods of premature infant skin care.[5–12] A summary related to daily topical ointment

---

Box 21.1 Reasons for increased risk of systemic toxicity from topically applied agents in infants

Increased surface area to body weight ratio

Differences in drug excretion

Differences in drug metabolism

Differences in drug protein binding

Differences in drug distribution

Fig. 21.1 Dry, flaking skin on term infant 36 hours old.

Fig. 21.2 Dry fine desquamation on leg of postmature infant.

Fig. 21.3 Postmature infant. Long fingernails and peeling of the palms can be seen this 2-day-old infant.

Box 21.2 Care of the premature infant's skin

Gentle handling

Use adhesive tape sparingly, in the smallest possible area

Infrequent cardiac monitor changes

Sparing use of antibacterial cleansing solutions

Avoid frictional trauma to the skin

Intervention

Humidify infant environment

Skin lubrication with awareness of possible absorption of preservatives and emulsifiers within the product used

Localized use of semipermeable wound dressings

therapy suggests that it improves infant skin condition, but because of a trend toward an increased risk of bacterial infections, it should not be used routinely.[13] Many ethnic cultures use topical oils and one study suggested that in a mouse model, sunflower seed oil accelerated epidermal barrier recovery better than mustard, olive, or soybean oils.[14] Control trials in Egypt and Bangladesh documented that sunflower seed oil treatment of the skin of preterm infants protected the infants from nosocomial infections and improved the infant's skin condition.[9,11] Future studies will continue to improve on current protocols. At this time, the dry, flaking, fissured skin of premature infants should be treated with sunflower seed oil or preservative-free ointments. Ointments placed on an infant's skin under an infrared warmer will not cause cutaneous burns. Semipermeable wound dressings may offer additional cutaneous pain relief and protection, but additional studies must be done to analyze the potential for associated risk with bacterial growth under the dressings.[7]

TRANSIENT SKIN DISEASE

Milia

Clinical features

Milia are multiple, white, 1–2 mm papules seen over the forehead, cheeks, and nose of infants (Fig. 21.4). They may be present in the oral cavity as well, where they are called Epstein's pearls. Approximately 40% of newborns have milia on the skin, and 60% on the palate.[15] The cystic spheres rupture onto the skin surface and exfoliate their contents within a few weeks of birth.

Differential diagnosis

Molluscum contagiosum, an acquired viral infection, may mimic milia but does not usually appear in the immediate neonatal period. Sebaceous gland hyper-

Fig. 21.4 Milia. Multiple white papules seen over the forehead of an infant.

plasia also occurs over the nose and cheeks of infants, but it is yellow rather than whitish.

Pathogenesis

On histologic examination, milia appear as superficial epithelial cysts in the upper dermis, just beneath the epidermis. The cyst cavity is filled with keratin.

Sebaceous Gland Hyperplasia

Clinical features

Tiny (1 mm) yellow macules or yellow papules are seen at the opening of each pilosebaceous follicle over the nose and cheeks of newborns (Figs 21.5, 21.6). These occur in about 50% of infants.[15] They recede completely by 4–6 months of age.

Differential diagnosis

Milia may mimic sebaceous hyperplasia but are white and cystic in appearance.

Pathogenesis

Maternal androgenic stimulation is responsible for the increase in sebaceous gland volume, sebaceous cell size, and the total number of sebaceous cells.

Mottling

Clinical features

A lacelike pattern of dusky erythema appears over the extremities and trunk of neonates when exposed to a temperature decrease. This phenomenon may be

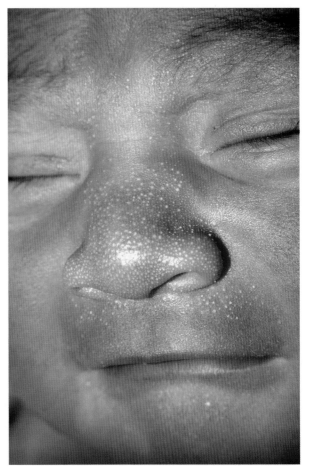

Fig. 21.5 Sebaceous gland hyperplasia on the nose and upper lip of a neonate.

Fig. 21.6 Sebaceous gland hyperplasia on nose of infant.

sensitive to small increments of temperature change. The mottling disappears on rewarming. Mottling that persists beyond 6 months of age may be a sign of hypothyroidism or the vascular malformation cutis marmorata telangiectatica congenita, which can be associated with musculoskeletal or vascular abnormalities.[16] Occasionally, it can be seen associated with large areas of dermal melanocytosis.[17]

Differential diagnosis

Certain birthmarks, such as cutis marmorata telangiectatica congenita, may mimic mottling, but the color change will not disappear with rewarming. Similarly, the livedo reticularis seen with collagen vascular diseases, such as neonatal lupus erythematosus, will persist when the skin is warmed.

Pathogenesis

The cause of cutis marmorata telangiectatica congenita is not known.

Harlequin Color Change

Clinical features

When a low-birth-weight infant is placed on one side, an erythematous flush with a sharp demarcation at the midline develops on the dependent side. The upper half of the body becomes pale. The color change usually subsides within a few seconds of placing the baby in the supine position, but may persist for as long as 20 minutes.

Differential diagnosis

The color change is seldom confused with other vascular problems.

Pathogenesis

The exact mechanism of this unusual phenomenon is not known, but the immaturity of autonomic vasomotor control is believed to be responsible. Recently, this condition was associated with the dose of systemic prostaglandin E_1 infusion.[18]

Subcutaneous Fat Necrosis

Clinical features

In subcutaneous fat necrosis of the newborn, firm, sharply circumscribed, reddish or purple nodules appear over the cheeks, buttocks, arms, and thighs (Figs 21.7, 21.8).[19–21] The lesions usually begin within the first 2 weeks of life and resolve spontaneously

Fig. 21.7 Subcutaneous fat necrosis. Multiple firm indurated nodules on the back of an infant.

Fig. 21.8 Subcutaneous fat necrosis. Red plaques of immobile skin on back of infant.

over several weeks to months. Occasionally, the lesions can heal with atrophy, leaving a skin depression (Fig. 21.9). Infrequently, hypercalcemia can occur with or without associated irritability, vomiting, weight

Fig. 21.9 Subcutaneous fat necrosis. Dusky, depressed area of atrophy after redness cleared.

loss, and failure to thrive.[20,21] Occasionally, hypocalcemia can occur.[22] Serum calcium evaluations should be repeated weekly until the lesions have totally resolved for a month or more in infants who have multiple large plaques of involved skin or have renal disease.[21]

Differential diagnosis

Bacterial cellulitis or septicemic lesions may be confused with subcutaneous fat necrosis at the onset. The infant with fat necrosis often appears healthy and nurses vigorously, in contrast to those with bacterial infections. Several separate lesion sites are often seen with subcutaneous fat necrosis and would be extremely unusual with cellulitis. Ultrasound, computed tomography (CT) or magnetic resonance imaging (MRI) imaging may be helpful in confirming the diagnosis if a skin biopsy is not done.[23]

Pathogenesis

These lesions are usually seen in infants with perinatal stress or asphxia.[21] Cold injury may also be related to subcutaneous fat necrosis. The fat of the neonate contains more saturated fatty acids, which have a higher melting point.[19] Once the temperature of the skin drops below the melting point of the fat, crystallization occurs within the fat of the subcutaneous fat cells and is followed by a granulomatous reaction.

Sclerema

Clinical features

Premature newborns who suffer hypothermia are susceptible to the development of sclerema, a diffuse har-dening of the skin. The skin becomes tight, immobile, yellow, and shiny. Sclerema appears in severely ill newborns who have suffered sepsis, hypoglycemia, metabolic acidosis, or other severe metabolic abnormalities.[19] Temperature control, nutritional replacement, correction of metabolic acidosis, and possibly repeated exchange transfusions will arrest the process. Infant mortality in sclerema is high.

Differential diagnosis

The thickening and hardening of the skin are so characteristic of sclerema that it is not confused with other disorders.

Pathogenesis

The susceptibility of the subcutaneous fat to cold injury is believed to be the cause of sclerema. Edema of fibrous septa surrounding fat lobules, without fat necrosis, is found.

Sucking Blisters

Clinical features

Sucking blisters are usually solitary intact oval blisters or erosions on noninflamed skin in the newborn.[24] They occur on the forearms, wrists, fingers (Fig. 21.10), or upper lip and resolve within a few days.

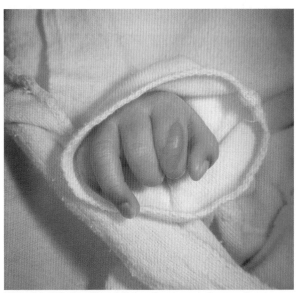

Fig. 21.10 Sucking blister. Oval noninflammatory blister on the finger of a newborn.

Differential diagnosis

Herpes virus infection or bullous impetigo should be considered when sucking blisters are encountered, but these lesions appear on an erythematous base. In incontinentia pigmenti, multiple linear blisters are present, in contrast to the solitary sucking blister. Epidermolysis bullosa usually presents with multiple new blisters that develop after birth.

Pathogenesis

Vigorous sucking in utero has been postulated as the cause of these blisters.

Erythema Toxicum

Clinical features

Blotchy, erythematous macules 2–3 cm in diameter, with a tiny 1 –4 mm central vesicle or pustule, are seen in erythema toxicum (Figs 21.11–21.13). They

Fig. 21.11 Erythema toxicum. Blotchy erythematous macules and plaques with multiple papules and pustules.

Fig. 21.12 Erythema toxicum. Vesicles and pustules which are with or without an erythematous base.

Fig. 21.13 Erythema toxicum. Typical lesions on leg of newborn.

usually begin at 24–48 hours of age. They occur in about 50% of term infants and less commonly in premature infants.[25] Lesions are seen on the chest, back, face, and proximal extremities, sparing the palms and soles. The individual lesions clear in 4–5 days and new lesions may occur from birth to the tenth day of life. Smear of the central vesicle or pustule contents will reveal numerous eosinophils on Wright-stained preparations. A peripheral blood eosinophilia up to 20% may accompany the tissue eosinophil accumulation, particularly in infants with numerous lesions. Recent studies suggest that normal bacterial flora gain entry into the skin tissue through the hair canal. The erythematous lesions are a local immune system response. The early neonatal microbial exposure may be important for the maturation of the immune system.[25]

Transient Neonatal Pustular Melanosis

Clinical features

The lesions of transient neonatal pustular melanosis present at birth as vesicles, pustules, or ruptured vesicles or pustules with a collarette of surrounding scale. Many of the lesions will have a base that does not have surrounding erythema.[26] Pigmented macules are also often present at birth, or they develop at the sites of resolving pustules or vesicles (Fig. 21.14). The vesicles and pustules usually disappear by 5 days of age, whereas the pigmented macules resolve over 3 weeks to 3 months. These lesions are more common on black infants, and they can occur on the palms and soles. Smear of the vesicle or pustule contents will reveal numerous neutrophils and an occasional eosinophil on Wright-stained preparations.[26]

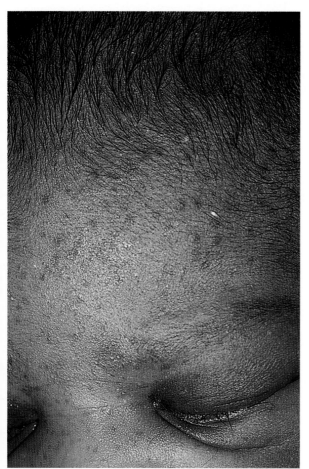

Fig. 21.14 Transient neonatal pustular melanosis. Multiple macules at sites of previous pustules on a 10-day-old infant.

Differential diagnosis

Miliaria rubra is frequently confused with erythema toxicum. The erythema around miliaria rubra is small in area (1–2 mm versus 20–30 mm in erythema toxicum). The central vesicle or pustule may mimic herpes simplex or bacterial folliculitis lesions. A Gram's stain of the pustules of erythema toxicum or transient neonatal pustular melanosis will be negative. The Wright-stained slide from a pustule of erythema toxicum will show a predominance of eosinophils, whereas the slide of a pustule of transient neonatal pustular melanosis will usually show a predominance of neutrophils.

Pathogenesis

Erythema toxicum is believed to be associated with normal bacterial flora in the pilosebaceous orifice. The

cause of transient neonatal pustular melanosis is not known.

Pustules in the Newborn

Clinical features

Pustules are discrete, yellow, 1–9 mm raised lesions that frequently display a red base. The appearance of pustules in the newborn should immediately bring to mind the possibility of bacterial sepsis. Pustules on the newborn skin in association with other signs or symptoms of sepsis, or when prolonged rupture of maternal membranes has occurred, should make one suspect bacterial sepsis. Bacterial culture of pustules of other body fluids, such as blood, urine, and cerebrospinal fluid, should be performed. There is no rapid, completely reliable method of determining whether a baby has bacterial sepsis, and one should always maintain a high index of suspicion. The incidence of bacterial sepsis is higher in the preterm infant than in the full-term infant, and overall sepsis is an uncommon cause of pustules in the newborn. However, the high mortality rate of unrecognized bacterial sepsis makes it imperative for the clinician to consider this possibility.

Differential diagnosis

Other causes of pustules in the newborn may be considered after bacterial sepsis is eliminated as a possibility. Erythema toxicum may occasionally be pustular, particularly if skin involvement is extensive. Transient neonatal pustular melanosis mimics erythema toxicum and is characterized by pustules present at birth. Herpes simplex skin infections may be pustular but are usually characterized as a grouping of vesicular lesions. Acne neonatorum is usually not present in the first 14 days of life, and evolution to the pustular stage may require several more weeks. Candidiasis, particularly of the diaper area or of other intertriginous areas, may be pustular, and satellite pustules are characteristically found at a distance from the margins of confluent areas of candidiasis. Congenital candidiasis, acquired in utero, may also be pustular, with discrete pustules at birth and subsequent development of diffusely eczematous skin. Infantile acropustulosis may begin at birth or within the newborn period and present with discrete pustules limited to the distal extremities, with prominent involvement of the palms and soles. Nevus comedonicus is a birthmark consisting of patulous follicular openings in which pustule formation, or even deeper abscesses, may occur, but not usually in the newborn period. Psoriasis rarely occurs in the newborn period, but it also may be extensive and pustular.

Pathogenesis

In bacterial infections, pustules arise as the result of accumulation of neutrophils within the skin after dissemination of bacteria from the blood to the skin or direct bacterial invasion of the skin.

Acne Neonatorum

Clinical features

Neonatal acne (see also Ch. 3) is rarely present at birth but may appear as multiple, discrete papules at 2–4 weeks of age. The face, chest, back, and groin are the usual areas for cutaneous lesions (Figs 21.15, 21.16). Papules evolve into pustules after a few weeks. Neonatal acne may persist up to 8 months of age. There is some suggestion that infants with extensive neonatal acne may experience severe acne as adolescents.

Differential diagnosis

The differential diagnosis of acne neonatorum is the same as for pustules in the newborn. In addition, neonatal cephalic pustulosis is associated with *Malassezia*, but the infants demonstrate pustules and no comedones.[27,28]

Pathogenesis

Neonatal acne may be a part of the so-called miniature puberty of the newborn. Neonatal sebaceous

Fig. 21.16 Acne papules and pustules on cheek of 2-week-old infant.

glands are hyperplastic, and hydroxysteroid dehydrogenase activity in these structures is high in the 2 months just before birth and at birth. There is evidence that newborns with acne experience transient increases in circulating androgens.

Treatment

Neonatal acne usually resolves spontaneously without treatment. If the involvement is severe, topical therapy with 2.5% benzoyl peroxide gel can be used.

Acropustulosis of Infancy

Clinical features

Acropustulosis of infancy presents as pustules or vesicles on the palms and soles (Figs 21.17–21.19). The lesions may be present at birth or occur up to age 3.[29] The lesions occur in recurrent crops of erythematous papules that rapidly become pruritic pustules.[30] Pruritus in the neonate or infant may be expressed as an irritable, fretful child who does not demonstrate the coordination to scratch. The pustules resolve with scale, and eventually lichenification may develop in the affected area. The lesions may recur until 2–3 years of age.

Differential diagnosis

Lesions caused by scabies can be very similar to the lesions of acropustulosis of infancy.[31] All infants should be examined for scabies by scraping the involved area and looking for mites. A history of pruritus in family members is strongly suggestive for scabies, and if mites are not found on the infant, the family mem-

Fig. 21.15 Acne neonatorum. Multiple small inflammatory papules on the face of a 1-month-old infant.

Fig. 21.18 Infantile acropustulosis. Vesicles and pustules on infant's heel.

Fig. 21.17 Pustules, scaling, and lichenification on the hand of an infant with infantile acropustulosis.

Fig. 21.19 Infantile acropustulosis. Vesicles and pustules on foot of 3-week-old.

bers should be examined and scraped. Dyshidrotic eczema usually occurs in older children and adults and presents with smaller vesicles.

Pathogenesis

Bacterial cultures of the lesions should be sterile. The histology will demonstrate edema between keratinocytes and an infiltrate of mononuclear cells, neutrophils, or possibly eosinophils. The cause of this condition is unknown, and once scabies is excluded, biopsy or culture is unnecessary because of the characteristic presentation of the lesions.

Treatment

Moderate-potency topical steroids may be required to decrease the intensity of pruritus. Occasionally,

oral antihistamines (hydroxyzine 2 mg/kg/day) may also be required. The lesions continue to recur until 2–3 years of age.

Patient education

Reassessment and continued suspicion of scabies is important because of the long-term nature of this condition. Long-term therapy for the pruritus should be monitored on a quarterly basis.

Congenital and Neonatal Candidiasis
Clinical features

Candida albicans can present in the neonate as a congenital infection acquired before birth or as a neonatal infection acquired during the birth process.[32,33] Infants with congenital cutaneous candidiasis have scaling lesions, erythematous papules, and pustules at birth (Fig. 21.20). Invasion into follicular structures may be seen as yellowish plaques in premature infants (Fig. 21.21). A skin scraping prepared with potassium hydroxide (KOH) should document the pseudo-hyphae and/or budding yeast, and a skin culture should document C. *albicans*. Infants with neonatal candidiasis will develop lesions several days or weeks after birth. The infants may have a diffuse scaling dermatitis or present with typical satellite pustules in the intertriginous areas. The KOH preparation and cutaneous culture should document the cause of the cutaneous eruption.

Differential diagnosis

Erythema toxicum, miliaria, transient neonatal pustular melanosis, and herpes virus infections can cause blisters and pustules in the neonate. The KOH preparation will document a yeast infection, and a cutaneous culture will confirm *Candida albicans*. Low-birth-weight infants may develop systemic candidiasis.[33]

Pathogenesis

C. *albicans* can penetrate through the amnion and chorion to cause congenital infections.[32,33] The neonatal infection appears to be acquired during the birth process through the vagina colonized with *Candida*.

Treatment

Topical treatment with an antifungal such as nystatin, miconazole, or ketoconazole is effective for infants with only cutaneous lesions. Systemic infections in

Fig. 21.20 Pustules and erythematous papules noted at birth in an infant with congenital cutaneous candidiasis.

Fig. 21.21 Congenital candidiasis. Closeup view of yellowish plaques of candidiasis and adjacent normal premature infant skin.

low-birth-weight infants require intensive antifungal intravenous therapy.

Herpes Simplex Infection

Clinical features

Grouped vesicles on an erythematous base should bring to mind neonatal herpes simplex virus (HSV) infection (Figs 21.22, 21.23). Any area of skin may be involved, but vesicles on the scalp or buttock are particularly common (Fig. 21.24). Monitoring electrodes may produce sufficient skin trauma on involved skin sites to allow invasion by the virus and to induce herpes simplex virus skin lesions.[34] Vesicles may be present immediately at birth, but the onset after birth is more likely, with 6 days as the mean age of onset. Visible lesions are diagnosed in over half of infants diagnosed clinically and in less that 25% of the infants diagnosed at postmortem.[35] Mucous membrane involvement is common. The majority of neonatal herpes simplex infections are type 2.[35]

Differential diagnosis

Other blistering diseases of the newborn, such as congenital varicella, bullous impetigo, and incontinentia pigmenti, may be considered in a differential diagnosis. A Wright-stained smear of cells scraped from a vesicle base will demonstrate multinucleated giant cells and balloon cells in herpes simplex virus infection. Fluorescein-tagged antiherpes simplex virus-specific antibody may be used to examine vesicle smears or snap-frozen biopsy sections of skin to make a rapid diagnosis. Viral culture of herpes simplex virus

Fig. 21.22 Neonatal herpes simplex. Grouped vesicles on an erythematous base in this 9-day-old infant.

Fig. 21.23 Neonatal herpes simplex. Grouped vesicles on red base on trunk of newborn.

Fig. 21.24 Neonatal herpes simplex. Many groups of vesicles on skin of newborn.

requires 12–120 hours to grow, and in all infected or suspected neonates, cultures of skin lesions, urine, nasopharynx, eyes, and cerebrospinal fluid are indicated. Serum antibodies for herpes simplex virus are of little assistance in making the diagnosis accurately. Rapid diagnosis of herpes simplex virus is essential, and a high index of suspicion should be maintained.

Pathogenesis

Herpes simplex virus is usually related to maternal infection in the birth canal.[34] Infected infants are likely to have had a premature birth, may have signs that mimic bacterial sepsis, and may develop psychomotor retardation even if obvious signs of dissemination of herpes simplex virus are not evident in the newborn period.[35] Infants born to mothers with a primary herpes genital infection at the time of delivery are more likely to develop neonatal herpes simplex than infants born to mothers with recurrent genital lesions.[34,35]

Treatment

High-dose acyclovir, administered intravenously, is the treatment of choice.[35] Early recognition and early therapeutic intervention appear to lead to an improved outcome in the infected infant. Caesarean delivery may be effective in prevention of neonatal herpes simplex infections.[34] Prevention of acquisition of genital HSV-1 and HSV-2 near term will be the therapy of the future.[34]

Varicella

Clinical features

Congenital varicella is quite rare but may mimic herpes simplex virus in the newborn (see Ch. 8). The congenital varicella syndrome is different in that it is a varicella infection associated with intrauterine infection in the first 20 weeks of gestation resulting in cutaneous, musculoskeletal, and neurological lesions.[36] Congenital varicella is associated with maternal chickenpox 2–3 weeks before delivery. Lesions appear as crops of macules and papules that evolve into vesicles and then crust. Age of onset is within the first 10 days after birth, and mortality has been reported in infants who develop skin lesions between 5 and 10 days of age. A Wright-stained smear of cells from a blister base or a skin biopsy demonstrates the same changes seen in herpes simplex virus. Maternal history of varicella and cutaneous lesions in the infant compatible with varicella are most useful in making the diagnosis. Varicella can also develop in neonates infected postnatally. This could result in a severe infection, especially in premature infants.[37]

Differential diagnosis

Herpes simplex virus infection and bullous impetigo are the two most important considerations in the differential diagnosis of congenital varicella. Fluorescein-tagged antiherpes zoster virus-specific antibody may be used to examine vesicle smears or snap-frozen biopsy sections of skin to make a rapid diagnosis. Culture identification of the virus from the vesicles may require 7–14 days.

Pathogenesis

Maternal infection with varicella-zoster virus results in dissemination of the virus to the newborn. Maternal infection may be unrecognized.

Treatment

Immediate administration of zoster immune globulin to the infant is recommended if maternal infection is present from 5 days before to 2 days after delivery.[38] Infected infants require therapy with intravenous acyclovir. Passive immunization with varicella-zoster immunoglobulin should be considered for premature and term infants who have had postnatal exposure to varicella.

Impetigo
Clinical features

Bacterial impetigo may be observed in the newborn period (see Ch. 5). Flaccid, well-demarcated bullae that evolve into erosions may be seen. Any area of skin may be involved, but the scalp, face, and diaper areas are the most common sites of infection. A collarette of scale around the erosion is characteristic of *Staphylococcus aureus* (Fig. 21.25).[39]

Differential diagnosis

Bacterial culture of skin lesions and culture of the nasopharynx will yield the organism within 24 hours. Smear of vesicle contents and a Gram's stain will demonstrate the bacteria.

Fig. 21.25 Impetigo over the suprapubic area of a neonate. A collarette of scale around erythematous erosions is characteristic of *Staphylococcus aureus* impetigo.

Pathogenesis

S. aureus is a predominant organism producing impetigo, including those strains capable of producing the staphylococcal scalded skin syndrome (SSSS); therefore, prompt recognition and treatment are necessary. Occasionally group A streptococci or Gram-negative bacteria can cause impetigo in the newborn period.

Treatment

The appropriate systemic antibiotic should be administered promptly to prevent sepsis and diminish spread of bacteria to other patients and hospital personnel.

Staphylococcal Scalded Skin Syndrome (Ritter's Disease)
Clinical features

Infants 2–30 days old may develop an abrupt onset of generalized erythema followed in 24 hours by bullae, with subsequent exfoliation of large sheets of skin within 48 hours. The lesions are commonly around the head, neck, buttocks, groin, axillae, and periumbilical area of the abdomen.[40]

Differential diagnosis

Toxic shock syndrome (TSS) and toxic epidermal necrolysis (TEN) should be considered in the differential diagnosis of SSSS. However, these conditions are rarely observed in the newborn period.

Pathogenesis

Skin injury in SSSS is the result of an intraepidermal cleavage through the granular layer of epidermis caused by circulating exotoxin produced by *S. aureus*. Both bullous impetigo and SSSS are caused by an exfoliative toxin (ET) elaborated by certain strains of *S. aureus*. The toxin is a serine proteases which causes proteolysis of desmoglein 1, a protein associated with desmosomes.[41] Culture of the nasopharynx, rectum, and skin lesions are likely to yield the organism.[42]

Treatment

Isolation of the affected newborn to prevent nursery epidemics is essential. Antistaphylococcal antibiotics should be administered systemically, and fluid and electrolyte replacement provided, much like that provided for burn therapy. Topical lubrication will decrease the pain and associated discomfort.

Breast Abscess
Clinical features

Swelling, erythema, and fluctuance in one breast of a newborn infant may signify a breast abscess. Onset usually begins 5–20 days after birth. Fever may be present, but the infant is usually asymptomatic otherwise.

Differential diagnosis

Breast hyperplasia caused by miniature puberty of the newborn may produce asymmetric enlargement of one breast without erythema.

Pathogenesis

S. aureus and Gram-negative organisms are the most likely pathogens for breast abscess. A needle aspiration of the infection may be necessary to obtain a positive bacterial culture.

Treatment

Systemic antibiotic therapy with the appropriate antistaphylococcal agent is usually necessary.

Omphalitis
Clinical features

Redness and induration of the umbilical region is characteristic of omphalitis (Fig. 21.26). Often, the redness is not well localized and diffusely spreads beyond the umbilicus.

Differential diagnosis

An irritant dermatitis produced by treatment of the umbilicus with various bacteriostatic agents may sometimes mimic omphalitis.

Pathogenesis

Bacterial infection through the cut surface of the umbilical cord is the usual cause of omphalitis. It is predominantly caused by *S. aureus* and, if untreated, may progress to bacterial sepsis.

Treatment

Prophylactic bacteriostatic agents applied to the cord in the newborn period may not reduce the likelihood

Fig. 21.26 Omphalitis. Swelling and redness of umbilicus in 7-day-old infant.

of this infection in nurseries in high-intake settings.[43] The frequency of omphalitis and neonatal mortality was reduced in a developing country using chlorhexidine cord care.[44] Administration of systemic antistaphylococcal antibiotic is the treatment of choice if infection develops.

Caput Succedaneum and Cephalohematoma
Clinical features

Caput succedaneum is subcutaneous edema over the presenting part of the head.[45] Cephalohematoma is a subperiosteal collection of blood.[45] Edema or hemorrhage of the scalp appears as deep swelling, with or without purpura. The swelling occurs primarily in vertex deliveries, particularly those with prolonged labor, and resolves spontaneously in 7–10 days. If the purpura is extensive, it can serve as a source of hyperbilirubinemia. Secondary bacterial infection of cephalohematoma may rarely occur, resulting in cellulitis.

Differential diagnosis

The caput succedaneum tends to feel soft and lacks a well-defined outline. The cephalohematoma is bounded by the suture lines of the skull and often feels fluctuant. Both lesions can mimic cellulitis or bacterial abscess. Appropriate cultures may assist in the differential diagnosis.

Pathogenesis

Both lesions are caused by shearing forces on the scalp skin and skull during labor.

Petechiae and Purpura
Clinical features

Petechiae and purpura may be presenting features of congenital infection, particularly when the newborn is small for gestational age and has hepatosplenomegaly. An acronym used for these infections is the TORCH (*t*oxoplasmosis, *o*ther (syphilis), *r*ubella, *c*ytomegalovirus, and congenital *h*erpes simplex virus infections) syndrome. Petechiae and purpura are the most common cutaneous symptoms for this group of congenital infections and may be important clues to the diagnosis. Newborns with congenital infection may also demonstrate other features, such as microphthalmia, congenital heart defects, cataracts, and psychomotor retardation.

Differential diagnosis

Toxoplasmosis, syphilis (see also Ch. 5), rubella, cytomegalovirus, and congenital herpes simplex virus infections are the usual congenital infections responsible for the production of petechiae and purpura. Serologic tests and viral cultures for these infections should be performed. Other causes of petechiae and purpura in the newborn include trauma, with face and scalp petechiae common in difficult vertex deliveries or in deliveries by caesarean section (Fig. 21.27). Neonatal thrombocytopenia caused by maternal autoantibodies, as in idiopathic thrombocytopenic purpura or systemic lupus erythematosus, may also produce neonatal petechiae a few hours after birth. Hypoprothrombinemia may result in purpura in the newborn older than 2 or 3 days because of vitamin K deficiency. Protein C deficiency can also cause severe purpura in the neonate. Neonatal petechiae and purpura are unusual in the hemophilias, but bleeding from circumcision sites may be the first manifestation of hemophilia in the newborn period. Neonatal purpura secondary to platelet dysfunction may be observed in von Willebrand's disease or Wiskott-Aldrich syndrome.

BIRTHMARKS

Birthmarks represent an excess of one or more of the normal components of skin per unit area: blood vessels, lymph vessels, pigment cells, hair follicles, sebaceous glands, epidermis, collagen, or elastin. Birthmarks

Fig. 21.27 Petechiae in a newborn. Multiple petechiae on the forehead of a neonate after a difficult vertex delivery.

are collections of highly differentiated cells in tissue. Vascular birthmarks are the most common.

Congenital malformations are most frequently observed in skin. The two most commonly seen are the so-called salmon patch and mongolian spots. Salmon patches are observed in about 70% of white infants and 60% of black infants.[46] Mongolian spots are more frequently observed in Asian infants (80%) and black infants (95%) but are less common in white infants.[47] Mongolian spots and salmon patches are observed at least 100 times more frequently than any other skin birthmark.[46]

Vascular Birthmarks: Salmon Patches and Port Wine Stains

See Chapter 13 for detailed description of diagnosis and treatment of the individual conditions.

The salmon patch appears as a light-red macule over the nape of the neck, the upper eyelids, and the glabella (Figs 21.28, 21.29). A salmon patch is present over the back of the neck in over 40% of infants. Salmon patches fade with time, but remnants may persist well into adult life. Generally, the eyelid lesions fade by 6–12 months of age and the glabellar lesions by 5–6 years of age. Lesions on the nape of the neck are more likely to persist.

Port-wine stains appear as deep-red or purple-red macules over the face or extremities (Figs 21.30–21.32). They are usually unilateral. Occasionally, they are extensive and cover large areas of skin. A port-wine stain over the face may be a clue to Sturge-

Fig. 21.29 Salmon-patch (capillary malformation) lesion on the glabella and upper eyelids.

Weber syndrome (Figs 21.33, 21.34). Port-wine stains over the face or an extremity may be associated with soft tissue and bony hypertrophy (Fig. 21.35). Some may develop inflammation and scaling (Fig. 21.36).

Vascular Birthmarks: Hemangiomas

Hemangiomas may not be observed at birth (see Ch. 13), but a circumscribed area of blanched skin with a few fine telangiectases may be present, representing a developing hemangioma (Fig. 21.37). By 2 to 4 weeks of age, the skin becomes raised, with red or purple nodules (Fig. 21.38). The lesions grow out of proportion to the baby for the first 8 to 12 months

Fig. 21.28 Salmon-patch lesion (port-wine stain, capillary malformation) on the nape of the neck. Also called a stork bite because in mythology this is where the stork carries the baby before it is delivered.

Fig. 21.30 Port-wine stain (capillary malformation) on cheek of newborn.

Fig. 21-31 Port-wine stain (capillary malformation) over mandibular skin and ear in newborn. No evidence of Sturge-Weber syndrome.

Fig. 21.32 Port-wine stain (capillary malformation) over back of newborn.

Fig. 21.33 Port-wine stain (capillary malformation) on face and scalp of infant with Sturge-Weber syndrome.

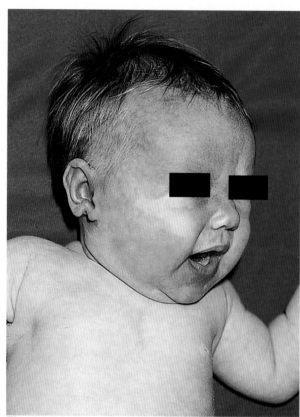

Fig. 21.34 Port-wine stain on infant who subsequently developed seizures associated with Sturge-Weber syndrome.

Fig. 21.35 Port-wine stain and hypertrophy of leg in neonate with Klippel-Trenaunay-Weber syndrome.

Fig. 21.37 Precursor to raised hemangioma. Blanched skin with fine telangiectasia is present at birth. Later the lesion will become raised.

Fig. 21.36 Redness and scaling overlying port-wine stain in inflammatory nuchal-occipital port-wine stain. Vascular laser treatment eradicated inflammatory change.

Fig. 21.38 Hemangioma on a 2-week-old. This lesion is raised with a blue-red color.

of life. Hemangiomas begin to show signs of involution around 15 months of age, when pale gray areas appear within the red nodule. Soon the first sign of flattening appears. In hemangiomas, ulceration of the epithelial surface may be associated with secondary S. aureus bacterial superinfection (Figs 21.39, 21.40).

Cutis Marmorata Telangiectatica Congenita

In cutis marmorata telangiectatica congenita, a mottled pattern of blue or dusky-red erythema is seen from birth (see Ch. 13). Often, a single extremity is involved, but the lesions may occur bilaterally on the extrem-

Fig. 21.39 Hemangioma of upper lip with early ulceration interfering with feeding in 3-week-old.

Fig. 21.40 Ulceration of buttocks hemangioma.

Fig. 21.42 Superficial hemangioma in neonate.

ities or on the trunk. The skin surface overlying such areas may be depressed. A gradual increase in the size of lesions is expected over the first few years of life, but most fade by adult life. Rigorous natural history studies of cutis marmorata telangiectatica congenita are not available. Associations with musculoskeletal or vascular abnormalities occur and are discussed in Chapter 13.

Diffuse Neonatal Hemangiomatosis

In the rare syndrome called diffuse neonatal hemangiomatosis (see Ch. 13), multiple, small, raised, cutaneous hemangiomas are noted that may be associated with hemangiomas in the liver, lungs, gastrointestinal tract, and central nervous system (Figs 21.41–21.44). The raised hemangiomas may be present at birth and more develop with time. The hemangiomas range 2–15 mm in diameter. Spontaneous involution of the lesions has been reported. Bleeding may occur into the gastrointestinal tract.

Fig. 21.41 Disseminated neonatal hemangiomatosis. Multiple small red papules on trunk of neonate.

Fig. 21.43 Diffuse neonatal hemangiomatosis in an 18-day-old infant.

Lymph Vessel Birthmarks: Lymphangiomas

Lymphangiomas may be circumscribed, superficial skin papules (Figs 21.45, 21.46) or deep, cavernous nodules (see Ch. 13). Circumscribed lymphangiomas

Fig. 21.44 Infant in Figure 21.43 at 30 days of age. Note rapid enlargement of the size of the lesions and the multiple lesions on the back and arm.

Fig. 21.46 Lymphangioma circumscriptum. After minor trauma the lesions may darken secondary to bleeding into the lesion.

appear as a solitary group of 2–4 mm, gelatinous, skin-colored papules limited to a skin area less than 10 cm. They are often connected to underlying venous channels, and hemorrhage into one or more papules may occur, producing sudden darkening. They may be present at birth, but are often not noticed until late infancy or childhood.

Pigment Cell Birthmarks: Mongolian Spots

An infant's skin is always light at birth and becomes progressively darker with increasing age. Hyperpigmentation of the scrotum and of the linea alba is common in dark-skinned infants at birth. The most commonly observed pigmentary abnormality of infants is the *mongolian spot* (see Ch. 17).

Mongolian spots are blue-black macules commonly located over the lumbosacral area (Fig. 21.47). They are occasionally noted over the shoulders and back and may extend over the buttocks and extremities. Mongolian spots fade somewhat with time, and the difference in pigmentation from normal skin pigment becomes less obvious as the newborn's pigment darkens. Some traces of mongolian spots may persist into adult life.

Pigment Cell Birthmarks: Café-au-lait Spots

Light-brown oval macules that may appear more dark brown on black skin are found anywhere on the body and are called café-au-lait spots. Black infants are far more likely (12%) than white infants (0.3%) to have

Fig. 21.45 Lymphangioma circumscriptum. Grouping of gelatinous skin-colored papules on the abdomen.

Fig. 21.47 Mongolian spot on the buttock of a neonate.

a solitary café-au-lait spot.[48] Café-au-lait spots persist through childhood and may increase in number with age (see Ch. 17).

Pigment Cell Birthmarks: Junctional Nevocellular Nevi

Dark-brown or black macules with distinct borders represent clones of melanocytes found at the junction of the epidermis and dermis and are called junctional nevocellular nevi. As an infant ages, these nevi may become slightly raised and papular and develop intra-dermal melanocytes, creating a compound nevus. Often, the surface of the lesion at birth is slightly irregular.

Pigment Cell Birthmarks: Raised Nevocellular Nevi

Skin-colored to tan or brown solitary papules with smooth surfaces represent intradermal nevi (see Ch. 17). Most nevi are small, measuring less than 1.5 cm at their greatest diameter. When these localized, raised pigment cell lesions are greater than 5% of the body surface area, there is a concern about their cancer potential (Figs 21.48, 21.49).

Hypopigmentation: Phenylketonuria

Clinical features

Newborns with phenylketonuria have blond hair, blue eyes, and light-colored skin. Routine screening tests for the presence of excessive amounts of phenylalanine in the blood will help detect this syndrome.

Fig. 21.48 Giant melanocytic congenital nevus in a bathing-trunk distribution.

Fig. 21.49 Congenital melanocytic nevus on the hand of an infant.

Differential diagnosis

Phenylketonuria should be distinguished from albinism and Chediak-Higashi syndrome. Analysis of blood for phenylalanine is the most useful differentiating test.

Pathogenesis

Patients with phenylketonuria lack the enzymes needed to utilize phenylalanine. Their hypopigmentation is thought to be related to the tight binding of phenylalanine to the receptor sites of tyrosinase such that the enzyme cannot oxidize phenylalanine to melanin.

Epidermal Birthmarks: Epidermal Nevi

Increases in mature epidermal cells, hair follicles, or sebaceous glands may appear as birthmarks. They are curvilinear and follow the lines of Blaschko (Fig. 21.50, also see Fig 4.18A). The majority of lesions are present at birth but new lesions can develop into adolescence.

Clinical features

Epidermal nevi have a warty surface and appear anywhere on the body (Fig. 21.51). They are often linear or oval, with the long axis of the lesion parallel to the long axis of the dermatome. The majority of lesions are present at birth and up to 95% of the lesions are present by 7 years of age.[49] Initially, the lesion is barely palpable and may be a confluence of smooth-topped papules. In time, the lesion becomes more wartlike and scaly (Fig. 21.52). Most are 2–5 cm in length, but occasionally they may appear as long, unilateral streaks involving an entire extremity or one side of the trunk (nevus unius lateris). The lesions may be so extensive

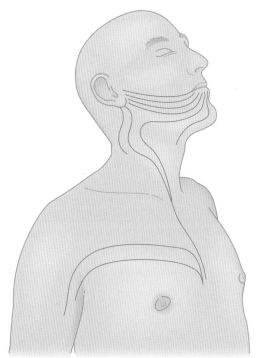

Fig. 21.50 Lines of Blaschko. (From Bolognia J, Jorrizo J, Rapini R, eds. Dermatology. Mosby: London; 2003:Fig. 62 A, with permission.)

Fig. 21.52 Epidermal nevus. Linear hyperpigmented lesion on the dorsum of the hand.

Patients with epidermal nevi may have associated abnormalities. They have an increased number of cutaneous lesions, including café-au-lait spots, congenital hypopigmented macules, and congenital nevocellular nevi. They may have associated skeletal defects, seizure disorders, mental retardation, and ocular abnormalities.[50,51] Patients with more extensive skin involvement have a higher association of other abnormalities than those with limited skin involvement.

Differential diagnosis

Warts are commonly confused with epidermal nevi. The presence from birth and the linear arrangement will help distinguish epidermal nevi from warts. Extensive lesions may be confused with ichthyosis, and certain features of congenital bullous ichthyosiform erythroderma may exactly mimic epidermal nevi. Some epidermal nevi may have keratin abnormalities as seen in epidermolytic hyperkeratosis.[52] Inflammatory linear epidermal nevi may be confused with the warty stage of incontinentia pigmenti, with lichen striatus, or with a dermatitis.

Pathogenesis

Epidermal nevi show thickening of the epidermis and hyperkeratosis. In some lesions, a peculiar vacuolization of the granular layer appears, with separation of the cells in that layer, resulting in a microscopic blister cavity. This process is called epidermolytic hyperkeratosis and it may be associated with genetic mosaicism.[50,52] In inflammatory lesions, dermal accumulation of inflammatory cells and alternating bands of parakeratosis

Fig. 21.51 Epidermal nevus. Unilateral lesion on the right side of the penis, scrotum, and pubic skin.

as to involve most of the body. The terms ichthyosis hystrix or benign congenital acanthosis nigricans have been applied to such extensive epidermal nevi. Epidermal nevi may become erythematous and itchy, with episodes of redness and inflammation, and may be called inflammatory linear verrucous epidermal nevi (ILVEN).

are described. Overgrowth of sebaceous glands and apocrine glands may be found underlying the epidermal proliferation.

Treatment

For small lesions, surgical excision is the best treatment. Extensive lesions may be improved with the use of mild keratolytics (see Ch. 22) or with bland lubricant therapy. The lesions revert to their hyperkeratotic state when treatments are discontinued.

Patient education

It should be emphasized to parents that this birthmark may be a clue to internal problems. Infants with extensive lesions should have careful neurologic examinations and bone radiographic studies to detect skeletal lesions. A birth defect clinic may be a good referral source for a multidisciplinary approach to such infants. Most infants have no other abnormalities.[49]

Follow-up visits

The frequency of follow-up visits is determined by the severity of the associated problems.

Epidermal Birthmarks: Sebaceous Nevi

Clinical features

Jadassohn's sebaceous nevus appears at birth as a slightly raised oval or linear area with a yellow or orange color (Figs 21.53–21.57). These nevi are common on the scalp and are devoid of hair, producing a congenital circumscribed hair loss. They may be seen on the face as well. Sebaceous nevus may be contiguous with an epidermal nevus and constitute part of the epidermal nevus syndrome. At puberty, or with androgenic stimulation, the nevi enlarge and become warty on the surface and raised (Fig. 21.58). Basal cell carcinomas arise in these tumors. Recent studies have suggested that trichoblastoma can be confused with basal cell carcinoma in a sebaceous nevus. Basal cell carcinomas and other types of benign tumors occur in about 15–20% of these lesions.[53-55]

Differential diagnosis

Juvenile xanthogranulomas and xanthomas are yellow or orange lesions that may mimic sebaceous nevus. Skin biopsy will distinguish these lesions.

Fig. 21.53 Epidermal nevus on the plantar aspect of foot.

Fig. 21.54 Nevus sebaceous. Orange-colored lesion on the scalp of an infant.

Pathogenesis

Sebaceous nevus is a birthmark with an increased number of sebaceous glands without hair follicles. Such lesions often have an increased number of apocrine glands as well.

Treatment

Surgical excision is often the treatment of choice for these lesions because of the potential for tumor growth. For lesions in the scalp, the excision can often be done after puberty with local anesthesia. Cosmetically less attractive lesions on the face may require earlier excision.

Patient education

The nature of this birthmark should be explained. The possibility of future benign or malignant skin growth should be explained.

Fig. 21.55 Nevus sebaceous. Linear, yellow-colored hairless lesion on the scalp of an infant.

Fig. 21.56 Nevus sebaceous in curvilinear arrangement on neck and ear of infant.

Follow-up visits

Follow-up visits should be as usual for newborn care.

Epidermal Birthmarks: Nevus Comedonicus

Clinical features

In nevus comedonicus, linear or oval groups of widely dilated follicular openings plugged with keratin are present at birth on the face and scalp (Fig. 21.59).[50] They may become inflamed and pustular as the child ages and mimic acne. Bilateral and widespread lesions occur rarely.

Fig. 21.57 Nevus sebaceous. Hairless orange lesion on the scalp of a newborn.

Differential diagnosis

In contrast to nevus comedonicus, neonatal acne begins at 1 month of age and involves discrete, single lesions rather than grouped arrangements of lesions.

Pathogenesis

Nevus comedonicus is a birthmark consisting of pilosebaceous follicles with patulous openings.

Fig. 21.58 Nevus sebaceous after puberty. Warty, raised growth in the scalp.

Treatment

In small lesions, simple surgical excision is the treatment of choice. Large or extensive lesions may be controlled with the application of topical retinoic acid cream once or twice daily.

Fig. 21.59 Nevus comedonicus on the cheek of a child.

Patient education

The clinician should explain to the family that this is a birthmark containing pilosebaceous follicles and it is not necessarily related to acne.

Follow-up visits

Follow-up can be made on routine neonatal care visits.

Aplasia Cutis Congenita

Clinical features

In aplasia cutis congenita, oval, sharply marginated, 1–2 cm depressed areas are seen primarily in the midline of the posterior scalp (Fig. 21.60). They are hairless, may appear as an ulcer, or are covered by a smooth, finely wrinkled epithelial membrane. A collar of hair may surround them (Fig. 21.61) Ulcerated defects heal with scar formation. Aplasia cutis congenita is a developmental defect rather than a true birthmark.[56] It occurs in about 1 per 5000 live births.[46] Aplasia cutis most commonly appears as an isolated lesion without associated defects. Other developmental defects, such as cleft palate or lip, syndactyly, absence of digits, and congenital heart disease may be associated. It may be seen as an autosomal dominant trait in some families. Although the majority of lesions appear on the scalp, lesions may be found on the trunk, face, or proximal extremities. Medical evaluation should include imaging studies when suspicion exists of underlying bone or brain involvement.

Differential diagnosis

Scalp ulcers at birth may be mistaken for obstetric trauma, although a careful history will distinguish between the two. Other forms of

Fig. 21.60 Aplasia cutis congenita. Two oval lesions on the scalp of a newborn.

Fig. 21.61 Aplasia cutis congenita. Two scalp lesions with long hairs in surrounding skin (hair collar sign).

congenital circumscribed hair loss should be considered.

Pathogenesis

Aplasia cutis congenita represents a developmental failure of skin fusion. Dermis, epidermis, and fat all may be missing, or single layers may be absent.

Treatment

If the lesion is small, surgical excision, with mobilization of the scalp and simple closure, will correct the hairless defect. Hair transplantation has been successful into large defects.

Patient education

Explanation of the failure to form certain layers of skin will help parents understand that this lesion does not represent mishandling of the child during the birth process.

Follow-up visits

Follow-up visits as necessary for routine newborn care are advised.

Connective Tissue Birthmarks

Connective tissue nevi are skin lesions consisting predominantly of the elements of extracellular collagen tissue and products of fibroblasts, such as collagen, elastin, and proteoglycans.[57] All connective tissue nevi are quite rare, although the precise incidence is not known.

Clinical features

Connective tissue nevi are localized areas of thickened skin appearing as multiple skin-colored papules and plaques (Fig. 21.62). Stretching the overlying skin will give a yellowish discoloration to the areas. They may occasionally have increased vascularity and appear red. Collagenomas are localized areas of thickened skin with multiple skin-colored papules or plaques. They may be solitary or appear in a zosteriform segmental pattern. Elastomas are solitary plaques that are present at birth and contain increases in both elastic tissue and proteoglycans. Elastomas may be solitary or they may be multiple in the Buschke-Ollendorff syndrome. This autosomal dominant

Fig. 21.62 Connective tissue nevus. Raised, skin-colored papules grouped over the sacrum.

syndrome appears as symmetrically distributed skin-colored papules or nodules with a predilection for the lower trunk or for the extremities. Lesions may assume a thickened appearance of skin and develop a lacy pattern over the trunk. Radiographs may show sclerotic densities of the ends of long bones, pelvis, and hands, although such lesions are often asymptomatic. The shagreen patch of tuberous sclerosis is a connective tissue nevus. The nevi are subtle at birth and may go unnoticed. They tend to persist throughout life.

Differential diagnosis

The lesions of connective tissue birthmarks are so characteristic that they are seldom misdiagnosed. Examinations for possible associated systemic disease such as Proteus syndrome[50] or tuberous sclerosis[58] may be necessary.

Pathogenesis

Connective tissue nevi show thickened, abundant collagen bundles with or without associated increases in elastic tissue. Such histologic changes are difficult to appreciate unless the skin biopsy includes adjacent normal skin for comparison.

Treatment

Treatment is unnecessary.

Patient education

Connective tissue nevus is a birthmark consisting of collagen and/or elastin, and it should be emphasized that such lesions may be related to systemic or genetic disease. In the absence of associated disease, the connective tissue nevus does not represent a serious problem.

Follow-up visits

Follow-up visits are unnecessary except for routine neonatal visits.

COMMON CONGENITAL MALFORMATIONS THAT INVOLVE SKIN

Congenital malformations involving the skin are frequently observed in newborns. They are observed in 7 per 100 live births.

Ear Anomalies

Minor abnormalities in the formation of the ear constitute the most common congenital malformations. Loss of the fold of the skin in the superior part of the helix is the most common abnormality. Low-set ears that angle away from the eye, periauricular skin tags, accessory tragus (Figs 21.63, 21.64), auricular or preauricular pits (Fig. 21.65), or auricular sinuses and/or small ears are less common. Deafness may accompany congenital malformations of the external ear, or they may be associated with hemifacial microsomia (Goldenhar's syndrome).

Digital Abnormalities

A single crease on one or both upper palms, called a simian crease, occurs in 2 per 100 live births. It is one feature of Down syndrome, but it also may be observed

Fig. 21.63 Preauricular skin tag (accessory tragus) on an infant.

Fig. 21.64 Accessory tragus on mandibular skin of infant.

Fig. 21.65 Ear pit in neonate.

in a variety of other syndromes, including trisomy 13, Cornelia de Lange syndrome, Seckel's syndrome, and cri du chat syndrome. Clinodactyly with inward curvature of a digit is often observed in the fifth finger, and overlapping of the second and third toes is also a frequently observed malformation. Partial or complete fusion (syndactyly) of the second or third toes and clubfoot also occur with relative frequency.

Genital Abnormalities

Hydrocele of one testis and hypospadias are the most common genital anomalies and malformations observed. Malformations of the external genitalia may be clues to urinary tract anomalies, and investigation of the urinary tract may be indicated. They may also be clues to chromosomal abnormalities and may be associated with undescended testes.

Epicanthal Folds

Epicanthal folds of skin on the inner aspect of each eye are frequently observed. They are present in chromosomal abnormalities such as Down, Turner's, and Klinefelter's syndromes.

Supernumerary Nipples

Supernumerary nipples occur in approximately 2.5–4% of newborns.[59,60] These lesions may enlarge during puberty. In the past, an association with renal abnormalities was suggested, but recent studies suggest that supernumerary nipples are not associated with renal abnormalities.[61]

Neural Tube Defects

Primary defects in neural tube closures, such as meningomyelocele, encephalocele, and anencephaly are fortunately rare congenital malformations. Occult spinal dysraphism can be missed if a cutaneous clue to an underlying neural tube defect is not noticed. The clue is a midline lipoma, dimple, hairy patch, deviation of the gluteal furrow; or vascular abnormality or a combination of lesions.[62] Early diagnosis by ultrasound or MRI may identify a surgically correctable lesion before neurologic damage.

Abnormalities of the Lip and Mouth

Pits in the lips have been described in 2 per 100 live births (Fig. 21.66). Cleft lip and palate, or cleft lip alone, are less common. The finding of lip pits or cleft lips and/or cleft palate may be a clue to the so-called first arch syndrome, which includes a small jaw and ocular hypertelorism. A number of syndromes are associated with first arch syndrome, including Pierre Robin syndrome, orodigitofacial syndromes, and Treacher Collins syndrome.

Skin Dimpling

Infants may develop small dimple-like depressed scars secondary to injury during amniocentesis procedures. The skin over the lesion appears to be pulled in by absent dermis. The lesion may not be noticed until the infant is several months old and has developed additional subcutaneous fat. Midline dimpling is of more serious concern, as mentioned above.

Fig. 21.66 Lip pits present since birth.

MAJOR CHROMOSOMAL ABNORMALITIES

Chromosomal abnormalities occur in 1 of 200 live births, in a higher percentage of births resulting in perinatal death, and in up to 50% of spontaneous abortions.

Trisomy 21 (Down Syndrome)

Trisomy 21 is seen in 1 per 800 live births. Mothers over 40 years of age have an increased chance of giving birth to a child with Down syndrome. Cutaneous features are most useful in the recognition of this syndrome. These include prominent epicanthal folds, eyes slanting upward, small ears, simian palmar crease, excessive skin over the back of the neck, and clinodactyly of the fifth fingers. The presence of these cutaneous features, plus muscular hypotonia and evidence of congenital heart disease, is the major clinical characteristic. Chromosomal analysis will confirm the diagnosis. Mental retardation may be severe, and growth failure associated with congenital heart disease makes the prognosis poor.

Trisomies 18 and 13–15

Trisomy 18 is observed in 1 per 3000 live births; trisomy 13–15 occurs in 1 per 5000 live births. In both of these chromosomal abnormalities, increased parental age has been an associated feature. Babies with trisomies 18 or 13–15 are small for gestational age, have low-set ears, simian creases, congenital heart disease, and severe mental retardation. The presence of a cleft lip and palate associated with these features makes trisomy 13–15 more likely, whereas rocker-bottom feet and flexion contractures of the fingers make trisomy 18 the more likely diagnosis. Chromosomal analysis is required for precise diagnosis.

Turner's Syndrome

The most common sex chromosome anomaly is Turner's syndrome, in which only one X chromosome is present (XO). Newborns with Turner's syndrome exhibit webbing of the neck and marked edema of the hands and feet. The neck is often quite short. Coarctation of the aorta may be associated. Chromosomal analysis is necessary to confirm the diagnosis.

Klinefelter's Syndrome

Extra sex chromosomes are characteristic of Klinefelter's syndrome (XXY, XXXY, XXXXY). A low birth weight, undescended testes, and a small penis lead to suspicion of this syndrome. Hypotonia and a variety of other anomalies may also be observed. Mental deficiency is usually severe in this syndrome, and chromosomal analysis is required to confirm the diagnosis.

MISCELLANEOUS SKIN CONDITIONS IN THE NEWBORN

The Red, Scaly Newborn

Physiologic scaling and redness

A scaling and often red newborn may be an enigma to the inexperienced observer.[63] A postmature baby may exhibit desquamation that is marked over the hands, feet, and lower trunk, and, if observed during the first day of life when the newborn skin is quite red, may result in an erroneous diagnosis of one of the ichthyoses. Similarly, preterm infants born at 32 weeks of gestational age or earlier will have red or glistening skin that similarly may be confused with ichthyosis. Such changes are transient and are often resolved within the newborn period.

Collodion baby

Newborns with an encasement of shiny, tight, inelastic scale are said to have a collodion membrane (Fig. 21.67). The membrane is composed of greatly thickened stratum corneum that has been saturated with water. As the water content evaporates in extrauterine life, large fissures appear in the membrane and the membrane is shed, revealing red skin underneath.

Fig. 21.67 Collodion baby. Thick membrane encases skin.

The presence of a collodion membrane does not allow one to predict that the affected baby will necessarily develop ichthyosis, and spontaneous healing may occur.[64] The collodion membrane may be seen in autosomal recessive lamellar ichthyosis cause by mutations in transglutaminase-1 gene TGM1 and an ATP-binding cassette transporter defect in ABCA12 gene.[65] It can be seen in autosomal recessive nonbullous congenital ichthyosiform erythroderma caused by mutations in transglutaminase-1 gene TGM1 and also in novel lipoxygenases genes ALOXE3 orALOX12B.[65] It can also be seen in an autosomal dominant form of nonbullous congenital ichthyosiform erythroderma caused by mutations in loricrin gene LOR.[65] Skin biopsy of the collodion membrane is usually not diagnostic. Most collodion babies do have a form of ichthyosis, and the majority of them develop features of lamellar ichthyosis. Infants with bullous ichthyosis, X-linked ichthyosis, Netherton's syndrome, or Gaucher's disease have also been reported to present as collodion babies. Collodion babies should be observed closely for dehydration associated with high transepidermal water loss.[66]

Harlequin fetus

Harlequin ichthyosis (or the harlequin fetus) is caused by a defect in a keratinocyte lipid transporter associated with lipid transport in lamellar granules and loss of function of the gene, ABCA12, which leads to a defective lipid barrier in the stratum corneum.[67] Harlequin fetus is usually incompatible with extra-uterine life; infants have massive, dense, platelike scales, which produce severe deformities of skeletal and soft tissues that restrict respiration. Recently, infants treated with oral retinoids have survived, with residual severe ichthyosis.[68]

Atopic Dermatitis and Seborrheic Dermatitis

Atopic dermatitis is said to have its onset after the newborn period, with the most frequently observed age of onset being 2–3 months. If a dermatitis begins within the newborn period, many authorities designate it seborrheic dermatitis. It has now become clear, however, that infants who later develop typical atopic dermatitis may have the onset of their skin eruption within the newborn period, possibly associated with ichthyosis vulgaris.[69] There is significant overlap in infants who have seborrheic and atopic dermatitis,

both in distributions of the lesions, which involve the scalp, diaper area, and extensor area, and in the history of pruritus, feeding patterns, food intolerance, and family members with atopic disease. Physiologic overproduction of sebum occurs in the newborn period, giving any dermatitis a greasy feel to the skin surface. It is advisable to designate dermatitis seen in newborns simply as dermatitis (see also Ch. 4).

Diaper Dermatitis

Diaper dermatitis occurring in the newborn period is primarily perianal in location and is related to the irritant substances found in stool.[70] Superinfection with C. albicans is frequent in any diaper dermatitis present for more than 72 hours.

Scabies

Infants with scabies may present with a generalized dermatitis. They may have only a few or as many as thousands of lesions. Infants usually have involvement of the head and neck. Individual burrows may be obscured and difficult to detect because of the confluence of dermatitis. The scabies mite can be recovered from papules or burrows, with the hands and feet the best sites of recovery.

Histiocytosis X

A generalized dermatitis, particularly that with purpuric papules or petechiae within the dermatitis and involvement of the head and neck, is characteristic of histiocytosis X. The skin eruption may be present at birth, and the presence of chronic draining ears and enlargement of the liver and spleen are useful additional clues in the diagnosis. Skin biopsy will demonstrate the characteristic infiltration with histiocytic cells containing Langerhans-like granules (see also Ch. 12).

REFERENCES

1. Lane AT. Development and care of the premature infant's skin. Pediatr Dermatol 1987; 4(1):1–5.
2. Lund CH, Osborne JW, Kuller J, et al. Neonatal skin care: clinical outcomes of the AWHONN/NANN evidence-based clinical practice guideline. Association of Women's Health, Obstetric and Neonatal Nurses and the National Association of Neonatal Nurses. J Obstet Gynecol Neonatal Nurs 2001; 30(1):41–51.
3. Darmstadt GL, Dinulos JG. Neonatal skin care. Pediatr Clin North Am 2000; 47(4):757–782.

4. Kaufman D, Fairchild KD. Clinical microbiology of bacterial and fungal sepsis in very-low-birth-weight infants. Clin Microbiol Rev 2004; 17(3):638–680, table of contents.

5. Vernon HJ, Lane AT, Wischerath LJ, et al. Semipermeable dressing and transepidermal water loss in premature infants. Pediatrics 1990; 86(3):357–362.

6. Lane AT, Drost SS. Effects of repeated application of emollient cream to premature neonates' skin. Pediatrics 1993; 92(3):415–419.

7. Mancini AJ, Sookdeo-Drost S, Madison KC, et al. Semipermeable dressings improve epidermal barrier function in premature infants. Pediatr Res 1994; 36(3):306–314.

8. Nopper AJ, Horii KA, Sookdeo-Drost S, et al. Topical ointment therapy benefits premature infants. J Pediatrics 1996; 128(5 Pt 1):660–669.

9. Darmstadt GL, Badrawi N, Law PA, et al. Topically applied sunflower seed oil prevents invasive bacterial infections in preterm infants in Egypt: a randomized, controlled clinical trial. Pediatr Infect Dis J 2004; 23(8):719–725.

10. Darmstadt GL, Nawshad Uddin Ahmed AS, Saha SK, et al. Infection control practices reduce nosocomial infections and mortality in preterm infants in Bangladesh. J Perinatol 2005; 25(5):331–335.

11. Darmstadt GL, Saha SK, Ahmed AS, et al. Effect of topical treatment with skin barrier-enhancing emollients on nosocomial infections in preterm infants in Bangladesh: a randomised controlled trial. Lancet 2005; 365(9464):1039–1045.

12. Edwards WH, Conner JM, Soll RF. The effect of prophylactic ointment therapy on nosocomial sepsis rates and skin integrity in infants with birth weights of 501 to 1000 g. Pediatrics 2004; 113(5):1195–1203.

13. Conner JM, Soll RF, Edwards WH. Topical ointment for preventing infection in preterm infants. Cochrane Database Syst Rev 2004(1):CD001150.

14. Darmstadt GL, Mao-Qiang M, Chi E, et al. Impact of topical oils on the skin barrier: possible implications for neonatal health in developing countries. Acta Paediatr. 2002; 91(5):546–554.

15. Rivers JK, Frederiksen PC, Dibdin C. A prevalence survey of dermatoses in the Australian neonate. J Am Acad Dermatol 1990; 23(1):77–81.

16. Garzon MC, Schweiger E. Cutis marmorata telangiectatica congenita. Semin Cutan Med Surg 2004; 23(2):99–106.

17. Happle R. Phacomatosis pigmentovascularis revisited and reclassified. Arch Dermatol 2005; 141(3):385–388.

18. Rao J, Campbell ME, Krol A. The harlequin color change and association with prostaglandin E_1. Pediatr Dermatol. 2004; 21(5):573–576.

19. Fretzin DF, Arias AM. Sclerema neonatorum and subcutaneous fat necrosis of the newborn. Pediatr Dermatol 1987; 4(2):112–122.

20. Tran JT, Sheth AP. Complications of subcutaneous fat necrosis of the newborn: a case report and review of the literature. Pediatr Dermatol 2003; 20(3):257–261.

21. Burden AD, Krafchik BR. Subcutaneous fat necrosis of the newborn: a review of 11 cases. Pediatr Dermatol 1999; 16(5):384–387.

22. Karochristou K, Siahanidou T, Kakourou-Tsivitanidou T, et al. Subcutaneous fat necrosis associated with severe hypocalcaemia in a neonate. J Perinatol 2006; 26(1):64–66.

23. Srinath G, Cohen M. Imaging findings in subcutaneous fat necrosis in a newborn. Pediatr Radiol 2006; 36(4):361–363.

24. Libow LF, Reinmann JG. Symmetrical erosions in a neonate: a case of neonatal sucking blisters. Cutis 1998; 62(1):16–17.

25. Marchini G, Nelson A, Edner J, et al. Erythema toxicum neonatorum is an innate immune response to commensal microbes penetrated into the skin of the newborn infant. Pediatr Res 2005; 58(3):613–616.

26. Van Praag MC, Van Rooij RW, Folkers E, et al. Diagnosis and treatment of pustular disorders in the neonate. Pediatr Dermatol 1997; 14(2):131–143.

27. Bernier V, Weill FX, Hirigoyen V, et al. Skin colonization by *Malassezia* species in neonates: a prospective study and relationship with neonatal cephalic pustulosis. Arch Dermatol 2002; 138(2):215–218.

28. Bergman JN, Eichenfield LF. Neonatal acne and cephalic pustulosis: is *Malassezia* the whole story? Arch Dermatol 2002; 138(2):255–257.

29. Dromy R, Raz A, Metzker A. Infantile acropustulosis. Pediatr Dermatol 1991; 8(4):284–287.

30. Vignon-Pennamen MD, Wallach D. Infantile acropustulosis. A clinicopathologic study of six cases. Arch Dermatol 1986; 122(10):1155–1160.

31. Mancini AJ, Frieden IJ, Paller AS. Infantile acropustulosis revisited: history of scabies and response to topical corticosteroids. Pediatr Dermatol 1998; 15(5):337–341.

32. Aldana-Valenzuela C, Morales-Marquec M, Castellanos-Martinez J, et al. Congenital candidiasis: a rare and unpredictable disease. J Perinatol. 2005; 25(10):680–682.

33. Darmstadt GL, Dinulos JG, Miller Z. Congenital cutaneous candidiasis: clinical presentation, pathogenesis, and management guidelines. Pediatrics 2000; 105(2):438–444.

34. Brown ZA, Wald A, Morrow RA, et al. Effect of serologic status and cesarean delivery on transmission rates of herpes simplex virus from mother to infant. JAMA 2003; 289(2):203–209.

35. Nahmias AJ. Neonatal HSV infection Part I: continuing challenges. Herpes 2004; 11(2):33–37.

36. Sauerbrei A, Wutzler P. The congenital varicella syndrome. J Perinatol 2000; 20(8 Pt 1):548–554.

37. Lipton SV, Brunell PA. Management of varicella exposure in a neonatal intensive care unit. JAMA. 1989;261(12):1782–1784.

38. Diseases CoI. Red Book 2003, Varicella zoster infections, 26th edn. Elk Grove Village, IL: American Academy of Pediatrics; 2003:672–686.

39. Darmstadt GL, Lane AT. Impetigo: an overview. Pediatr Dermatol 1994; 11(4):293–303.

40. Ladhani S, Joannou CL, Lochrie DP, et al. Clinical, microbial, and biochemical aspects of the exfoliative toxins causing staphylococcal scalded-skin syndrome. Clin Microbiol Rev 1999; 12(2):224–242.

41. Payne AS, Hanakawa Y, Amagai M, et al. Desmosomes and disease: pemphigus and bullous impetigo. Curr Opin Cell Biol 2004; 16(5):536–543.

42. Hedrick J. Acute bacterial skin infections in pediatric medicine: current issues in presentation and treatment. Paediatr Drugs 2003; 5(Suppl 1):35–46.

43. Zupan J, Garner P, Omari AA. Topical umbilical cord care at birth. Cochrane Database Syst Rev. 2004(3):CD001057.

44. Mullany LC, Darmstadt GL, Khatry SK, et al. Topical applications of chlorhexidine to the umbilical cord for prevention of omphalitis and neonatal mortality in southern Nepal: a community-based, cluster-randomised trial. Lancet 2006; 367(9514):910–918.

45. Parker LA. Part 1: early recognition and treatment of birth trauma: injuries to the head and face. Adv Neonatal Care 2005; 5(6):288–297; quiz 298–300.

46. Alper JC, Holmes LB. The incidence and significance of birthmarks in a cohort of 4,641 newborns. Pediatr Dermatol 1983; 1(1):58–68.

47. Jacobs AH, Walton RG. The incidence of birthmarks in the neonate. Pediatrics 1976; 58(2):218–222.

48. Alper J, Holmes LB, Mihm MC Jr. Birthmarks with serious medical significance: nevocellular nevi, sebaceous nevi, and multiple café au lait spots. J Pediatr 1979; 95(5 Pt 1):696–700.

49. Rogers M. Epidermal nevi and the epidermal nevus syndromes: a review of 233 cases. Pediatr Dermatol 1992; 9(4):342–344.

50. Sugarman JL. Epidermal nevus syndromes. Semin Cutan Med Surg 2004; 23(2):145–157.

51. Vujevich JJ, Mancini AJ. The epidermal nevus syndromes: multisystem disorders. J Am Acad Dermatol 2004; 50(6):957–961.

52. Paller AS, Syder AJ, Chan YM, et al. Genetic and clinical mosaicism in a type of epidermal nevus. N Engl J Med 1994; 331(21):1408–1415.

53. Munoz-Perez MA, Garcia-Hernandez MJ, Rios JJ, et al. Sebaceus naevi: a clinicopathologic study. J Eur Acad Dermatol Venereol 2002; 16(4):319–324.

54. Cribier B, Scrivener Y, Grosshans E. Tumors arising in nevus sebaceus: A study of 596 cases. J Am Acad Dermatol 2000; 42(2 Pt 1):263–268.

55. Jaqueti G, Requena L, Sanchez Yus E. Trichoblastoma is the most common neoplasm developed in nevus sebaceus of Jadassohn: a clinicopathologic study of a series of 155 cases. Am J Dermatopathol 2000; 22(2):108–118.

56. Frieden IJ. Aplasia cutis congenita: a clinical review and proposal for classification. J Am Acad Dermatol 1986; 14(4):646–660.

57. Uitto J, Santa Cruz DJ, Eisen AZ. Connective tissue nevi of the skin. Clinical, genetic, and histopathologic classification of hamartomas of the collagen, elastin, and proteoglycan type. J Am Acad Dermatol 1980; 3(5):441–461.

58. Korf BR. The phakomatoses. Clin Dermatol 2005; 23(1):78–84.

59. Mimouni F, Merlob P, Reisner SH. Occurrence of supernumerary nipples in newborns. Am J Dis Child 1983; 137(10):952–953.

60. Jojart G, Seres E. Supernumerary nipples and renal anomalies. Int Urol Nephrol 1994; 26(2):141–144.

61. Adams BB. Supernumerary nipples a risk factor? Pediatr Dermatol. 2002; 19(5):463–464; author reply 4.

62. Guggisberg D, Hadj-Rabia S, Viney C, et al. Skin markers of occult spinal dysraphism in children: a review of 54 cases. Arch Dermatol 2004; 140(9):1109–1115.

63. Shwayder T, Akland T. Neonatal skin barrier: structure, function, and disorders. Dermatol Ther 2005; 18(2):87–103.

64. Frenk E, de Techtermann F. Self-healing collodion baby: evidence for autosomal recessive inheritance. Pediatr Dermatol 1992; 9(2):95–97.

65. Richard G. Molecular genetics of the ichthyoses. Am J Med Genet C Semin Med Genet 2004; 131C(1):32–44.

66. Buyse L, Graves C, Marks R, et al. Collodion baby dehydration: the danger of high transepidermal water loss. Br J Dermatol 1993; 129(1):86–88.

67. Akiyama M. Harlequin ichthyosis and other autosomal recessive congenital ichthyoses: the underlying genetic defects and pathomechanisms. J Dermatol Sci. 2006; 42(2):83–89.

68. Singh S, Bhura M, Maheshwari A, et al. Successful treatment of harlequin ichthyosis with acitretin. Int J Dermatol 2001; 40(7):472–473.

69. Palmer CN, Irvine AD, Terron-Kwiatkowski A, et al. Common loss-of-function variants of the epidermal barrier protein filaggrin are a major predisposing factor for atopic dermatitis. Nat Genet 2006; 38(4):441–446.

70. Lane AT, Rehder PA, Helm K. Evaluations of diapers containing absorbent gelling material with conventional disposable diapers in newborn infants. Am J Dis Child 1990; 144(3):315–38.

Chapter 22
Dermatopharmacology and Topical Formulary

A great variety of topical preparations are available to treat the skin of pediatric patients. However, the majority of these preparations have not been rigorously investigated as to their efficacy and risk–benefit ratio in infants and children. This chapter reviews the principles and rationale for use of topical preparations. Specific treatment programs are discussed in the other chapters on each skin disease.

Treatment should be simple and aimed at preserving or restoring the normal physiologic state of the skin. Topical therapy is often preferred because topical medication can be delivered in optimal concentrations at the exact site where it is needed, and effects on internal organs can be minimized. Compounding of preparations or adding medications to commercially available topical preparations is not advised because the ingredients may lose their bioavailability.[1]

PERCUTANEOUS ABSORPTION

Development and repair of the epidermal barrier involves complex interaction of many processes.[2–4] Absorption of topical medications through the epidermal barrier into the dermis is a complex process.[2–4] However, for clinical purposes, percutaneous absorption may be simplified and related to skin hydration. In the normal state of hydration of the stratum corneum, the epidermal barrier may be penetrated only by medications passing through a tight lipid barrier between cells.

Hydration of the skin allows binding of water molecules to hydrophilic lipids between stratum corneum cells, so that water-soluble medications may pass between cells. Thus, any of the factors that enhance hydration of the skin increase percutaneous absorption (e.g. plastic wrap, airtight occlusion, the use of oils or ointments, urea compounds, propylene glycol). Excessive hydration increases permeability.[5] The mechanism of action of occlusive substances is prevention of evaporation of the 200–300 mL of body water that normally moves through the stratum corneum daily and would ordinarily evaporate had it not been for those occlusive coverings. Urea compounds and propylene glycol interact with the lipids between stratum corneum cells. The factors that enhance percutaneous absorption are listed in Box 22.1.

When choosing a topical medication for a child, one selects a preparation that contains two major components, the active medication and the vehicle. Each is important in determining the success or failure of the therapeutic regimen. Selection of the correct active medication and incorrect vehicle may cause failure of the treatment program.

Water and the Skin

The outermost layer of the epidermis, the stratum corneum, forms a barrier, the epidermal barrier (see Ch. 1), to the penetration of active medication into the skin. Both excessive environmental humidity and low environmental humidity result in changes of the integrity of the epidermal barrier.[6]

Environmental humidity

Environmental conditions markedly influence epidermal structure and function.[7] Mice maintained in a dry environment have less daily water loss through their skin than mice maintained in a humid environment.[7] In addition, the improved barrier function was associated with a thicker stratum corneum.[7] Abrupt changes from a humid to a dry environment causes deterioration of the normal barrier function, even

Box 22.1 Factors enhancing percutaneous absorption
Epidermal injury
Heat
Increased water content of stratum corneum
Inflammation

in normal skin.[6] Excessive water exposure results in replacement of lipid covalent bonds between the stratum corneum cells by weak hydrogen (water) bonds, and the stratum corneum cells separate. We see this clinically as maceration. Maceration occurs in naturally occluded areas in which evaporation of water is usually retarded, such as in the axillae, under the breasts, and in the perineum, scalp, and interdigital webs. Preventing evaporation of water from the skin surface with plastic occlusive wraps, ointments, or oils will also result in maceration. Excessively dry skin may have a rough feel and may be seen as thin scales with erythema around the borders (eczema craquelé), and dry, inspissated plugs of scale in follicular openings (keratosis pilaris).

Substances Designed to Retain Water on the Skin Surface (Moisturizers)

The terms lubricant, emollient, and moisturizer are often interchanged. Emollients are materials designed to soften and smooth the surface of the skin while moisturizers contain humectants which attract water into the skin.[8–10] On dry, exposed areas of skin, such as the dorsum of the hands and arms, it is desirable to retain water in the stratum corneum. Moisturization is often all that is necessary to treat chronic dryness and inflammation of the skin successfully (Box 22.2).[11] Moisturizers are complex mixtures of either water-in-oil emulsions or oil-in-water emulsions.[8] The individual ingredients are combined to make them more efficient at hydrating the skin and enable them to give a more pleasing cosmetic appearance when applied.[12] Creams are the most common types of delivery systems use for moisturizing.[8] Moisturizers are composed

Box 22.2 Function of moisturizers
Impede water loss
Retain heat
Increase percutaneous absorption
Reduce scaling
Promote epidermal repair

Box 22.3 Useful moisturizing lotions
Petrolatum based
Dermasil
DML Lotion
Moisturel Lotion
Nutraderm Lotion
Replenaderm Lotion
Mixtures of lanolin and petrolatum
Eucerin Lotion
Lubriderm Lotion
Keri Lotion
Nivea Moisturizing Lotion
Without lanolin or petrolatum
Complex 15 Lotion
Corn Huskers Lotion
Cetaphil Lotion

Box 22.4 Useful moisturizing creams
Petrolatum based
DML Forte
Purpose Dry Skin Cream
Replenaderm Cream
Cetaphil Cream
Dermasil Cream
Mixtures of lanolin and petrolatum
Eucerin Creme
Without lanolin or petrolatum
Neutrogena Norwegian Formula Hand Cream

Box 22.5 Useful moisturizing ointments
Petrolatum based
White petrolatum (Petrolatum White, Vaseline Pure Petroleum Jelly)
Mixtures of lanolin and petrolatum
Aquaphor Natural Healing Ointment

of varying concentrations and types of fats, emulsifiers, humectants, preservatives, chelating substances, antioxidants, and fragrances.[8] Lists of useful moisturizers are found in Boxes 22.3–22.5.

Components of moisturizers and vehicles and their function

The functions of frequently used ingredients of moisturizers and of medicated creams and lotions are listed in Table 22.1. One should not recommend a skin preparation unless he or she is familiar with its ingredients

Table 22.1 Components of lubricants and vehicles and their function

Component	Function
Cetyl alcohol, stearates, cholesterol	Additional water binding
Polyethylene glycol (Carbowax)	Dispersants
Yellow wax, white wax	Stiffness
Parabens, formaldehyde releasers	Preservatives
Propylene glycol, alcohol	Solvent
Essential oils	Fragrance
Cholesterol, polysaccharide polymers (Tween, Span)	Emulsifiers

and its therapeutic indications. Petrolatum, the base for most moisturizers, is prepared from the residue remaining in stills after the distillation of petroleum. It usually is a colored solid and must be decolorized to make white petrolatum (petroleum jelly, white soft paraffin). Petrolatum contains a mixture of hydrocarbons, including triglycerides, and is insoluble in water. It retains heat, impedes water loss from the skin surface, and increases percutaneous absorption. It has minor vasoconstrictive activity when applied to the skin and may enhance reepithelialization of wounds. Petrolatum alone is cosmetically disagreeable, leaving a greasy film on the skin surface that frequently results in overheating of the skin and sweat obstruction. The mixing of substances to allow the addition of water to petrolatum will result in a more efficient moisturizing capacity of the skin with a less greasy feel and more cosmetic acceptance. Substances added to moisturizers to increase water-binding capacity include cetyl alcohol, stearyl alcohol, and other stearates. Addition of cetyl alcohol to petrolatum will increase its water-binding capability from 10% to 50%. Other additives include polyethylene glycol (PEG) of low molecular weight (PEG 300–400) or of high molecular weight (PEG 1540, 4000) (Carbowax) as an agent to uniformly disperse the mixture or for its solvent properties. Addition of cholesterol or polysaccharide macromolecules such as polysorbate (Tween 20 or 80) as emulsifiers and the addition of yellow or white wax (beeswax) for stiffness of the product are common practices. Glycerin, a fatty alcohol derived from triglycerides as a byproduct of the manufacture of soap, is a clear, colorless, sticky liquid that takes up water from the skin surface. Its role as an additive to certain creams is unclear.

Bacteriostatic and fungistatic agents are added to preparations that contain water to prolong the life of the product. Popular preservatives include parabens, formaldehyde, or formaldehyde-releasing agents (imidazolinylureas); oxyquinoline sulfate; organic quaternary ammonium compounds; chlorobutanol; and hexachlorophene. Fragrances are added to cover any unpleasant smell from the basic product. The added preservatives and fragrances can be responsible for irritant or allergic reactions to these moisturizers in children.

Liquid petrolatum (mineral oil, liquid paraffin) is a fluid phase of petrolatum obtained by distilling the residual petroleum liquid at 330°F and decolorizing it. It is composed of 15–20 carbon hydrocarbons and, because it is in a fluid form at room temperature, it is added to skin preparations in which easy spread on the skin surface is desirable.

Lanolin is a purified fatlike substance obtained from the wool of sheep. It consists of cholesterol esters and oxycholesterol esters called wool fat or wool wax alcohol. Ordinary lanolin contains 25–30% water and is a yellowish-white solid. It must be mixed with other agents such as mineral oil or cetyl alcohol so that it can be spread smoothly on the skin. Lanolin is found in a number of skin moisturizers. Fragrance-, lanolin-, and preservative-free preparations are listed in Box 22.6.

Ointments: Ointments spread easily on the skin and are more cosmetically pleasing if they contain some water. White petrolatum, mineral oil, and liquid paraffin are completely water insoluble and have maximal water-retaining (occlusive) properties. However, they

---

Box 22.6 Skin lubricants that are fragrance, lanolin, and preservative free

Fragrance free
DML Lotion

Eucerin Creme and Lotion

Fragrance free, lanolin free
Moisturel Lotion

Replenaderm Cream and Lotion

Vanicream

Fragrance free, preservative free
Aquaphor Natural Healing Ointment

Fragrance free, preservative free, and lanolin free
White petrolatum (Vaseline Pure Petroleum Jelly, Petrolatum White)

often leave a greasy film on the skin and cause excessive heat retention, which make them unacceptable to many patients.

Mixing ointments or oils with water and an emulsifier makes them spread on the skin more easily and give less of a greasy feel. Most of the moisturizers in clinical use are emulsified with water and contain mostly ointment, with a small amount of water. The water stays in droplet form in the ointment phase, making such moisturizers water-in-oil emulsions.

These preparations should be applied to the skin two or three times per day for maximal lubrication. Some patients prefer to wet the skin with a 5- or 10-minute bath and then apply the moisturizers to the wet skin before drying it. This adds additional time necessary to complete the daily therapy and may not be necessary. These preparations are used successfully on most regions of the skin except the scalp and axillae.

Creams and lotions (oil-in-water emulsions): When environmental humidity is high and in naturally occluded areas, the use of moisturizers that contain more water than oil is desirable. These are the lubricating creams and lotions, which contain oil in droplet form in water (oil-in-water emulsions). Creams are viscous and do not pour, whereas lotions are less viscous and pour slowly.[9] Such preparations are easily washed from skin surfaces and are cosmetically pleasing. Lubricant creams and lotions must be applied more frequently to achieve the same lubricant effect obtained with every 12-hour application of ointment. Microemulsions, created by uniform lipid droplet size, significantly enlarge the absorptive surface.

Skin-hydrating agents: Certain chemicals act as skin-hydrating agents by adding extra water-binding sites to the skin rather than by simple occlusion. Alphahydroxy acids and urea remove excess adherent scales and make the skin more pliable. Commercially available urea and alphahydroxy acid moisturizers are listed in the formulary at the end of this chapter.

The urea creams dissolve hydrogen bonds and add water-binding sites. To make a cream, the urea must first be dissolved in water before mixing with oil. High concentrations of urea (20% or more) or improper mixing may result in urea crystals in the preparation, causing severe irritation when applied to the skin.

Lactic acid is one of the alphahydroxy acids and may act as a moisturizer by loosening the dry surface layer of dead cells. Lactic acid-containing preparations

may burn or sting when applied to the skin, limiting their usefulness in children. Combinations of lower concentrations of lactic acid and urea may decrease the incidence of discomfort and increase effectiveness as a moisturizer.

Caution must be observed if using a salicylic acid- or lactic acid-containing product when treating large surface areas in children. Both products can be absorbed and can be toxic.[13–15]

Gels: Gels are colorless semicolloids that liquefy on contact with the skin. Because of their alcoholic base, they may burn and sting. They permit good penetration of steroids and other medications and are useful in medications applied to the scalp and in acne preparations. They are the most effective delivery system for benzoyl peroxides for use in acne (see Ch. 3) and the clear, colorless, odorless tar preparations used for psoriasis.

Foams: Recently, foam formulations have been developed that offer a cosmetically appealing treatment option as they are easy to spread and lack any residue. They are easier to use in hairy areas.

Amount to dispense and patient education

Therapy often fails because patients apply the topical medication incorrectly. In a comparison of medication application by trained technicians and by patients, it was found that trained technicians applied 1.8 g/m^2 of body surface, but the self-application group averaged 16.3 g/m^2, with a range of 0.4 to 44.3 g/m^2.[16] Overmedication is common and expensive for the patient.

Table 22.2 presents guidelines for the amount of topical therapy to dispense. Box 22.7 lists important rules for prescribing topical medication that will result in therapeutic success when followed by the patient. One way to estimate the amount of topical therapy to apply is to use the fingertip unit (FTU).[17] Most topical prescription preparations have a tube orifice of about 5 mm. One FTU is the amount of ointment that is expressed from a tube, which reaches from the distal tip of an adult finger to the crease on the skin over the distal interphalangeal (DIP) joint (see Fig. 4.20). Two FTUs are equivalent to about 1 g of ointment. One FTU covers the approximate area of two times the surface area of one flat adult hand with the fingers held together.[17] As a result of these calculations, the surface area of four adult hands requires two FTUs, which equals 1 g of topical product. Table 22.2 is based

Table 22.2 Amount to dispense in grams

	One application (g)	Approximate twice-daily application for 2 weeks (g)
3- to 6-month old		
Face and neck	$\frac{1}{2}$	15
Arm and hand	$\frac{1}{2}$	15
Leg and foot	$\frac{3}{4}$	20
Chest and abdomen	$\frac{1}{2}$	15
Back and buttocks	$\frac{3}{4}$	20
1- to 2-year-old		
Face and neck	$\frac{3}{4}$	20
Arm and hand	$\frac{3}{4}$	20
Leg and foot	1	30
Chest and abdomen	1	30
Back and buttocks	$1\frac{1}{2}$	45
3- to 5-year-old		
Face and neck	$\frac{3}{4}$	20
Arm and hand	1	30
Leg and foot	$1\frac{1}{2}$	45
Chest and abdomen	$1\frac{1}{2}$	45
Back and buttocks	$1\frac{3}{4}$	50
6- to 10-year-old		
Face and neck	1	30
Arm and hand	$1\frac{1}{4}$	35
Leg and foot	$2\frac{1}{4}$	65
Chest and abdomen	$1\frac{3}{4}$	50
Back and buttocks	$2\frac{1}{2}$	70

Box 22.7 Rules for prescribing topical medication

1. Prescribe enough medication
2. Demonstrate to the patient how to apply the medication
3. Apply moisturizer liberally to wet skin
4. Substitute moisturizer therapy for topical steroids whenever possible; do not allow the patient to use the steroid for the moisturizer properties of the vehicle when the vehicle alone would suffice
5. Apply ointments to exposed dry areas, creams to naturally occluded moist areas
6. Use medications twice daily
7. Avoid Class 1 and 2 steroids in prepubertal children
8. Use only Class 6 and 7 steroids in diaper area and face
9. Monitor the quantity of the steroids used and growth parameters in children who have used steroids for long periods

on estimates of the amount of product to dispense for different ages of children using the FTU.[17]

ANTIINFLAMMATORY AGENTS

Wet Dressings

Water is an important therapeutic tool, but it is often forgotten that it is also an antiinflammatory agent. The evaporation of water from the skin surface results in vasoconstriction, relief of pruritus, and debridement of crusts from the skin surface. Water is also the active ingredient in the drying lotions. Wet dressings can be used in acute dermatitis from any cause. Pruritus is relieved by placing the skin in an environment in which the humidity is 90% and allowing it to evaporate to 60%. This slow evaporation of water from the skin surface occurring over a 4–6-hour period is the basis of the wet-dressing technique. The methods for wet dressings are described in Box 4.6 and in the Patient Information Sheets. Relief of pruritus from wet dressings is dramatic, as is reduction of erythema. After 24 hours the patient is greatly improved, with maximal benefit occurring at 48–72 hours. Treatment beyond this period is of little benefit. Topical steroid creams or ointments applied to the skin before the application of wet dressings enhances the wet-dressing technique considerably.

Topical Glucocorticosteroids

Topical glucocorticosteroids are the mainstay of therapy of many inflammatory and hyperproliferative skin diseases.[1,18,19] Glucocorticosteroids applied to the skin reduce inflammation by causing vasoconstriction and preventing the egress of inflammatory cells (neutrophils, lymphocytes, monocyte/macrophages, eosinophils) from the bloodstream to tissue sites. Maximal glucocorticosteroid penetration is achieved from ointment vehicles, followed by gels and creams. Penetration is poor with lotions or sprays. A cutaneous antiinflammatory effect can be achieved with topical glucocorticosteroids without adrenal suppression, which is not the case with systemic steroids. Many parents are fearful of topical steroid use.[20] Better information needs to be given regarding the safety, potency, and appropriate use of topical corticosteroids. Moderate-potency topical steroids used daily in infants and children for months to years are efficacious and safe.[21]

Box 22.8 Potency of topical glucocorticosteroids

Class 1 – Superpotent
Betamethasone dipropionate, 0.05% gel, ointment
Clobetasol propionate cream, ointment, 0.05%

Class 2 – Potent
Betamethasone dipropionate cream, 0.05%
Desoximetasone cream, ointment, gel 0.05% and 0.25%
Fluocinonide cream, ointment, gel, 0.05%

Class 3 – Upper midstrength
Betamethasone dipropionate cream, 0.05%
Betamethasone valerate ointment, 0.1%
Fluticasone propionate ointment, 0.005%
Mometasone furoate ointment, 0.1%
Triamcinolone acetonide cream, 0.5%

Class 4 – Midstrength
Desoximetasone cream, 0.05%
Fluocinolone acetonide ointment, 0.025%
Triamcinolone acetonide ointment, 0.1%

Class 5 – Lower mid-strength
Betamethasone valerate cream/lotion, 0.1%
Fluocinolone acetonide cream, 0.025%
Fluticasone propionate cream, 0.05%
Triamcinolone acetonide cream/lotion, 0.1%

Class 6 – Mild strength
Desonide cream, 0.05%

Class 7 – Least potent
Topicals with hydrocortisone, dexamethasone, flumethasone, methylprednisolone, and prednisolone

Potency of topical steroids

The potency of a topical steroid is evaluated by vasoconstriction (blanching) of the skin, which roughly correlates with its antiinflammatory effects. Glucocorticosteroid potency is commonly subdivided into seven categories related to potency. Box 22.8 (modified from Del Rosso and Friedlander) lists generic preparations that are available in the identified potency.[19] Numerous glucocorticosteroids are available in many of the potency classifications, including less expensive generics. The different products are often available in creams, ointments, and possibly lotions and gels. Some vehicles may increase the potency of a corticosteroid by increasing penetration through the epidermis. The clinician should usually select topical steroids from Class 3 through 7 for children with inflammatory skin diseases. Rarely are Class 1 or 2 glucocorticosteroids necessary in children.

Guidelines for use of topical steroids

For most acute, subacute, and chronic dermatitides, the physician should select a preparation from Class 3 to 5 and instruct the patient and family to apply twice daily for 3–10 days or until symptoms have subsided. Bland moisturizers should also be applied twice daily. As the patient improves, the topical glucocorticosteroid can be applied once daily and the moisturizer continued twice daily. Topical glucocorticosteroid use should be eliminated as soon as possible. There are no indications for Class 1 and 2 topical glucocorticosteroid use in children, except for pulse-dose therapy under the direction of an experienced dermatologist.

On the face and scrotum, only Class 6 or 7 glucocorticosteroids should be used, because the epidermis is thin in these areas and the side effects may be severe (Figs 22.1, 22.2; Box 22.9).

Fig. 22.1 Steroid atrophy secondary to long-term application of a moderate-potency steroid (triamcinolone) and mycostatin combination (Mycolog).

Fig. 22.2 Steroid atrophy secondary to long-term use of topical steroids for atopic dermatitis.

Box 22.9 Side effects of topical steroids

Local

Striae (especially in genital area and axillae)

Persistent erythema and telangiectasia (face)

Pustular acneiform eruption (face) (steroid rosacea)

Atrophic, shiny, erythematous skin

Telangiectasia, purpura

Granuloma gluteal infantum

Folliculitis, miliaria

Hypertrichosis

Steroid addiction syndrome

Allergic contact dermatitis

Systemic

Suppression of hypothalamic–pituitary–adrenal axis

Stunted growth in children

Cataracts and glaucoma

Glycosuria

Cushing's syndrome

Fig. 22.3 Steroid addiction appearing to be acne. This condition was caused by long-term application of a moderate-potency steroid (triamcinolone) and mycostatin combination (Mycolog).

Fig 22.4 Steroid atrophy injection.

Fig 22.5 Linear steroid striae (mycolog).

When applied to the skin, high-potency glucocorticosteroids and some moderate-potency glucocorticosteroids may cause tachyphylaxis. That is, after 1–3 days of application, maximal vasoconstriction has been achieved and further application results in a rebound vasodilatation, manifested by diffuse erythema on the child's face. This is particularly true with the superpotent topical steroids. The clinician should simply substitute bland moisturizers for such patients, and their skin will return to normal in 1–2 weeks.

Systemic side effects have been noted with use of potent topical glucocorticosteroids on small surface areas in children.[22]

Topical steroid addiction

Because potent and superpotent topical glucocorticosteroids have become available, a syndrome of topical steroid addiction has been recognized (Figs 22.3, 22.4). The syndrome is the result of chronic daily application for greater than a 1-month period of a potent or moderately potent glucocorticosteroid preparation to the facial skin. As treatment continues, the patient experiences a rebound vasodilatation of the facial skin 2–6 hours after the application. The face becomes red, and the patient applies the steroid more frequently. Soon, burning of the skin is experienced and is only relieved by further steroid applications. Permanent redness of the facial skin eventuates, with thinning and fine wrinkling of the skin observed. It is

difficult to withdraw the steroid because the patient cannot tolerate the burning sensation, which is relieved only by topical steroids. Substitution of a bland ointment for the topical steroid, plus administration of oral erythromycin, will result in progressive improvement over a 4-week period.[23] In susceptible infants and children, application of potent or moderately potent glucocorticosteroid preparations to the facial skin may also result in redness and acneiform papules and pustules located on the nose, chin, cheeks, and lower eyelids. This is known as steroid rosacea or perioral dermatitis (Fig. 22.5). Abruptly stopping the topical steroid preparation will result in increased numbers of papules and pustules over the subsequent 7 days. Treatment with oral or topical erythromycin is usually effective.[23]

Coal Tar Preparations

Coal tars are byproducts of the destructive distillation of coal. Coal tar preparations are available in emulsions, shampoos, gels, lotions, and solutions. They contain hydrocarbons and benzene, toluene, naphthalene, anthracene, xylene, phenol, cresols, pyridine ammonia, peroxides, and other aromatic compounds. They are black, stain the skin and clothing, and are malodorous. Their mechanism of action is unknown, but they restore normal keratinization in eczematous and hyperplastic epidermis. Most tar compounds are derived from coal tars, but oil shale tars (ichthammol), juniper tars (cade oil), or pine tars are sometimes used.

Crude coal tar, 1–10% in petrolatum, was commonly used in the past for hospitalized patients or in outpatient psoriasis daycare centers. Because of the staining properties, usually commercial preparations listed in the formulary are used.

Tars are applied twice daily and always with a downward motion rather than a circular or up-and-down motion, to avoid tar folliculitis. The tar may concentrate in follicular openings, resulting in a superficial chemical folliculitis. Such chemical folliculitis is rapidly responsive to benzoyl peroxide gels applied twice daily. New colorless and relatively odorless tar preparations have increased the acceptability of tar therapy and made it a viable alternative to topical steroids. The tar gels are clear and colorless vehicles that allow penetration into the skin. They are applied twice daily and are immediately covered with a lubricant because gels are drying. Tar gels are equivalent to crude coal tar 5%. Coal tar shampoos are useful on the scalp to treat scalp psoriasis. Coal tar solution, liquor carbonis detergens (LCD), is an alcoholic extract of coal tar. LCD 5% equals crude coal tar 1% in potency. It is used as a shampoo in tincture of green soap or as a bath additive.

Calcipotriene

Calcipotriene is a synthetic analogue of vitamin D_3, which is helpful in treatment of psoriasis. Applied twice a day, it improves the majority of patients who use it. The side effects include burning and itching, and its high cost is detrimental when used to treat large surface areas of involved skin. The safety of calcipotriene in children has not been documented.[24]

Nonsteroidal Topical Immunomodulators

Many new pharmacologic agents are being developed to modulate the immune response in disease conditions. Two relatively new therapies are topical calcineurin inhibitors. Topical tacrolimus and pimecrolimus are topical calcineurin inhibitors currently available for use in children over 2 years of age with atopic dermatitis.[25] Topical calcineurin inhibitors are potent immunosuppressive agents that suppresses cytokine production. In some children, the topical preparation is irritating to the skin. Topical pimecrolimus and tacrolimus are indicated for the short-term or intermittent treatment of mild to moderate (pimecrolimus) or moderate to severe (tacrolimus) atopic dermatitis. They are not indicated as first-line therapies, but are to be used in patients who are unresponsive to or intolerant of other conventional therapies.[25] Because of the potential of increases absorption, the use of topical calcineurin inhibitors to treat patients with diseases of cornification is consequently relatively contraindicated.[25] Part of the concern for these therapies is the theoretical risk of inducing cancer.[25]

A BRIEF FORMULARY FOR COMMON PEDIATRIC DERMATOLOGY CONDITIONS

This formulary is designed to provide information regarding a number of classifications of useful skin preparations, but it is not intended to be encyclopedic. Formulas for compounding skin mixtures are omitted because low-cost and high-quality preparations from pharmaceutical manufacturers are readily available and are often superior to compounded mixtures. Many internet search systems are available to expand the list of preparations listed and to identify the most economical preparation that is available.

I. Skin Moisturizers and Cleansers

Creams and lotions contain water, requiring the addition of preservatives, which are potential allergens.

They must be applied more frequently than ointments but are aesthetically more pleasing to apply. Many different products are available and the ingredients of the brand-name products may change. Many brand-name manufactures market several products that may have properties that are fragrance free, preservative free, or lanolin free, whereas other products with a similar name will have different ingredients. Boxes 22.3, 22.4, 22.5, and 22.6 list commonly used products.

A. Urea creams and lotions
  1. Cream 10% (Aquacare, Nutraplus)
  2. Cream 20% (Carmol 20)
  3. Lotion 10% (Aquacare, Nutraplus, Carmol 10)
B. Lactic acid-containing lotions
  1. 5% (LactiCare)
  2. 12% (Lac-Hydrin) (prescription product)
     Lac-Hydrin is a prescription moisturizer that contains 12% lactic acid. Lactic acid-containing preparations, especially LacHydrin, may frequently burn or sting when applied to the skin, limiting usefulness in children. By combining lower concentrations of lactic acid and urea, moisturizers may reduce the incidence of discomfort and increased effectiveness.
C. Lactic acid and urea
  1. Eucerin Plus Cream and Lotion
D. Soaps and soap substitutes[26]
   NOTE: For children with sensitive skin, soap substitutes are preferred. If soap is to be used, it should be neutral pH.
  1. Cetyl alcohol cleanser (Cetaphil lotion, Aquanil lotion). These are soap substitutes that can be massaged into skin and then patted dry and not rinsed off.
  2. Moisturel Sensitive Skin Cleanser
  3. Purpose Gentle Cleansing Wash
  4. Dove 4.75 oz bar

II. Hair and Scalp Preparations

The therapeutic shampoos are generally massaged for several minutes into a wet scalp. The shampoo should remain in contact with the scalp for several minutes before it is rinsed out with water.

A. Antimicrobial shampoos
  1. Selenium sulfide suspension 1% (Selsun Blue), 2.5% (Exsel, Selsun)
  2. Zinc pyrithione (Denorex, Head & Shoulders, Sebulon)
  3. Ketoconazole 1% shampoo
B. Tar shampoos
  1. 0.5– 2% (Sebutone, T-Gel, DHS-T, Zetar)
C. Keratolytic shampoos
  1. Salicylic acid-sulfur (Sebulex, Ionil, Vanseb, P&S) (salicylic acid 2%, sulfur 2% in detergent shampoo)
D. Detergent shampoos
   A large variety of commercial over-the-counter shampoos are available. Their main ingredients are water, sodium lauryl sulfate as an emulsifier and dispersing agent, and fragrance. The sodium lauryl sulfate may act as an irritant. For dry scalp or cradle cap, such preparations may be used daily. Massage the shampoo in for 20 minutes, then rinse out.

III. Keratolytic Agents

These preparations are used for excessive thickening of the palms and soles, the ichthyoses, and follicular plugging states. The mechanism of action is unknown, but faulty cell-to-cell adherence is the major effect.

A. Retinoic acid, tretinoin (Retin-A)
   Available in:
  1. 0.01%, 0.025% gel; 15 g, 45 g tubes
  2. 0.025%, 0.05%, 0.1% cream; 20 g, 45 g tubes
B. Lactic acid (see I. B and 1.C above)
C. Salicylic acid: 3–6% ointment
  1. Keralyt Gel (salicylic acid 6%, propylene glycol 60% in alcohol)

IV. Agents that Reduce Sweating

A. Aluminum chloride solutions
  1. Aluminum chloride hexahydratein alcohol (20%, Drysol or 6.25%, Xerac AC)
  2. Aluminum chlorohydrate spray (Arrid Extra Dry, Unscented)
B. Glutaraldehyde 10% solution (must be compounded)
   NOTE: Restricted for use on feet only. Stains skin brown. Allergic contact dermatitis may occasionally result.

V. Sunscreens

The potency of sunscreens is determined by a sun protection factor (SPF), which represents the multiples of time to sunburn. At least SPF 15 or higher should be recommended. Waterproof sunscreens are also suggested for children. A large number of sunscreens are available. Sunscreens that are fragrance free and nonstinging to children's skin are preferred. As with moisturizers, the manufacture may change ingredients of a given sunscreen brand, or a given brand name may have variations of ingredients with different SPF factors.

VI. Coal Tars

    A. Coal tar 1% ointment USP and 5% lotion
    B. Tar gels (Estar [5%], PsoriGel [17.5%])

REFERENCES

1. Metry DW, Hebert AA. Topical therapies and medications in the pediatric patient. Pediatr Clin North Am 2000; 47(4):867–876.
2. Segre JA. Epidermal barrier formation and recovery in skin disorders. J Clin Invest 2006; 116(5):1150–1158.
3. Madison KC. Barrier function of the skin: 'la raison d'etre' of the epidermis. J Invest Dermatol 2003; 121(2):231–241.
4. Rawlings AV, Matts PJ. Stratum corneum moisturization at the molecular level: an update in relation to the dry skin cycle. J Invest Dermatol 2005; 124(6):1099–1110.
5. Blank IH, Moloney J 3rd, Emslie AG, et al. The diffusion of water across the stratum corneum as a function of its water content. J Invest Dermatol 1984; 82(2):188–194.
6. Sato J, Denda M, Chang S, et al. Abrupt decreases in environmental humidity induce abnormalities in permeability barrier homeostasis. J Invest Dermatol 2002; 119(4):900–04.
7. Denda M, Sato J, Masuda Y, et al. Exposure to a dry environment enhances epidermal permeability barrier function. J Invest Dermatol 1998; 111(5):858–863.
8. Loden M. Role of topical emollients and moisturizers in the treatment of dry skin barrier disorders. Am J Clin Dermatol 2003; 4(11):771–788.
9. Jackson EM. Latest information on how moisturizers work. Cosmetic Dermatol 1992; 5:35.
10. Orchard D, Weston WL. The importance of vehicle in pediatric topical therapy. Pediatr Ann 2001; 30(4):208–210.
11. Hannuksela A, Kinnunen T. Moisturizers prevent irritant dermatitis. Acta Derm Venereol 1992; 72(1):42–44.
12. Draelos ZD. Therapeutic moisturizers. Dermatol Clin 2000; 18(4):597–607.
13. Goldsmith LA. Salicylic acid. Int J Dermatol 1979; 18(1):32–36.
14. Chiaretti A, Schembri Wismayer D, Tortorolo L, et al. Salicylate intoxication using a skin ointment. Acta Paediatr 1997; 86(3):330–331.
15. Abdel-Magid EH, el-Awad Ahmed FR. Salicylate intoxication in an infant with ichthyosis transmitted through skin ointment – a case report. Pediatrics 1994; 94(6 Pt 1):939–940.
16. Schlagel CA, Sanborn EC. The weights of topical preparations required for total and partial body inunction. J Invest Dermatol 1964; 42:253–256.
17. Long CC, Mills CM, Finlay AY. A practical guide to topical therapy in children. Br J Dermatol 1998; 138(2):293–296.
18. Hepburn D, Yohn JJ, Weston WL. Topical steroid treatment in infants, children, and adolescents. Adv Dermatol 1994; 9:225–254; discussion 255.
19. Del Rosso J, Friedlander SF. Corticosteroids: options in the era of steroid-sparing therapy. J Am Acad Dermatol 2005; 53(1 Suppl 1):S50–S58.
20. Charman C, Williams H. The use of corticosteroids and corticosteroid phobia in atopic dermatitis. Clin Dermatol 2003; 21(3):193–200.
21. Ellison JA, Patel L, Ray DW, et al. Hypothalamic-pituitary-adrenal function and glucocorticoid sensitivity in atopic dermatitis. Pediatrics 2000; 105(4 Pt 1):794–799.
22. Siklar Z, Bostanci I, Atli O, et al. An infantile Cushing syndrome due to misuse of topical steroid. Pediatr Dermatol 2004; 21(5):561–563.
23. Weston WL, Morelli JG. Steroid rosacea in prepubertal children. Arch Pediatr Adolesc Med 2000; 154(1):62–64.
24. Scott LJ, Dunn CJ, Goa KL. Calcipotriol ointment. A review of its use in the management of psoriasis. Am J Clin Dermatol 2001; 2(2):95–120.
25. Berger TG, Duvic M, Van Voorhees AS, et al. The use of topical calcineurin inhibitors in dermatology: safety concerns. Report of the American Academy of Dermatology Association Task Force. J Am Acad Dermatol 2006; 54(5):818–823.
26. Morelli JG, Weston WL. Soaps and shampoos in pediatric practice. Pediatrics 1987; 80(5):634–637.

Index

Page numbers followed by b indicate boxes; f, figures; t, tables.

A

ABCA12, 345, 409
Abscess
  cutaneous, 68–70
  lymph node, cat-scratch disease, 73, 74
  neonatal breast, 393
Absorption, percutaneous, 413–414, 415
Acantholytic cells, 23
Acanthosis nigricans, 331f, 331–332
  benign congenital, 401
Accessory tragus, 406f, 406
Acetaminophen, fixed drug eruptions, 374
Acetylsalicylic acid, erythema nodosum treatment, 271
Acidosis
  following topical therapy over large surface area, 347
  neonatal sclerema, 385
Acne congoblata, 34
Acne fulminans, 34
Acne vulgaris, 6, 25–33, 58, 69, 218
  aggravating factors, 32
  clinical features, 25–26, 26f, 27f, 28f
  comedonal, 25, 27f, 30
  comedones/microcomedones, 25, 26f, 27f, 29, 37
  differential diagnosis, 29b, 29
  drug-induced, 36f, 36
  follow-up visits, 32–33
  grading, 32, 33t
  infantile, 35–36
  inflammatory, 25, 27f, 28f, 29, 30, 31, 32
  neonatorum, 34f, 34–35, 203, 387, 388f, 388, 403
  nodulocystic, 25, 28f, 31
  papulopustular, 25, 27f
  pathogenesis, 29

  patient education, 32
  scarring, 25, 28f, 33
  treatment, 29t, 29–32, 30t
    response evaluation, 32–33
Acrodermatitis enteropathica, 95, 361f, 361–362
  human immunodeficiency virus infection, 137
Acropustulosis of infancy, 94, 387, 388–389, 389f
Actinic cheilitis, 186f, 186
Actinic keratosis, 183
  xeroderma pigmentosum, 191, 192f
Actinic prurigo, 185f, 185–186, 186f, 187
  treatment, 188
Acute generalized erythematous pustulosis, 365, 374f, 374, 377
  associated drugs, 374b
Acyclovir
  erythema multiforme prophylaxis, 197
  herpes simplex, 132
    neonatal infection, 391
  infectious mononucleosis, 123
  varicella, 135
    congenital infection, 391
Adapalene, 30
Adenovirus infection, 199
  exanthems, 113
  keratoconjunctivitis, 131
Adnexal tumors, 217–219
Adolescents
  acanthosis nigricans, 331
  acne vulgaris, 25–33, 26f, 27f, 28f
  athlete's foot (tinea pedis), 87
  atopic dermatitis, 40f, 40, 43
  Becker's nevus, 328f, 328
  chronic pigmented purpuras, 278–280, 279f
  delayed-pressure urticaria, 263
  dermatitis herpetiformis, 204f, 204
  epithelial cysts, 213, 215f

  heat- and exercise-induced urticaria, 263
  herpes progenitalis, 129
  human immunodeficiency virus infection, 138
  infectious mononucleosis, 122–124
  lichen sclerosus, 339
  lupus erythematosus, 166, 167, 168
  malignant melanoma, 329, 331
  mycobacterial granulomas, 78
  pityriasis rosea, 158, 159
  psoriasis, 158
  seborrheic dermatitis, 55, 56
  sun protection, 184
  syphilis, 76, 77
  syringomas, 218
  toxic shock syndrome, 72, 73
  trichoepitheliomas, 218
  vulvovaginal candidiasis, 94, 95
Adrenal insufficiency, 332
Adrenocorticotrophic hormone, drug-induced acne, 36
AIDS, 137
  see also Human immunodeficiency virus (HIV)
Airway involvement
  angioedema, 259, 261, 372
  infantile hemangiomas, 240, 241f
Albinism, 319f, 319–320, 400
  classification, 319b
Albuterol, angioedema-related airway obstruction, 261
Allergic contact dermatitis, 51–55, 52f, 53f, 55f, 190, 195, 210
Allergens, 52–53, 53b, 54t
  elicitation phase, 54
  epicutaneous (patch) testing, 54f, 54–55
  id reaction, 53
  sensitization phase, 53–54
  treatment, 54
Allergic eczema see Atopic dermatitis

Allergic reactions
  drug eruptions, 378
  moisturizer components, 415
  sun protection agents, 184
Alopecia
  acquired circumscribed, 285, 286b
  acquired diffuse, 292–293
    differential diagnosis, 293b
  androgenetic, 294
  congenital circumscribed, 286, 290f,
    290, 402, 404
    differential diagnosis, 290b
  congenital diffuse, 291f, 291–292,
    292f, 293b
  marginal, 289
  neonatal occipital, 289
  scarring forms, 285, 290–291, 292f
    differential diagnosis, 291b
    recessive dystrophic epidermolysis
      bullosa, 351
  secondary syphilis, 160
  traction, 289f, 289
  traumatic, 288–289
Alopecia areata, 84, 156, 285–287,
  286f, 288
  nail abnormalities, 285, 286f, 299,
    300f, 300, 303
Alopecia mucinosis (follicular mucinosis),
  57, 58f, 58, 59
Alopecia totalis, 285, 286f, 287f, 287
Alopecia universalis, 285
ALOX12, 345
ALOX12B, 409
ALOXE3, 345, 409
α-fucosidosis, 249, 253–254
Alpha-hydroxy acid moisurizers, 416
Alternative therapies, atopic dermatitis,
  47–48
Amikacin, mycobacterial granulomas,
  79
Ammonium lactate solution, ichthyoses
  management, 347
Amoxicillin
  acute generalized erythematous
    pustulosis, 374
  Lyme disease, 76
Ampicillin
  cellulitis, 66
  morbilliform eruptions induction with
    infectious mononucleosis, 122,
    123, 378
Anaemia, human parvovirus B19
  induction in immunosupressed
  children, 119
Anagen:telogen ratio, 23
Alopecia areata, 287
Anagen effluvium, 294
Anagen hair stage, 5, 6
Anaphylactoid purpura, 272
Anaphylaxis, 365
  drug reactions management, 379
Anaplasmosis, 102
Ancylostoma braziliensis, cutaneous
  larva migrans, 109

Androgenetic alopecia (male pattern hair
  loss), 6, 294
Androgens
  acne vulgaris pathogenesis, 29
    drug-induced acne, 36
    female adolescents, 31
    neonates, 35, 388
  hirsutism pathogenesis, 297
  milia pathogenesis, 383
  neonatal sebaceous gland hyperplasia
    pathogenesis, 383
  pubertal hair changes, 6
  sebaceous gland function
    dependence, 6
  sebaceous nevi response, 402, 404f
Anencephaly, 407
Angioedema, 257–261, 259f, 365
  airway involvement, 259, 261, 372
  C1 esterase inhibitor deficiency, 259,
    261
  differential diagnosis, 260b, 260
  drug-induced, 372, 379
  hereditary, 257–226
Angiofibromas, 29, 219, 311f, 311
Angiogenic factors, hemangiomas
  pathogenesis, 243
Angiogenin, 243
Angiokeratoma circumscriptum, 247,
  249
Angiokeratomas, 247f, 247, 249
  diffuse, 253–254
Angiolipomas, 222, 223
Angiomas
  cherry, 253f, 253–254
  tufted, 242f, 242
Angiosarcomas, 249
Angular cheilitis, 93, 95, 161
Annular erythemas, 268–269
  differential diagnosis, 269b, 269
Annular lesions, 21f, 21
Anogenital lesions
  lichen sclerosus, 338, 339
  perianal cellulitis, 49, 64, 65f
  see also Genital lesions
Anonychia, 304
Anthralin
  alopecia areata, 287
  psoriasis, short contact protocol, 157
Anthrax, cutaneous, 61, 104
Antibiotics, systemic
  acne vulgaris, 30t, 31, 32–33
    infantile, 36
  atopic dermatitis secondary infection,
    45b, 46, 47, 48
  breast abscess in neonate, 393
  cat-scratch disease, 74
  cellulitis, 66
  ecthyma, 63
  furunculosis, 70
  guttate psoriasis-related streptococcal
    infection, 157, 158
  impetigo, 63, 64
    neonatal, 392
  intertrigo, 63

  Lyme disease, 76
  miliaria secondary infection, 203f,
    203
  mycobacterial granulomas, 79
  necrotizing fasciitis, 67
  omphalitis, 394
  staphylococcal scalded skin syndrome
    (Ritter's disease), 393
  toxic shock syndrome, 73
Antibiotics, topical
  acne vulgaris, 30t, 30, 31, 33
  folliculitis, 70
  perioral dermatitis, 38
  steroid rosacea, 38
Anticonvulsants, drug reactions, 368,
  370, 372
  acne, 36
  relative risk, 366t
Antifungal agents, 84, 85, 90
  side effects, 84–85, 90, 91
  topical, 88–89, 89t, 95
Antigen-processing cells, 5
Anti-gliadin antibodies, dermatitis
  herpetiformis, 205
Antihistamines
  acropustulosis of infancy, 389
  anaphylactic drug reactions, 379
  atopic dermatitis, 45b, 46, 47, 48
  erythema multiforme, 197
  erythema nodosum, 271
  erythropoietic protoporphyria, 189
  nummular dermatitis, 57
  papular urticaria prevention, 107
  physical urticarias, 264
  seabather's eruption, 110
  transient urticaria, 261
  urticarial drug eruptions, 379
  urticarial vasculitis, 264
  varicella, 135
Antiinflammatory agents, topical
  preparations, 417
Antimicrobial shampoos, 421
Antinuclear antibodies
  dermatomyositis, 173
  lupus erythematosus, 167, 169
  morphea, 335
  polyarteritis nodosa, 276
Antiproliferative agents, warts, 142
Antituberculous drugs, drug-induced
  acne, 36
AP3B1, 320
Aphthous stomatitis, 94, 131, 161, 165,
  200f, 200–202, 201f
Aphthous ulcers, 195, 197, 200f,
  200–202, 201f, 208
  differential diagnosis, 201b, 201
  genitals, 210
  recurrence, 200, 201
Aplasia cutis congenita, 358
  associated defects, 404
  congenital circumscribed alopecia,
    286, 290f, 290
  neonates, 404–405, 405f
  treatment, 290

Apocrine glands, 6
  development, 7
Apoptosis, 1
APT2A2, 360
Arrangement of lesions, 19, 20f, 21
Arterial embolism, 67
Arteriovenous malformations (fistulae),
    248
Arthralgia
  Lyme disease, 75
  morbilliform drug eruptions, 371
  morphea, 335
  secondary syphilis, 160
  serum-sickness-like drug reaction,
    373
  toxic shock syndrome, 73
Arthritis
  Henoch-Schönlein purpura, 273
  human parvovirus B19 (erythema
    infectiosum), 118–119, 121
  Lyme disease, 75
  palpable purpuras, 273
  psoriasis, 154, 155f, 156
  rubella, 116
Aseptic meningitis, echovirus infections,
    121, 122
Ash-leaf macules, 310–311, 311f
Aspirin
  drug reactions, 378
  sunburn treatment, 183
  urticaria induction, 261
Asymmetric periflexural exanthem, 113,
    114f
Athlete's foot (tinea pedis), 51, 87f, 87,
    90
Atopic dermatitis, 39–48, 49, 50, 55, 58,
    84, 87, 88, 98, 125, 156, 187
  age-dependent distribution, 40f, 40
  aggravating factors, 44b, 44
  clinical features, 39–44, 41f, 42f, 43f
  diagnosis, 39b, 39
  differential diagnosis, 45
  dry skin, 43f, 43, 46
  eczema herpeticum (Kaposi's
    varicelliform eruption), 130f, 130,
    132
  ichthyosis vulgaris association, 343
  itching, 40, 42f, 43, 44, 47, 48
  neonates, 409
  Netherton's syndrome, 347–348
  pathogenesis, 45
  patient education, 48
  pityriasis alba, 43f, 43
  secondary skin infection, 44f, 44, 46
  treatment, 45b, 45–47, 46b
    alternative therapies, 47–48
    long-term management, 46b, 46,
      47b, 47
    maintenance care, 45b, 46b, 46
    specialist referral, 47
    stress management, 46–47
    topical calcineurin inhibitors, 420
    wet dressings, 46b, 46, 47
  urticaria association, 257

Atopic eczema see Atopic dermatitis
Atrophic changes, 14, 17f
  morphea, 335, 336f, 338
Atrophic nails, 303–304
Atrophoderma, 336
Atropine, scarlatiniform drug eruptions,
    68
Atypical (dysplastic) melanocytic nevi,
    328–329, 329f, 331
Auricular pits, 406, 407f
Auspitz sign, 154, 155f
Autoantibodies
  dermatomyositis, 173
  immunobullous diseases, 204
  paraneoplastic pemphigus, 211
  pemphigoid, 210
  pemphigus foliaceous, 208
Autoimmune blistering (immunobullous)
    diseases, 204b, 204–211
Autoimmune disorders
  generalized vitiligo association, 316
  morphea, 337
  thyroiditis, 268
Automated reagin test (ART), 77
Axillary hair, 6
Azaleic acid, acne vulgaris, 30, 31
Azathioprine
  dermatomyositis, 173
  necrotizing venulitis, 275
  polyarteritis nodosa, 276
Azithromcyin
  cat-scratch disease, 74
  morbilliform eruptions induction with
    infectious mononucleosis, 122

B

B lymphocytes, 5
Bacillary angiomatosis, 74
Bacterial infections (pyoderma), 61–74,
    84
  congenital, 394
  human immunodeficiency virus-
    related, 137
  pustules in neonate, 387, 388
Bacterial intertrigo, 61–64, 62f, 63f, 94
  differential diagnosis, 61, 63
  treatment, 63
Bacterial ulcer, 79
Bartonella henselae, 74
Basal cell carcinoma
  associated syndromes, 219t
  chronic ultraviolet light exposure
    association, 183
  clinical features, 218
  pathogenesis, 219
  sebaceous nevi changes, 402
  xeroderma pigmentosum patients,
    192
Basal cell nevus syndrome, 192, 218,
    219
Basement membrane, 3–4
Basic fibroblast gowth factor, 243
Bazex's syndrome, 192, 218, 219

Beau's lines, 299
Becker's nevus, 328f, 328, 331
Beeswax, moisturizer composition, 415
Behçet's disease, 201, 210
  erythema nodosum association, 270
Benign cephalic histiocytosis, 231, 232f,
    232
Benign congenital acanthosis nigricans,
    401
Benzathine penicillin
  cellulitis, 66
  syphilis, 77
Benzoyl peroxide
  acne vulgaris treatment, 30, 31, 33
    neonates, 35, 388
  gel preparations, 416
Besnier's prurigo see Atopic dermatitis
Beta blockers, lichenoid drug eruptions,
    374
Betacarotene, 2
  erythropoietic protoporphyria therapy,
    189, 190
  photoprotective function, 3
Biliary obstruction, 11
Biopsy, 23
  aphthous ulcers, 201
  atypical urticaria, 260
  calcified nodules, 228
  cutaneous T-cell lymphoma (mycosis
    fungoides), 234
  dermatomyositis, 173
  DRESS syndrome, 368
  epidermolysis bullosa, 348, 353
  erythema annulare, 269
  erythema multiforme, 197
  erythropoietic protoporphyria, 189
  follicular mucinosis, 59
  histiocytosis, 232
  hypopigmented lesions, 309
  ichthyosis, 346, 347
  immunobullous disease, 205
  incontinentia pigmenti, 356
  infantile hemangiomas, 243
  juvenile xanthogranulomas, 226
  keratosis pilaris, 59
  lichen planus, 165
  lupus erythematosus, 169, 170
  mastocytosis, 267
  morphea, 336
  mycobacterial granulomas, 79
  nail disorders, 302–303
  neurofibromas, 222
  nodules, 213
  panniculitis, 228
  pernio, 277
  pityriasis lichenoides, 162
  polyarteritis nodosa, 276
  porokeratosis of Mibelli, 176
  purpuric papules (palpable purpura),
    274
  pyoderma gangrenosum, 281
  pyogenic granuloma, 227
  sarcoidosis, 229
  sebaceous nevi, 402

Biopsy (cont'd)
  Stevens-Johnson syndrome, 368
  tinea versicolor, 92
  toxic epidermal necrolysis, 368
  xeroderma pigmentosum, 192
Biotin-responsive dermatoses, 55, 56
Birth injury
  caput succedaneum, 394
  cephalohematoma, 394
  neonatal petechiae/purpura, 394f,
    394
  scalp ulceration, 404
Birthmarks, neonates, 394–406
  connective tissue, 405–406
  epidermal, 400–404
  pigment cell, 399–400
  vascular, 394–399
Black widow spider bite, 103–104
Black-dot ringworm, 81, 82f
Blanching, 15
Blaschko's lines, 19, 20f, 401f
  epidermal nevi, 400
  Goltz syndrome (focal dermal
    hypoplasia), 358
  hypomelanosis of Ito, 315
  incontinentia pigmenti, 355
  lichen striatus, 173f, 174
  linear and whorled nevoid
    hypermelanosis, 323
Blistering conditions, 22–23
  exfoliative cytology, 23
  immunobullous diseases, 204b,
    204–211
  spontaneous vesicobullous eruptions,
    195b, 195–196, 353
  see also Bullous disease
Blistering dactylitis, 64f, 64
Blue nevus, 328, 329f, 331
Body temperature regulation, 4–5, 6
Body-louse (Pediculus humanus
    humanus) infestation, 104, 105
Bone
  lytic lesions, pustular psoriasis, 154
  malformations, Goltz syndrome, 358f,
    358
Borrelia burgdorferi
  Lyme disease, 75
  morphea pathogenesis, 337
  tick vector, 102
Boston exanthem, 121, 122
Botulinum toxin injection, gustatory
    flushing, 272
BP180, 353
Bradykinin, 269
Braid alopecia, 289
Branchial cleft cysts, 213, 215f, 216
Breast abscess, neonatal, 393
Brown lesions, 23, 320–332
  circumscribed flat, 320–324
    differential diagnosis, 324b
  melanocytic nevi, 324–331
    acquired, differential diagnosis,
      330b, 330
  see also Hyperpigmentation

Brown recluse spider (Loxosceles
    reclusa) bite, 104
Buccal cellulitis, 65
Bulla, 12, 15f
Bullous disease, 195–211
  spontaneous vesicobullous eruptions,
    195b, 195–196
Bullous drug eruptions, 365, 375f, 375,
    377–378
  associated drugs, 375b
Bullous ichthyosiform erythroderma,
    congenital, 346, 401
Bullous ichthyosis, 343, 346f, 346, 347,
    409
  of Siemens, 346
Bullous impetigo, 61, 62f, 70, 195, 356
  neonates, 386, 390, 392
Bullous pemphigoid, 61, 197, 209f,
    209–210
Bullous pemphigoid antigen 1, 4
Bullous pemphigoid antigen 2, 4
Burns, 61, 94
  desquamation, 11
  vesicobullous eruptions, 195
Buschke-Ollendorff syndrome, 405–406
Butterfly rash
  lupus erythematosus, 166f, 166
  pemphigus foliaceus, 207

C

C1 esterase inhibitor deficiency, 259,
    261
c-kit, 267, 310
Café-au-lait spots, 222, 226, 309, 321f,
    321, 322f, 323, 324, 401
  neonates, 399–400
Calcified nodules, 227–228, 228f
Calcineurin inhibitors, topical, 420
  atopic dermatitis, 47
Calcinosis, dermatomyositis, 172, 173
Calcipotriene
  juvenile pityriasis rubra pilaris, 178
  morphea, 337
  psoriasis, 157, 420
  side effects, 420
  topical preparations, 420
Calcipotriol, vitiligo, 317
Calluses, 229
Candida albicans (candidiasis), 69, 88,
    92–95, 203, 339
  acrodermatitis enteropathica, 362
  angular cheilitis, 93, 95
  chronic mucocutaneous, 93f, 94,
    362
  clinical features, 92f, 92–93, 93f
  diaper dermatitis secondary infection,
    49f, 49, 93f, 93, 95, 409
    management, 50
  differential diagnosis, 94–95
  granulomas, 94
  intertriginous, 63, 93–94, 94f
  neonatal/congenital, 93, 94, 389–390,
    390f

pustular lesions, 387
systemic infection, 390
paronychia, 93f, 93, 95, 131, 305f,
    305
pathogenesis, 95
thrush, 92f, 93, 95, 137
treatment, 95
vulvovaginal, 94, 95
Canine scabies mite infestation, 101
Cantharidin
  molluscum contagiosum, 145
  warts, 142
Capillary malformations (port-wine
    stains), 246f, 246–247
  hyperkeratotic (angiokeratomas),
    247f, 247
  treatment, 249–250, 250f
Caput succadaneum, 394
Carbon dioxide laser therapy, warts,
    142
Cardiac disease
  infantile hemangioma associations,
    239, 244
  Kawasaki disease, 199
  Lyme disease, 75
  neonatal lupus erythematosus
    syndrome, 168
Carney complex (NAME syndrome),
    192, 321, 324
Carotenemia, dark-skinned infants, 17
Carrier treatment
  furunculosis, 70
  staphylococcal scalded skin
    syndrome, 72
  see also Contacts treatment
Castleman's tumor, 211
Cat-scratch disease, 73–74, 74f
Catagen hair stage, 5, 6
Cathelicidins, 5
CDCN2A, 330
CDK4, 331
Cefotaxime, cellulitis, 66
Cefoxitin, mycobacterial granulomas, 79
Ceftriaxone
  cellulitis, 66
  Lyme disease, 76
Cell-mediated immunity, allergic contact
    dermatitis, 53
Cellulitis, 64f, 64–66, 67, 131, 260
  blue, 64, 66
  buccal, 65
  human immunodeficiency virus
    infection, 137
  neonates, 385
    cephalohematoma seconady
      infection, 394
  perianal/perivaginal, 64, 65f
  periorbital, 65, 66
  treatment, 66
Central nervous system disorders
  epidermal nevi, 401
  Goltz syndrome, 358
  incontinentia pigmenti, 356
  infantile hemangiomas, 238

infectious mononucleosis, 122, 124
Lyme disease, 75
morphea en coup de sabre, 335
neonatal herpes simplex, 129
neurocutaneous melanosis, 324,
    326
    scalp whorl location abnormalities,
        298
    Sturge-Weber syndrome, 246
    toxic shock syndrome, 73
Cephalexin
    furunculosis, 70
    pyodermas, 63
Cephalic pustulosis, neonatal, 388
Cephalohematoma, 394
Cephalosporins
    serum-sickness-like reactions, 373
    urticaria induction, 261
Cetrizine
    papular urticaria prevention, 107
    urticaria, 261
        physical, 264
Cetyl alcohol, moisturizer composition,
    415
Chancre, 76f, 76, 77
Chancroid, 77
Chediak-Higashi syndrome, 319, 320,
    400
Chemical folliculitis, 69
Chemical vaginitis, 95
Chemotherapy
    acquired diffuse alopecia, 292, 294
    drug eruptions, 378
    Kasabach-Merrit syndrome, 245
    mucositis, 368
    nail surface ridging (Beau's lines), 299
    rhabdomyosarcoma, 233
Cherry angiomas, 253f, 253–254
Chickenpox see Varicella
Chiggers (harvest mite) infestation, 101
Child abuse, 307f, 307
    traction alopecia, 289
Chloramphenicol, cellulitis, 66
Chlorobutanol, 415
Cholesterol, moisturizer composition,
    415
Cholineric urticaria, 263
Chromosomal abnormalities, 408
Chronic infantile neurologic cutaneous
        and articular syndrome, 263
CHS1, 320
Ciclopirox, tinea versicolor, 92
Cicloporaxamine nail lacquer,
        onychomycosis, 91
Ciclosporin
    atopic dermatitis, 47
    pyoderma gangrenosum, 281
Cimetidine
    dermatitis herpetiformis, 205
    molluscum contagiosum, 145
    warts, 142
Ciprofloxacin
    cat-scratch disease, 74
    mycobacterial granulomas, 79

Circumscribed neurodermatitis see
        Atopic dermatitis
Clarithromycin, mycobacterial
        granulomas, 79
Cleansers, 420–421
Cleft lip and palate, 407, 408
Clindamycin
    methicillin-resistant Staphylococcus
        aureus cellulitis, 66
    necrotizing fasciitis, 67
    topical, acne vulgaris treatment,
        30
    toxic shock syndrome, 73
Clinodactyly, 407
Clobetasol propionate
    pemphigoid, 210
    pemphigus foliaceous, 209
Clotrimazole
    angular cheilitis, 95
    thrush (oral candidiasis), 95
    tinea versicolor, 92
Cloxacillin, pyodermas, 63
Clutton's joints, 77
Coal tars see Tar preparations
Coccidioidomycosis, erythema
        nodosum, 269
Colchicine
    dermatitis herpetiformis, 206
    pyoderma gangrenosum, 281
    urticarial vasculitis, 264
Cold exposure
    cheek injury (popsicle panniculitis), 65
    mottling reponse, 276
    neonate, 383–384
    pernio, 277
    polyarteritis nodosa exacerbation,
        276
    sclerema, 385
    subcutaneous fat necrosis, 385
Cold urticaria, 261, 263, 264
    differential diagnosis, 263b
Collagen type I, 4, 8
Collagen type III, 4, 8
Collagen type IV, 4
Collagen type V, 8
Collagen type VII, 4, 353
Collagen type 17, 207, 210
Collagen vascular disease, 87, 120,
        170, 173, 227, 249, 268
    livido reticularis, 384
    purpuric papules (palpable purpura),
        273–274
    urticaria, 257
Collagenomas, 405
Collagens, 4
    defects in Ehlers-Danlos syndrome,
        341
    fetal dermis development, 8
Collodion baby/collodion membrane,
        343, 408f, 408–409
    congenital nonbullous ichthyosiform
        erythroderma, 345
    ichthyosis, 409
    lamellar, 345

Color changes, 11
    nails, 306b, 307
Color, examination of skin, 15, 17
Comedonal acne, 25, 27f
Comedones, 25, 26f, 27f, 144
    closed, 25
    open (blackheads), 25, 26f, 27f
Complement deficiency
    neonatal lupus erythematosus
        syndrome, 169
    subacute cutaneous lupus
        erythematosus, 167, 169
Compound melanocytic nevi, 327f, 327,
        330, 400
Computed tomography, subcutaneous
        fat necrosis, 385
Condylomata acuminata (venereal
        warts), 140f, 141f, 141
Condylomata lata, 160, 161
Congenital acanthosis nigricans, benign,
        401
Congenital circumscribed alopecia, 286,
        290f, 290
    differential diagnosis, 290b
Congenital diffuse alopecia, 291f,
        291–292, 292f, 293f
    differential diagnosis, 293b
Congenital hypertrichosis, 295f,
        295–296, 296f
Congenital ichthyosiform erythroderma
    bullous, 346, 401
    nonbullous, 345
Congenital malformations involving skin,
        406–407
Congenital nevocellular nevi, 401
Congenital self-healing
        reticulohistiocytosis, 229, 231f,
        232
Conjunctivitis, 131
    cat-scratch disease, 73
    human parvovirus B19 (erythema
        infectiosum), 119–120
    Kawasaki disease, 198
    measles, 113
Connective tissue nevi, 405f, 405–406
Conradi-Hunerman ichthyosis, 19
Consumption coagulopathy, Kaposiform
        hemangioendothelioma, 241f,
        241
Contact dermatitis, 37, 45, 48–55, 65,
        88, 92, 125, 187, 260
    allergic, 51–55
    primary irritant, 48–51
Contacts treatment
    impetigo/ecthyma, 64
    pediculoses (louse infestations),
        106
    scabies, 100
    tinea capitis, 85
    see also Carrier treatment
Cool compresses, sunburn, 183
Cornelia de Lange syndrome, 407
Cornrow alopecia, 289
Corns, 229f, 229

Corticosteroids, intralesional
  alopecia areata, 287
  infantile hemangiomas, 244
  keloids, 221
Corticosteroids, systemic
  acne fulminans, 34
  allergic contact dermatitis, 54
  alopecia areata, 287
  dermatomyositis, 173
  infantile hemangiomas, 244
  infectious mononucleosis, 123
  Kaposiform hemangioendothelioma,
    245
  Kasabach-Merrit syndrome, 245
  Langerhans cell histiocytosis, 232
  morphea, 338
  paraneoplastic pemphigus, 211
  pemphigoid, 210
  pemphigus foliaceous/pemphigus
    vulgaris, 209
  polyarteritis nodosa, 276
  pyoderma gangrenosum, 281
  venomous spider bites, 104
Corticosteroids, topical
  acropustulosis of infancy, 389
  addiction, 419f, 419–420
  allergic contact dermatitis, 54
  alopecia areata, 287
  antiinflammatory activity, 417–420
  aphthous ulcers, 201
  atopic dermatitis, 45b, 45, 46, 47
  drug-induced acne, 36
  finger tip unit, 48f, 48
  follicular mucinosis, 59
  gel preparations, 416
  guidelines for use, 418–419
  juvenile plantar dermatosis, 51
  lichen planus, 166
  lichen sclerosus, 339
  lichen spinulosus, 59
  lupus erythematosus, 171
  nummular dermatitis, 57
  patient education, 48
  pemphigoid, 210
  pemphigus foliaceous, 209
  phytophotodermatitis, 191
  polymorphous light eruption, 187
  potency, 418b, 418
  psoriasis, 157
  safety, 417
  seabather's eruption, 110
  seborrheic dermatitis, 56
  side effects, 418f, 419b
    systemic, 419b, 419
  solitary mastocytoma, 267
  steroid rosacea, 29, 37f, 37–38
  tinea corporis appearance following
    inappropriate treatment, 86f, 86
  vitiligo, 317
Corynebacterium minutissimum, 88
Cosmetic appearance, 11
Cosmetics
  allergic contact dermatitis, 52, 53f
  noncomedogenic, 32t

Coxsackievirus A5, 201
Coxsackievirus A10, 201
Coxsackievirus A16, 136, 201
  papular acrodermatitis, 125
Coxsackieviruses, 122
  hand-foot-and-mouth disease, 136f,
    136–137
Cradle cap, 56
Creams
  moisturizers, 414b, 414, 416
    urea-containing, 416
  topical glucocorticosteroids, 417
Creeping eruption (cutaneous larva
    migrans), 108f, 108–109
Cri du chat syndrome, 407
Crusting, 14, 15, 17f
  dermatitis, 39
Cryoglobulins
  cold urticaria, 263, 264
  polyarteritis nodosa, 276
Cryotherapy
  porokeratosis of Mibelli, 176
  warts, 142
Curvilinear lesions, 19, 20f
Cutaneous larva migrans (creeping
    eruption), 108f, 108–109
Cutaneous T-cell lymphoma (mycosis
    fungoides), 162, 233–234, 234f
  erythema annulare association, 268,
    269
Cutis laxa, 4
Cutis marmorata telangiectatica
    congenita, 248–249, 249f, 276,
    383–384
  neonates, 397–398
Cyanosis, dark-skinned infants, 17
Cyclic neutropenia, 200
Cyclophosphamide
  necrotizing venulitis, 275
  pemphigus foliaceous/pemphigus
    vulgaris, 209
  polyarteritis nodosa, 276
  side effects, 209
Cyproheptidine, cold urticaria, 264
Cystic fibrosis, 362
Cysts, 12, 16f, 213–217
  types, 214t
Cytodestructive therapy, warts, 141,
    142
Cytomegalovirus, 74, 118
  congenital infection, 116, 394
  erythema multiforme, 197
  infectious mononucleosis, 122–124
  papular acrodermatitis, 125

D

Danazol
  drug-induced acne, 36
  hereditary angioedema, 261
Dandruff, 84
Dandy-Walker malformations, 238
Dapsone
  dermatitis herpetiformis, 205

linear IgA dermatosis, 207
  pyoderma gangrenosum, 281
  side effects, 205, 206
  urticarial vasculitis, 264
Darier-White disease (keratosis
    follicularis), 354, 359f, 359–360,
    360f
Darier's sign, 226, 266f, 266
Deafness *see* Hearing loss
Defensins, 5
Delayed hypersensitivity reactions,
    papular urticaria, 106f, 106–108,
    107f
Delayed-pressure urticaria, 261, 263, 264
Delta gene, 6
Dengue, 122
Deodorant, allergic contact dermatitis,
    52, 53f
Dermal nevi, 3, 328, 330
Dermatitis, 11, 39–59
  acute, 39
  atopic *see* Atopic dermatitis
  chronic, 39
  contact *see* Contact dermatitis
  diaper *see* Diaper dermatitis
  moisturizer use, 418
  nail surface abnormalities, 299, 301,
    302f
  neonates, 409
  paronychia, 305
  secondary impetigo, 63
  subacute, 39, 61
  topical glucocorticosteroids, 418
  wet dressings, 417
Dermatitis herpetiformis, 98, 104, 135,
    204f, 204–206, 205f, 249
  gluten sensitivity, 205
  treatment, 205–206
Dermatofibromas, 220f, 220, 221
Dermatographism, 261–263, 262f, 264
  mastocytosis association, 266, 267
Dermatomyositis, 156, 169, 170f, 170,
    171f, 171–173, 172f, 378
  calcified nodules, 227
  muscle symptoms, 172
  treatment, 173
Dermatophyte infections, 11, 23, 69,
    81–91, 187, 224, 269
  athlete's foot (tinea pedis), 51, 87f,
    87, 90
  hair *see* Tinea capitis
  human immunodeficiency virus
    infection, 137
  kerion, 61, 74
  nail infection *see* Onychomycosis;
    Tinea unguium
  skin only *see* Tinea corporis
  tinea cruris, 88–89
  tinea faciei, 37, 87f, 87–88, 88f, 137,
    170
  topical antifungal agents, 88–89, 89t
Dermis, 4–5
  development, 8
  epidermal interactions, 8

Dermoid cysts, 213, 214f, 216
Desloratidine, cold urticaria, 264
Desmoglein, 1, 359, 393
  pemphigus foliaceous associated
    autoantibodies, 208
Desmoglein 3, pemphigus vulgaris
    associated autoantibodies, 208
Desmogleins, 1
Desmosomes, 1
Desquamation, 14
  sunburn, 181
  toxic shock syndrome, 72, 73
Detergent shampoos, 421
Development, skin, 7–8
Diabetes mellitus, 11
  candidiasis susceptibility, 94
  chronic paronychia, 305
  necrobiosis lipoidica diabeticorum,
    225
  necrotizing fasciitis, 66f, 66, 67
Diaper dermatitis, 48–50, 49f, 65, 88,
    94, 231
  Candida albicans infection, 93f, 93,
    95, 409
  neonates, 409
  treatment, 49–50
Diarrhea
  acrodermatitis enteropathica, 361,
    362
  toxic shock syndrome, 72
Dicloxacillin
  bullous varicella, 135
  cellulitis, 66
  furunculosis, 70
  pyodermas, 63
  scarlet fever, 68
  staphylococcal scalded skin
    syndrome, 72
Diffuse cutaneous mastocytosis, 72,
    195
Diffuse neonatal hemangiomatosis,
    398f, 398, 399f
Diffuse palmoplantar keratoderma, 358f
Digits
  fetal development, 7–8
  fibrous tumors, 221
Dimpling malformations, 407
Diphenhydramine hydrochloride,
    urticaria, 261
Diphtheria, cutaneous, 61, 104
Discrete lesions, 19f, 19
Disruption of skin surface, 15
  dermatitis, 39
Disseminated intravascular coagulation,
    278f, 278
Distribution of lesions, 21
Disulfiram, drug-induced acne, 36
Diuretics, lichenoid drug eruptions, 374
DLX transcription factor, 6
DNA repair, xeroderma pigmentosum,
    192
Down syndrome see Trisomy 21
Doxycycline
  acne vulgaris, 31

Lyme disease, 76
  mycobacterial granulomas, 79
  syphilis, 77
Drug eruptions, 68, 113, 156,
    365–379
  acute generalized erythematous
    pustulosis, 365, 374, 377
  allergic, 378
  bullous, 195, 365, 375f, 375,
    377–378
    thin/atrophic nails, 304
  diagnosis, 365–366
  differential diagnosis, 377–378
  fixed eruptions, 365, 373–374, 377
  history profile, 365b, 365
  human immunodeficiency virus
    infection, 137
  information for parents/patient, 379
  juvenile pityriasis rubra pilaris-like,
    178
  lichen planus-like, 165
  lichenoid, 365, 374, 375f, 377
  lupus-like syndromes, 170b, 170
  morbilliform (maculopapular), 365,
    370–371, 377, 378, 379
  onset following ingestion of medicine,
    365t
  pathogenesis, 378–379
  photosensitive, 3, 189, 365, 375–376,
    378–379
  serum-sickness-like reaction, 373,
    378
  Sweet's syndrome, 376, 378
  treatment, 379
  urticarial, 257, 261, 365, 371–373,
    377, 378, 379
  vasculitic, 365, 374, 377, 378
Drug rash, eosinophilia, systemic
    symptoms (DRESS) syndrome,
    365, 366, 368, 369f, 369–370, 377
  associated drugs, 370b
Drug reactions
  acne, 36f, 36
  erythema nodosum, 270, 365, 375,
    377
  linear IgA dermatosis, 206, 207
  necrotizing venulitis, 275
  Stevens-Johnson syndrome, 366f,
    366–369
  toxic epidermal necrolysis, 366–369,
    367f
  see also Drug rash, eosinophilia,
    systemic symptoms (DRESS)
    syndrome
Dry skin, 414
  atopic dermatitis, 43f, 43, 46
  ichthyosis vulgaris, 343
  juvenile plantar dermatosis, 51
  keratosis pilaris, 58, 59
  moisturizer treatment, 414
  topical retinoid side effects, 30
Dry-skin dermatitis, 48, 50f, 50–51, 162
DTNBP1, 320
Dyshidrotic eczema, 389

E

Ear, congenital malformations, 406f,
    406, 407f
Ecchymoses, 272
Eccrine sweat glands, 4, 5, 6
  development, 7, 8
  obstruction in miliaria, 203f, 203
Echovirus 2, 122
Echovirus 4, 122
Echovirus 6, 122
Echovirus 9, 115, 121–122
Echovirus 11, 122
Echovirus 16, 118, 121, 122
Echovirus 25, 122
Echovirus 30, 122
Echovirus exanthems, 121f, 121–122
Econazole, candidiasis, 95
Ecthyma, 61–64, 62f
  depth of invasion, 63f, 63
  differential diagnosis, 61
  treatment, 63
Ecthyma gangrenosum, 104, 281
Ectodermal dysplasias, 6, 156, 293b,
    354–360
  congenital diffuse alopecia, 291
  hidrotic, 354, 356–357
  hypohidrotic, 354, 356f, 356–357
  nail surface abnormalities, 299
  thin/atrophic nails, 303f, 303
Ectodysplasin, 6, 357
Eczema craquelé, 414
Eczema herpeticum (Kaposi's
    varicelliform eruption), 44f, 44,
    130f, 130, 132
  treatment, 45b, 46
Eczema/eczematous lesions, 15, 23, 39
  see also Dermatitis
Edema
  acute hemorrhagic of infancy, 273f,
    273
  angioedema, airway involvement, 259
  transient urticaria, 257
  vascular reactions, 257
EDN3, 310
EDNRB, 310
Ehlers-Danlos syndrome, 4, 15, 335,
    339–342
  blood vessel fragility, 341
  hyperextensible joints, 339, 340f,
    340
  skin fragility/healing problems,
    339–340, 341f
  subtypes, 339, 340t
Ehrlichiosis, 102
Elastin, 4, 8
Elastomas, 405
Electrocautery, pyogenic granuloma,
    252
Electrodesiccation, warts, 142
Electron microscopy, epidermolysis
    bullosa, 348, 353
Emollients, 414
  see also Moisturizers

Emulsifiers, moisturizer composition, 415, 416
Emulsions
  coal tar preparations, 420
  oil-in-water, 414, 416
  water-in-oil, 414, 416
Encephalitis, 102
  cat-scratch disease, 74
Encephalocele, 407
  circumscribed occipital hypertrichosis association, 295
Enterotoxin C, 73
Enterovirus 71, hand-foot-and-mouth disease, 136, 137
Enterovirus exanthems, 113, 115
  see also Echovirus exanthems
Enzyme-linked immunosorbent assay (ELISA), syphilis, 77
Eosinophilic cellulitis, 271
Eosinophilic fasciitis, 335
Eosinophilic folliculitis, 137
Eosinophils, erythema toxicum pathogenesis, 386, 387
Epicanthic folds, 407
Epicutaneous (patch) testing, allergic contact dermatitis, 54f, 54–55
Epidermal appendages, 5–6
  development, 7–8
    dermal influences, 8
Epidermal barrier, 1–2, 5, 381
  environmental humidity effects, 413–414
  topical preparations absorption, 413–414
Epidermal cysts, 144
Epidermal giant cells, 23
  herpes simplex virus infection, 130, 131f, 132
Epidermal nevi, 19, 176
  associated abnormalities, 401
  congenital circumscribed alopecia, 290
  inflammatory linear, 401
  neonates, 400–402, 401f
  treatment, 290
Epidermis, 1–4, 2f
  basement membrane, 3–4
  development, 7
    dermal influences, 8
  nutrition, 4
  water content, 2
    neonate, 381
Epidermolysis bullosa, 94, 195, 197, 210, 267, 348–354, 358, 386
  albopapuloid form, 353
  differential diagnosis, 353
  dominant dystrophic, 351, 352f
  gene mutations, 353f, 353
  junctional, 350f, 350, 353
    Herlitz form, 350
  milia, 213, 353
  nonscarring types, 348–350
  nursing care, 354
  pathogenesis, 353–354

recessive dystrophic, 4, 350–351, 351f, 352f, 353
  scarring types, 348, 350–353
  simplex, 348f, 348–350, 349f, 353
    Dowling-Meara type, 349f, 350, 354
    Koebner type, 349f, 349
  thin/atrophic nails, 303
Epidermolytic hyperkeratosis, 346f, 346, 347
  epidermal nevi pathogenesis, 401
Epidermophyton floccosum
  tinea corporis, 86
  tinea cruris, 88
Epiligrin, 1
Epinephrine, agioedema-related airway obstruction, 261
Epithelial cysts, 213, 214f, 216, 222
Epithelioid melanocytic nevi, 226, 330
Epstein-Barr virus, 74, 122
  erythema multiforme, 197
  erythema nodosum, 269
  hydroa vacciniforme-like eruption, 186
  infectious mononucleosis, 122f, 122–124
  papular acrodermatitis, 125
Epstein's pearls, 382
Erosions, 14, 17f, 195
Erysipelas, 260
Erythema, 5, 257
  dark-skinned infants, 17
  pressure, 65
  reactive, 268–272
    annular, 268–269, 269b
  sunburn, 181, 183
Erythema annulare, 268f, 268
Erythema annulare centrifugum, 268
Erythema chronicum migrans, 74–75, 75f, 76, 102
Erythema infectiosum see Human parvovirus B19
Erythema marginatum, 75, 268f, 268–269
Erythema multiforme, 75, 94, 131, 195, 196f, 196–198, 197f, 201, 257, 260, 367, 377
  bullous forms, 61
  isomorphic (Koebner) phenomenon, 196f, 196
  recurrent oral, 367
  target/iris lesions, 196f, 196, 197f
  thin/atrophic nails, 304
Erythema nodosum, 269–271, 270f
  cat-scratch disease, 74
  drug reactions, 365, 375f, 375, 377
    associated drugs, 375b
  treatment, 271
Erythema toxicum, 94, 390
  neonates, 386f, 386, 387
Erythrasma, 88
Erythroderma, congenital ichthyosiform bullous, 346, 401
  nonbullous, 345–346

Erythromycin
  acne vulgaris, 30, 31
    infantile, 36
    neonatal, 35
  linear IgA dermatosis, 207
  perioral dermatitis, 38
  pityriasis lichenoides, 163
  pityriasis rosea, 159
  pyodermas, 63
  scarlet fever, 68
  steroid rosacea, 38
  topical corticosteroid addiction, 420
Erythropoietic protoporphyria, 181, 187, 188f, 188–190, 378
  chronic skin changes, 188f, 189f, 189
Escherichia coli septicemia, disseminated intravascular coagulation, 278
Etretinate, juvenile pityriasis rubra pilaris, 178
Evaluation procedure, 11–23
  documentation, 21
  examination see Examination of skin
  laboratory findings, 23
  medical history, 11
  problem-oriented algorithm, 21–23, 22f, 22t
Examination of skin, 11–12
  arrangement of lesions, 19, 20f, 21
  color, 15, 17
  distribution of lesions, 21
  mobility, 15
  primary skin lesions, 12f, 12, 13f, 14f, 15f, 16f
  secondary skin changes, 12, 14, 17f, 18f
  surface disruption, 15
Exanthem
  cat-scratch disease, 73
  scarlet fever, 67f, 67
  viral see Viral exanthems
Exanthem subitum (roseola), 113, 117f, 117–118, 122
Excoriations, 14, 15, 18f
  dermatitis, 39
Exercise-induced urticaria, 261, 262f, 264
Exfoliatin A, 72
Exfoliative cytology, 23
Exfoliative dermatitis, 365
Exfoliative toxin, 393
Eye lesions see Ophthalmic disorders
Eyelid discoloration, dermatomyositis, 172f, 172

F

Fabry's disease, 249, 253, 254
Facial palsy, herpes zoster, 134f, 135
Facial telangiectasia, keratosis pilaris association, 57, 58f
  treatment, 59
Failure to thrive
  acrodermatitis enteropathica, 361

epidermolysis bullosa
  junctional, 350
  recessive dystrophic, 351
human immunodeficiency virus
    infection, 137
Netherton's syndrome, 348
subcutaneous fat necrosis, 385
Famciclovir
  herpes simplex, 132
  varicella, 135
Familial cold urticaria, 261, 263,
    264
Familial melanoma syndrome, 328, 329,
    330–331
FAPA syndrome, 200–201
Febrile convulsions
  human herpesvirus 6 or 7 infection,
    118
  roseola, 118
Feet
  acrodermatitis enteropathica, 361f,
    362
  acropustulosis of infancy, 388–389,
    389f
  calluses, 229
  congenital toe malformations, 407
  corns, 229f, 229
  diffuse palmoplantar keratoderma,
    358f, 359
  epidermolysis bullosa
    dystrophic, 351f, 351, 352f
    simplex, 348, 349f
  infantile pemphigoid, 209
  juvenile pityriasis rubra pilaris, 176,
    177f
  Kawasaki disease, 198
  pernio, 277f, 277
  piezogenic pedal papules, 228f, 228
Fetal skin development, 7–8
Fever
  acute pityriasis lichenoides (Mucha-
    Habermann disease), 161
  cat-scratch disease, 73
  dermatomyositis, 172
  disseminated intravascular
    coagulation, 278
  drug rash, eosinophilia, systemic
    symptoms (DRESS) syndrome,
    369
  echovirus 9 infection, 122
  hypohidrotic ectodermal dysplasias,
    356, 357
  infectious mononucleosis, 122
  Kawasaki disease, 198, 199
  Lyme disease, 75
  measles, 113
  morbilliform (maculopapular) drug
    eruptions, 371
  polyarteritis nodosa, 275
  roseola, 117, 118
  serum-sickness-like reaction, 373
  Stevens-Johnson syndrome, 368
  sunburn, 181
  toxic epidermal necrolysis, 368

toxic shock syndrome, 72, 73
  varicella (chickenpox), 133
Fialaggrin, 45
Fibromas, 220–221
Fifth disease see Human parvovirus
    B19
Figurate erythemas, 86
Finasteride, androgenetic alopecia, 294
Finger tip unit, 48f, 48, 416–417
Fingers see Hands/fingers
First arch syndrome, 407
Fissures (cracking), 14, 15, 18f
  dermatitis, 39
Fixed drug eruptions, 61, 365, 373f,
    373–374, 377
  associated drugs, 373b
Flea bites, papular urticaria, 107, 108
Fluconazole
  candidiasis, 95
  tinea cruris, 88
  tinea versicolor, 92
Fluorescein-tagged antiherpes zoster
    virus-specific antibody, 391
Fluorescent antinuclear antibody test,
    lupus erythematosus, 169
Fluorescent treponemal antibody
    absorption test, 77
5-Fluorouracil, porokeratosis of Mibelli,
    176
Flushing, mastocytosis, 267
Foams, 416
Focal dermal hypoplasia see Goltz
    syndrome
Fogo selvaem, 207
Follicular mucinosis (alopecia
    mucinosis), 57, 58f, 58
  treatment, 59
Follicular occlusion triad, acne
    congobata, 34
Folliculitis, 58
  bacterial, 68–70, 69f
  chemical, 69
    tar preparation-related, 420
Food-related urticaria, 257, 261
Foreign-body granuloma, 78
Formaldehyde, 415
Formulary, topical preparations,
    420–422
Foscarnet, varicella, 135
Fowl mite infestation, 101
Fragrance-free moisturizers, 415b
Fragrances, moisturizer components,
    415
Freckles, 320f, 320, 323, 324, 326
  xeroderma pigmentosum association,
    192
Free oxygen radicals, 3
Frey syndrome (gustatory flushing),
    271f, 271–272
Friction blisters, 353
Fried egg mole, 327f, 328
Fungal culture, tinea capitis, 83
Fungal infections, 74
  palpable purpuras, 273

see also Dermatophyte infections;
    Yeast infections
Fungal scraping, 23
Fungal ulcer, 79
Furunculosis, 68–70, 69f

G

Gaft-versus-host disease, 368
Gamma benzene hexachloride
  pediculoses, 105–106
  scabies, 100
Ganciclovir, roseola, 118
Gardner's syndrome, 213, 216, 217
Garifloxacin linezolid, mycobacterial
    granulomas, 79
Gaucher's disease, 409
Gels, 416
  coal tar preparations, 420
  topical glucocorticosteroids, 417
Genetic mosaicism, 19
Genital lesions
  aphthous ulcers, 200
  pemphigus vulgaris, 207
  psoriasis, 149, 152f
Genital malformations, 407
Genodermatoses, 343–362
Gentamicin, cat-scratch disease, 74
Geographic tongue, 94, 161, 195, 202f,
    202
Gianotti-Crosti syndrome (papular
    acrodermatitis), 124f, 124–125
Giant urticaria, 65
Gingivostomatitis, herpes simplex, 127f,
    127, 128f, 131, 132
Glomus tumor, 227, 251
Glucagonoma, 362
Glucose-6-phosphate dehydrogenase
    deficiency, 205
Gluten sensitivity, dermatitis
    herpetiformis, 205
Gluten-free diet, dermatitis
    herpetiformis, 205, 206
Glycerin, moisturizer composition, 415
Goldenhar's syndrome (hemifacial
    microsomia), 406
Goltz syndrome (focal dermal
    hypoplasia), 19, 354, 357f,
    357–359
  bony malformations, 358f, 358
Gonorrhea, 94, 131
  palpable purpuras, 273
Granulocytic leukemia, 226
Granuloma annulare, 21, 86, 87, 223f,
    223–224, 224f, 269
Granulomas
  candidiasis, 94
  mycobacterial, 78f, 78–79
Griseofulvin
  onycomycosis (tinea unguium), 90
  side effects, 84–85
  tinea capitis, 84, 85
  tinea cruris, 88
Grotton's papules, 170f, 171

GUJB6, 357
Gustatory flushing, 271f, 271–272

H

Haemophilus influenzae, cellulitis, 64, 65
Hair
  dermatophyte infection (tinea capitis), 81–85
  growth, 5–6
  microscopic examination, 23
  telogen/anagen counts, 23, 287
  transplantation, 405
Hair disorders, 23, 285–298
  ectodermal dysplasias, 354
    hidrotic/hypohidrotic forms, 356
  structural defects, 291f, 291–292, 292f
  unmanageable hair, 297f, 297
Hair excess, 294–294
  acquired, 296–297, 297b
  congenital, 295–296
Hair follicles
  bacterial infections, 68–70, 69f
  congenital hamartomas, 326
  development, 7
  hair growth, 5–6
Hair loss, 285–294, 402
  acrodermatitis enteropathica, 362
  aplasia cutis congenita, 404–405, 405f
  diagnostic categories, 285, 286b, 290
  lichen planus, 163
  lupus erythematosus, 166, 167f
  morphea (en coup de sabre), 335, 336f
  sebaceous nevi, 402
  tinea capitis, 81, 84f, 84, 285, 287
  uncommon forms, 289–290
  see also Alopecia
Hair pulling, 84, 285, 288f, 288–289
Halo nevus, 328f, 328
Halogens, drug-induced acne, 36
Haloprogin, candidiasis, 95
Hamartin, 312
Hand-foot-and-mouth disease, 135, 136f, 136–137, 210
  nail surface ridging (Beau's lines), 299
Hands/fingers
  acrodermatitis enteropathica, 362
  acropustulosis of infancy, 388–389, 389f
  blistering dactylitis, 64f, 64
  calluses, 229
  congenital malformations, 406–407
  dermatitis herpetiformis, 205f
  dermatomyositis, 170f, 171f, 171, 172f
  digital fibrous tumors, 221
  epidermolysis bullosa
    dystrophic, 351, 352f
    simplex, 348f, 348
  erythema multiforme, 196

erythropoietic protoporphyria, 188f, 189f
fetal development, 7–8
granuloma annulare, 223f, 223
herpes simplex virus infection, 129, 131
infantile pemphigoid, 209
juvenile pityriasis rubra pilaris, 176, 177f
Kawasaki disease, 198f, 198, 199f
knuckle pads, 228f, 228
lichen striatus, 173f
lupus erythematosus, 167f, 167, 168f, 170
palmoplantar keratodermas, 358f, 359f, 359
pernio, 277
psoriasis, 150, 153f, 154f, 155f
pyogenic granuloma, 227
sucking blisters, 385, 386f
Haptens, 53
Harlequin color change, neonates, 384
Harlequin fetus/harlequin ichthyosis, 343, 409
Harvest mite (chiggers) infestation, 101
Head-louse *Pediculus humanus capitis* infestation, 104, 105f, 106
  treatment, 105–106
Hearing loss
  external ear congenital malformation association, 406
  Golz syndrome, 358
  keratitis-ichthyosis deafness syndrome, 354
  palmoplantar keratodermas association, 359
Heat rash *see* Miliaria rubra
Heat sensitivity, keratosis follicularis (Darier-White disease), 360
Heat-induced urticaria, 261, 262f
Heatstroke, 181, 183f, 184
Helminth (parasitic worm) infestation, 108f, 108–109
Hemangiomas, infantile, 227, 237–243
  classification, 238b
  complications, 238–240, 240b, 240f, 241f
  congenital, 243f, 243, 245
  deep, 237, 239f, 241f, 245
  differential diagnosis, 243, 249, 251
  follow-up, 245
  growth phase, 237
  high output cardiac failure, 241
  Kaposiform hemangioendothelioma, 241f, 241, 243, 245
  lumbosacral, 238, 239
  mixed, 237, 239f, 240f
  neonates, 395, 397f, 397
    diffuse hemangiomatosis, 398f, 398, 399f
  periorbital, 238, 241f, 245
  presentation, 237, 238b, 238f, 239f
  regression phase, 237, 240f, 243, 397

residual post-regression hypopigmentation/telangiectasia, 237, 240f
  superficial, 237, 239f
  treatment, 244–245
    indications, 244b
    options, 244b
  tufted angiomas, 242f, 242, 243, 245
  ulceration/bacterial superinfection, 244f, 244–245, 397f, 397, 398f
Hemidesmosomes, 4
Hemifacial atrophy, morphea, 335, 336f, 338
Hemifacial microsomia (Goldenhar's syndrome), 406
Hemophilia, 394
Hemorrhagic edema of infancy, acute, 273f, 273
Henoch-Schönlein purpura, 272, 273f, 273, 274, 275
Hepatitis A, 125, 126
  morbilliform/urticarial eruption, 125
  post-exposure vaccination, 126
Hepatitis B, 126f, 126–127, 275
  erythema nodosum, 269
  papular acrodermatitis association, 125
  polyarteritis nodosa association, 276
  skin eruptions, 125, 126, 127
  treatment, 127
  vaccination, 127
Hepatitis B immunoglobulin, 127
Hepatitis C, 126–127, 275
  lichen planus association, 166
  polyarteritis nodosa association, 276
  skin eruptions, 125, 126
Hepatitis D, 126–127
Hepatitis E, 125, 126
  morbilliform eruption, 125
Hepatitis, viral exanthems, 122, 125–127
Hereditary angioedema
  erythema marginatum, 269
  management, 261
Hereditary hemorrhagic telangiectasia (Osler-Weber-Rendu syndrome), 252f, 252, 253f
Hereditary immunodeficiencies, 45, 49
  seborrheic dermatitis, 55
Hereditary mechanobullous disorders, 195
Hereditary periodic fever syndromes, erythema nodosum association, 270
Hermansky-Pudlak syndrome, 319, 320
Herpangina, 131
Herpes facialis, 128, 129f, 129, 131
Herpes gingivostomatitis, 127f, 127, 128f, 131, 132, 137, 208
Herpes gladiatorum, 128
Herpes keratitis, 128f, 128, 132
Herpes labialis, 128f, 128, 131
  erythema multiforme association, 196f, 196, 197f

Continued from inside front cover.

2. Nonblanching (purpuric)
   A. Coagulation disorders
      i. Idiopathic thrombocytopenic purpura, 123
      ii. Leukemia, 233-234
      iii. Hemophilia, 394
   B. Trauma, 394
   C. Progressive pigmentary purpura, 278-280
   D. Erythema nodosum, 269-271
   E. Meningococcemia, 115, 122, 273
   F. Rocky Mountain spotted fever, 115, 122
   G. Atypical measles, 115, 122
   H. Herpes simplex purpura, 127-132
   I. Gonococcemia, 273
   J. Staphylococcal sepsis, 68, 273
   K. Subacute bacterial endocarditis, 273
   L. Pseudomonas sepsis, 273
   M. Infectious mononucleosis, 122-124
   N. Echovirus, 121-122

Papulosquamous Disorders

Newborns
1. Candidiasis, 93, 94, 389-390
2. Epidermal nevus, 400-402
3. Tinea corporis, 85-86
4. Ichthyosis, 343-347
5. Psoriasis, 149-158
6. Congenital rubella, 116, 117, 394
7. Pityriasis rubra pilaris, 176-178
8. Dermatitis, 39-59, 409

Infants and Children
1. Pityriasis rosea, 158-160
2. Psoriasis, 149-158
3. Tinea corporis or tinea faciei, 85-86, 87-88
4. Keratosis pilaris, 57-59
5. Dermatitis, 39-59
6. Scabies, 97-100
7. Lichen planus, 163-166
8. Lupus erythematosus, 166-171
9. Pityriasis lichenoides, 161-163
10. Ichthyosis, 343-347
11. Pityriasis rubra pilaris, 176-178
12. Porokeratosis of Mibelli, 175-176
13. Dermatomyositis, 171-173
14. Secondary syphilis, 76, 77, 160-161
15. Darier's disease, 359-360

Eczematous Disorders

Newborns
1. Diaper dermatitis, 48-50, 409
2. Atopic dermatitis, 39-48, 409
3. Contact dermatitis, 48-55
4. Scabies, 97-100, 388-389, 409
5. Candidiasis, 93, 94, 389-390
6. Langerhans cell histiocytosis, 229-232
7. Acrodermatitis enteropathica, 361-362
8. Ichthyoses (Netherton's, EHK, lamellar), 343-347
9. Leiner's disease, 55
10. Multiple carboxylase deficiency (biotin-responsive dermatoses), 55

11. Severe combined immunodeficiency, 55
12. HIV, 137, 138

Infants and Children
1. Atopic dermatitis, 39-48
2. Contact dermatitis, 48-55
3. Nummular eczematous dermatitis, 56-57
4. Polymorphous light eruption, 185
5. Drug eruption, 365-379
6. Tinea corporis, 85-86
7. Scabies, 97-100
8. Sunburn, 181-184
9. Juvenile plantar dermatosis, 51
10. Candidiasis, 92-95
11. HIV, 137-138
12. Seborrheic dermatitis, 55-56
13. Langerhan's cell histiocytosis, 229-232
14. Lichen planus, 163-166
15. Dermatitis herpetiformis, 204-206

Hair Disorders

Newborns
1. Congenital circumscribed hair loss, 286, 290
   A. Sebaceous nevus, 286, 290, 402-403
   B. Epidermal nevus, 290, 400-402
   C. Hair follicle hamartomas, 326
   D. Aplasia cutis congenita, 286, 290, 404-405
   E. Conradi's disease, 17
   F. Sutural alopecia of Hallermann-Streiff syndrome, 356
   G. Triangular alopecia of frontal scalp, 290t
2. Congenital diffuse hair loss, 291-292
   A. Trichorrhexis nodosa, 291, 292, 293t
   B. Pili torti, 293t
   C. Monilethrix, 292, 293t
   D. Trichorrhexis invaginata, 293t, 347
   E. Ectodermal dysplasia, 293, 254-260
   F. Progeria, 293t
   G. Congenital hypothyroidism, 295
   H. Atrichia congenita, 293t
   I. Congenital alopecia with papules, 291
   J. Down syndrome, 298

Infants and Children
1. Acquired circumscribed hair loss
   A. Alopecia areata, 285-287
   B. Tinea capitis, 81-85
   C. Traction alopecia, (includes trichotillomania), 288-289
   D. Kerion, 83-84
   E. Pyoderma, 61-74
   F. Varicella, 132-133
   G. Lichen planus, 163-166
   H. Lupus erythematosus, 166-171
   I. Darier's disease, 226, 266
   J. Porokeratosis of Mibelli, 175-176
   K. Physical trauma (abrasions, cuts), 289
   L. Chemical or thermal burns, 195
   M. Radiation injury, 290

   N. Psoriasis, 149-158
   O. Secondary syphilis, 76, 77, 160-161
2. Acquired diffuse hair loss
   A. Hypothyroidism, 293t
   B. Hypopituitarism, 293t
   C. Hypoparathyroidism, 293t
   D. Diabetes mellitus, 293t
   E. Androgenetic alopecia (male-pattern baldness), 293t, 294
   F. Hypervitaminosis A, 293t
   G. Acrodermatitis enteropathica, 361-362, 293t
   H. Marasmus, 293t
   I. Heparin or coumarin therapy, 293t
   J. Antithyroid drugs, 293t
   K. Antimetabolites, 293t
   L. Thallium poisoning, 293t
   M. Telogen effluvium, 293

Nail Disease

Newborns
1. Thick nails
   A. Pachyonycia congenita, 301, 303
   B. Ectodermal dysplasia, 303, 354-360
   C. Congenital malaligned nails, 299
2. Thin or atrophic nails
   A. Ectodermal dysplasia, 303, 354-360
   B. Epidermolysis bullosa, 303, 351
   C. Incontinentia pigmenti, 355-356
   D. Nail-patella syndrome, 304
   E. Acrodermatitis enteropathica, 361-362
   F. Anonychia with or without ectrodactyly, 304
   G. Focal dermal hypoplasia, 303b, 357-359
   H. Ellis-van Creveld syndrome, 304b
   I. Turner's syndrome, 407, 408
   J. Dyskeratosis congenita, 303b, 304b,
   K. Trisomy, 13, 18
   L. Periodic shedding of nails, 304
   M. Coffin-Siris syndrome, 304b
   N. Hallermann-Streiff syndrome, 304b
   O. Progeria, 304b

Infants and Children
1. Thick nails, 299
   A. Psoriasis, 150, 156, 299, 300
   B. Lichen planus, 163-165, 300, 301
   C. Onychomycosis, 301-302
   D. Trachyonychia, 163-165, 299, 300
   E. Pachyonychia congenita, 301, 303
   F. Ectodermal dysplasia, 303, 354-360
   G. Norwegian scabies, 97, 100
   H. Dermatitis, 299, 301
   I. Palmoplantar keratodermas (hereditary forms), 359
2. Thin or atrophic nails, 303
   A. Trauma, 304
   B. Lichen planus, 163-165, 300, 301
   C. Raynaud's phenomenon, 304
   D. Drug eruptions, 365-379
   E. Trachyonychia, 163-165, 299, 300

Herpes progenitalis, 129, 131
Herpes simplex, 21, 23, 61, 77, 94, 104,
    113, 127–132, 135, 165, 195, 196,
    197, 201, 249, 281, 356, 386
  differential diagnosis, 130–131, 131b
  eczema herpeticum (Kaposi's
    varicelliform eruption), 44f, 44,
    45b, 46, 130f, 130, 132
  erythema multiforme pathogenesis,
    197, 198
  hand/finger infections, 129f, 129, 131
  herpes facialis, 128, 129f, 129, 131
  herpes keratitis, 128f, 128, 131, 132
  herpes labialis, 128f, 128, 131
  herpes progenitalis, 129, 131
  immunosupressed children, 130
  neonates, 39, 116–117, 129, 130f,
    131, 132, 387, 390–391, 391f, 394
    prevention, 391
  pathogenesis, 132
  primary gingivostomatitis, 127f, 127,
    128f, 131, 132, 208
  recurrent infection, 127–128, 128f,
    131
  treatment, 132
  type 1, 127, 128, 129, 130, 132, 391
  type 2, 129, 130, 132, 390, 391
  whitlow, 65, 305
Herpes zoster, 21, 23, 104, 131, 133f,
    133–136, 134f, 195, 249
  differential diagnosis, 135
  distribution, 134f, 134
  human immunodeficiency virus
    infection, 137f, 137
  keratitis, 134, 135
Herpetic whitlow, 128, 129f
Hexachlorophene, 415
Hidrotic ectodermal dysplasia, 354,
    356–357
Hirsutism, 296–297, 297b
  acne vulgaris/hyperandrogenism
    association in female
    adolescents, 31
Histamine, 5, 263
  drugs producing release in
    mastocytosis, 266b, 267–268
  transient urticaria pathogenesis, 260
Histiocytosis, 226, 229–232, 230f,
    267
  differential diagnosis, 231
Histiocytosis X, 231, 362
  neonates, 409
Histoplasmosis, erythema nodosum,
    269
Hives see Urticaria
Hodgkin's disease, erythema nodosum
  association, 270
Hookworm, cutaneous larva migrans,
    109
Hot-comb alopecia, 289
Human herpesvirus 1 see Herpes
  simplex
Human herpesvirus 2 see Herpes
  simplex

Human herpesvirus 3 see Herpes zoster;
    Varicella (chickenpox)
Human herpesvirus 4 see Epstein-Barr
    virus
Human herpesvirus 5 see
    Cytomegalovirus
Human herpesvirus 6, 122
  infectious mononucleosis, 122–124
  Langerhans cell histiocytosis
    association, 232
  papular acrodermatitis, 125
  see also Roseola
Human herpesvirus 7, 118, 122
  infectious mononucleosis, 122–124
  pityriasis rosea association, 159
Human immunodeficiency virus (HIV),
    45, 49, 74, 77, 137f, 137–138
  acrodermatitis
    enteropathica/nutritional zinc
    deficiency, 137
  candidiasis, 93
  cellulitis, 137
  congenital infection, 137, 138
  dermatophyte infections, 137
  drug eruptions, 137
  eosinophilic folliculitis, 137
  Epstein-Barr virus-related infectious
    mononucleosis, 123
  herpes gingivostomatitis, 137
  herpes zoster, 137f, 137
  molluscum contagiosum, 137, 144
  Norwegian scabies, 137
  progression to AIDS, 137
  pyodermas, 137
  seborrheic dermatitis, 55, 56, 137
  thrush (oral candidiasis), 94, 137
  type 1, 137
Human papillomavirus infection, warts,
    138t, 138–143
Human parvovirus B19 (erythema
    infectiosum), 113, 116, 118–121,
    119f, 123, 126, 170, 275
  infection in pregnancy, 120, 121
  polyarteritis nodosa association, 276
  purpuric hand and foot eruption, 118,
    120f
  slapped-cheek appearance, 118,
    119f
Humectants, 414
Humidification
  dry-skin dermatitis management, 51
  wet dressings antiinflammatory
    activity, 417
  see also Hydration
Humidity, effects on epidermal barrier,
    413–414
Hutchinson's summer prurigo see
    Actinic prurigo
Hutchinson's teeth, 77
Hydralazine, necrotizing venulitis
  association, 275
Hydration
  enhancing agents, moisturizer
    components, 416

influence on topical preparations
    absorption, 413
  see also Humidification
Hydroa vacciniforme, 186, 187f
Hydrocele, 407
Hydrops fetalis, congenital syphilis, 77
Hydroxychloroquine
  dermatomyositis, 173
  lupus erythematosus, 171
Hydroxyzine
  acropustulosis of infancy, 389
  mastocytosis, 267
  urticaria, 261
    physical, 264
Hygiene measures
  anogenital lichen sclerosus, 339
  bacterial intertrigo, 63, 64
  ecthyma, 63, 64
  hair follicle infections, 70
  impetigo, 63, 64
  necrotizing fasciitis, 67
  viral hepatitis, 126
Hyperandrogenism, acne vulgaris in
    female adolescents, 31
Hypermobile skin, 335, 339–342
Hyperpigmentation, 309
  circumscribed flat lesions, 320–324
    differential diagnosis, 324b
  diffuse, 332
    differential diagnosis, 332b
  photosensitive drug reactions, 376,
    379
  phytophotodermatitis, 190f, 190, 191
  postinflammatory, 323, 324
Hyperthyroidism, 11
Hypertrichosis
  circumscribed, 295
    differential diagnosis, 295, 296b
    midline with nervous system
      abnormalities, 295
  congenital, 295–296
  lanuginosa, 295f, 295
  nevoid, 295, 296f
  syndromic associations, 296b
Hypertrophic scars, 220f, 220, 221
  acne, 25
Hypohidrotic ectodermal dysplasia, 5,
    293f, 354, 356f, 356–357
Hypomelanosis of Ito, 19, 92, 312, 314f,
    315
Hypopigmentation, diffuse (albinism),
    319b, 319f, 319–320
Hypopigmented lesions, 309
  acquired circumscribed flat, 316–319
  congenital circumscribed flat,
    309–315
    differential diagnosis, 311–312
  lichen striatus, 174f, 174
  neonates, 400
  patchy pigment loss, 314b
  postinflammatory, 318f, 318–319
Hypospadias, 407
Hypotension, toxic shock syndrome, 72,
    73

Hypothyroidism
  drug rash, eosinophilia, systemic
    symptoms (DRESS) syndrome,
    370
  neonates
    excessive body hair association,
      295
    skin mottling, 383

I

Ichthyosiform erythroderma, 94
  congenital bullous, 346
  congenital nonbullous, 345–346, 409
Ichthyosis, 50, 343–347, 401, 409
  bullous, 343, 346f, 346, 347, 409
  collodion membrane association, 343,
    345, 409
  differential diagnosis, 346–347
  ectodermal dysplasias, 354
  harlequin/harlequin fetus, 343, 409
  lamellar, 343, 345f, 345–346, 347, 409
  X-linked, 343–345, 344f, 347, 409
Ichthyosis hystrix, 401
Ichthyosis vulgaris, 58, 343, 344f, 347
  atopic dermatitis association, 409
Idiopathic photodermatoses, 181,
    185–188, 378
  differential diagnosis, 187
  types, 184b, 185–186
Idiopathic scrotal edema, 260
Idiopathic thrombocytopenic purpura,
    123
Idiopathic trachyonychia, 299, 300,
    301f, 301, 302f
IKKg, 355
Imidazole, candidiasis with diaper
    dermatitis, 50
Imidazolinylureas, 415
Imipenem, mycobacterial granulomas,
    79
Imiquimod, topical
  molluscum contagiosum, 145
  morphea, 337
  porokeratosis of Mibelli, 176
  warts, 142
Immediate pigment darkening, 3
Immobile skin, 335–339
Immune complexes
  cold urticaria, 263
  lupus erythematosus, 170
  purpuric papules (palpable purpura),
    274, 275
  urticarial vasculitis, 264
Immune response, 5
Immunobullous diseases, 195, 204b,
    204–211, 377
Immunofluorescence examination, 23
  dermatitis herpetiformis, 205
  epidermolysis bullosa, 348
  erythropoietic protoporphyria, 189
  immunobullous diseases, 205
  Stevens-Johnson syndrome, 368
  toxic epidermal necrolysis, 368

Immunoglobulin, intravenous
  dermatomyositis, 173
  Kawasaki disease, 199
  necrotizing fasciitis, 67
Immunosupressed children
  candidiasis, 93f, 93, 95
    chronic mucocutaneous, 93f, 94
    oral thrush, 94
  herpes simplex, 127, 130
  herpes zoster, 135
  human parvovirus B19 (erythema
    infectiosum), 119, 120, 121
  necrotizing fasciitis association, 66
  scabies, 97, 99, 100
  tinea corporis, 86
  varicella (chickenpox), 133, 135
  warts, 141
Immunosupressive therapy
  immunobullous diseases, 204
  pemphigus foliaceous/pemphigus
    vulgaris, 208–209
  pyoderma gangrenosum, 281
Impetigo, 5, 57, 61–64, 62f, 68, 95, 131,
    135, 208
  bullous, 61, 62f, 70, 195, 356, 386,
    390, 392
  depth of invasion, 63f, 63
  differential diagnosis, 61
  neonates, 386, 390, 392f, 392
  secondary, 97
  treatment, 63, 64
Incision/drainage
  abscesses, 70
  furunculosis, 70
Incontinentia pigmenti, 19, 190, 315,
    354, 355f, 355–356
  blistering episodes, 355f, 355, 356
  neonates, 386, 390
  pigmented lesions, 355f, 355
  warty lesions, 355f, 355, 356, 401
Indomethacin
  erythema nodosum, 271
  urticarial vasculitis, 264
Infantile acne, 35–36
Infants
  blistering dactylitis, 64f, 64
  cellulitis, 64–65
  diaper dermatitis, 48–50, 49f
  heatstroke susceptibility, 184
  newborn see Neonates
  popsicle panniculitis, 65
  preterm see Preterm infants
  roseola, 117–118
  seborrheic dermatitis, 55
Infectious mononucleosis, 68, 77, 118,
    122f, 122–124
  laboratory findings, 123t, 123
  viral agents, 125b
Infestations, 97–110
Inflammatory bowel disease
  erythema nodosum association, 270
  pyoderma gangrenosum association,
    182, 280
Inflammatory linear epidermal nevi, 401

Inflammatory papules/nodules, 23
Inflammatory response, 5
Infliximab
  dermatitis herpetiformis, 206
  pyoderma gangrenosum, 281
Ingrown toenails, 305–307, 306f
Insect bites, 110, 135, 136, 162, 270,
    281
  urticaria, 106–107, 257
Insect repellents, 101t, 103, 107
  DEET-containing, 108
Insulin resistance, acanthosis nigricans
    association, 331, 332
Insulin-like growth factor, 243
Integrins, 4
  mutations, 353
Interferon alpha
  infantile hemangiomas, 244, 245
  side effects, 244
  warts, 142
Interferon inducers, warts, 142
Intertrigo
  bacterial, 61–64, 62f, 63f, 94, 339
    treatment, 63
  candidal, 63, 93–94, 94f
Involucrin, 1
5-Iodo-2-deoxyuridine, herpes keratitis,
    132
Irritant contact dermatitis, 48–51
Isomorphic (Koebner) phenomenon,
    149, 153f, 175
  erythema multiforme, 196f, 196
  lichen nitidus, 165
  lichen planus, 163, 164f, 165f
  lichen sclerosus, 339
Isotretinoin
  acne congoblata, 34
  acne fulminans, 34
  acne vulgaris, 31
  infantile acne, 36
  juvenile pityriasis rubra pilaris, 178
  side effects, 31
  teratogenicity, 31
Itch sensation, 5
  see also Pruritus
Itraconazole
  candidiasis, 95
  onycomycosis (tinea unguium), 90,
    303
  side effects, 90
  tinea capitis, 84
  tinea cruris, 88
  tinea versicolor, 92
Ivermectin
  cutaneous larva migrans, 109
  scabies, 100

J

Jadassohn's sebaceous nevus, 402f,
    402, 403f
Jaundice
  dark-skinned infants, 17
  viral hepatitis, 125, 126

Jellyfish eruption, 109f, 109–110
Joints, cellulitis involvement, 64, 65
Junctional epidermolysis bullosa, 350f, 350
    Herlitz form, 350
Junctional melanocytic nevi, 327f, 327, 330
    neonates, 400
Juvenile pityriasis rubra pilaris, 176–178, 177f
    islands of sparing, 177, 178f
Juvenile plantar dermatosis, 43, 45, 48, 51f, 51, 87
Juvenile rheumatoid arthritis, 260
    purpuric papules (palpable purpura), 274
    transient urticaria, 269
    urticarial vasculitis, 264
Juvenile spring eruptiom, 185f, 185
Juvenile xanthogranulomas, 225f, 226f, 226, 231, 251, 402

K

Kaposiform hemangioendothelioma, 241f, 241, 243
    treatment, 245
Kaposi's sarcoma, 249
Kaposi's varicelliform eruption see Eczema herpeticum
Kasabach-Merrit syndrome, 241f, 241, 242
    treatment, 245
Kawasaki disease (mucocutaneous lymph node syndrome), 68, 73, 195–196, 198–199, 275, 368
    clinical features, 198f, 198, 199f
    human parvovirus B19 association, 121
Keloids, 220f, 220–221, 221f
    acne, 25, 28f
    treatment, 221
Keratin 1, 1, 346, 359
Keratin 5, 1, 353
Keratin 6a/b, 303, 359
Keratin 9, 359
Keratin 10, 1, 346
Keratin 14, 1, 353, 359
Keratin 16, 303, 359
Keratin 17, 214, 303, 359
Keratin K2e, 346
Keratinization, 1
Keratinocyte-cultured autografts, 354
Keratinocytes, 1
    melanin response to ultraviolet light exposure, 3
Keratins, 1, 4
Keratitis
    herpes simplex, 128f, 128, 131
    herpes zoster, 134
Keratitis-ichthyosis deafness syndrome, 354
Keratohyaline granules, 1
Keratolytic agents, 421

epidermal nevi management, 402
keratosis pilaris, 59
shampoos, 421
Keratosis follicularis (Darier-White disease), 354, 359f, 359–360, 360f
Keratosis pilaris, 57f, 57–59, 58f, 165, 360, 414
    atopic dermatitis, 43
    dry-skin dermatitis, 50
    ichthyosis vulgaris association, 343
    treatment, 59
Kerion, 61, 74, 85
    tinea capitis, 81, 82f, 83f, 83–84
Ketoconazole
    neonatal/congenital candidiasis, 390
    onycomycosis (tinea unguium), 90
    tinea capitis, 84, 85
    tinea versicolor, 92
Kibes, 277
Klinefelter's syndrome, 407, 408
Klippel-Trenaunay syndrome, 246f, 247f, 247, 250
Klippel-Trenaunay-Weber syndrome, 397f
Knuckle pads, 228f, 228
Koebner phenomenon see Isomorphic phenomenon
Koplik's spots, 114f, 114

L

Laboratory findings, 23
Lactic acid-containing moisturizers, 416
    ichthyoses, 347
    keratosis pilaris, 59
    lotions, 421
Lamellar ichthyosis, 343, 345f, 345–346, 347, 409
Laminin 1, 4
Laminin 5, 4, 353
Laminin 6, 4
Langerhans cell histiocytosis, 49, 55, 79, 98, 229, 230f, 231f, 231
    chemotherapy, 232
    pathogenesis, 231–232
Langerhans cells, 5, 7, 53
Lanolin, 415
Lanolin-free moisturizers, 415b
Lanugo overgrowth, transient, 295
Laser therapy see Carbon dioxide laser therapy; Pulsed dye laser therapy
Leiner's disease, 55
Leishmaniasis, 79
LEKTI, 348
Lentigenes, 320f, 321f, 321, 323, 324
LEOPARD syndrome, 192, 321f, 321, 324
Leptospirosis, 73, 199
Letterer-Siwe disease, 94
Leukemia, 170, 233–234, 234f
Leukoplakia, 165, 339
Lichen nitidus, 141, 165f, 165
    bullous, 165

Lichen planus, 84, 90, 94, 98, 141, 156, 163–166, 170
    clinical features, 163b, 163f, 163–165, 164f, 165f
    hypertrophic, 163, 164f
    isomorphic phenomenon, 163, 164f, 165f
    nail abnormalities, 163–165, 165f, 299, 300, 301f, 301, 303, 304
    pruritus, 165
    treatment, 166
Lichen sclerosus, 317, 336, 338f, 338–339
    anogenital lesions, 338f, 338–339
    extragenital lesions, 338f, 339
    malignant potential, 339
    morphea concurrent lesions, 335, 339
Lichen spinulosus, 57, 58f, 58
    treatment, 59
Lichen striatus, 19, 156, 173f, 174f, 174–175, 176, 401
    nail abnormalities, 299
Lichenoid drug eruptions, 125, 365, 374, 375f, 377
    associated drugs, 375b
Lindane, scabies, 100
Linear epidermal nevi, 156
Linear immunoglobulin A (IgA) dermatosis, 61, 94, 206f, 206–207
Linear lesions, 19f, 19
Lipids, skin, 1
Lipocytes, 6
Lipomas, 222f, 222–223, 249
    midline, 407
Lips
    congenital malformations, 407
    pits, 407f, 407
Liquid petrolatum/liquid paraffin, 415
Liquor carbonis detergens, 420
Lithium, drug-induced acne, 36, 378
Liver function, erythropoietic protoporphyria, 189, 190
Livido reticularis, 270, 384
    chronic cutaneous polyarteritis nodosa, 275f, 275, 276f
    dermatomyositis, 172, 173
    lupus erythematosus, 167, 170
LKB1, 324
LMX1B, 304
LOR, 409
Loricin, 359
Lotions
    coal tar preparations, 420
    moisturizers, 414b, 416
    topical glucocorticosteroids, 417
Louse infestations (pediculoses), 104–106, 105f
Loxosceles reclusa (brown recluse spider) bite, 104
Lubricants see Moisturizers
Lues see Syphilis, secondary
Lunula, 6

Lupus erythematosus, 84, 86, 87–88, 123, 156, 166–171, 172, 173, 189, 269, 378
  bullous, 167f, 167
  butterfly erythematous maculopapular eruption, 166f, 166
  clinical features, 166f, 166–169, 167f, 168f
  differential diagnosis, 169–170
  discoid lesions, 166f, 166, 167f, 170, 171
  laboratory evaluation, 169b, 169
  neonatal syndrome, 117, 168f, 168, 169f, 169
  panniculitis, 168f, 168, 170, 171
  pathogenesis, 170–171
  photosensitivity, 167f, 167, 168, 181, 187
  purpuric papules (palpable purpura), 274
  subacute cutaneous, 167
  treatment, 171
  urticarial vasculitis association, 264
Lyme disease, 74–76, 102, 103
  erythema chronicum migrans, 74–75, 75f, 76
  vaccination, 103
Lymphadenopathy
  cat-scratch disease, 73, 74
  cellulitis, 64
  drug rash, eosinophilia, systemic symptoms (DRESS) syndrome, 369
  echovirus exanthems, 121
  herpes simplex, 128
  human immunodeficiency virus infection, 137
  infectious mononucleosis, 122
  Kawasaki disease, 198
  Lyme disease, 75
  measles, 114
  pityriasis rosea, 158
  rubella, 116
  scarlet fever, 67–68
  Stevens-Johnson syndrome, 368
  syphilis, 76, 160
  tinea capitis, 81
  toxic epidermal necrolysis, 368
Lymphangiomas see Lymphatic malformations
Lymphatic malformations (lymphangiomas), 223, 248
  deep, 248
  neonates, 398–399, 399f
  superficial, 248f, 248, 249
Lymphedema, 260
Lymphogranuoma venereum, 77
Lymphoid malignancy, hydroa vacciniforme-like eruption, 186
Lymphoma, 11, 74, 170, 233–234, 234f, 277, 370
  dermatitis herpetiformis association, 205
Lymphomatoid papulosis, 162

M

McCune-Albright syndrome, 323, 324
Maceration, 414
Macrophages, 5, 53
Macule, 12f, 12
Magnetic resonance imaging
  dermatomyositis, 172–173
  infantile hemangiomas, 243, 245
    lumbosacral, 239
  necrotizing fasciitis, 66
  neural tube defects, 407
  neurocutaneous melanosis, 324
  subcutaneous fat necrosis, 385
Majocchi's granulomas, 86f, 86
Malassezia
  neonatal cephalic pustulosis, 388
  tinea versicolor, 92
Malathion, pediculoses, 106
Marginal alopecia, 289
Massage alopecia, 289
Mast cells, 5
  angioedema, 260
  transient urticaria, 260
Mastocytoma, solitary, 226, 227, 265f, 265, 267
Mastocytosis, 195, 265–268
  bullous (diffuse cutaneous), 195, 265, 266–267, 267f
  dermatographism association, 263, 266, 267
  differential diagnosis, 260
  drugs producing histamine release, 266b, 267–268
  systemic, 266
MATP, 320
Measles, 113–116, 199
  atypical, 114, 115f, 115, 116, 122
  classic, 113–114
  complications, 114, 116
  Koplik's spots, 114f, 114
Mechanical sensitivity, 5
Median nail dystrophy, 299, 300f
Median raphe cysts, 213, 215f
Medical history, 11
Melanin, 2–3, 3f, 7, 17, 181
  photoprotective function, 3
  phytophotodermatitis-related production, 191
  ultraviolet light exposure-related increase, 3
Melanocortin-1 receptor, 324
Melanocyte–keratinocyte unit, 2f, 2
Melanocytes, 2, 7
  hypofunctional, 314, 315
  transplantation, 317
Melanocytic nevi, 227
  acquired see Moles, common
  congenital, 324, 325f, 325–326, 326f
    management, 326
    nevus spilus, 325, 326f
    neonates, 400f, 400
Melanoma, malignant, 227, 251, 329–331, 330f
  atypical (dysplastic) nevi relationship, 328, 330
  clinical features, 329b, 329–330
  common moles (acquired melanocytic nevi) association, 326, 327
  congenital melanocytic nevi association, 326
  differential diagnosis, 330b, 330
  pathogenesis, 330
  sunburn history, 183
  treatment, 331
  xeroderma pigmentosum patients, 192
Melanosis
  neurocutaneous, 324, 326
  transient neonatal pustular, 386–387, 387f, 390
Melanosomes, 2, 3f, 7
Melkersson-Rosenthal syndrome, 260
Meningocele, circumscribed occipital hypertrichosis association, 295
Meningococcemia, 73, 115, 122
  disseminated intravascular coagulation, 278
  palpable purpuras, 273
Meningomyelocele, 407
Merkel cells, 7
Metastatic calcification, 67
Methicillin-resistant Staphylococcus aureus (MRSA)
  antibiotic therapy, 63, 66, 70
  atopic dermatitis secondary infection, 46
  bullous varicella, 133, 135
  cellulitis, 65, 66
  folliculitis, 69–70
  impetigo, 63
Methotrexate
  dermatomyositis, 173
  juvenile pityriasis rubra pilaris, 178
  morphea, 338
  polyarteritis nodosa, 276
  psoriasis, 157
Methoxsalen photochemotherapy, psoriasis, 157
Methylprednisone, necrotizing venulitis, 275
Metronidazole, topical
  perioral dermatitis, 38
  steroid rosacea, 38
Miconazole
  candidiasis, 95
  neonatal/congenital candidiasis, 390
  tinea versicolor, 92
Microcomedones, 25, 29
Microemulsions, moisturizing creams/lotions, 416
Microsporum canis, 84t, 84
  tinea capitis, 81, 82f, 84, 85
  tinea corporis, 86
  tinea faciei, 87
Microsporum gypseum, tinea corporis, 86

Midline
  circumscribed hypertrichosis, nervous
    system abnormalities, 295
  dimpling, 407
Milia, 58, 213, 215f, 216
  dystrophic epidermolysis bullosa scar
    borders, 351f, 351, 353
  neonates, 382–383, 383f
Miliaria, 35, 94, 195, 202–203, 203f,
  390
  crystallina, 202
  pustulosa, 202
  rubra (heat rash), 202, 203f, 387
Miniature puberty of the newborn
  breast abscess, 393
  neonatal acne, 388
Minocycline
  acne vulgaris, 31
  drug reactions, 370
Minoxidil
  alopecia areata, 287
  androgenetic alopecia, 294
Mite infestations, 97–101
  non-human sources, 101
    papular urticaria, 107, 108
MITF, 310
Mobility, skin, 15, 19f, 23
Moisturizers, 414–416
  atopic dermatitis, 45b, 45, 46, 47b,
    47, 48
  components, 414–415, 415t
  creams, 414b, 414, 416
  dermatitis treatment, 418
  diaper dermatitis, 49, 50
  dry-skin dermatitis, 50–51
  epidermal nevi, 402
  formulary, 420–421
  fragrance-free, 415b
  fragrances, 415
  function, 414b
  ichthyosis vulgaris, 347
  juvenile plantar dermatosis, 51
  keratosis pilaris, 59
  lanolin-free, 415b
  lichen spinulosus, 59
  lotions, 414b, 416
    neonatal skin care, 381
  neonatal staphylococcal scalded skin
    syndrome (Ritter's disease), 393
  noncomedogenic, 30, 32t
  ointments, 414b, 415–416
  preservative-free, 415b
  preservatives, 415
  toxic shock syndrome, 73
  water-binding capacity enhancement,
    415
  X-linked ichthyosis, 347
Moles, common (acquired melanocytic
  nevi), 324, 326–331, 327f
  atypical (dysplastic), 328–329, 329f,
    330, 331
  Becker's nevus, 328f, 328, 331
  blue nevus, 328, 329f, 331
  compound, 327, 330

  fried egg mole, 327f, 328
  skin colored, 327f, 328
  dermal, 328, 330
  developmental changes, 327, 328
  halo nevus, 328f, 328
  junctional, 327f, 327, 330
  malignant change see Melanoma,
    malignant
  Spitz nevus, 328f, 328, 329f, 330
  treatment, 331
Molluscum contagiosum, 45, 58, 138,
  143f, 143–145, 144f, 227, 251,
  382
  differential diagnosis, 29, 144
  giant lesions, 143, 144f
  human immunodeficiency virus
    infection, 137, 144
  treatment, 145
Mongolian spots, 309, 322f, 323, 324
  neonates, 395, 399f, 399
Monilethrix, 292f, 293b
Monocytes, 5
Mononucleosis syndromes, 113
Montelukast, urticaria, 261
Morbilliform eruptions, 113–127
  differential diagnosis, 114b, 115b
  drug eruptions, 159, 365, 370f,
    370–371, 371f, 377, 378, 379
    associated drugs, 371b
    frequency with antibiotic treatment,
      371t
  exanthems, 156
    with petechiae, 120b, 120
Morphea, 317, 335–338, 336f, 339
  classification, 335, 336b
  deep, 335
  en coup de sabre, 335, 336f
  guttate, 335, 337f
  inflammatory phase, 337
  lichen sclerosus concurrent lesions,
    335, 339
  linear, 335, 336f
  sclerotic phase, 337
  treatment, 337–338
Morphologic groups of skin diseases,
  11
  problem-oriented algorithm, 21–23,
    22f, 22t
Mosquitoes
  bites, papular urticaria, 107
  repellents, 107–108
Mottling, neonates, 383–384
Mucha-Habermann disease (pityriasis
  lichenoides et varioliformis acuta),
  161f, 161
Muckle-Wells syndrome, 263
Mucocutaneous lymph node syndrome
  see Kawasaki disease
Mucocutaneous syndromes, 195
Mucopolysaccharides, 4
Multiple carboxylase deficiency, 55
Multiple lentigenes syndromes, 192
Mupirocin
  furunculosis, carrier treatment, 70

methicillin-resistant *Staphylococcus
  aureus* infection, 63
Myalgia
  Lyme disease, 75
  toxic shock syndrome, 73
Mycobacterial disease, 74, 78–79
Mycobacterial granulomas, 78f, 78–79
Mycobacterium avium-intercellulare, 78
Mycobacterium chelonei, 78, 79
Mycobacterium marinum, 78f, 78, 79
Mycophenolate mofetil
  atopic dermatitis, 47
  dermatomyositis, 173
  linear IgA dermatosis, 207
  paraneoplastic pemphigus, 211
  pemphigus foliaceous/pemphigus
    vulgaris, 209
  therapeutic monitoring, 209
Mycosis fungoides see Cutaneous T-cell
  lymphoma
Myelodysplastic disease, pyoderma
  gangrenosum association, 280,
  281

N

Nail disorders, 23, 299–307
  central splitting, 299, 300f
  color changes, 306b, 307
  dermatophyte infection see
    Onycomycosis
  dystrophic epidermolysis bullosa,
    351f, 351, 352f
  ectodermal dysplasias, 354
    Goltz syndrome, 358
    hidrotic form, 356, 357
  hemorrhage into nail, 307f, 307
  ingrown toenails, 305–307, 306f
  keratosis follicularis (Darier-White
    disease), 360
  paraneoplastic pemphigus, 210f, 210
  paronychia see Paronychia
  pitting, 299, 300f
    alopecia areata, 285, 286f
    psoriasis, 150, 154b, 154f, 154, 155f,
      156
  self-trauma, 299, 300f
  surface disruption, 299
  thickening, 299–303
    differential diagnosis, 302–303,
      303b
  thinning/atrophy, 303–304
    differential diagnosis, 304b, 304
  trachyonychia, 156, 299, 300f, 300
    lichen planus, 163–165, 165f
Nail matrix, 6
Nail plate, 6, 8
Nail-patella syndrome, 304, 305f
Nails, 6
  development, 7–8
NAME syndrome (Carney complex),
  192, 321, 324
Necrobiosis lipoidica diabeticorum,
  225f, 225

Necrolytic migratory erythema, 362
Necrotizing fasciitis (streptococcal gangrene), 66f, 66–67, 104
Necrotizing vasculitis, 162
Necrotizing venulitis, 272, 273f, 273, 274
  drug-induced, 275
NEMO, 355
Neonates, 381–409
  acne, 34f, 34–35, 203, 387, 388f, 388, 403
    differential diagnosis, 34–35
  aplasia cutis congenita, 404–405, 405f
  atopic dermatitis, 409
  birthmarks, 394–406
    connective tissue, 405–406
    epidermal, 400–404
    pigment cell, 399–400
    vascular, 394–399
  breast abscess, 393
  café-au-lait spots, 399–400
  candidiasis, 387, 389–390
    congenital, 94
    thrush, 93
  caput succadaneum, 394
  cephalic pustulosis, 35, 388
  cephalohematoma, 394
  chromosomal abnormalities, 408
  collodion membrane, 408f, 408–409
  congenital infections, 77, 116, 390, 391–392, 394
  congenital malformations involving skin, 406–407
  connective tissue nevi, 405f, 405–406
  cord care, 393–394
  cutis marmorata telangiectatica, 397–398
  diaper dermatitis, 409
  diffuse cutaneous mastocytosis, 72
  epidermal nevi, 400–402, 401f
  epidermolysis bullosa, 348, 350, 354
  epithelial cysts, 213, 214f
  erythema toxicum, 386f, 386, 387, 390
  harlequin color change, 384
  hemangiomas, 395, 397f, 397
    congenital infantile, 243f, 243
  herpes simplex, 129, 130f, 131, 132, 390–391, 391f, 392
  histiocytosis X, 409
  hypopigmentation, 309, 400
  impetigo, 392f, 392
    bullous, 386, 390, 392
  junctional nevocellular nevi, 400
  lupus erythematosus syndrome, 117, 168f, 168, 169f, 169
  lymphangiomas, 398–399, 399f
  milia, 213, 382–383, 383f
  miliaria, 390
    crystallina, 202
  miniature puberty, 388, 393
  Mongolian spots, 395, 399f, 399
  mottling, 383–384

necrotizing fasciitis of abdominal wall, 66
nevus comedonicus, 403–404, 404f
occipital alopecia, 289
omphalitis, 393f, 393–394
petechiae, 394
phenylketonuria, 400
platelet dysfunction, 394
port-wine stains, 395f, 395, 396f, 397f
postmature, 382f, 408
protein C deficiency, 394
psoriasis, 388
pubic-louse infestation, 104
purpuras, 272b, 394
pustules, 387–388
raised nevocellular nevi, 400f, 400
red scaly skin, 408
rubella, congenital, 116
salmon patches, 395f, 395
scabies, 409
sclerema, 385
sebaceous gland hyperplasia, 382–383, 383f
sebaceous nevi, 402f, 402–403, 403f
seborrheic dermatitis, 55, 409
skin appearance, 381, 382f
skin care, 381–382
staphylococcal scalded skin syndrome (Ritter's disease), 70, 71f, 72, 392–393
subcutaneous fat necrosis, 384f, 384–385, 385f
sucking blisters, 385–386, 386f
syphilis, congenital, 77
systemic toxicity of topically applied compounds, 347, 381b, 381
thrombocytopenia, 394
tinea capitis, 81
TORCH syndrome, 394
transient pustular melanosis, 386–387, 387f, 390
transient skin diseases, 382–394
varicella, congenital, 390, 391–392
vascular malformations, 246–250
vitamin K deficiency, 394
Nerves, cutaneous, 5
Netherton's syndrome, 292f, 293f, 347f, 347–348, 348f, 354, 409
Neural tube defects, 407
Neuroblastoma, 233–234, 234f
Neurocutaneous melanosis, 324, 326
Neurofibromas, 222f, 222
  differential diagnosis, 222b, 222
  neurofibromatosis type 1, 322f, 323
  plexiform, 222, 249
Neurofibromatosis type 1, 222, 309, 324
  café-au-lait spots, 321f, 321, 322f, 323
  diagnostic criteria, 321b
  soft cutaneous neurofibromas, 322f, 323
Neurofibromin, 324
Neutrophils, 5

neonatal bacterial infection with pustules, 388
neonatal transiennt pustular melanosis, 386, 387
pyoderma gangrenosum pathogenesis, 281
Nevoid hypermelanosis, linear and whorled, 323f, 323, 324
Nevoid hypertrichosis, 295, 296f
Nevus anemicus, 309, 311, 315f, 315
Nevus comedonicus, 34f, 34, 387
  neonates, 403–404, 404f
Nevus depigmentosus, 309, 311, 312, 313f, 313–315
Nevus of Ito, 323, 324
Nevus of Ota, 323f, 323, 324
Nevus spilus, 324, 325f
Nevus unius lateris, 400
Nickel, allergic contact dermatitis, 52f, 52, 53f, 53, 54
Nikolsky sign, 73
Nipples, supernumerary, 407
Nits, 104–105, 105f
  removal, 106
Nodular vasculitis, 275f, 275
Nodules, 12, 13f, 23, 213–234
  adnexal tumors, 217–219
  calcified, 227–228, 228f
  grouped, 21
  orange/brown lesions, differential diagnosis, 226b
  types, 214t
Nonbullous ichthyosiform erythroderma, congenital, 345–346, 409
Noninvoluting congenital infantile hemangioma (NICH), 243, 244, 245, 249
Nonsteroidal antiinflammatory agents, drug reactions, 368, 378
Nonsteroidal immunomodulators, topical preparations, 420
Norwegian scabies, 97, 99f, 100
  human immunodeficiency virus infection, 137
Notch, 6
Nummular dermatitis, 45, 56f, 56–57, 57f, 61, 159, 162
  treatment, 57
Nystatin, candidiasis, 50, 95, 390

O

Obesity, acanthosis nigricans association, 331, 332
Occlusive coverings
  influence on topical preparations absorption, 413
  maceration association, 414
Ocular albinism, 319
Oculocutaneous albinism, 319f, 319
Oil-in-water emulsions, 414
  creams/lotions, 416

Oils, topical
  influence on topical preparations
    absorption, 413
  maceration association, 414
  preterm infant skin care, 382
Ointments
  application, 416
  glucocorticosteroids, 417
  influence on topical preparations
    absorption, 413
  maceration association, 414
  moisturizers, 414b, 415–416
  preterm infant skin care, 381–382
Omphalitis, 393f, 393–394
Onycholysis, psoriasis, 300
Onycomycosis (tinea unguium), 89f,
    89–91, 90f, 299
  human immunodeficiency virus
    infection, 137
  nail thickening, 301–302, 302f
  treatment, 303
Oozing (weeping), 14, 15, 17f
  dermatitis, 39
Ophiasis, 285, 286f, 287f, 287
Ophthalmic disorders
  Ehlers-Danlos syndrome, 341, 342
  epidermal nevi, 401
  Goltz syndrome, 358
  incontinentia pigmenti, 356
  infantile hemangiomas, 238, 239,
    241f, 244
  juvenile xanthogranulomas, 226
  morphea en coup de sabre, 335
  Stevens-Johnson syndrome, 367f,
    367–368, 369
  Sturge-Weber syndrome, 246
  xeroderma pigmentosum, 192
Oral contraceptives
  acne vulgaris management in female
    adolescents, 31
  drug-induced acne, 36
  erythema nodosum reaction, 270, 375
Oral lesions
  aphthous ulcers, 200f, 200–202,
    201f
  epidermolysis bullosa
    junctional, 350f, 350
    recessive dystrophic, 351
  erythema multiforme, 196, 197f, 197
  juvenile pityriasis rubra pilaris, 178
  Kawasaki disease, 198
  lichen planus, 163, 164f
  milia (Epstein's pearls), 382
  paraneoplastic pemphigus, 210
  pemphigus vulgaris, 207
  pityriasis rosea, 159
  Stevens-Johnson syndrome, 366f,
    367
  syphilis, secondary, 160, 161
Orf, 143, 144f
Orodigitofacial syndrome, 407
Osler-Weber-Rendu syndrome
    (hereditary hemorrhagic
    telangiectasia), 252f, 252, 253f

Oval and linear palmoplantar
    keratoderma, 358f, 359f, 359
Overdressing, miliaria pathogenesis,
    203
'Owl-eye' appearance, neonatal lupus
    erythematosus syndrome, 168,
    169f
Oxiconazole, candidiasis, 95
Oxyhemoglobin, 2, 15
Oxyquinoline sulfate, 415

P

Pachyonychia congenita, 90, 301, 302f,
    303
  type 2, 214
Pain
  abdominal
    Henoch-Schönlein purpura, 273
    hereditary angioedema, 258–259
    mastocytosis, 267
  angiolipomas, 222, 223
  aphthous ulcers, 200, 201
  herpes simplex hand/finger infections,
    129
  herpes zoster, 133, 134
  localized vulvar pemphigoid, 209
  pemphigus vulgaris oral lesions,
    207
  preterm infant skin care, 381, 382
  staphylococcal scalded skin
    syndrome, 72
  sunburn, 181, 183
Pain sensation, 5
Palatal clefts, 407
Palmoplantar keratodermas, 229, 354,
    358f, 359f, 359
Panniculitis, 228, 270
  cold injury, 65
  lupus erythematosus, 168f, 168, 170,
    171
Papular acrodermatitis (Gianotti-Crosti
    syndrome), 124f, 124–125
  viral agents, 125b
Papular urticaria, 101, 106f, 106–108,
    107f, 110, 135
Papules, 12, 13f, 23
  grouped, 21
Papulosquamous disorders, 15, 23,
    149–178
  differential diagnosis, 155b
Parabens, 415
Parallel linear lesions, 19, 20f
Paraneoplastic pemphigus, 197, 210f,
    210–211, 368
Parapsoriasis, 86
  guttate, 178
Parinaud's oculoglandular syndrome, 74
Paronychia, 305
  acrodermatitis enteropathica, 362
  candidiasis, 93f, 93, 95, 131, 305f,
    305
  congenital, 94
  Proteus, 305

Pseudomonas, 305
  Staphylococcus aureus, 94, 305
Parry-Romberg syndrome, 335
Parvovirus B19 see Human parvovirus
    B19
Pastia's sign, 67
Patch (epicutaneous) testing, allergic
    contact dermatitis, 54f, 54–55
Paul-Bunnel (heterophil) test, 123
pax-3, 310
Pediculoses (louse infestations),
    104–106, 105f
Pediculus humanus capitis (head louse),
    104, 105, 106
Pediculus humanus humanus (body
    louse), 104, 105
Pemphigoid, 61, 197, 209–210
  infantile, 209f, 209
  localized childhood vulvar, 209f, 209
Pemphigus, 23, 197, 201
  paraneoplastic, 197, 210f, 210–211,
    368
Pemphigus erythematosus, 207
Pemphigus foliaceous, 207f, 207–209
  endemic form (fogo selvaem), 207
  treatment, 208–209
Pemphigus vulgaris, 207–209, 208f
  treatment, 208–209
  vegetans variant, 208f, 208
Penicillin
  drug eruptions, 68, 261, 379
  Lyme disease, 76
  morbilliform eruptions induction with
    infectious mononucleosis, 122,
    123
  scarlet fever, 68
  syphilis, 77
Penicillin G
  Lyme disease, 76
  syphilis, 77
Penicillin V
  cellulitis, 66
  pyodermas, 63
Penis
  lichen planus, 163, 164f
  psoriasis, 149, 152f
  see also Genital lesions
Pentoxifylline, actinic prurigo, 188
Percutaneous absorption, 413–414
  effects of occlusive substances, 413
  enhancement by moisturizers, 415
  factors enhancing, 414b
Perianal cellulitis, 49, 64, 65f
Periarteritis nodosa see Polyarteritis
    nodosa
Periderm, 7
Periodic fever syndrome, aphthous
    ulcers, 201
Perioral dermatitis, 37f, 37–38, 419f,
    420
Periorbital cellulitis, 65
Periorbital infantile hemangiomas, 238,
    241f, 245
Periungual warts, 138–139, 139f

Perivaginal cellulitis, 64, 65f
Permethrins
    pediculoses, 106
    scabies, 100
Pernio, 277f, 277–278
Petechiae, 272
    infectious mononucleosis, 122
    neonates, 394
Petrolatum, moisturizer composition, 415
Petroleum jelly, moisturizer composition, 415
Peutz-Jeghers syndrome, lentigenes, 320f, 321, 324
PHACE syndrome, 239, 240f, 240
Phenylketonuria, 400
Phenytoin, linear IgA dermatosis induction, 206
Phlebectasia, congenital, 249f, 249
Photoactivation, herpes simplex infections, 127, 128
Photoallergic drug eruptions, 3, 365, 375–376, 378
    associated drugs, 376b
Photochemotherapy
    atopic dermatitis, 47
    psoriasis, 157
Photoprotection/sun avoidance
    albinism, 320
    erythema multiforme prevention, 198
    erythropoietic protoporphyria, 188
    hypopigmented lesions, 313, 314, 315
    idiopathic photodermatoses, 187–188
    lupus erythematosus, 171
    malignant melanoma prevention, 331
    sunburn prevention, 183, 184
    vitiligo, 317
    xeroderma pigmentosum, 192, 193
    see also Sun blocks; Sunscreens
Photoprotective pigments, 3
Photosensitivity/sun sensitivity, 181–193
    dermatomyositis, 169–170, 172
    differential diagnosis, 183b
    drug eruptions, 365, 375–376, 378–379
    erythropoietic protoporphyria, 188, 189
    laboratory evaluation, 181, 183b
    lupus erythematosus, 167f, 167, 168, 171, 181, 187
Photosensitizing agents, 181
Phototherapy see Ultraviolet light therapy
Phototoxic lesions
    drug eruptions, 3, 365, 375–376, 376f, 378
        associated drugs, 376b
    lupus erythematosus, 167f, 167
Phototypes, sun sensitivity, 182b
Physical urticarias, 261–264
    differential diagnosis, 263
Phytophotodermatitis, 110, 190f, 190–191

Piebaldism, 309–310, 310f, 317
Pierre Robin syndrome, 407
Piezogenic pedal papules, 228f, 228
Pigmentation, 2–3
    ultraviolet light exposure-related increase, 3
Pigmentation disorders, 309–332
    brown lesions, 320–332
    ectodermal dysplasias, 354
    incontinentia pigmenti, 355f, 355
    white lesions, 309–320
Pigmented nevi, congenital, 295
Pigmented purpuras, chronic, 278–280, 279f
Pilar hamartomas, congenital, 326
Pili triangulati et cabaliculi (uncombable hair syndrome), 297f, 297
Pilomatricomas (calcifying epithelioma), 217f, 217, 218, 219
Pimecrolimus, topical, 420
    atopic dermatitis, 47
    vitiligo, 317
Pityriasis, 11
Pityriasis alba, 43f, 43, 317, 318f, 318
Pityriasis lichenoides, 135, 161–163
    acute (Mucha-Habermann disease), 161f, 161, 162
    chronic, 161, 162f, 163
    treatment, 163
Pityriasis rosea, 77, 86, 149, 156, 158f, 158–160, 159f, 160f, 162, 170, 260, 269
    herald patch, 158f, 158, 159
Pityrosporum orbicularis, 56
Plantar warts, 140f, 140, 229
Plaque, 12
Platelet dysfunction, neonates, 394
Pleconaril, hand-foot-and-mouth disease, 137
Plectin, 353
Plexiform neurofibromas, 249
Pneumocystis carinii pneumonia, 137
Podophyllum
    molluscum contagiosum, 145
    warts, 143
Poison ivy/poison oak, 190
    allergic contact dermatitis, 51f, 52, 54
Polyarteritis nodosa (periarteritis nodosa), 173, 274, 275f, 275–277, 276f
    chronic cutaneous, 275
    infantile, 275
    livido reticularis, 275f, 275, 276f
Polyethylene glycol, moisturizer composition, 415
Polymorphous light eruption, 45, 170, 184f, 185f, 185, 189
    treatment, 187–188
Polysorbate, moisturizer composition, 415
Ponytail alopecia, 289
Popsicle panniculitis, 65

Porokeratosis of Mibelli, 84, 175f, 175–176, 176f
    malignant degeneration, 176
Porphyria cutanea tarda, 353, 378
Porphyrias, 377, 378
Port-wine stains, 246f, 246–247
    neonates, 395f, 395, 396f, 397f
    treatment, 249–250, 250f
Post-bone marrow transplantation eruption, 159
Postinflammatory hyperpigmentation, 323, 324
Postinflammatory hypopigmentation, 318f, 318–319
Postmature newborns, 408
    skin appearance, 382f
Poststreptococcal glomerulonephritis, 63
Potassium hydroxide examination
    candidiasis, 94, 390
    tinea capitis, 82–83, 83f, 285
    tinea corporis, 86
    tinea cruris, 88
    tinea faciei, 87, 170
    tinea unguium (onychomycosis), 90f, 90
    tinea versicolor, 91f, 92
Potassium hydroxide, molluscum contagiosum treatment, 145
Prader-Willi syndrome, scalp whorl location, 298
Preauricular pits, 406, 407f
Preauricular skin tags, 406f, 406
Prednisone
    allergic contact dermatitis, 54
    antireflux medication, 209
    aphthous ulcers, 201
    erythema nodosum, 271
    infectious mononucleosis, 123
    lichen planus, 166
    necrotizing venulitis, 275
    pemphigoid, 210
    pemphigus foliaceus/pemphigus vulgaris, 209
    polyarteritis nodosa, 276
    spider bite, 104
    urticarial vasculitis, 264
Pregnancy
    human parvovirus B19 infection, 120, 121
    rubella exposure, 117
Preservative-free moisturizers, 415b
Preservatives, moisturizer components, 415
Pressure erythema, 65
Preterm infants
    epidermal barrier function, 7
    erythema toxicum, 386
    excessive hair, 295
    infantile hemangiomas, 243
    red scaly skin, 408
    sclerema, 385
    sepsis, 387
    skin care, 381–382, 382b

subcutaneous fat, 7
systemic toxicity of topically applied compounds, 381
zinc deficiency, 362
Primary irritant contact dermatitis, 48–51
Primary skin lesions, 12f, 12, 13f, 14f, 15f, 16f
size, 12
PRKAR1A, 324
Problem-oriented algorithm, 21–23, 22f, 22t
Profilaggrin, 1
Propionibacterium acnes, 29
Propylene glycol, influence on topical preparations absorption, 413
Propylthiouracil, necrotizing venulitis association, 275
Prostaglandins, 3
Protein C deficiency, neonatal pupura, 394
Proteus paronychia, 305
Proteus syndrome, 315, 322f, 323, 406
Protoporphyrin IX, 189
Pruritus, 11
    acropustulosis of infancy, 388, 389
    actinic prurigo, 185
    atopic dermatitis, 40, 42f, 43, 44, 47, 48
    cutaneous larva migrans, 108
    dermatitis herpetiformis, 204–205
    erythropoietic protoporphyria, 188
    herpes zoster, 134
    lichen planus, 165
    lichen sclerosus, 339
    morbilliform (maculopapular) drug eruptions, 371
    nummular dermatitis, 56, 57
    papular urticaria, 106
    pediculoses, 104
    photoallergic drug reactions, 376
    pityriasis rosea, 159
    psoriasis, 154
    scabies, 97, 99, 100
    serum-sickness-like reaction, 373
    swimmer's/seabather's eruption, 109–110
    tick bites, 102
    urticaria
        drug eruptions, 377
        transient, 257
    viral hepatitis, 126
    wet dressings, 417
Pseudoepherdrine, angioedema, 261
Pseudomonas, 104
    folliculitis, 69, 70
    infantile hemangiomas infection, 238
    palpable purpuras, 273
    paronychia, 305
Psoralen/ultraviolet A-range therapy (PUVA)
    atopic dermatitis, 47
    mastocytosis, 267
    morphea, 337

polymorphous light eruption, 188
psoriasis, 157
vitiligo, 317f, 317
Psoralens, 3
    phytophotodermatitis, 191
Psoriasis, 11, 49, 58, 78, 84, 86, 87, 90, 94, 95, 149–158, 165, 170, 173, 178, 260
    arthritis association, 154, 155f, 156
    Auspitz sign, 154, 155f
    clinical features, 149–150, 150f, 151f, 152f, 153f, 154f
    differential diagnosis, 155b, 156
    distribution, 149, 150f
    drug reactions, 378
    emotional support for patients, 158
    erythroderma, 157
    guttate, 19, 149, 152f, 153f, 156, 157, 158, 159, 162
    isomorphic (Koebner) phenomenon, 149, 153f
    nails involvement, 150, 154b, 154f, 155f, 156, 299, 300f, 300, 301f, 301, 303
    neonates, 388
    pathogenesis, 156
    patient education, 157–158
    pruritus, 154
    pustular, 154, 155f, 157
    secondary impetigo, 63
    treatment, 156–157
        calcipotriene, 420
        tar preparations, 420
    vulgaris, 149, 151f, 152f
Psoriasis susceptibility genes (PSORS), 156
Psychotherapy, warts management, 143
PTCH gene, 218
Pthirus pubis (pubic-louse) infestation, 104, 105
PTPN11, 324
Puberty
    acne vulgaris, 25
    hair changes, 6
    sebaceous nevi changes, 402, 404f
Pubic hair, 6
Pubic-louse (*Pthirus pubis*) infestation, 104
Pulsed dye laser therapy
    cherry angioma, 254
    infantile hemangioma, 244–245, 245f
    pyogenic granuloma, 227, 252
    spider telangiectasia, 253
    vascular malformations, 249–250, 250f, 251f
Punch biopsy, 23
Punctate palmoplantar keratoderma, 359f
Puncture wounds, cellulitis complicating, 64
Purpuras, 272–281
    anaphylactoid, 272
    chronic pigmented, 278–280, 279f
    dissecting, 278

drug eruptions, 365
flat acral, 272b
flat generalized, 272b
Henoch-Schönlein, 272, 273f, 273
neonatal, 272b, 394
nodular
    with livido, 275–277
    pernio, 277–278
palpable (purpuric papules), 272–275, 273f
    acute hemorrhagic edema of infancy, 273f, 273
    cutaneous necrotizing venulitis, 272, 273f, 273, 274, 275
    differential diagnosis, 274b, 274
Pustules, 11, 12, 16f
    neonates, 387–388
Pyoderma see Bacterial infections
Pyoderma gangrenosum, 104, 280f, 280–281
    pathergy, 280f, 280
Pyogenic granuloma, 227f, 227, 229, 250–252, 251f
Pyrethrin shampoo, pediculoses, 106

Q

Quaternary ammonium compounds, 415
Quinine, scarlatiniform drug eruptions, 68

R

Radiotherapy, rhabdomyosarcoma, 233
Ramsay Hunt syndrome, 134f, 135, 136
Rapid plasma reagin (RPR) test, 77
Rapidly involuting congenital infantile hemangioma (RICH), 243f, 243, 244, 249
Rash, 11
Raynaud's disease, thin/atrophic nails, 304
Raynaud's phenomenon, 170
    lupus erythematosus association, 168
Reactive erythemas, 268–272
Records, 21
    drug-associated eruptions, 379
Recurrent digital fibrous tumors, 221
Recurrent oral erythema multiforme, 367
Red-cell aplasia, human parvovirus B19 infection in immunosupressed children, 119, 120
Red/red-brown lesions, 23
    blanching, 15
Renal disease
    Henoch-Schönlein purpura, 273
    polyarteritis nodosa, 275
Reticuloendothelial neoplasms, candidiasis association, 94
Reticulohistiocytosis, congenital self-healing, 229, 231f, 232

Retinoic acid, topical, 421
  nevus comedonicus, 404
  warts, 142
Retinoids, systemic
  acne vulgaris, 31
  ichthyoses, 347
  juvenile pityriasis rubra pilaris, 178
  keratosis follicularis (Darier-White
    disease), 360
  psoriasis, 157
Retinoids, topical
  acne vulgaris, 29–30, 30t, 31, 33
  neonatal acne, 35
  psoriasis, 157
  side effects, 30
Reye's syndrome, complicating varicella,
    133
Rhabdomyosarcoma, 233f, 233
Rheumatic fever, 68
  erythema marginatum, 268–269
Rheumatoid arthritis, pyoderma
    gangrenosum association, 280,
    281
Rheumatoid nodules, 224–225
Rickettsial-pox, 135
Rifampin
  cat-scratch disease, 74
  methicillin-resistant Staphylococcus
    aureus infection, 63
    cellulitis, 66
    furunculosis, 70
  mycobacterial granulomas, 79
Ringworm see Tinea capitis
Ritter's disease see Staphylococcal
    scalded skin syndrome
Rocky Mountain spotted fever, 73, 102,
    115, 122
  disseminated intravascular
    coagulation, 278
Rosacea, 29
  topical steroid-induced, 37f, 37–38,
    420
Roseola (exanthem subitum; human
    herpesvirus 6 infection), 113,
    117f, 117–118, 122
Rubella, 68, 113, 116–117, 122, 123,
    126, 136
  congenital, 116, 117, 394
  exposure in pregnancy, 117
Rubeola see Measles
Rubinstein-Taybi syndrome, scalp whorl
    location, 298

S

Sabouraud dextrose agar, 83, 94
Salicylic acid, 421
  corns/calluses, 229
  porokeratosis of Mibelli, 176
  precautions with topical use, 416
  psoriasis, scalp involvement
    management, 157
  warts, 142
Salmon patches, 395f, 395

SAPHO syndrome, acne fulminans, 34
Sarcoidosis, 78, 86, 269
  erythema nodosum, 269
  granulomas, 229
Sarcoptes scabei, 100
Scabies, 11, 45, 50, 55, 87, 97–100,
    98f, 99f, 100f, 101, 104, 110,
    231
  neonates/infants, 388–389, 409
  Norwegian, 97, 99f, 100
  pruritus, 97, 99, 100
  secondary impetigo, 63, 97
  treatment, 100
Scaling, 11, 14, 18f
  red lesions, 23
Scalp involvement
  juvenile pityriasis rubra pilaris, 178
  lupus erythematosus, 166, 167f
  psoriasis, 150f, 150, 151f, 153f
Scalp whorls, 298
Scarlatiniform eruptions, 68, 113
  drug eruptions, 365
  toxic shock syndrome, 72
Scarlet fever, 61, 67f, 67–68, 68f, 199
  rheumatic fever association, 68
Sclerema, neonates, 385
Scleroderma, 15, 84, 170
  localised see Morphea
Seabather's eruption, 109–110
Sebaceous cysts, 216
  see also Epithelial cysts
Sebaceous glands, 6
  androgen sensitivity, 29
  function in neonate, 35
  hyperplasia, 382–383, 383f
Sebaceous nevi, 19
  congenital circumscribed alopecia,
    286, 290f, 290
  malignant potential, 402
  neonates, 402f, 402–403, 403f
  puberty-related changes, 402, 404f
  treatment, 290
Seborrhea capitis, 55, 56
Seborrheic dermatitis, 37, 45, 55f,
    55–56, 84, 88, 92, 99, 156, 231
  human immunodeficiency virus
    infection, 137
  neonates, 409
  tinea capitis, 81, 83f
Seborrheic keratosis, 141
Sebum, 6
Seckel's syndrome, 407
Secondary infection
  atopic dermatitis, 44f, 44
  candidiasis in diaper dermatitis, 49f,
    49, 50, 93f, 93, 95, 409
  epidermolytic hyperkeratosis, 346
  hemangiomas, 238, 397f, 397,
    398f
  impetigo, 97
    scabies lesions, 63, 97
  varicella, 63, 133, 135
Secondary skin changes, 12, 14, 17f,
    18f

Selenium sulfide shampoo
  tinea capitis, 85
  tinea versicolor, 92
Self-haircutting, 288
Sensory nerve endings, 5, 7
Sepsis, neonatal
  pustules, 387
  sclerema, 385
Septicemia
  complicating cellulitis, 65
  disseminated intravascular
    coagulation, 278
  palpable purpuras, 273, 274
  scarlet fever, 68
Serum-sickness-like drug reaction, 373,
    378
Severe combined immunodeficiency, 55
Sexual abuse, 78, 143, 339
Sexual transmission, herpes progenitalis,
    129
Shagreen patch, 311f, 311
Shampoos/shampooing
  antifungal
    tinea capitis, 85
    tinea versicolor, 92
  antimicrobial, 421
  detergent, 421
  formulary, 421
  keratolytic, 421
  pediculoses, 105–106
  psoriasis, 157
  seborrheic dermatitis, 56
  tar preparations, 420, 421
  traction alopecia, 289
Shave biopsy, 23
Shoe dermatitis, 52f, 52
SHP-2, 324
Simian crease, 406–407, 408
Sjögren's syndrome, 268
Skin, 1–8
  body temperature regulation, 4–5
  defensive functions, 5
  development, 7–8
  nerve supply, 5
  pigmentation, 2–3
  vasculature, 4
Skin biopsy see Biopsy
Skin cancer
  chronic ultraviolet light exposure
    association, 183
  xeroderma pigmentosum patients,
    191–192
Skin fragility/healing problems,
    Ehlers-Danlos syndrome,
    339–340, 341f
Skin tags
  acanthosis nigricans, 331
  preauricular, 406f, 406
Skin-colored lesions, 23
Slapped-cheek appearance, human
    parvovirus B19 infection, 118,
    119f
SLC39A4, 362
SLUG, 310

Smooth muscle nevus, 295
Smooth-muscle hamartoma, 227, 326
Soap substitutes, 421
   atopic dermatitis, 46, 47, 48
Solar urticaria, 186, 187
Soles see Feet
SOX10, 310
Spider bite, 103f, 103–104, 281
Spider telangiectasia, 252f, 252–253
Spina bifida, circumscribed midline
      hypertrichosis association, 295
Spinal dyraphism, occult, 407
Spindle nevus, 226, 330
SPINK5, 45, 348
Spirochetal diseases, 74–79
Spitz nevus, 251, 328f, 328, 329f, 330
Sporotrichosis, 79
Squamous cell carcinoma
   chronic ultraviolet light exposure
      association, 183
   in dystrophic epidermolysis bullosa
      atrophic scars, 351, 352f
   xeroderma pigmentosum patients, 192
Stanozolol, hereditary angioedema, 261
Staphylococcal infection
   cellulitis, 65, 66
   folliculitis, 69
   furunculosis, 70
   palpable purpuras, 273
   scarlet fever, 67
Staphylococcal scalded skin syndrome
      (Ritter's disease), 61, 70f, 70–72,
      71f, 73, 267, 368
   neonates, 392–393
Staphylococcus aureus, 61, 84
   abscess, 68
      neonatal breast, 393
   atopic dermatitis secondary infection,
      44f, 44, 46
   bullous varicella, 133f, 133
   cellulitis, 65
   epidermolytic hyperkeratosis
      secondary infection, 346
   furunculosis, 68
   hemangiomas superinfection, 238,
      397f, 397, 398f
   human immunodeficiency virus-related
      pyodermas, 137
   impetigo, 63
      neonates, 392
   miliaria pustulosa, 202
   omphalitis, 393
   paronychia, 94, 305
   psoriasis-related skin overgrowth, 158
   toxic shock syndrome, 73
   toxins, 72, 73, 393
STAR complex, 116, 118, 121, 123
   differential diagnosis, 115b
Stearyl alcohol, moisturizer composition,
   415
Steatocystoma multiplex, 214, 215f, 216
Steroid rosacea, 37f, 37–38, 420
Stevens-Johnson syndrome, 195, 199,
   208, 211, 365

drug reactions, 366f, 366–369
   mucous membrane involvement, 367,
      368
   toxic epidermal necrolysis overlap,
      368
   treatment, 369
   types, 368
STK11, 324
Stratum corneum, 1
   development, 7
   friction-related thickening, 2
   shedding, 2
   see also Epidermal barrier
Strawberry tongue
   Kawasaki disease, 198
   scarlet fever, 67, 68f
Streptococcal infection, 122
   cellulitis, 64, 65, 66
   disseminated intravascular
      coagulation, 278
   erythema marginatum, 269
   erythema nodosum, 269, 270
   guttate psoriasis, 149, 156, 157, 158
   necrotizing fasciitis (streptococcal
      gangrene), 66f, 66–67, 104
   nephritogenic, 63
   scarlet fever, 67, 68f, 68
   toxins, 68
Streptococcus group A
   ecthyma, 63
   necrotizing fasciitis, 66
   neonatal impetigo, 392
Streptococcus pyogenes, 61
   atopic dermatitis secondary infection,
      46
Streptomycin, scarlatiniform drug
      eruptions, 68
Striate palmoplantar keratoderma, 359f,
   359
Strongyloides stercoralis, cutaneous
      larva migrans, 109
Sturge-Weber syndrome, 246f,
   246–247, 250, 395, 396f
Subacute bacterial endocarditis, 273
Subcutaneous fat, 6–7
   necrosis, neonates, 384f, 384–385,
   385f
Sucking blisters, 385–386, 386f
Sucralfate, aphthous ulcers, 201
Sulfasalazine, dermatitis herpetiformis,
   205–206
Sulfonamides, drug reactions, 368, 370
   fixed drug eruptions, 374
   scarlatiniform eruptions, 68
Sun avoidance see Photoprotection/sun
   avoidance
Sun blocks, 184
Sun exposure
   common mole (acquired melanocytic
      nevi) development, 326, 330
   malignant melanoma association,
      330, 331
   photosensitive drug eruptions, 375–376
   see also Ultraviolet light

Sun protection agents see Sunscreens
Sun protection factors, 184b, 184, 421
Sun sensitivity see Photosensitivity/sun
   sensitivity
Sunburn, 3, 181–184, 182f, 183f, 189
   common moles (acquired melanocytic
      nevi) association, 327
   desquamation, 11
   miliaria crystallina association, 202
   pathogenesis, 181–183
   prevention, 183–184, 184b
   rapid onset, 181
   skin phototype susceptibility, 182b
   treatment, 183
   xeroderma pigmentosum patients,
      191f, 191
Sunburn cells, 183
Sunflower seed oil, preterm infant skin
   care, 382
Sunlight, 3
   see also Ultraviolet light
Sunscreens (sun protection agents),
   184b, 184
   allergic reactions, 184
   formulary, 421–422
   sun protection factors, 184b, 184, 421
   see also Photoprotection/sun
      avoidance
Supernumerary nipples, 407
Surface disruption of skin, 23
Sweating, 4, 6, 8
   agents reducing, 421
Sweating abnormalities
   diagnosis, 357
   ectodermal dysplasias, 354
   hypohidrotic ectodermal dysplasia,
      356
Sweet's syndrome, 365, 376f, 376, 378
   associated drugs, 377b
Swimmer's eruption, 109–110
Syncope, mastocytosis, 267
Syndactyly, 407
Syphilis, 76–78, 131, 269
   chancre, 76f, 76, 77
   condylomata lata, 141, 160, 161
   congenital, 77, 78, 94, 116, 394
   differential diagnosis, 160
   primary, 76
   secondary, 76f, 76, 77, 86, 156, 159,
      162
      cutaneous signs, 160b, 160–161
   serological diagnosis, 77
Syringocystadenoma papilliferum, 218f,
   218
Syringomas, 218f, 218
Systemic sclerosis, 335, 336

T

T lymphocytes, 5
   allergic contact dermatitis, 53, 54
   alopecia areata pathogenesis, 287
   psoriasis pathogenesis, 156
   vitiligo pathogenesis, 317

Tacrolimus, 420
  atopic dermatitis, 47
  pyoderma gangrenosum, 281
  vitiligo, 317
Tanning, 3, 182, 183–184
Tar preparations, 420, 421
  atopic dermatitis, 47
  folliculitis, 69
  gels, 416
  psoriasis, 157, 420
  shampoos, 157, 421
Tazarotene, 30
  psoriasis, 157
    nail disease, 303
Teeth defects
  ectodermal dysplasias, 354
    Goltz syndrome, 358
    hypohidrotic form, 356
    incontinentia pigmenti, 355f
    recessive dystrophic epidermolysis
      bullosa, 351, 352f
Telangiectasia macularis eruptiva
    perstans, 265
Telangiectatic malformations, 247, 249
  treatment, 250, 251f
Telogen (club) hairs, 6
Telogen effluvium, 6, 292, 293–294,
    294f
Tepid bathing, roseola, 118
Terbinafine
  onycomycosis (tinea unguium), 90,
    303
  tinea capitis, 84, 85
  tinea cruris, 88
  tinea versicolor, 92
Terminal hair, 6
Testicular maldescent, 407
Testosterone 5α-reductase, 29
Tetracycline
  acne vulgaris, 31
  syphilis, 77
TGM1, 345, 409
Thalidomide
  actinic prurigo, 188
  erythema nodosum, 271
Thermal sensitivity, 5
Thiabendazole, cutaneous larva migrans,
    109
Thickened skin, 335
  see also Morphea
Thrombocytopenia, neonates, 394
Thrush (oral candidiasis), 92f, 93, 94,
    137
  treatment, 95
Thyroiditis, urticaria, 257
Tick bites, 102f, 102–103
Tick necrosis and adenopathy
    syndrome, 102
Tick paralysis, 102
Tick-borne infections, 102
  Lyme disease, 74–76
Ticks removal, 102f, 102–103
Tinea capitis, 56, 81–85, 156, 288
  clinical features, 81, 82f, 83f

differential diagnosis, 84
fugal culture, 83
hair loss, 285, 287
kerions, 81, 82f, 83f, 83–84, 85
organisms, 84t, 84
potassium hydroxide examination,
    82–83, 83f
treatment, 84–85
Wood's light examination, 81
Tinea corporis, 57, 85f, 85–86, 92, 159,
    162, 170, 224
  organisms, 86
Tinea cruris, 88–89
Tinea faciei, 37, 87f, 87–88, 88f, 170
  human immunodeficiency virus
    infection, 137
Tinea gladiatorum, 86
Tinea incognito, 86f, 86
Tinea pedis (athlete's foot), 51, 87f, 87,
    90
Tinea unguium see Onycomycosis
Tinea versicolor, 91f, 91–92, 317, 318
Tongue changes
  Kawasaki disease, 198
  scarlet fever, 67, 68f
Topical preparations, 413–420
  ammount to dispense, 416–417, 417t
  antiinflammatory agents, 417
    glucocorticoids, 417–420
  application, 416–417
  calcipotriene, 420
  finger tip unit, 48f, 48, 416–417
  foams, 416
  formulary, 420–422
  gels, 416
  nonsteroidal immunomodulators, 420
  patient education, 48
  percutaneous absorption, 413–414
    surface area considerations, 347
  prescribing rules, 417b
  skin-hydrating agents, 416
  systemic toxicity in neonates, 347,
    381b, 381
  tars, 420
  water retention in skin surface
    (moisturizers), 414–416
TORCH complex, 131, 394
Tourniquet test, scarlet fever, 67
Touton giant cell, 226
Toxic epidermal necrolysis, 71, 72, 195,
    365, 392
  complications, 368
  drug reactions, 366–369, 367f, 368f
  Stevens-Johnson syndrome overlap,
    368
  treatment, 369
  types, 368
Toxic shock syndrome, 61, 68, 72–73,
    199, 392
  diagnostic criteria, 72b, 72
Toxoplasmosis, 74
  congenital, 116, 394
Trachyonychia, 156, 299, 300f, 300
  lichen planus, 163–165, 165f

Traction alopecia, 84, 289f, 289
Transient neonatal pustular melanosis,
    94, 386–387, 387f, 390
Trauma
  alopecia, 288–289
  blisters, 195
  nails
    hemorrhage into, 307f, 307
    surface abnormalities, 299
    thickening, 302, 303f
    thinning/atrophy, 304
    neonatal petechiae/purpura, 394
Traumatic alopecia, 288–289
Treacher Collins syndrome, 407
Treponema pallidum, 77
Tretinoin, 30, 421
  keratosis pilaris, 59
  porokeratosis of Mibelli, 176
Triamcinolone acetonide
  aphthous ulcers, 201
  keloids, 221
Trichoblastoma, sebaceous nevi
    changes, 402
Trichoepithelioma, 218f, 218, 219
Trichogram, 294
Trichomonas vaginalis, 94
Trichophyton mentagrophytes
  tinea corporis, 86
  tinea cruris, 88
  tinea pedis (athlete's foot), 87
Trichophyton rubrum
  tinea corporis, 86
  tinea pedis (athlete's foot), 87
Trichophyton soudanese, tinea capitis,
    81
Trichophyton tonsurans, 56, 84t, 84
  culture, 83
  tinea capitis, 81, 84, 85
  tinea corporis, 86
Trichophyton verrucosum
  tinea corporis, 86
  tinea faciei, 87
Trichophyton violaceum, tinea capitis,
    81
Trichorrhexis invaginata, Netherton's
    syndrome, 293f, 347
Trichorrhexis nodosa, 291f, 292f, 293b
Trichotillomania, 288f, 288–289
Trifluridine, herpes keratitis, 132
Trimethoprim-sulfamethoxazole
  cat-scratch disease, 74
  drug eruptions
    fixed eruptions, 374
    human immunodeficiency virus
      infection, 137
  methicillin-resistant Staphylococcus
      aureus infection, 63
    cellulitis, 66
    furunculosis, 70
    morbilliform drug eruption, 370f, 371f
    mycobacterial granulomas, 79
Trisomy 13, 407, 408
  scalp whorl location, 298
Trisomy 14-15, 408

Trisomy 18, 408
Trisomy 21 (Down syndrome), 408
 epicanthic folds, 407
 scalp whorl location, 298
 simian crease, 406
TS1, 312
TS2, 312
TSS-1 toxin, 73
Tuberculosis, 78
 erythema nodosum, 269
Tuberin, 312
Tuberous sclerosis, 309, 312f, 312, 313,
 406
 angiofibromas, 29, 219, 311f, 311
 ash-leaf macules, 310–311, 311f
 diagnostic criteria, 313b
 fibrous forehead plaque, 311, 312f
 shagreen patch, 311f, 311
Tufted angiomas, 242f, 242, 243, 249
 treatment, 245
Tularemia, 102
 erythema nodosum, 269
Tumor, 12
Tumor necrosis factor blockers
 polyarteritis nodosa, 276
 psoriasis, 157
Turner's syndrome, 407, 408
Typhus, 122
Tyrosinase, 2
 defects, 319–320
Tzanck smear, herpes simplex, 130,
 131f, 132

U

Ulcer, 14, 17f
Ultrasound
 neural tube defects, 407
 subcutaneous fat necrosis, 385
Ultraviolet light, 3
 biologic effects, 3t
 blocking agents see Sunscreens
 freckles induction, 320f, 320, 324
 linear IgA dermatosis induction, 206
 long-term effects on skin, 183
 skin damage pathogenesis, 181–183
 xeroderma pigmentosum, 192
 sunburn, 3, 181
 tanning response, 182, 183–184
 see also Sun exposure; Sunlight
Ultraviolet light therapy (phototherapy)
 acne vulgaris, 32
 atopic dermatitis, 47
 erythropoietic protoporphyria, 189
 mastocytosis, 267
 morphea, 337
 pityriasis lichenoides, 163
 pityriasis rosea, 159, 160f
 polymorphous light eruption, 188
 psoriasis, 157, 158
 vitiligo, 317
Umbilical cord care, 393–394
Uncombable hair syndrome (pili
 triangulati et cabaliculi), 297f, 297

Unmanageable hair, 297f, 297
Urea compounds
 influence on topical preparations
 absorption, 413
 keratosis pilaris, 59
 moisturizer components, 416
Urea creams/lotions, 421
Uremia, 11
Urinary tract anomalies, 407
Urticaria, 156, 159, 197, 257–268
 dermatitis herpetiformis, 204
 differential diagnosis, 260b, 260
 giant lesions, 65, 257, 260
 infectious mononucleosis, 122
 persistent, 261–268
 physical, 261–264
 transient, 257–261, 258b, 258f, 259f
Urticaria pigmentosa, 265f, 265–266,
 266f, 267
Urticarial drug eruptions, 365, 371–373,
 372f, 377, 378, 379
 associated drugs, 372b
 serum-sickness-like reaction, 373
Urticarial vasculitis, 264f, 264–265
UVA, 3
UVB, 3
UVC, 3

V

Vaginitis, chemical, 95
Valaciclovir
 herpes simplex, 132
 varicella, 135
Vancomycin
 bullous drug eruptions, 375f, 375
 linear IgA dermatosis induction, 206
 methicillin-resistant Staphylococcus
 aureus cellulitis, 66
Varicella (chickenpox), 19, 132f,
 132–133, 133f, 135, 162
 bullous, 133f, 133
 complications, 133
 congenital infection, 390, 391–392
 congenital syndrome, 391
 differential diagnosis, 135
 disseminated intravascular
 coagulation, 278
 postvaricella scarring, 135
 secondary bacterial infection, 63,
 133, 135
 vaccine, 135
Vascular birthmarks, 237
 classification, 238b
 differential diagnosis, 238t
Vascular endothelial growth factor, 227,
 243
Vascular lesions, 23, 237–254
 acquired, 250–254
Vascular malformations, 246–250
 arteriovenous (fistulae), 248, 249
 capillary (port-wine stains), 246f,
 246–247, 249, 250f, 250
 classification, 238b, 246

 differential diagnosis, 249
 hyperkeratotic (angiokeratomas), 247
 lymphatic, 248f, 248, 249
 telangiectatic, 247, 249, 250, 251f
 treatment, 249–250, 250f
 venous, 247–248, 248f, 249
 see also Vascular birthmarks
Vascular plexuses, skin, 4
Vascular reactions, 23, 257–281
Vascular tumors, 170, 237–245
 clinical features, 237–242
Vasculitis, 104, 260, 267, 271
 drug eruptions, 365, 374f, 374, 377,
 378
 associated drugs, 374b
 urticarial, 264f, 264–265
Vellus hairs, 6
 eruptive cysts, 215, 216f, 216
Venereal Disease Research Laboratory
 (VDRL) test, 77, 159, 160, 161
Venereal warts (condylomata acuminata),
 140f, 141f, 141, 143
Venomous spider bite, 103–104
Vernix caseosa, 7
Verruca plana (flat wart), 139f, 139, 141
Verruca vulgaris (common wart), 138f,
 138, 139f, 142
Vesicant therapy, warts, 142
Vesicles, 11, 12, 15f
 grouped, 21
Vesicobullous eruptions
 spontaneous, 195b, 195–196
 viral exanthems, 127–137, 131b
Vidarabine, herpes keratitis, 132
Vincristine, Kaposiform
 hemangioendothelioma, 245
Viral exanthems, 113–138, 159, 181,
 203
 morbilliform eruptions, 113–127
 patterns, 113
 photoactivation, 113
 vesicobullous eruptions, 127–137,
 131b
Viral hepatitis, 68, 125–127
Viral infection
 congenital, 394
 spontaneous vesicobullous eruptions,
 195
Virus-induced tumors, 138–145
Vitamin A, measles management, 116
Vitamin B2, drug-induced acne, 36
Vitamin B6, drug-induced acne, 36
Vitamin B12, drug-induced acne, 36
Vitamin deficiency, 95
Vitamin K deficiency, neonatal pupura,
 394
Vitiligo, 316f, 316–318
 generalized, 316f, 316
 halo nevus association, 328
 segmental, 316, 317f
 therapy, 317f, 317
Vogt-Koyanagi-Harada syndrome, 316f,
 316
Volar pads development, 7–8

Vomiting
    cat-scratch disease, 73
    Henoch-Schönlein purpura, 273
    Lyme disease, 75
    mastocytosis, 267
    toxic shock syndrome, 72
Von Willebrand's disease, 394
Vulvar lichen sclerosus, 338f, 338, 339
Vulvar pemphigoid, localized childhood, 209f, 209
Vulvar ulcers
    differential diagnosis, 209b
    localized childhood pemphigoid, 209f, 209
Vulvovaginitis, candidiasis, 94, 95

W

Waardenburg's syndrome, 309–310
    types, 309
Warthin-Finkeldy cells, 115
Warts, 58, 78, 138–143, 144, 227, 251, 356, 401
    clinical types, associated human papillomavirus type, 138t
    common (verruca vulgaris), 138f, 138, 139f, 142
    differential diagnosis, 141
    filiform, 139f, 139
    flat (verruca plana), 29, 139f, 139, 141, 142, 156
    mucosal, 139f, 139
    partial removal ('fairy ring'), 140f, 140
    pathogenesis, 141
    periungual, 138–139, 139f, 142
    plantar, 140f, 140, 142, 229
    treatment, 141t, 141–143

antiproliferative agents, 142
    cytodestructive therapy, 141, 142
    immunologic, 142
    psychotherapy, 143
    surgical excision, 142
    venereal (condylomata acuminata), 140f, 141f, 141, 142
Water exposure
    epidermal barrier effects, 413–414
    see also Humidification; Hydration
Water-in-oil emulsions, 414
    ointments, 416
Wax, moisturizer composition, 415
Weber-Cockayne disease, 348
Wet dressings, 417
    allergic contact dermatitis, 54
    atopic dermatitis, 46b, 46, 47
    erythema multiforme, 197
    keratosis follicularis (Darier-White disease), 360
    polymorphous light eruptions, 187
    roseola, 118
    sunburn, 183
    varicella, 135
Wheal, 12, 14f
White lesions, 23, 309–320
White soft paraffin, moisturizer composition, 415
White sponge nevus, 165
Whorled lesions, 19, 20f
Wigs, 287
Wiskott-Aldrich syndrome, 117, 394
Wood's light examination
    ash-leaf macules, 310
    erythrasma, 88
    piebaldism, 309
    tinea capitis, 81
    tinea versicolor, 92

Wool fat, 415
Wool wax alcohol, 415
Woolly hair, 297
Woolly hair nevus, 297
Wound dressings, epidermolysis bullosa, 354

X

X-linked ichthyosis, 343–345, 344f, 347, 409
X-ray therapy, warts, 142
Xanthomas, 226, 402
Xeroderma pigmentosum, 181, 191f, 191–193, 192f, 218

Y

Yeast infections, 91–95
    tinea versicolor, 91f, 91–92
Yellow lesions, 23
Yersinia infection, erythema nodosum, 269

Z

Zafirlukast
    necrotizing venulitis association, 275
    urticaria, 261
Zinc deficiency, 95
    acquired, 362
    acrodermatitis enteropathica, 361
    human immunodeficiency virus infection, 137
    laboratory assessment, 362
Zinc sulfate suplements, 362
Zoster immune globulin, 135
    congenital varicella, 391